Intraocular Tumors

Vikas Khetan
Editor

Intraocular Tumors

Springer

Editor
Vikas Khetan
Sankara Nethralaya
Chennai, Tamil Nadu
India

ISBN 978-981-15-0394-8 ISBN 978-981-15-0395-5 (eBook)
https://doi.org/10.1007/978-981-15-0395-5

This Springer imprint is published by the registered company Springer Nature Singapore Pte Ltd.
The registered company address is: 152 Beach Road, #21-01/04 Gateway East, Singapore 189721, Singapore

Foreword by Brenda Gallie

Dr. Khetan has assembled strong leaders in ocular oncology, representing the multidisciplinary teams required for optimal care of intraocular tumors. The chapters show various approaches, with input from many geographic regions addressing the major intraocular tumors, that are biologically the same, no matter where the patients live.

Readers at all levels of expertise, ranging from general ophthalmologists and trainees to expert consultants, can find useful details in this book. The knowledge provided ranges from the very earliest history of these cancers to envisioning incorporation of personalized genomic knowledge into care, the future that is arriving quickly.

Several of the chapters describe the same elements, illustrating different approaches. Major differences are of interest, for example, the retinoblastoma prognosis to save an eye: different chapters cite systems that are significantly different, but generally they all recognize the difficulties this creates and welcome the newest, evidence-based, TNMH standard classification, developed by international collaboration and published in 2017 in the major Tumor, Node, Metastasis cancer staging manual. Incorporation of "H" for heritability shows the leadership of the field of ocular oncology in cancer in general; retinoblastoma is the first cancer in which heritability is recognized to influence outcome.

Against the historic background of the Cooperative Ocular Melanoma Study, which demonstrated that multicenter collaboration works, the current concern about accurately counseling the patient on prognosis emerges as a hot topic with many viewpoints that may best be resolved by good data and evidence.

Consistent in all chapters is support for collaborative research to generate a sound basis for treatment of ocular cancers! This book provides a good base to achieve high-quality evidence in support of the best care for our patients.

This book is not to be read from beginning to end. Rather, the reader can focus on finding details for their clinical or scientific issue at hand. Many chapters may be relevant, and frequently authors cross-reference so that the reviewer can also consider information in a different chapter.

Congratulations to Dr. Khetan! You have succeeded in leading a large multidisciplinary team, who have all contributed to produce a novel and useful book on intraocular tumors.

Brenda Gallie
Hospital for Sick Children
Toronto ON Canada

Alberta Children's Hospital
Calgary AB Canada

Techna Institute, University Health Network
Toronto ON Canada

Department of Ophthalmology
University of Toronto
Toronto ON Canada

Department of Medical Biophysics
University of Toronto
Toronto ON Canada

Department of Molecular Genetics
University of Toronto
Toronto ON Canada

Foreword by Lingam Gopal

Subspecialization (or super specialization) is at the same time a boon and a bane. Very rapidly what was within the competence of a general ophthalmologist becomes the domain of the specialist (of course) with better quality of care being delivered. Ocular oncology has grown to be a distinct subspecialty in ophthalmology, courtesy some landmark developments in the management of common intraocular tumors. The developments in the field of imaging, chemotherapy, and genetics have been nothing short of being phenomenal. The force that drives these rapid strides is passion for the specialty and the ardent desire to make a difference.

Vikas Khetan has that passion. Ever since he became a vitreo-retinal fellow first, and then a fellow with the legendary Dr. Brenda Galle, this passion has been evident. In addition to making a difference to the way the specialty is practiced in his place of work, he strived to bring together like-minded people across the region to create forums for interaction.

It is this desire to disseminate knowledge that made him to bring together luminaries in the field and make them contribute to this textbook. This book does not pretend to be an all-encompassing encyclopedia of ocular oncology, but concentrates on the more common intraocular tumors. Retinoblastoma and choroidal melanoma take the center stage with detailed exposition of the diagnostic, genetic, and therapeutic aspects. General topics include imaging of ocular tumors (from ophthalmologist's and radiologist's perspective), pathology of intraocular tumors, management of the anophthalmic socket, and the art of counseling. Most of the chapters were written by internationally renowned ocular oncologists with decades of experience in the art and science of treating patients with intraocular tumors.

I am sure this textbook will be a good addendum to the practitioners of ocular oncology in delivering quality care, utilizing all available tools to control the tumors.

Singapore
September 2018

Lingam Gopal

Preface

Ocular oncology is an emerging subspecialty in ophthalmology that is gradually making a place for itself. At the time of writing this text book, it is estimated that there are about 200–250 ocular oncologists all over the world. In India, until a few years ago there were only a handful of trained ocular oncologists; however, there is an encouraging trend and a lot of youngsters are now taking up this specialty. The world of ocular oncology is developing at a very rapid pace, and newer treatment modalities are emerging every other day.

The aim of the book is to provide the readers with a basic, yet detailed reference for a variety of intraocular tumors. Most of the chapters in the book are written by world experts. I hope it helps our readers in understanding the nuances of intraocular tumors.

I would like to offer my deepest thanks to the families and children who allowed us the privilege of participating in their care.

This work would not have been possible without the support of my family and friends. The time that I spent on this project was taken out the time from my spouse and child, and I am thankful to them for letting me do this.

I would also like to thank my parents and siblings for their constant and endless support.

I dedicate this book to the Founder of Sankara Nethralaya—Dr S S Badrinath. I sincerely hope that the world has many more visionaries like him.

Chennai, India — Vikas Khetan

Acknowledgements

This book has been a wonderful journey, made possible by many beautiful people from around the globe, all coming together to make this happen.

I would like to thank all the contributors for their time, diligence and hard work in preparing the individual chapters and help enhance the knowledge with the readers.

I would like to especially thank my two mentors Drs Brenda Gallie and Lingam Gopal for their constant support and guidance in my career. I would also like to thank them for writing the forewords for this book.

A word of mention to my other mentor Dr Alex V Levin, who taught me the art of examining the patient as a whole.

I would also like to thank my family members for their understanding and support. It is the sacrifice of personal time that enable me to indulge in this book editing.

I am grateful to Springer Nature and their associates especially Mr Naren Aggarwal, Rakesh Kumar Jotheeswaran and Vignesh Manohar for their help with the book.

Last but not the least, I am grateful to Sankara Nethralaya and all the patients that I have cared for who have allowed me to share the information with the readers.

Wishing you happy reading…

Contents

About the Editor

Vikas Khetan is a specialist in vitreoretina, ocular oncology and ocular genetics. He is an alumnus of Sankara Nethralaya, Chennai, Hospital for SickKids, Toronto and Wills Eye Hospital, Philadelphia. He is a well-published author with articles in both national and international journals and has contributed chapters in many books. He is a well-known speaker at various conferences and a reviewer for many journals. He is currently the section editor of Ocular Genetics for *Indian Journal of Ophthalmology* and is also a section editor for *Nepalese Journal of Ophthalmology*.

He is the recipient of many awards including the prestigious JM Pahwa award at VRSI meeting, IJO Gold award for paper published in IJO for the year 2012 and IJO best reviewer award. He is also the recipient of many travel grants for various meetings like APAO, APVRS, etc. Last year he received the P Siva Reddy International award at the AIOS meeting. He also received SAO (SAARC Academy of Ophthalmology) excellence award at the SAO meeting in Kathmandu last year.

1 Retinoblastoma: Diagnosis, Classification and Management

Bhavna Chawla

1.1 Introduction

Retinoblastoma is the most common primary intraocular malignancy of childhood. It contributes to approximately 4% of all pediatric cancers. The incidence is around 1 in 18,000 live births [1]. The tumour was initially described as fungus haematodes in 1809 [2]. It was renamed as Retinoblastoma in 1926 by the American Ophthalmological Society after a general consensus was reached that the tumour originated from retinoblasts [3]. The retinoblastoma gene (RB1), encoded on chromosome 13q14, was the first described tumor suppressor gene. Constitutional loss of one RB1 allele causes cancer predisposition, and loss of the second allele in a developing retinal cell leads to retinoblastoma. Retinoblastoma can be sporadic or inherited. Older age and unilateral presentation is usually seen in sporadic tumours, whereas younger age and bilateral presentation is observed in inherited tumours. All cases of bilateral tumours are heritable and carry a germline mutation of the RB1 gene. They account for approximately one third of all the RB cases. Only a small proportion of unilateral retinoblastoma cases are heritable.

B. Chawla (✉)
Ocular Oncology Service, Rajendra Prasad Centre for Ophthalmic Sciences, All India Institute of Medical Sciences, New Delhi, India

National Eye Institute, National Institutes of Health, Bethesda, MD, USA

1.2 Diagnosis

The average age for diagnosis of retinoblastoma is 18 months and 95% of children are diagnosed by the age of 5 years. Bilateral disease is diagnosed earlier then unilateral disease. Germline tumors can present as early as the first month while sporadic cases are diagnosed later, usually by 24 months of age [4].

A whitish pupillary reflex or leucocoria is the most common presenting symptom. Other signs include strabismus, poor vision and redness of the eye. In some instances, retinoblastoma may also present as buphthalmos, aseptic orbital cellulitis or phthisis bulbi. Proptosis and fungating orbital masses are signs of advanced disease, which may be accompanied by metastasis in the bone, bone marrow, lymph nodes, and central nervous system [5].

Figure 1.1 shows some of the clinical presentations of this tumour. Typically, the diagnosis of retinoblastoma is established by characteristic ophthalmic findings, often requiring general anaesthesia, and B-scan ultrasonography. A dilated fundus examination of both eyes with 360° scleral depression should be undertaken in all suspected cases. The tumour appears as an elevated mass in the fundus (Fig. 1.2). There may be multiple tumours in the same eye (Fig. 1.3). RetCAM is a wide angled fundus camera which helps to document the tumor and assess response to therapy. Other findings may be present such as the presence of vitreous and/or sub-retinal seeds, vitreous

V. Khetan (ed.), *Intraocular Tumors*, https://doi.org/10.1007/978-981-15-0395-5_1

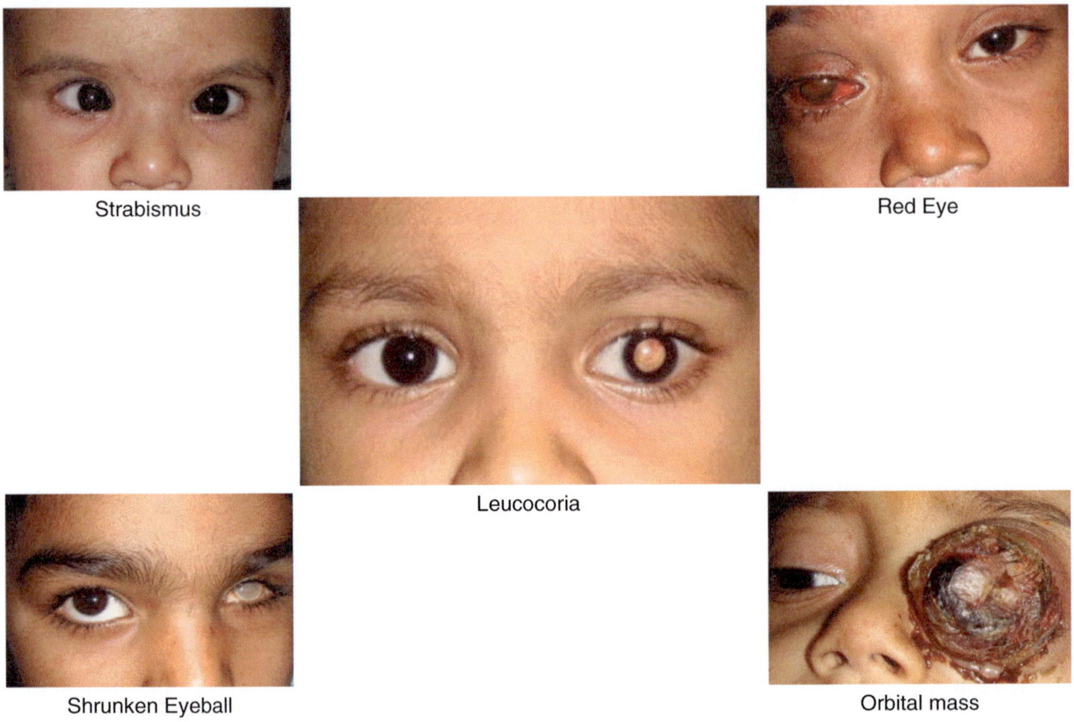

Fig. 1.1 Various clinical presentations of retinoblastoma

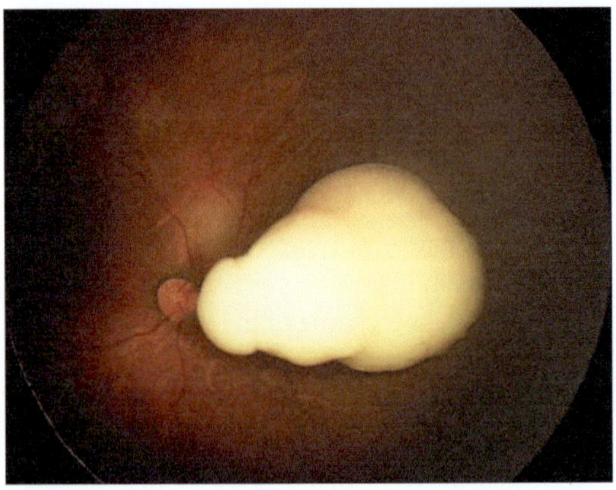

Fig. 1.2 Fundus picture showing the elevated tumour

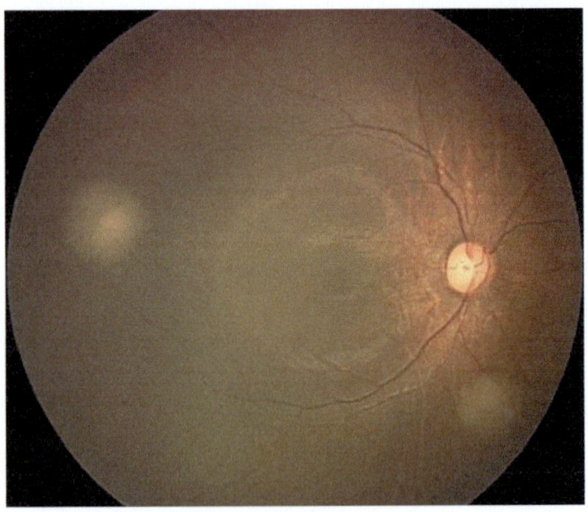

Fig. 1.3 RetCAM image of the right eye showing two tumours

haemorrhage, sub-retinal fluid, retinal detachment etc. It is also important to evaluate the anterior segment and look for abnormal findings such as neovascularization of the iris, pseudohypopyon, cataract, ectropion uveae, hyphaema, iris seeding by tumor cells, buphthalmos or other abnormalities (Fig. 1.4). Measurement of intraocular pressure should be done. Some of these eyes may have elevated intraocular pressure, that could be due to neo-vascular glaucoma, anterior shift of the lens with resultant pupillary block and angle closure or the obstruction of the outflow of aqueous humour

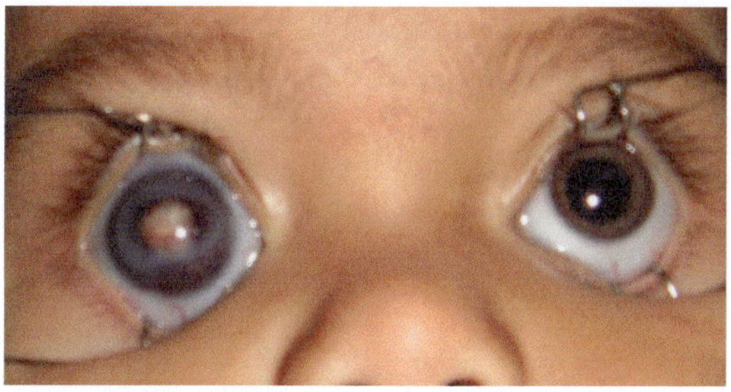

Fig. 1.4 Examination under anaesthesia

through the trabecular meshwork by the tumour cells [6].

Imaging plays an important role in confirming the diagnosis and in differentiating retinoblastoma from other simulating conditions. Imaging also helps in staging the disease and assessing the tumour response to treatment. When considering a diagnosis of retinoblastoma, there are several other diseases which need to be differentiated. These include congenital cataract, Coats' disease, persistent fetal vasculature, retinopathy of prematurity, retinal detachment, vitreous hemorrhage, Toxocariasis and coloboma and endogenous endophthalmitis. A misdiagnosis, although rare, can occur as some diseases, particularly end-stage conditions, may simulate retinoblastoma closely, resulting in a diagnostic dilemma [7, 8].

The various imaging modalities available include B scan ultrasonography, ultrasound biomicroscopy (UBM), fluorescein angiography (FA), optical coherence tomography (OCT), computed tomography (CT) scan and magnetic resonance imaging (MRI) [9]. Along with clinical examination, B-scan ultrasonography helps to establish the diagnosis in the majority of cases. On ultrasonography, retinoblastoma appears as an elevated mass in the posterior segment of the eye, with areas of high internal reflectivity due to calcification within the mass. It is also very useful in cases of diagnostic dilemma, to differentiate retinoblastoma from other common conditions that may present with leucocoria. Other advantages of ultrasound include its wide availability, simplicity of use by an ophthalmologist, no requirement for anaesthesia and lack of exposure to radiation. High-frequency UBM provides high-resolution in vivo imaging of the anterior segment in a non-invasive fashion. In addition to the tissues easily seen such as the cornea, iris, and sclera, structures hidden from clinical observation, like the ciliary body and angle, can be imaged and their morphology assessed (Fig. 1.5). Ultrasound bio-microscopy imaging has been shown to document anterior disease and contribute to the management of children affected with retinoblastoma [10, 11]. It is also used prior to intra-vitreal chemotherapy to look for tumour extension. Fluorescein angiography can be done for smaller tumors which show minimally dilated feeding vessels in the arterial phase, blotchy hyperfluorescence in the venous phase and late staining. Hand-held high-resolution spectral domain optical coherence tomography has been evaluated in retinoblastoma and found to be useful [12]. CT scan is most sensitive to detect calcification within the tumour (Fig. 1.6) and aids in identifying extraocular extension. However, it should be used sparingly due to the risk of exposure to ionizing radiation, especially in cases with germline mutation. It is usually reserved for cases that do not demonstrate calcification on ultrasound and/or cases of diagnostic dilemma with atypical presentation. Neuroimaging with contrast MRI is the imaging modality of choice in advanced cases with suspected extraocular extension for assessment of orbital, optic nerve and intracranial extension (Fig. 1.7). MRI has the advantage of superior soft tissue resolution as compared to CT scan and does not expose the child to radiation. There are several

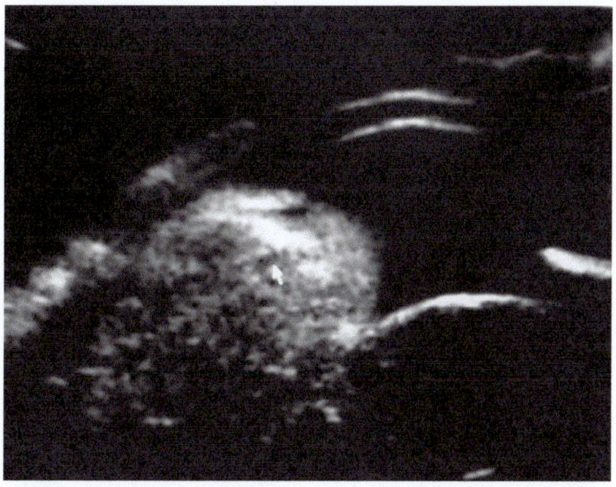

Fig. 1.5 Ultrasound biomicroscopy for anterior segment invasion

studies on the diagnostic accuracy of MRI in predicting optic nerve invasion [13, 14]. Rarely, children with retinoblastoma have a pineal tumour (trilateral retinoblastoma)that may be found on imaging. MRI has also been helpful in tumor staging of patients who present with orbital cellulitis and in differentiating between inflammation of the coats and extra-ocular invasion [15]. Cerebrospinal fluid and bone marrow evaluation are not performed routinely and should only be undertaken if indicated clinically or by imaging studies.

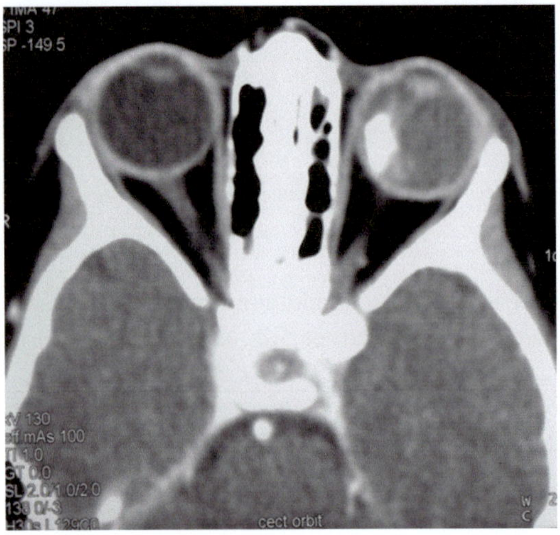

Fig. 1.6 CT scan showing intralesional calcification in the left eye

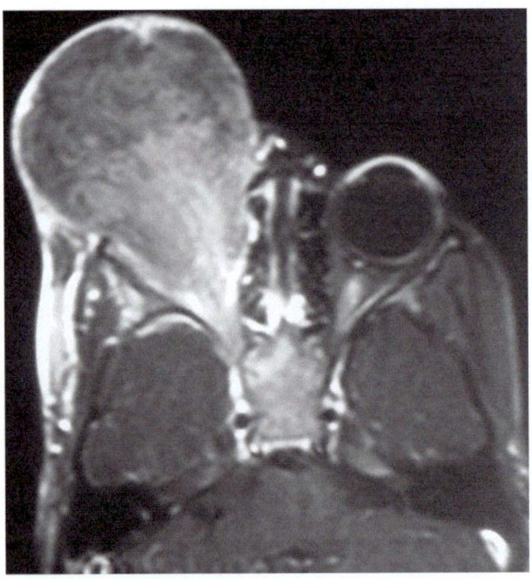

Fig. 1.7 T1 weighted MR image showing extensive orbital invasion by the tumour

1.3 Classification and Staging

Retinoblastoma may be intra-ocular (Fig. 1.8) or extra-ocular at presentation.

Appropriate management requires correct staging of the tumour at the time of diagnosis. Hence, a knowledge of the classification systems for staging of retinoblastoma is essential.

In the 1960s, the primary treatment modalities for retinoblastoma were surgery and external beam radiotherapy (EBRT). It was during this period that Dr. Algernon Reese and Dr. Robert Ellsworth developed a classification system for intraocular retinoblastoma that had prognostic significance for maintenance of sight and control of local disease (Table 1.1) [16].

The Reese Ellsworth classification system had a few drawbacks. These included:

a. A worse ocular prognosis for peripheral, large and multi-focal tumours as they were presumed to be more aggressive in the EBRT era.

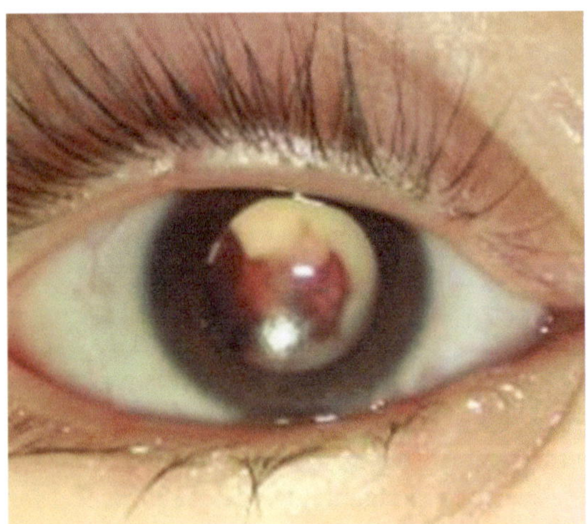

Fig. 1.8 Intraocular tumour

Table 1.1 Reese-Ellsworth classification for retinoblastoma

Group	Likelihood of salvage	Features
I	Very favorable for maintenance of sight	a. Solitary tumor, <4 DD, at or behind the equator b. Multiple tumors, none >4 DD, at or behind the equator
II	Favorable for maintenance of sight	a. Solitary tumor, 4–10 DD, at or behind the equator b. Multiple tumors, 4–10 DD, behind the equator
III	Doubtful for maintenance of sight	a. Any lesion anterior to the equator b. Solitary tumor, >10 DD, behind the equator
IV	Unfavorable for maintenance of sight	a. Multiple tumors, some >10 DD b. Any lesion extending anteriorly to the ora serrata
V	Very unfavorable for maintenance of sight	a. Massive tumor involving more than one half of the retina b. Vitreous seeding

DD disc diameters

Table 1.2 International Classification System for retinoblastoma [17]

Group	Clinical features
A Very low risk	All tumors are 3 mm or smaller, confined to the retina, and located at least 3 mm from the foveola and 1.5 mm from the optic nerve.
B Low risk	Retinal tumors may be of any size or location not in Group A. No vitreous or subretinal seeding allowed. A small cuff of subretinal fluid extending no more than 5 mm from the base of the tumor is allowed.
C Moderate risk	Eyes with only focal vitreous or subretinal seeding and discrete retinal tumors of any size and location. Vitreous or subretinal seeding may extend no more than 3 mm from tumor. Upto one quadrant of sub-retinal fluid may be present.
D High risk	Eyes with diffuse vitreous or sub-retinal seeding and/or massive, non-discrete endophytic or exophytic disease.
E Very high risk eyes	*Eyes with one or more of the following* • Neo-vascular glaucoma • Massive intraocular hemorrhage • Aseptic orbital cellulites • Phthisis or pre-phthisis • Tumor anterior to anterior vitreous face • Tumor touching the lens • Diffuse infiltrating retinoblastoma

b. No distinction was made between sub-retinal and vitreous seeds in the classification system and the presence of sub-retinal seeding was not addressed.

In the 1990s, systemic chemotherapy started becoming popular as a primary treatment for retinoblastoma. Therefore, a new classification system that could predict the results of chemotherapy with more accuracy was needed (Table 1.2). Thus, the International Classification System for intraocular retinoblastoma was introduced, and it was found to be a good predictor of chemoreduction success [17, 18].

Recently, the American Joint Committee on Cancer has formulated the 8th edition of retinoblastoma staging, with the view to define the extent of disease at the time of diagnosis and to predict eye survival, metastatic risk, and patient survival [19]. Unique to the 8th edition tumour node metastasis (TNM) staging for retinoblastoma, is the inclusion of germ line cancer predisposition, which incurs a high risk for new post-diagnosis tumors and second primary tumours such as osteosarcoma and cutaneous melanoma, thus affecting overall patient survival. It has introduced the stage category H to indicate the germ line status of RB1 gene (H1) inferred clinically by bilateral retinoblastoma, reti-

Table 1.3 The International Retinoblastoma Staging System

Stage	Description	
Stage 0	Eye has not been enucleated	
	Conservative treatment	
Stage I	Eye enucleated, completely resected histologically	
Stage II	Eye enucleated, microscopic residual tumor in the form of	
	1. Tumor invasion into extrascleral space	
	2. Tumor invasion into the cut end of optic nerve	
Stage III	Regional extension	a. Overt orbital disease
		b. Pre-auricular or cervical lymph node extension
Stage IV	Metastatic disease	a. Hematogenous metastasis
		1. Single lesion
		2. Multiple lesions
		b. CNS extension
		1. Pre-chiasmatic lesion
		2. CNS mass
		3. Leptomeningeal and CSF disease

noblastoma with an intracranial primitive neuroectodermal tumor (i.e., trilateral Rb), patient with family history of retinoblastoma, or molecular definition of a constitutional RB1 gene mutation. For extra-ocular retinoblastoma, the International Retinoblastoma Staging System proposed by Chantada et al. is used to stage the tumour (Table 1.3) [20]. The tumour is staged from Stage 0 to Stage IV, depending upon the extent of invasion, taking histopathology and imaging findings into account.

1.4 Management

The management of retinoblastoma depends on several factors such as age of the child, laterality and stage of the disease at presentation, and visual potential of the affected eye. The primary aim of treatment is survival of the child, with globe preservation and maintenance of vision being secondary goals. In the past, the tumour was associated with a high mortality but with the introduction of enucleation, the survival rate improved dramatically. While enucleation remains the standard of care for advanced intraocular tumours, conservative treatment which can result in globe salvage and preservation of useful vision is being successfully used for less advanced disease. These therapies include focal consolidation with trans-pupillary thermotherapy, laser photocoagulation and cryotherapy, systemic chemotherapy, radiation treatment with plaque brachytherapy or external beam radiotherapy, and local injections of chemotherapeutic agents through the sub-tenon or subconjunctival route, as an adjunct to systemic chemotherapy. In the following section, each of these treatment modalities will be discussed in detail.

1.5 Trans-pupillary Thermotherapy

Transpupillary thermotherapy (TTT) is used for local control of the tumour, alone or in conjunction with systemic chemotherapy. The procedure is usually carried out under general anaesthesia using an infra-red diode laser (810 nm) mounted on an indirect ophthalmoscope (Fig. 1.9). The laser is applied directly to the tumour under wide pupillary dilation. The target temperature ranges between 45 and 60 °C, which spares the retinal vessels from coagulation as it is below their coagulative threshold [21, 22]. A spot size of 1.2 mm and a mean power of 300–600 mW is used to cover the tumour. Initially, the power is started at 200 mW and increased or decreased at 5 mW increments until an adequate take is observed in the mass [21, 22]. Effective therapy usually requires multiple sessions at monthly intervals. Various mechanisms of action for TTT have been described which include a direct

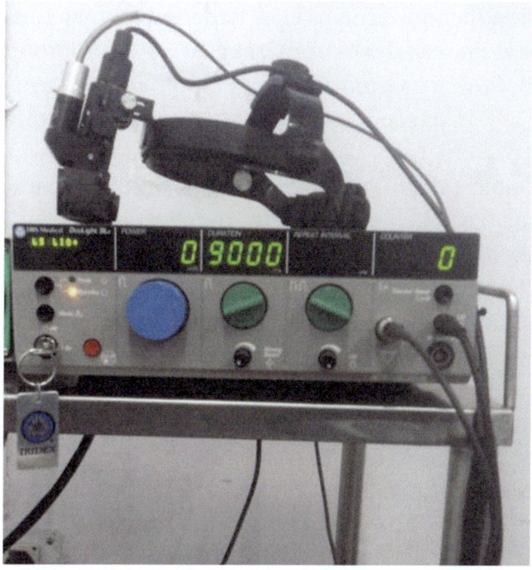

Fig. 1.9 Trans-pupillary thermotherapy

cytotoxic effect of heat on tumour cells, induction of apoptosis, heat-induced alteration of tumour microenvironment, modulation of drug resistance of tumour cells and increased uptake of carboplatin into tumour cells at temperatures above 44 °C [23, 24].

There are several studies on the role of TTT in retinoblastoma. Abramson et al. proposed that tumours <1.5 DD in base diameter can be treated with TTT alone [21]. Shields et al. treated 188 tumours (80 eyes) with TTT and reported complete regression in 161 (85.6%) tumours and recurrence in 27 (14.4%) tumours [22]. Complications reported included focal iris atrophy (36%) and peripheral focal lens opacity (24%).

1.6 Laser Photocoagulation

The purpose of argon laser photocoagulation (532 nm) is to coagulate all the blood supply to the tumour. Feeder vessels are obliterated at a mean power of 350 mW over a duration of 1–4 s. Only small and posterior tumours located away from the fovea and optic disc are managed by laser photocoagulation. Complications include retinal detachment, vascular occlusions, retinal traction, and preretinal fibrosis [25–27].

While TTT can be used for tumours adjacent to the fovea or optic nerve, laser photocoagulation can damage these vital areas. Thermotherapy causes a lower rise in temperature and its higher wavelength (810 nm) as compared to argon laser helps it to act directly on the retina so that the blood vessels are not damaged. On the contrary, during laser therapy (532 nm), the blood vessels are coagulated, leading to retinal ischemia [26, 27].

1.7 Cryotherapy

Cryotherapy alone may be used as primary therapy for small peripheral tumours located anterior to the equator. Cryotherapy induces the tumor tissue to freeze rapidly, and a temperature upto −90 °C causes intracellular ice crystal formation, protein denaturation, pH changes, and cell rupture, resulting in damage to the vascular endothelium with secondary thrombosis and infarction of the tumour tissue. Tumors are typically treated three times (triple freeze and thaw technique) per session trans-conjunctivally, with one or two sessions at monthly intervals [28, 29]. It is most effective for tumours <4 mm in basal diameter and 2 mm in thickness It can also be used as an adjunct to systemic chemotherapy and has synergistic effect when applied within 2–3 hours of intravenous chemotherapy. The complications are few and rarely serious, and include lid edema, transient conjunctival edema, serous retinal detachments and retinal tears. Vitreous hemorrhage can be observed in large or previously irradiated tumours [30, 31].

1.8 Systemic Chemotherapy

It was in the 1990s that systemic chemotherapy was used to treat intraocular retinoblastoma after observing good tumour control and ocular salvage rates of 30–70% when intravenous chemotherapy was given prior to EBRT [32]. The recognition of increased risk of second non-ocular cancers with EBRT further led to more extensive use of chemotherapy. Today, it is one of the most widely used treatment modalities for retinoblastoma.

The main objectives of chemotherapy for intraocular retinoblastoma are eye salvage and avoidance of enucleation or EBRT.

Systemic chemotherapy is indicated for large tumours that cannot be treated with local therapy alone, recurrent lesions, relapsed tumours, and as adjuvant therapy to enucleation surgery in cases with high risk histopathology features [33–35]. Systemic chemotherapy is also used as a part of multi-modal treatment for extra-ocular retinoblastoma. The various chemotherapeutic drugs used in treatment include carboplatin, etoposide, vincristine, methotrexate, cyclophosphamide, melphalan, doxorubicin, and triethylene melamine in various combinations. The most commonly used intravenous chemotherapy drugs are vincristine, etoposide, and carboplatin (VEC) [36]. Table 1.4 shows the standard dosage and schedule of drugs that are recommended for use. Cyclosporine has also been used to overcome the problem of drug resistance [37]. Other drug combinations such as two-drug therapy of vincristine and carboplatin have also been proposed so that the side effects of etoposide can be avoided [38].

Systemic chemotherapy combined with focal therapy has been the mainstay of globe-preserving treatment for less advanced disease [39]. The tumour size undergoes reduction following chemotherapy, and local therapies such as cryotherapy, laser photocoagulation, or TTT are used to eradicate the remaining disease. This combined treatment approach has been shown to be more efficacious for tumour control than chemotherapy alone. By employing combination therapy, Shields et al. reported tumour control rates of 100% for Group A, 93% for Group B, 90% for Group C, and 47% for Group D eyes [18]. In a recent study from our centre, systemic chemotherapy and focal consolidation was found to achieve outcomes that were comparable to those reported from the West [40]. Close monitoring by a paediatric oncologist is essential during therapy to look for any signs of drug toxicity. Although the VEC regimen is usually well tolerated, side effects include myelosuppression, neutropenia, infections, liver toxicity, and increased risk of second malignancy [41, 42]. Ototoxicity and nephrotoxicity may be rarely observed.

1.9 Local Chemotherapy

Although systemic chemotherapy in combination with focal therapy has achieved good outcomes, intravenous chemotherapy can lead to serious toxic side effects including myelosuppression and infection. As a result, newer treatment approaches have focused on localized delivery of chemotherapy to minimize the systemic side effects of intravenous chemotherapy. Routes of local chemotherapy delivery include subconjunctival or sub-tenon injections that are given as an adjunct to systemic chemotherapy. In recent years, targeted forms of drug delivery such as intra-arterial and intra-vitreal chemotherapy have shown promising results and gained popularity.

Table 1.4 Intravenous chemotherapy for retinoblastoma [5]

Drug	Dosage/route	Schedule	Side effect/remarks
Carboplatin Platinum coordinator compound which cross-links DNA	560 mg/m^2/day 18.6 mg/kg/day for children <3 years	Day 0	Nephrotoxicity, ototoxicity, neurotoxicity, hypomagnesemia Escalation of dose is done depending on stage of disease.
Etoposide Inhibits DNA	150 mg/m^2/day 5 mg/kg/day for children <3 years	Days 0 and 1	Allergic reactions, hepatotoxicity, CNS toxicity, hypotension, AML, mucositis. Escalation of dose is done depending on stage of disease.
Vincristine Vinca alkaloid	1.5 mg/m^2/day (0.05 mg/kg/day for children <3 years) maximum dose 2 mg	Day 0	Neurotoxicity, myelosuppression. Avoid extravasation.

1.9.1 Sub-conjunctival/Sub-tenon Chemotherapy

It has been observed that systemic chemotherapy alone may not be sufficient to treat Groups C and D eyes. Friedman et al. reported that only 53% of Reese Ellsworth Group V eyes could be controlled with chemotherapy alone [35]. Chan et al. and Villablanca et al. reported that approximately 40% of group C and 70% of group D eyes failed systemic chemotherapy alone [43, 44]. Therefore, local injections of chemotherapeutic agents have been used with varying degrees of success, usually as an adjuvant to systemic chemotherapy to avoid enucleation and external beam radiotherapy in these cases. Sub-conjunctival carboplatin has been noted to result in favourable outcomes in those tumours that progressed despite ablative therapy [45]. The trial proposed by the Children's Oncology Group (COG) involved the use of systemic chemotherapy with carboplatin, vincristine, and etoposide, along with subtenon carboplatin for group C and D eyes [46, 47]. The sub-tenon route, though slightly more invasive than the sub-conjunctival route, is associated with a decreased incidence of lid swelling and a rapid diffusion of drug. For Group C and D tumours, the use of 20 mg sub-tenon carboplatin along with chemo-reduction and focal consolidation has been recommended by the Children's Oncology Group [48]. Optic nerve ischaemic necrosis, reduced ocular motility due to fibrosis, orbital fat necrosis and pseudo-preseptal cellulitis are some of the reported side effects of treatment [49–51].

1.9.2 Super-Selective Intra-arterial Chemotherapy

In 2004, Japanese investigators described the technique of 'selective ophthalmic artery infusion' (SOAI), where a micro-balloon catheter was positioned by a trans-femoral artery approach at the cervical segment of the internal carotid artery, just distal to the orifice of the ophthalmic artery [52, 53]. Abramson and Gobin further modified the technique of SOAI into direct intra-arterial (Ophthalmic artery) infusion [54]. The technique, known as super-selective infusion, involved advancing a micro-catheter into the orifice of the ophthalmic artery through a trans-femoral artery approach (Fig. 1.10). In a Phase I/II clinical trial, Abramson et al. reported their

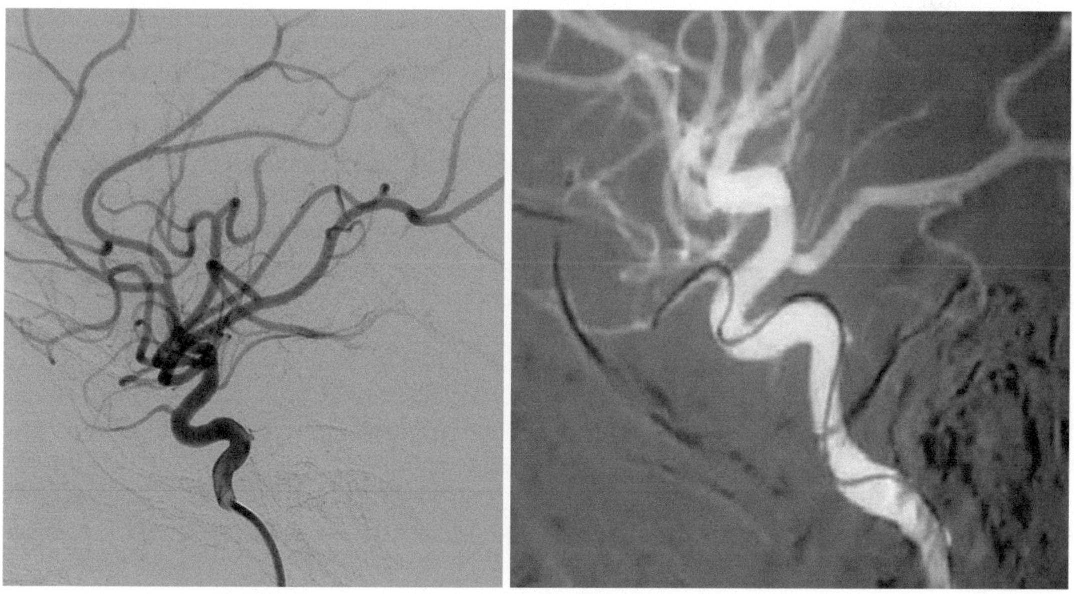

Fig. 1.10 Intra-arterial chemotherapy

initial experience with intra-arterial ophthalmic artery chemotherapy using melphalan in 10 children with advanced retinoblastoma who were indicated for enucleation [54]. Since then, several investigators have reported their experience with selective intra-arterial chemotherapy [55, 56]. Intra-arterial chemotherapy has been reported to be associated with an overall success rate of 55–100% in salvaging the globe, in addition to the advantage of very low systemic toxicity. The most commonly used agent is melphalan; topotecan and carboplatin can be used in recalcitrant cases.

Based on the encouraging results in preliminary studies, Selective Intra-arterial Chemotherapy (SIAC) has also been used as a first line treatment in less advanced cases of intraocular retinoblastoma [57]. Although more widely used for refractory cases, SIAC has also been investigated in treatment naive eyes [58–60]. Chen et al. have studied the effect of IAC in infants less than 3 months of age [60]. Their study suggests that IAC as primary therapy is a feasible and promising treatment for retinoblastoma in infants less than 3 months of age [60]. Simultaneous bilateral ophthalmic artery chemosurgery for bilateral retinoblastoma (tandem therapy) has also been reported [61].

Although intra-arterial chemotherapy has the advantage of fewer systemic side effects as compared to intravenous chemotherapy, there are concerns about retinal toxicity of melphalan. Exposure to fluoroscopy related radiation and ophthalmic artery occlusion are other concerns. Michaels and co-workers reported the toxicities and outcome of 19 eyes in 17 patients with retinoblastoma receiving SIAC treatment between 2008 and 2013 [62]. From the 87 treatments, mild local reactions were common. Myelosuppression was more common after triple-agent SIAC than single-agent melphalan. Further, SIAC is not always a straightforward procedure, and it may require an alternative approach [63, 64]. Alternative routes of intra-arterial chemotherapy for intraocular retinoblastoma appeared in the short term as effective and safe as the traditional drug infusion through the ophthalmic artery.

1.9.3 Intra-vitreal Chemotherapy

Intravenous chemotherapy has poor penetration in the avascular vitreous cavity. Hence, vitreous seeds remain the biggest challenge in the management of intraocular retinoblastoma. Intravitreal chemotherapy (IViC) has overcome this problem and found to be effective in the treatment of vitreous seeds. Similar to intra-arterial chemotherapy, melphalan remains the drug of choice for IViC. The use of melphalan is based on in vitro studies by Inomata and Kaneko [65]. Among the 12 anti cancer drugs that were studied, melphalan was found to be the most effective against retinoblastoma [65].

Munier et al. have described the technique of IViC injections with melphalan drug in a dose of 20–30 μg/0.1 mL [66]. The injection is given 3–3.5 mm away from limbus. The globe is shaken after the injection for uniform distribution of drug in the vitreous. After withdrawing the needle, triple freeze-thaw cryotherapy application is done at the injection site to avoid needle-track seeding. The procedure can be repeated every 7–10 days until a complete response is achieved [66]. Complete response is established if the seeds (1) completely disappear (vitreous seeding regression type 0), or are converted into (2) refringent and/or calcified residues (vitreous seeding regression type I), (3) amorphous, often non-spherical, inactive residues (vitreous seeding regression type II), or (4) a combination of the last two (vitreous seeding regression type III) [66]. With this technique, Munier et al. reported vitreous seed regression rate of 84% in eyes that had already been treated with intravenous and/or intra-arterial chemotherapy [66]. A localised peripheral salt-and-pepper retinopathy at the injection site was the only complication observed [66]. Another study by Shields et al. showed 100% (11/11) success rate with 1–4 cycles of monthly IViC (melphalan 20–30 μg) at 2 year follow-up [67].

Some investigators have also used topotecan as intravitreal injection [68]. Topotecan has a longer half life; it is used in a concentration of 8–20 μg/0.04 mL. Ghassemi et al. studied the effect of intravitreal topotecan (8–20 µg in 0.04 mL of balanced salt solution) combined with melphalan (40 µg in 0.04 mL of diluent) and found the combination to be safe and effective [68].

It is important to bear in mind that IViC is not a primary treatment modality but should be used as a salvage therapy in cases of recalcitrant and recurrent vitreous seeds.

Careful case selection and meticulous screening is very important. Contraindications for IViC include anterior segment or ciliary body invasion, group E retinoblastoma, presence of complete posterior vitreous detachment, diffuse vitreous seeds in all quadrants and total retinal detachment [69]. The risk of extra-ocular spread following IViC was evaluated by Smith et al. [70]. Of the 315 eyes of 304 patients who underwent 1300 injections, the proportion of patients with extra-ocular spread was found to be 0.003 [70]. Besides the risk of needle track seeding, the drug itself can have side effects on the retinal function. There have been some concerns about permanent melphalan induced retinal toxicity as evidenced by reduced ERG amplitude [69].

1.10 Radiotherapy

Radiation therapy has an established role in selected patients. It may be administered in the form of plaque brachytherapy or EBRT.

1.10.1 Plaque Brachytherapy

Plaque brachytherapy is mainly used as a secondary treatment option for recurrent and residual tumours after failure of systemic and focal therapies. The indications include unilateral solitary tumours <16 mm in base and <8 mm in thickness located anterior to the equator upto the ora serrata [71–74]. Larger tumours and those involving the macula are not suitable for plaque therapy. For tumours near the optic disc, special plaques with a notch are used. The most commonly used radioisotopes are Iodine (I^{125}) and Ruthenium (Ru^{106}) [75–77]. I^{125} seeds are inserted into a gold carrier to protect the normal surrounding tissue from radiation effects. A dose of 40 Gy is provided to the apex of the tumour with the help of dosimetry planning. The plaque is kept in situ for a period of 2–4 days, until the desired radiation dose has been delivered.

Radiation therapy may be associated with side effects that include dryness of eye, madarosis, cataract, scleral necrosis, retinopathy, papillopathy, optic neuropathy, and strabismus [71–74]. Second malignancies are not associated with local therapy. Shields et al. found plaque brachytherapy to be particularly useful for tumours that failed treatment with other conservative modalities. They observed tumour control in 79% of cases at 5-year follow-up, with young patients without vitreous or subretinal seeding showing the best long-term control [74]. Plaque brachytherapy has come up not only as a secondary treatment modality for recurrent or resistant tumours but also as a primary treatment. The American Brachytherapy Society Ophthalmic Oncology Task Force (ABS-OOTF) recommends primary brachytherapy for unilateral anterior lesions less than 15 mm in base and upto 10 mm in thickness in the absence of vitreous seeding [78].

1.10.2 External Beam Radiotherapy

External beam radiotherapy (EBRT) was extensively used for treatment of retinoblastoma prior to the chemotherapy era. Due to concerns about radiation induced growth deformities and second malignancies, the popularity of EBRT declined [79, 80]. Although it has limited use in intraocular retinoblastoma these days, EBRT is used as adjuvant therapy in cases with residual microscopic disease after enucleation, and as part of multi-modal therapy for orbital retinoblastoma. Side effects of EBRT include dryness, foreign body sensation, cataract, radiation retinopathy and papillopathy. Systemic complications like secondary malignancies in cases with germline mutations have been attributed to radiotherapy. Orbital hypoplasia is another side effect of EBRT (Fig. 1.11).

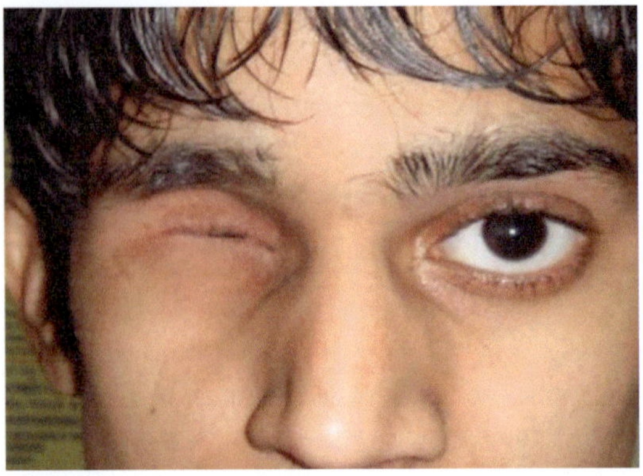

Fig. 1.11 Late effects of radiation therapy

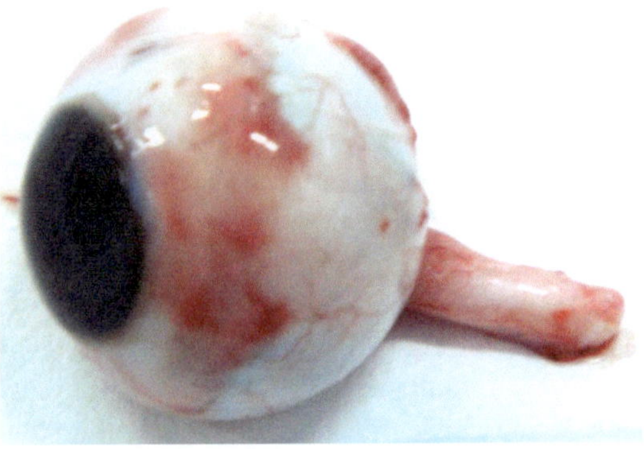

Fig. 1.12 Enucleated eyeball

The advent of newer radiotherapy techniques has led to improved radiation delivery to the target with better sparing of normal tissue. Stereotactic conformal radiotherapy (SCR) uses highly accurate positioning to deliver treatment with small beams. A recent study has shown that SCR provides more homogeneous dose within the target volume and similar or lower doses to the surrounding normal tissues [81]. However, its efficacy over plaque therapy has not been proven. Proton beam therapy also provides a uniform dose coverage of the target and unlike photon beams, does not distribute energy beyond the target. As a result, the incidence of late effects of radiation are minimized [82]. However, proton therapy is expensive and is not widely available. Sethi et al. compared the risk of second malignancies in retinoblastoma survivors treated with photon and proton radiation therapy [82]. A significant difference was observed in the 10 year cumulative incidence of radiotherapy induced second malignancies between the proton and photon modalities ($p = 0.015$) [82].

1.11 Enucleation

Although one of the oldest modalities of treatment, enucleation remains the standard of care for advanced intraocular retinoblastoma with poor visual potential. Most often, Group E tumours are treated by enucleation. Unilateral Group D tumours may also be offered enucleation, especially if the potential for vision is poor. Due to late presentation, enucleation is one of the most commonly performed procedures in the developing world [83]. The surgery is done using minimal manipulation, and an optic nerve stump of 15 mm is recommended, to minimize the chances of residual disease at the resected end of the optic nerve. Gross inspection of the enucleated globe should be done to look for any suspicious area (Fig. 1.12). An adequate sized implant should be placed in the socket to restore the lost volume at the time of surgery. Careful microscopic examination of the enucleated specimen should be performed to look for presence of high risk histopathological features. These include tumour infiltration into the iris, ciliary body, anterior chamber, massive choroidal invasion, scleral invasion and post-laminar optic nerve invasion [84]. Cases with one or more high risk features should be treated with six cycles of intravenous chemotherapy (VEC) as prophylactic treatment against local recurrence/systemic metastasis [85]. Presence of tumour cells in the extra-scleral tissues or at the resected end of optic nerve is indicative of residual microscopic disease, which should be treated with adjuvant chemotherapy and radiotherapy. An ocular prosthesis (artificial eye) is usually fitted at six weeks after surgery and every effort should be made to achieve a good cosmetic outcome.

1.12 Extraocular Retinoblastoma

Although extraocular disease is rare in the West, it is not an unusual feature in the developing world, where it constitutes 20–50% of all cases [83, 86, 87]. Extra-ocular disease is associated with a 10–27 times higher risk of metastasis and therefore demands a more aggressive treatment approach [87]. Extra-ocular disease may be non-metastatic (confined to the orbit and regional lymph-nodes) or metastatic. Figure 1.13 shows a child with tumour involving the right eye and extensive orbital invasion.

Orbital exenteration, a mutilating and disfiguring surgery, was used to treat patients with overt orbital disease in earlier days. Studies have shown that a multi-modal approach that consists of neo-adjuvant chemotherapy, surgery, EBRT, and adjuvant chemotherapy is effective in managing local orbital extension [88–90]. Treatment is initiated with 3–6 cycles of systemic chemotherapy. This induces tumour regression and makes enucleation surgery possible. After enucleation, orbital irradiation is administered followed by adjuvant chemotherapy for a total of 12 cycles.

Chantada et al. reported a 5-year EFS rate of 84% in 15 patients with orbital or preauricular disease treated with chemotherapy that included vincristine, doxorubicin, and cyclophosphamide or vincristine, idarubicin, cyclophosphamide, carboplatin, and etoposide [89]. These patients also received EBRT of 4500 cGy administered to the optic chiasma for patients with orbital disease and to the involved nodes for those with preauricular lymphadenopathy.

Recently, a prospective randomized comparative study on 54 cases of Stage III Retinoblastoma (International Retinoblastoma Staging System) was published from our centre [91]. For chemotherapy, patients were randomized into two groups; one group was treated with high-dose triple-drug chemotherapy consisting of VEC and the other group with carboplatin and etoposide, alternating with cyclophosphamide, idarubicin, and vincristine (five drugs). The study showed more effective tumour control and a better safety profile with the VEC protocol [91]. Central nervous system (CNS) metastasis was the most common cause of relapse and death. None of the cases needed orbital exenteration. Patients with metastatic extraocular disease have a poor prognosis when treated with regimens of conventional doses of chemotherapy. Recently, there has been encouraging data to suggest that patients with distant metastatic disease may benefit from high-dose chemotherapy and EBRT in conjunction with bone marrow stem cell transplantation. Metastasis to the CNS can occur in advanced, untreated cases (Fig. 1.14). It is rare for a patient with metastatic CNS involvement to survive using the therapies described above. Second malignant neoplasms are a major concern for survival. Osteosarcoma is the commonest second malignancy; other second neoplasms include rhabdomyosarcoma and melanoma.

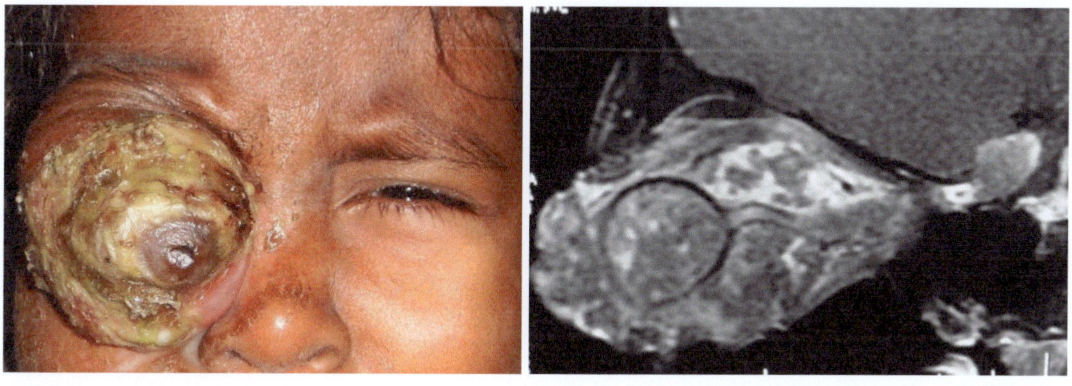

Fig. 1.13 Orbital retinoblastoma

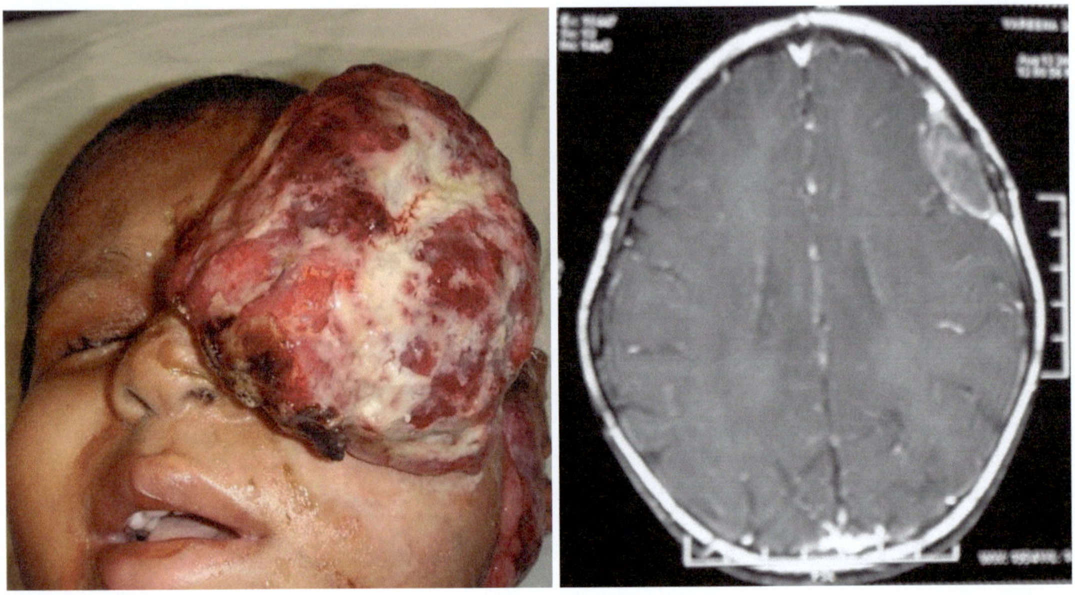

Fig. 1.14 Metastatic retinoblastoma

1.13 Regression Patterns

Differentiation of tumour regression from an incomplete response or recurrence is critical for appropriate management. Upon regression, the tumour usually assumes a smaller size and attains some degree of calcification. While some tumours become completely calcified, others may have minimal or no calcification, making assessment of regression challenging (Table 1.5). Regression patterns following systemic chemo-reduction have been described [92].

Table 1.5 Regression patterns in retinoblastoma following systemic chemotherapy

Type	Regression pattern
Type 0	No visible remnant
Type 1	Completely calcified remnant
Type 2	Completely noncalcified remnant
Type 3	Partially calcified remnant
Type 4	Atrophic chorioretinal flat scar

1.14 Prenatal Diagnosis

Advances in technology have facilitated pre-natal diagnosis of retinoblastoma [93]. Prenatal diagnosis can facilitate anticipatory planning for the child and the family. Both imaging as well as genetic testing can be used for prenatal diagnosis. Investigators have used high resolution ultrasound at 37 weeks of gestation to detect a 2–3 mm elevated lesion in a foetus at risk of heritable retinoblastoma [93]. Soliman et al. compared the conventional postnatal screening of familial retinoblastoma with prenatal RB1 mutation dentification followed by planned early-term delivery [94]. They concluded that in case of a parent having retinoblastoma, prenatal molecular diagnosis with early-term delivery increased the chances of infants having no detectable tumours at birth, better vision outcomes, and less invasive therapy [94].

To summarize, significant advances have been made in the diagnosis and management of retinoblastoma [95]. A clear understanding of these is essential for achieving the best outcome.

References

1. Bishop JO, Madsen EC. Retinoblastoma. Review of current status. Surv Ophthalmol. 1975;19:342–66.
2. Albert DM. Historic review of retinoblastoma. Ophthalmology. 1987;94:654–62.

3. Jackson E. Report of the committee to investigate and revise the classification of certain retinal conditions. Trans Am Ophthalmol Soc. 1926;24:38–9.
4. Shields CL, Schoenberg E, Kocher K, Shukla SY, Kaliki S, Shields JA. Lesions simulating retinoblastoma (pseudoretinoblastoma) in 604 cases: results based on age at presentation. Ophthalmology. 2013;120:311–6.
5. Chawla B, Seth R, Moksha L. Chemotherapy for ocular cancers. In: Pharmacology of ocular therapeutics. Cham: Springer; 2016. p. 333–58.
6. Yoshizumi MO, Thomas JV, Smith TR. Glaucoma-inducing mechanisms in eyes with retinoblastoma. Arch Ophthalmol. 1978;96:105–10.
7. Chawla B, Khurana S, Sen S, Sharma S. Clinical misdiagnosis of retinoblastoma in Indian children. Br J Ophthalmol. 2014;98:488–93.
8. Chawla B, Hada M, Seth R, Sen S, Gupta V, Kashyap S, et al. Trabeculectomy in eyes with unsuspected retinoblastoma. Ophthalmic Genet. 2016;12:1–4.
9. Shields J, Shields C. Retinoblastoma: diagnostic approaches. In: Shields J, Shields C, editors. Atlas of intraocular tumors. 3rd ed. Philadelphia: Lippincott, Wolters Kluwer; 2016.
10. Moulin AP, Gaillard MC, Balmer A, Munier FL. Ultrasound biomicroscopy evaluation of anterior extension in retinoblastoma: a clinicopathological study. Br J Ophthalmol. 2011;96:337–40.
11. Vasquez LM, Giuliari GP, Halliday W, Pavlin CJ, Gallie BL, Héon E. Ultrasound biomicroscopy in the management of retinoblastoma. Eye. 2011;25:141–7.
12. Rootman DB, Gonzalez E, Mallipatna A, Vandenhoven C, Hampton L, Dimaras H, et al. Hand-held high-resolution spectral domain optical coherence tomography in retinoblastoma: clinical and morphologic considerations. Br J Ophthalmol. 2013;97:59–65.
13. Chawla B, Sharma S, Sen S, Azad R, Bajaj MS, Kashyap S, et al. Correlation between clinical features, MRI and histopathologic findings in retinoblastoma: a prospective study. Ophthalmology. 2012;119:850–6.
14. de Jong MC, de Graaf P, Noij DP, Göricke S, Maeder P, Galluzzi P, et al. Diagnostic performance of magnetic resonance imaging and computed tomography for advanced retinoblastoma: a systematic review and meta-analysis. Ophthalmology. 2014;121:1109–18.
15. Chawla B, Duraipandi K, Sharma S. MRI in retinoblastoma associated orbital cellulitis. Ophthalmology. 2013;120:1308–9.
16. Reese AB, Ellsworth RM. The evaluation and current concept of retinoblastoma therapy. Trans Am Acad Ophthalmol Otolaryngol. 1963;67:164–72.
17. Linn Murphree A. Intraocular retinoblastoma: the case for a new group classification. Ophthalmol Clin N Am. 2005;18:41–53.
18. Shields CL, Mashayekhi A, Au AK, Czyz C, Leahey A, Meadows AT, et al. The International Classification of Retinoblastoma predicts chemoreduction success. Ophthalmology. 2006;113:2276–80.
19. Amin MB, Edge SB, Greene FL, Byrd DR, Brookland RK, Washington MK, et al., editors. Retinoblastoma. In: AJCC cancer staging manual. 8th ed. New York: Springer; 2017. p. 819–31.
20. Chantada G, Doz F, Antoneli CB, Grundy R, Clare Stannard FF, Dunkel IJ, et al. A proposal for an international retinoblastoma staging system. Pediatr Blood Cancer. 2006;47:801–5.
21. Abramson DH, Schefler AC. Transpupillary thermotherapy as initial treatment for small intraocular retinoblastoma: technique and predictors of success. Ophthalmology. 2004;111:984–91.
22. Shields CL, Santos MC, Diniz W, Gunduz K, Mercado G, Cater JR, et al. Thermotherapy for retinoblastoma. Arch Ophthalmol. 1999;117:885–93.
23. Hilderbrandt B, Wust P, Ahlers O, Dieing A, Sreenivasa G, Kerner T, et al. The cellular and molecular basis of hyperthermia. Crit Rev Oncol Hematol. 2002;43:33–56.
24. Ohtsubo T, Saito H, Tanaka N, Tsuzuki H, Saito T, Kano E. In vitro effect of hyperthermia on chemoenhancement and uptake of cisplatin in human pharyngeal carcinoma KB cells. Chemotherapy. 1997;43:43–50.
25. Shields JA, Shields CL, Parsons H, Giblin ME. The role of photocoagulation in the management of retinoblastoma. Arch Ophthalmol. 1990;108:205–8.
26. Shields JA. The expanding role of laser photocoagulation for intraocular tumors. The 1993 H. Christian Zweng Memorial Lecture. Retina. 1994;14:310–22.
27. Shields CL, Shields JA, Kiratli H, De Potter PV. Treatment of retinoblastoma with indirect ophthalmoscope laser photocoagulation. J Pediatr Ophthalmol Strabismus. 1995;32:317–22.
28. Murphree AL, Villablanca JG, Deegan WF, Sato JK, Malogolowin M, Fisher A, et al. Chemotherapy plus local treatment in the management of intraocular retinoblastoma. Arch Ophthalmol. 1996;114:1348–56.
29. Murphree AL, Munier FL. Retinoblastoma. In: Ryan SJ, editor. Retina. 2nd ed. St Louis: Mosby Year Book Inc.; 1994. p. 605–6.
30. Abramson DH, Ellsworth RM, Rozakis GW. Cryotherapy for retinoblastoma. Arch Ophthalmol. 1982;100:1253–6.
31. Shields JA, Parsons H, Shields CL, Giblin ME. The role of cryotherapy in the management of retinoblastoma. Am J Ophthalmol. 1989;108:260–4.
32. Kingston JE, Hungerford JL, Madreperla SA, Plowman PN. Results of combined chemotherapy and radiotherapy for advanced intraocular retinoblastoma. Arch Ophthalmol. 1996;114:1339–43.
33. Gallie BL, Budning A, DeBoer G, Thiessen JJ, Koren G, Verjee Z, et al. Chemotherapy with focal therapy can cure intraocular retinoblastoma without radiotherapy. Arch Ophthalmol. 1996;114:1321–8.
34. Shields CL, De Potter P, Himelstein BP, Shields JA, Meadows AT, Maris JM. Chemoreduction in the initial management of intraocular retinoblastoma. Arch Ophthalmol. 1996;114:1330–8.
35. Friedman DL, Himelstein B, Shields CL, Shields JA, Needle M, Miller D, et al. Chemoreduction and local ophthalmic therapy for intraocular retinoblastoma. J Clin Oncol. 2000;18:12–7.

36. Shields CL, Honavar SG, Meadows AT, Shields JA, Demirci H, Naduvilath TJ. Chemoreduction for unilateral retinoblastoma. Arch Ophthalmol. 2002;120:1653–8.
37. Chan HS, De Boer G, Thiessen JJ, Budning A, Kingston JE, O'Brien JM, et al. Combining cyclosporin with chemotherapy controls intraocular retinoblastoma without requiring radiation. Clin Cancer Res. 1996;2:1499–508.
38. Rodriguez-Galindo C, Wilson MW, Haik BG, Merchant TE, Billups CA, Shah N, et al. Treatment of intraocular retinoblastoma with vincristine and carboplatin. J Clin Oncol. 2003;21:2019–25.
39. Chawla B, Jain A, Azad R. Conservative treatment modalities in retinoblastoma. Indian J Ophthalmol. 2013;61:479–85.
40. Chawla B, Jain A, Seth R, Azad R, Mohan VK, Pushker N, et al. Clinical outcome and regression patterns of retinoblastoma treated with systemic chemoreduction and focal therapy: a prospective study. Indian J Ophthalmol. 2016;64:524–9.
41. Le Deley MC, Vassal G, Taibi A, Shamsaldin A, Leblanc T, Hartmann O. High cumulative rate of secondary leukemia after continuous etoposide treatment for solid tumors in children and young adults. Pediatr Blood Cancer. 2005;45:25–31.
42. Bayar E, Robinson MG, Kurczynski TW. Unilateral retinoblastoma with acquired monosomy 7 and secondary acute myelomonocytic leukemia. Cancer Genet Cytogenet. 1998;105:79–82.
43. Chan HS, Héon E, Budning A. Improvement of the cure rate of intraocular retinoblastoma without significantly increasing toxicity with higher dose carboplatin teniposide in a cyclosporine multidrug reversal regimen. In: Presented at the 10th international symposium on Retinoblastoma. Florida: Fort Lauderdale. p. 2001.
44. Villablanca JG. Clinical outcome of group V eyes treated with cyclosporine A/carboplatin/etoposide/vincristine. In: Presented at the 10th international symposium on Retinoblastoma. Florida: Fort Lauderdale. p. 2001.
45. Leng T, Cebulla CM, Schefler AC, Murray TG. Focal periocular carboplatin chemotherapy avoids systemic chemotherapy for unilateral, progressive retinoblastoma. Retina. 2010;30:S66–8.
46. Abramson DH, Frank CM, Dunkel IJ. A phase I/II study of subconjunctival carboplatin for intraocular retinoblastoma. Ophthalmology. 1999;106:1947–50.
47. Villablanca JG, Jubran RF, Murphree LA. Phase I study of subtenon carboplatin with systemic high dose carboplatin/etoposide/vincristine for eyes with disseminated intraocular Retinoblastoma. In: Presented at the 10th international symposium on retinoblastoma. Florida: Fort Lauderdale. p. 2001.
48. Shields CL, Shields JA. Retinoblastoma management: advances in enucleation, intravenous chemoreduction, and intra-arterial chemotherapy. Curr Opin Ophthalmol. 2010;21:203–12.
49. Mulvihill A, Budning A, Jay V, Vandenhoven C, Héon E, Gallie BL, et al. Ocular motility changes after subtenon carboplatin chemotherapy for retinoblastoma. Arch Ophthalmol. 2003;121:1120–4.
50. Schmack I, Hubbard GB, Kang SJ, Aaberg TM Jr, Grossniklaus HE. Ischemic necrosis and atrophy of the optic nerve after periocular carboplatin injection for intraocular retinoblastoma. Am J Ophthalmol. 2006;142:310–5.
51. Kiratli H, Kocabeyoglu S, Bilgic S. Severe pseudopreseptal cellulitis following sub-Tenon's carboplatin injection for intraocular retinoblastoma. J AAPOS. 2007;11:404–5.
52. Kaneko A, Suzuki S. Eye-preservation treatment of retinoblastoma with vitreous seeding. Jpn J Clin Oncol. 2003;33:601–7.
53. Suzuki S, Kaneko A. Management of intraocular retinoblastoma and ocular prognosis. Int J Clin Oncol. 2004;9:1–6.
54. Abramson DH, Dunkel IJ, Brodie SE, Kim JW, Gobin YP. A phase I/II study of direct intraarterial (ophthalmic artery) chemotherapy with melphalan for intraocular retinoblastoma initial results. Ophthalmology. 2008;115:1398–404.
55. Gobin YP, Dunkel IJ, Marr BP, Brodie SE, Abramson DH. Intra-arterial chemotherapy for the management of retinoblastoma: four-year experience. Arch Ophthalmol. 2011;129:732–7.
56. Shields CL, Bianciotto CG, Jabbour P, Ramasubramanian A, Lally SE, Griffin GC, et al. Intra-arterial chemotherapy for retinoblastoma: report No. 1, control of retinal tumors, sub-retinal seeds, and vitreous seeds. Arch Ophthalmol. 2011;129:1399–406.
57. Abramson DH, Marr BP, Brodie SE, Dunkel I, Palioura S, Gobin YP. Ophthalmic artery chemosurgery for less advanced intraocular retinoblastoma: five year review. PLoS One. 2012;7:e34120.
58. Thampi S, Hetts SW, Cooke DL, Stewart PJ, Robbins E, Banerjee A, et al. Superselective intra-arterial melphalan therapy for newly diagnosed and refractory retinoblastoma: results from a single institution. Clin Ophthalmol. 2013;7:981–9.
59. Tuncer S, Sencer S, Kebudi R, Tanyıldız B, Cebeci Z, Aydın K. Superselective intra-arterial chemotherapy in the primary management of advanced intra-ocular retinoblastoma: first 4-year experience from a single institution in Turkey. Acta Ophthalmol. 2016;94:e644–51.
60. Chen M, Zhao J, Xia J, Liu Z, Jiang H, Shen G, et al. Intra-arterial chemotherapy as primary therapy for retinoblastoma in infants less than 3 months of age: a series of 10 case-studies. PLoS One. 2016;11(8):e0160873.
61. Abramson DH, Marr BP, Francis JH, Dunkel IJ, Fabius AW, Brodie SE, et al. Simultaneous bilateral ophthalmic artery chemosurgery for bilateral retinoblastoma (tandem therapy). PLoS One. 2016;11(6):e0156806.
62. Michaels ST, Abruzzo TA, Augsburger JJ, Corrêa ZM, Lane A, Geller JI. Selective ophthalmic artery infusion chemotherapy for advanced intraocular retinoblastoma: CCHMC early experience. J Pediatr Hematol Oncol. 2016;38:65–9.

63. Bertelli E, Leonini S, Galimberti D, Moretti S, Tinturini R, Hadjistilianou T, et al. Hemodynamic and anatomic variations require an adaptable approach during intra-arterial chemotherapy for intraocular retinoblastoma: alternative routes, strategies, and follow-up. AJNR Am J Neuroradiol. 2016;37:1289–95.
64. Klufas MA, Gobin YP, Marr B, Brodie SE, Dunkel IJ, Abramson DH. Intra-arterial chemotherapy as a treatment for intraocular retinoblastoma: alternatives to direct ophthalmic artery catheterization. AJNR Am J Neuroradiol. 2012;33:1608–14.
65. Inomata M, Kaneko A. Chemosensitivity profiles of primary and cultured retinoblastoma cells in a human clonogenic assay. Jpn J Cancer Res. 1987;78:858–68.
66. Munier FL, Gaillard MC, Balmer A, Soliman S, Podilsky G, Moulin AP, et al. Intravitreal chemotherapy for vitreous disease in retinoblastoma revisited: from prohibition to conditional indications. Br J Ophthalmol. 2012;96:1078–83.
67. Shields CL, Manjandavida FP, Arepalli S, Kaliki S, Lally SE, Shields JA. Intravitreal melphalan for persistent or recurrent retinoblastoma vitreous seeds: preliminary results. JAMA Ophthalmol. 2014;132:319–25.
68. Ghassemi F, Shields CL, Ghadimi H, Khodabandeh A, Roohipoor R. Combined intravitreal melphalan and topotecan for refractory or recurrent vitreous seeding from retinoblastoma. JAMA Ophthalmol. 2014;132:936–41.
69. Francis JH, Schaiquevich P, Buitrago E, Del Sole MJ, Zapata G, Croxatto JO, et al. Local and systemic toxicity of intravitreal melphalan for vitreous seeding in retinoblastoma: a preclinical and clinical study. Ophthalmology. 2014;121:1810–7.
70. Smith SJ, Smith BD, Mohney BG. Ocular side effects following intravitreal injection therapy for retinoblastoma: a systematic review. Br J Ophthalmol. 2014;98:292–7.
71. Merchant TE, Gould CJ, Wilson MW, Hilton NE, Rodriguez-Galindo C, Haik BG. Episcleral plaque brachytherapy for retinoblastoma. Pediatr Blood Cancer. 2004;43:134–9.
72. Shields CL, Shields JA, De Potter P, Minelli S, Hernandez C, Brady LW, et al. Plaque radiotherapy in the management of retinoblastoma. Use as a primary and secondary treatment. Ophthalmology. 1993;100:216–24.
73. Hernandez JC, Brady LW, Shields CL, Shields JA, De Potter P. Conservative treatment of retinoblastoma. The use of plaque brachytherapy. Am J Clin Oncol. 1993;16:397–401.
74. Shields CL, Shields JA, Cater J, Othmane I, Singh AD, Micaily B. Plaque radiotherapy for retinoblastoma: long-term tumor control and treatment complications in 208 tumors. Ophthalmology. 2001;108:2116–21.
75. Shields CL, Mashayekhi A, Sun H, Uysal Y, Friere J, Komarnicky L, et al. Iodine 125 plaque radiotherapy as salvage treatment for retinoblastoma recurrence after chemoreduction in 84 tumors. Ophthalmology. 2006;113:2087–92.
76. Schueler AO, Fluhs D, Anastassiou G, Jurklies C, Sauerwein W, Bornfeld N. Beta-ray brachytherapy of retinoblastoma: feasibility of a new small-sized ruthenium-106 plaque. Ophthalmic Res. 2006;38:8–12.
77. Abouzeid H, Moeckli R, Gaillard MC, Beck-Popovic M, Pica A, Zografos L, et al. (106) Ruthenium brachytherapy for retinoblastoma. Int J Radiat Oncol Biol Phys. 2008;71:821–8.
78. American Brachytherapy Society - Ophthalmic Oncology Task Force. The American Brachytherapy Society consensus guidelines for plaque brachytherapy of uveal melanoma and retinoblastoma. Brachytherapy. 2014;13:1–14.
79. Marees T, Moll AC, Imhof SM, de Boer MR, Ringens PJ, van Leeuwen FE. Risk of second malignancies in survivors of retinoblastoma: more than 40 years of follow-up. J Natl Cancer Inst. 2008;100:1771–9.
80. Kleinerman RA, Tucker MA, Tarone RE, Abramson DH, Seddon JM, Stovall M, et al. Risk of new cancers after radiotherapy in long-term survivors of retinoblastoma: an extended follow-up. J Clin Oncol. 2005;23:2272–9.
81. Eldebawy E, Patrocinio H, Evans M, Hashem R, Nelson S, Sidi R, et al. Stereotactic radiotherapy as an alternative to plaque brachytherapy in retinoblastoma. Pediatr Blood Cancer. 2010;55:1210–2.
82. Sethi RV, Shih HA, Yeap BY, Mouw KW, Petersen R, Kim DY, et al. Second nonocular tumors among survivors of retinoblastoma treated with contemporary photon and proton radiotherapy. Cancer. 2014;120:126–33.
83. Chawla B, Hasan F, Azad R, Seth R, Upadhyay AD, Pathy S, et al. Clinical presentation and survival of retinoblastoma in Indian children. Br J Ophthalmol. 2016;100:172–8.
84. National Cancer Institute. Clinical Trials (PDQ). Phase III study of adjuvant vincristine, carboplatin and etoposide or observation only in patients with newly diagnosed retinoblastoma with or without histopathological high-risk features after enucleation. ClinicalTrials.gov registration NCT00335738. Last modified February 25, 2010. Available at http://www.cancer.gov/clinicaltrials/search/view?cdrid_483043&version_health_professional. Accessed August 2, 2011.
85. Honavar SG, Singh AD, Shields CL, Meadows AT, Demirci H, Cater J, et al. Post enucleation adjuvant therapy in high-risk retinoblastoma. Arch Ophthalmol. 2002;120:923–30.
86. Badhu B, Sah SP, Thakur SK, Dulal S, Kumar S, Sood A, et al. Clinical presentation of retinoblastoma in Eastern Nepal. Clin Exp Ophthalmol. 2005;33:386–9.
87. Gündüz K, Müftüoglu O, Günalp I, Unal E, Taçyildiz N. Metastatic retinoblastoma clinical features, treatment, and prognosis. Ophthalmology. 2006;113:1558–66.
88. Antoneli CB, Steinhorst F, de Cássia Braga Ribeiro K, Novaes PE, Chojniak MM, Arias V, et al. Extraocular retinoblastoma: a 13-year experience. Cancer. 2003;98:1292–8.

89. Chantada G, Fandiño A, Casak S, Manzitti J, Raslawski E, Schvartzman E. Treatment of overt extraocular retinoblastoma. Med Pediatr Oncol. 2003;40:158–61.
90. Chantada GL, Guitter MR, Fandiño AC, Raslawski EC, de Davila MT, Vaiani E, et al. Treatment results in patients with retinoblastoma and invasion to the cut end of the optic nerve. Pediatr Blood Cancer. 2009;52:218–22.
91. Chawla B, Hasan F, Seth R, Pathy S, Pattebahadur R, Sharma S, et al. Multimodal therapy for stage III retinoblastoma (international retinoblastoma staging system): a prospective comparative study. Ophthalmology. 2016;123:1933–9.
92. Shields CL, Palamar M, Sharma P, Ramasubramanian A, Leahey A, Meadows AT, et al. Retinoblastoma regression patterns following chemoreduction and adjuvant therapy in 557 tumors. Arch Ophthalmol. 2009;127:282–90.
93. Paquette LB, Miller D, Jackson HA, Lee T, Randolph L, Murphree AL, Panigrahy A. In utero detection of retinoblastoma with fetal magnetic resonance and ultrasound: initial experience. Am J Perinatol Rep. 2012;2:55–62.
94. Soliman SE, Dimaras H, Khetan V, Gardiner JA, Chan HS, Héon E, et al. Prenatal versus postnatal screening for familial retinoblastoma. Ophthalmology. 2016;123:2610–7.
95. Chawla B, Singh S. Recent advances and challenges in the management of retinoblastoma. Indian J Ophthalmol. 2017;65(2):133–9.

2 Genetics of Retinoblastoma for Patients and Their Families

Carol Lam Po Sang, Jaime Jessen, Hilary Racher, and Brenda L. Gallie

2.1 Introduction

Retinoblastoma is the most common intraocular cancer in children. The number of children affected each year in each country can be estimated from the population, live birth rate, and infant death rate. The global incidence rate for retinoblastoma is 1 in 16,000 to 18,000 affected children per live birth world wide and is not impacted by environment or race [1]. However, poverty impacts directly on outcomes, resulting in estimated 30% survival with vision in low-income countries through late diagnosis and poor awareness of parents and health care systems. High-income countries show survival greater than 95%.

Retinoblastoma is the first cancer recognized to be caused by genetic alterations. While " mutation" has been used extensively to mean the genetic change in the gene causing disease, this word is no longer considered appropriate in genetic counseling [2]. A high proportion of patients who are predisposed to retinoblastoma due to a constitutional change in the *RB1* gene, have no family history: the pathogenic variant is most commonly "new" to the affected child and the family. As explained below, the term "germline" is misleading to describe every patient who has retinoblastoma who carries an *RB1* pathogenic variant. The new staging classification [3] for retinoblastoma has a simpler and more accurate designation, H1, described in detail below.

Retinoblastoma is too rare for universal screening of all babies, but genetic testing of blood of each affected child for any *RB1* pathogenic variant in the predisposing tumor suppressor gene, *RB1*, supports family counseling and attention to H1 high risk relatives to optimize early diagnosis, safe eye salvage, and life-long surveillance for the secondary cancers in H1 persons carrying *RB1* pathogenic variants.

C. L. P. Sang
Hong Kong Eye Hospital, Ho Man Tin, Hong Kong

Chinese University of Hong Kong, Sha Tin, Hong Kong

J. Jessen · H. Racher
Impact Genetics, Bowmanville, ON, Canada
e-mail: JessenJ@dynacare.ca; hracher@impactgenetics.com

B. L. Gallie (✉)
Hospital for Sick Children, Toronto, ON, Canada

Techna Institute, University Health Network, Toronto, ON, Canada

Department of Ophthalmology, University of Toronto, Toronto, ON, Canada

Department of Medical Biophysics, University of Toronto, Toronto, ON, Canada

Department of Molecular Genetics, University of Toronto, Toronto, ON, Canada
e-mail: brenda@gallie.ca

V. Khetan (ed.), *Intraocular Tumors*, https://doi.org/10.1007/978-981-15-0395-5_2

2.2 Genetic Basis of Retinoblastoma

We have a rich understanding of the genetic basis and pathogenesis of retinoblastoma. In 1971, Knudson's observation that only two events ("hits") occurred to generate retinoblastoma was based on the simple observation of age at diagnosis of children with bilateral vs. unilateral retinoblastoma [4]. It had been observed that children with bilateral retinoblastoma were genetically susceptible to develop tumors in both eyes, and could pass this risk to their offspring. The location of this predisposition gene was suspected to be on chromosome 13q because children missing part of the "D" group of chromosomes [5–9], developed retinoblastoma. Studies of tumor and blood DNA then showed that when genomic markers could distinguish the two copies of chromosome 13 in blood, many retinoblastoma tumors showed only one, which was often duplicated [10, 11].

This observation led to the discovery of the first gene which encodes a protein that normally suppresses development of cancer. The *RB1* tumor suppressor gene is located at chromosome 13q14.2 [12, 13], and encodes the retinoblastoma protein (pRB), an important regulator of the cell division cycle and genomic stability in most cell types [1].

The first hit [4] that predisposes children to develop retinoblastoma is the functional loss of one of the two *RB1* alleles in most or all cells of the patient ($RB1^{+/-}$). Offspring of $RB1^{+/-}$ persons can inherit the pathogenic allele. The second hit is an acquired *RB1* somatic pathogenic variant that arises in one susceptible retinal cell and initiates cancer progression. Because only one additional hit is required, $RB1^{+/-}$ children usually develop multiple retinoblastoma tumors in both eyes, but may also have only unilateral disease.

Non-heritable retinoblastoma develops in a person with two normal *RB1* alleles in their constitutional cells ($RB1^{+/+}$). The two pathogenic variants or "hits" in both *RB1* alleles in the cancer are somatic, only in the retinal cell that becomes the tumor. Because $RB1^{+/+}$ persons are not predisposed, they develop only one unilateral tumor. In addition, a novel form of non-heritable unilateral retinoblastoma has been recognized: in 2% of unilateral patients with normal *RB1* alleles in the tumor ($RB1^{+/+}$), the *MYNC* oncogene is highly amplified, driving the retinal cells to proliferate out of control and cause aggressive cancer [14].

Commonly, the genomic instability induced by loss of *RB1* leads to other specific genomic alterations, including gains in oncogenes *MDM4*, *KIF14* (chromosome 1q32), *MYCN* (chromosome 2p24), *DEK* and *E2F3* (chromosome 6p22) and loss of the tumor suppressor gene *CDH11* (chromosome 16q22-24) [15, 16]. It is interesting that this "signature" of genomic chances in retinoblastoma tumors was first identified in 1985 by study of karyotypes of tumors [17], and is virtually unchanged in 2018 highly sophisticated "next generation" genomic analysis of retinoblastoma tumors [18].

The human retinal cell that is highly susceptible to become cancer when both *RB1* alleles are non-functional, shows properties of cone photoreceptor precursor cells [19]. Mature cones reside in the outer photoreceptor layer of retina, but the earliest identified very small retinoblastoma tumors in newborn predisposed ($RB1^{-/-}$) infants are clearly observed by optical coherent tomography to be located in the inner nuclear layer [20, 21]. It is speculated that a human $RB1^{-/-}$ cone precursor cell remains in, or mislocalizes to the inner nuclear layer [1, 21].

Loss of *RB1* is not sufficient for malignant transformation: rather, the $RB1^{-/-}$ developing retinal cell that has lost both copies of *RB1* ($RB1^{-/-}$) fails to complete differentiation, and instead forms a benign precursor tumor, retinoma [22]. Signature genomic changes characteristic of retinoblastoma were found in both retinoma and retinoblastoma in individual eyes, with adjacent retina normal. The extent and magnitude of the genomic copy number changes were less in retinoma, and increased in extent in adjacent retinoblastoma. The key genomic changes that push benign retinoma to malignant retinoblastoma are still unknown.

2.3 Cancer Staging

Cancer staging of retinoblastoma depends on the anatomic location of the tumor and extent of spread outside the retina, and is intended to help clinicians identify patients at high risk for metastases and assess the likelihood to safely treat and salvage the eye. Prognosis for the patient, eye and vision depend on the location of tumor origin, size of tumor, extent of subretinal fluid, presence of tumor seeds under the retina and in the vitreous, and features on pathology of the enucleated eye that suggest high risk that the tumor may have already metastasized. These children need further treatment before metastatic cells are ever detected (adjuvant chemotherapy). The 2017 AJCC 8th edition of cancer staging for retinoblastoma is based on international consensus and evidence from an international survey of 1728 eyes including data on the initial clinical and pathological features at first diagnosis and eye and life outcomes. Four previous eye staging systems [23–26] were compared for success to predict eye salvage without using external beam radiation. The same data was then analyzed by the new 8th edition retinoblastoma staging system, showing better separation of eye outcomes than any of the previous systems [3]. Retinoblastoma is the first cancer to recognize the importance of genetic status in patient outcome, including "H" for heritability (Table 2.1) [3, 8].

Patients with bilateral or trilateral tumor, positive family history or identification of a *RB1* pathogenic variant on high sensitivity genetic testing are considered H1. Unilateral patients who have not been tested, or who show a variant in *RB1* of unknown significance (which could be a normal polymorphism) are categorized HX. H0 applies to siblings and offspring of an H1 person who test negative for the known familial *RB1* pathogenic variant of their relative. H0∗ is proposed to categorize probands in which no *RB1* pathogenic variant is found in blood, and parents of affected children who test negative in blood for their child's known *RB1* pathogenic variant, but who remain at low risk (<1%) of undetectable mosaicism (the *RB1* pathogenic variant arose in only one cell of the developing embryo, which then affected the germline) [27]. However, offspring of H0∗ subjects who test negative for the known familial *RB1* pathogenic variant are truly H0; those who test positive are H1 and require

Table 2.1 AJCC 8th edition cancer staging includes H for heritability

Heritability	Definition	Examples
HX	Unknown or insufficient evidence of a constitutional *RB1* pathogenic variant	Unilateral without genetic testing
H0	Absence of familial *RB1* pathogenic variant in blood	Offspring who test negative for parent's *RB1* pathogenic variant
		Parents and siblings of proband who has homozygous methylation of *RB1* in tumor and not in blood
		Parents and siblings of proband who is negative in blood for both *RB1* pathogenic variants found in tumor
H0∗	Absence of familial *RB1* pathogenic variant in blood and residual <1% risk of undetectable mosaicism	Parents of H1 proband who test negative for proband's *RB1* pathogenic variant
		Proband who tests negative in blood for both *RB1* pathogenic variants found in tumor
H1	Presence in blood of *RB1* pathogenic variant	Bilateral retinoblastoma
		Trilateral retinoblastoma (retinoblastoma with intracranial CNS midline embryonic tumor)
		Retinoblastoma and close family history of retinoblastoma

intensive surveillance for retinoblastoma starting from birth and life-long for other cancers.

2.4 Genotype-Phenotype Correlations

The number of retinoblastoma tumors each person develops depends on the type of *RB1* pathogenic variant [28]. Nonsense and frame shift germline pathogenic variants that lead to absent or truncated dysfunctional *RB1* protein (pRB) result in almost complete penetrance (>95% of patients develop retinoblastoma) and high expressivity (more than 90% have bilateral disease). Partially functional *RB1* pathogenic variants show lower penetrance (more carriers of the pathogenic allele without retinoblastoma) and reduced expressivity (fewer tumors, more unilateral disease) with later onset of tumor [29]. Reduced penetrance *RB1* pathogenic variants include in-frame or missense changes, distinct splice and intronic pathogenic variants [30], pathogenic variants in the promoter region that reduce the level of *RB1* transcription [28], and methylation of the promoter reducing expression of that allele [31]. *RB1* pathogenic variants in exons 1 and 2, or exons 26–27, may be low penetrance because they can result in a truncated but otherwise normal, pRB. Large deletions encompassing *RB1* and the *MED4* gene result in only 30% of the number of tumors that full penetrance/expressivity pathogenic variants do, since loss of heterozygosity of such a deletion (the second hit in 70% of retinoblastoma [11]) results in 0 copies of the essential MED4 gene, and such cells cannot survive [32].

Some *RB1* mutant alleles show a parent-of-origin effect. Best characterized are the c.607+1G>T substitution affecting splicing [33, 34] and c.1981C>T (p.Arg661Trp) missense pathogenic variant [35]. Both skew *RB1* expression in favor of the maternal allele: if the mutated allele is inherited from the mother, expression of pRB is sufficient to suppress tumor development to as few as 10% of carriers; when inherited from the father, the low expression of the same mutated *RB1* allele leads to full penetrance retinoblastoma. The mechanism of reduced impact of these specific pathogenic variants when inherited from the mother is due to a differentially methylated region in intron 2 called CpG85 which shows parent-of-origin-specific DNA methylation [36], causing the preferential expression of maternal vs paternal allele [35].

2.5 Risks for Each Individual Depend on Genetic Test and Clinical Presentation

Genetic testing allows clinicians to select a surveillance program depending on the level of risk [37]. All bilaterally affected children carry a *RB1* pathogenic variant and are H1: in addition to treatment of their bilateral disease, they benefit from surveillance of the retinas to detect more developing retinoblastoma tumors in infancy, and lifelong surveillance for second cancers. Unilaterally affected children without a close family history have 15% to 19% [8] likelihood to carry an underlying *RB1* pathogenic variant; high sensitivity genetic testing can determine which of these children are H1 and at a high risk to develop bilateral disease, or if no *RB1* pathogenic variant is found they are H0∗ with <1% residual risk of an unidentified *RB1* pathogenic variant.

Once the *RB1* pathogenic variant is known in a H1 proband with bilateral or unilateral retinoblastoma, their offspring or siblings who test positive (also H1) for that specific *RB1* pathogenic variant have near 100% risk in infancy for retinoblastoma, and a lifelong risk for second cancers [38]. For patients with Li-Fraumeni cancer predisposition syndrome, a surveillance protocol including whole body MRI has been shown to detect asymptomatic cancers and improve 5-year survival rate [40]. A surveillance protocol to diagnose the types of second cancers common in retinoblastoma H1 persons is needed. Low penetrance/expressivity *RB1* pathogenic alleles have reduced risk for retinoblastoma, as described above, but no data is available on their lifelong risk for second cancers.

All bilateral probands are classified as H1, even in the event that no *RB1* pathogenic variant

Table 2.2 Checklist for genetic counseling for families affected by retinoblastoma

Retinoblastoma genetic counselling checklist	H1	H0	HX	H0∗
H status proband				
Eyes				
Early detection and regular monitoring for RB tumor by EUA	X		X	
Routine clinic exam to look for retinoma				(X)[a]
Risk of secondary malignancy				
Pathogenic RB1 variant increases risk of other cancers	X		X	(X)[a]
Regular surveillance (life long)	X		X	(X)[a]
Avoidance of direct sunlight	X		X	(X)[a]
H status parent				
Prenatal counselling				
Prenatal genetic diagnosis	X			
Early full term delivery at 36 weeks if fetus shown to be H1	X			
Genetic test for baby, confirm H1 status at birth	X		X	X[b]
Examination without anesthetic from birth until tumor found	X		X	X[b]
Examination under anaesthetic if tumor found and between 3 months and 3 years age	X		X	X[b]

[a]<1% risk to be H1; unknown second cancer risk
[b]Until genetic test determines if H0 or H1

is found in blood. The number of *RB1* pathogenic variants found divided by the number of bilateral probands tested is the clinical test sensitivity of a given testing lab, and is important to validate *RB1* pathogenic variant test in that laboratory (Table 2.2). Best practice recommends that the lab report include this clinical test sensitivity in order to guide families and clinicians in selecting a surveillance protocol for the relatives. Labs highly focused on detection of pathogenic *RB1* alleles currently have 97% clinical test sensitivity [8]. The missing 3% of bilateral patients with no identifiable *RB1* pathogenic allele are most likely to have low-level undetectable mosaicism and remain H1. Siblings and offspring of an H1 proband require regular examination as indicated in Table 2.2 and Skalet et al. [37].

Probands with unilateral retinoblastoma where no *RB1* pathogenic variant is found in blood and with no tumor available for testing, are scored H0∗, and carry a residual risk of undetectable mosaicism. The level of residual mosaicism risk will vary depending on the clinical *RB1* test sensitivity of the testing lab. Surveillance protocols to monitor for retinoblastoma development in the other eye, and in siblings and offspring are guided by these calculations [37].

When the blood test is negative for both *RB1* pathogenic variants identified in tumor of unilateral probands, the proband is still H0∗ with residual small risk of undetected mosaicism. However, since mosaicism cannot be inherited, the proband's parents, siblings and offspring who test negative for the two specific *RB1* pathogenic variants detected in the proband's tumor can be scored H0, and require no additional cancer surveillance. If an offspring of the unilateral H0∗ proband carries one of the pathogenic *RB1* alleles of the original tumor, the unilateral proband is proven to be H1 mosaic and will benefit from immediate retinal surveillance to facilitate early treatment [29].

2.6 Availability of Test

Molecular testing for *RB1* pathogenic variants in laboratories exhibiting high clinical sensitivity identifies the causative *RB1* variant in 97% of bilaterally affected patients [8]. This knowledge supports surveillance of infants and adults depending on their risk to be H1, and carry their family's pathogenic variant [37]. Clinicians can use these guidelines to determine the need for examination under anesthesia, frequency of visits, need for life long oncological surveillance, prenatal counseling and early treatment of H1 babies.

However, high sensitivity genetic testing is not available worldwide, particularly in developing countries, due to lack of reliable local expertise and cost barriers for testing abroad. In such circumstances, the clinicians' knowledge of retinoblastoma is of utmost importance, to identify individual family members at risk of retinoblastoma and lifetime risk of second malignancies. A future effective tumor surveillance program may decrease the morbidity and mortality of each at risk H1 individual.

Patients and their family also benefit from knowledge of the genetic basis of retinoblastoma so that they seek appropriate and prompt genetic counselling. Sometimes, even though parents were aware that retinoblastoma is heritable, they may not understand that their children need to be screened from birth. Early eye screening is associated with lower tumor burden, lower treatment burden, higher rate of ocular salvage and better visual outcome [40].

2.7 Genetic Counseling for Families with Retinoblastoma

"Genetic counseling is the process of providing individuals and families with information on the nature, inheritance, and implications of genetic disorders to help them make informed medical and personal decisions" [28]. Knowing the risk for each new baby in a family with history of retinoblastoma is very important to save vision, eyes, and life.

When either parent is H1 or H0∗ [8], two prenatal options are available to determine if the fetus has inherited the known *RB1* pathogenic variant: chorionic villus sampling (CVS) during the first trimester and amniocentesis during the second and third trimester. There is a low risk of miscarriage due to the procedures, 1% and 0.5% respectively. Parents can chose to use the fetal status (H1 or H0) information for pregnancy management decisions. They can opt to terminate or proceed with the pregnancy. Parents can also consider a third trimester amniocentesis when the fetus is more mature at which time the procedural risk is that of early premature delivery rather than miscarriage. If parents decline invasive procedures, they can opt for a series of third trimester fetal ultrasounds beginning at 30–32 weeks of pregnancy followed by a blood test from the baby at birth to test for the *RB1* pathogenic variant. However, only medium to large retinoblastoma will be detected by obstetrical ultrasound [29, 41].

If the fetus is negative for the parent's/familial *RB1* pathogenic variant (H0), there is no need for any intervention or examination after birth as the baby carries the same risk as the general population [37].

If the fetus is H1 and carries the parent's *RB1* pathogenic variant, early term delivery at 36 weeks gestation is shown to optimize vision and eye outcomes, supporting clinical examination at birth of both retinas [29]. Highest sensitivity to find tiny retinoblastoma before they even extend out of the inner nuclear of the retina is obtained by hand-held optical coherent tomography and wide-field retinal imaging without anaesthetic: early detection of a tumor increases the opportunity to optimize vision and chance to save the eye [42]. When a tumor is noted, EUA is necessary for full documentation and treatment. With the common type of pathogenic *RB1* gene, that produces no *RB1* tumor suppressor protein, there is >90% chance that the child will develop retinoblastoma tumors at some time in childhood. The infant needs regular examination without anesthesia, and after about 3 months of age under anaesthetic, even if no tumor has been noted on full clinic exams [37]. The H1 infant also carries a lifetime risk of developing second cancers [38].

2.8 Case Examples

2.8.1 Case 1

Age 1 year, only child, diagnosed with bilateral retinoblastoma, was treated with right eye enucleation (Stage T2b, pT1), showing tumor adherent to the optic nerve head. Genetic test showed *RB1* pathogenic deletion, confirming that the child is H1. The *RB1* pathogenic deletion was not found in either parent.

Risk to sibling

- Both parents do not show the pathogenic *RB1* deletion in blood and are H0∗.
- The likelihood of having another child with retinoblastoma is <1%, due to remaining risk of undetectable low-level mosaicism in either H0∗ parent.
- Each sibling can be tested at birth for the probands' *RB1* pathogenic variant. While the chances are low, this will ensure intense surveillance for tumors in infancy for only those siblings found to carry the proband's pathogenic variant and are H1.
- Sibs who test negative are H0, at population risk for retinoblastoma.

Risk to future offspring of proband

- Each offspring carries a 50% risk to inherit the *RB1* pathogenic variant.
- Prenatal diagnosis with early term delivery will optimize outcomes for any H1 fetus found to carry the *RB1* pathogenic variant.
- Offspring who test negative are H0, therefore at population risk for retinoblastoma.

Risk of secondary malignancy

- The *RB1* pathogenic variant in H1 persons imposes an increased lifetime risk of other cancers, specifically osteosarcoma, soft tissue sarcoma, melanoma and others.
  - Regular surveillance of signs and symptoms of secondary malignancies is suggested.
  - Protocols for surveillance for second cancers are being developed and may include whole body MRI.
  - Avoidance of excessive direct sunlight is recommended.

2.8.2 Case 2

The second child in a family with no history or prior knowledge of retinoblastoma was diagnosed at age 1.5 years with unilateral tumor, treated by enucleation (Stage cT3c, pT2). Genetic test showed the child is H1 with a *RB1* pathogenic variant (c.2086A>T). Blood test for the proband's *RB1* pathogenic variant revealed that the mother is H1 and has the same pathogenic *RB1* variant in 10% of her white blood cells (i.e. she is mosaic for the pathogenic variant).

Risk to sibling

- Mother carries a *RB1* pathogenic variant in 10% of her white blood cells (H1).
- For mosaic individuals, the proportion of cells with the *RB1* pathogenic variant in the various tissue types is dependent on the timing of the pathogenic event in embryogenesis. The maternal gonadal cells may or may not be affected, and if affected, may involve only a portion of the germ cells. Therefore, the risk to the proband's siblings of inheriting the pathogenic variant is between 0% and 50%. Each sibling can be tested for the pathogenic *RB1* variant at full term birth, or prenatally to facilitate early term delivery if H1.
- Siblings who test negative are H0, at population risk for retinoblastoma.

Risk to future offspring of proband

- Each offspring carries a 50% risk to inherit the pathogenic *RB1* variant.
- Prenatal diagnosis with early term delivery will optimize outcomes for any fetus found to carry the pathogenic *RB1* variant.
- Offspring who test negative are H0, at population risk for RB.

Risk of secondary malignancy

- The pathogenic *RB1* variant in H1 persons imposes an increased lifetime risk of other cancers, specifically osteosarcoma, soft tissue sarcoma, melanoma and others. The risk for mosaic H1 person is assumed to be less but no evidence yet confirms this.
- Regular surveillance of signs and symptoms of secondary malignancies is suggested.
- Protocols for surveillance for second cancers are being developed and may include whole body MRI.
- Avoidance of excessive direct sunlight is recommended.

2.8.3 Case 3

The H1 mosaic mother of the proband in case 2 is now pregnant.

Risk to the unborn child

- Test for the pathogenic *RB1* variant at full term birth, or prenatally to facilitate early term delivery if H1.

2.9 On the Horizon

Genetic testing undeniably helps to identify patients at risk and facilitates earlier treatment, increasing the probability of globe and life salvage for heritable retinoblastoma patients [40].

The analysis of cell free placental DNA (cfpDNA) in maternal plasma is an effective and less invasive method of screening for common fetal chromosomal defects. The concept that placental DNA could be found in maternal plasma was discovered in 1997 [43], and is now reality in clinical care [44]. Although prenatal cfpDNA genetic testing for *RB1* variants is not yet clinically available, this strategy could be a non-invasive tool in decreasing the risks of miscarriage associated with amniocentesis and chorionic villus sampling.

The quest for gene targeted therapies for retinoblastoma is ongoing [45]. Other genetic changes in retinoblastoma tumor cells are hopeful targets for novel, specific therapies [46], such as differential expression of specific microRNAs, recurrent pathogenic variants in the *BCOR* and *CREBBP* genes, up regulation of spleen tyrosine kinase (SYK oncogene) and epigenetic changes that promote increase expression of the SYK oncogene enhancing retinoblastoma cell survival [45].

However, the genomic instability resulting from loss of *RB1* [22] undermines successful gene targeted treatment, pointing to early diagnosis and definitive treatment while the tumor is intraocular without invasion of choroid and optic nerve, as the most effective way to save lives.

References

1. Dimaras H, Corson TW, Cobrinik D, White A, Zhao J, Munier FL, et al. Retinoblastoma. Nat Rev Dis Primers. 2015;1:15021.
2. den Dunnen JT, Dalgleish R, Maglott DR, Hart RK, Greenblatt MS, McGowan-Jordan J, et al. HGVS recommendations for the description of sequence variants: 2016 update. Hum Mutat. 2016;37(6):564–9.
3. Mallipatna A, Gallie BL, Chévez-Barrios P, Lumbroso-Le Rouic L, Chantada GL, Doz F, et al. Retinoblastoma. In: Amin MB, Edge SB, Greene FL, editors. AJCC cancer staging manual. 8th ed. New York: Springer; 2017. p. 819–31.
4. Knudson AG. Mutation and cancer: statistical study of retinoblastoma. Proc Natl Acad Sci U S A. 1971;68(4):820–3.
5. Knight LA, Gardner HA, Gallie BL. Segregation of chromosome 13 in retinoblastoma. Lancet. 1978;1(8071):989.
6. Yunis JJ, Ramsay N. Retinoblastoma and subband deletion of chromosome 13. Am J Dis Child. 1978;132(2):161–3.
7. Sparkes RS, Sparkes MC, Wilson MG, Towner JW, Benedict W, Murphree AL, et al. Regional assignment of genes for human esterase D and retinoblastoma to chromosome band 13q14. Science. 1980;208(4447):1042–4.
8. Soliman SE, Racher H, Zhang C, MacDonald H, Gallie BL. Genetics and molecular diagnostics in retinoblastomaDOUBLEHYPHENan update. Asia Pac J Ophthalmol. 2017;6(2):197–207.
9. Sparkes RS, Murphree AL, Lingua RW, Sparkes MC, Field LL, Funderburk SJ, et al. Gene for hereditary retinoblastoma assigned to human chromosome 13 by linkage to Esterase D. Science. 1983;219:971–2.
10. Godbout R, Dryja TP, Squire J, Gallie BL, Phillips RA. Somatic inactivation of genes on chromosome

13 is a common event in retinoblastoma. Nature. 1983;304(5925):451–3.
11. Cavenee WK, Dryja TP, Phillips RA, Benedict WF, Godbout R, Gallie BL, et al. Expression of recessive alleles by chromosomal mechanisms in retinoblastoma. Nature. 1983;305(5937):779–84.
12. Dryja TP, Rapaport JM, Joyce JM, Petersen RA. Molecular detection of deletions involving band q14 of chromosome 13 in retinoblastomas. Proc Natl Acad Sci U S A. 1986;83(19):7391–4.
13. Friend SH, Bernards R, Rogelj S, Weinberg RA, Rapaport JM, Albert DM, et al. A human DNA segment with properties of the gene that predisposes to retinoblastoma and osteosarcoma. Nature. 1986;323(6089):643–6.
14. Rushlow DE, Mol BM, Kennett JY, Yee S, Pajovic S, Theriault BL, et al. Characterisation of retinoblastomas without RB1 mutations: genomic, gene expression, and clinical studies. Lancet Oncol. 2013;14(4):327–34.
15. Corson TW, Gallie BL. One hit, two hits, three hits, more? Genomic changes in the development of retinoblastoma. Genes Chromosomes Cancer. 2007;46(7):617–34.
16. Theriault BL, Dimaras H, Gallie BL, Corson TW. The genomic landscape of retinoblastoma: a review. Clin Exp Ophthalmol. 2014;42(1):33–52.
17. Squire J, Gallie BL, Phillips RA. A detailed analysis of chromosomal changes in heritable and non-heritable retinoblastoma. Hum Genet. 1985;70(4):291–301.
18. Grobner SN, Worst BC, Weischenfeldt J, Buchhalter I, Kleinheinz K, Rudneva VA, et al. The landscape of genomic alterations across childhood cancers. Nature. 2018;555(7696):321–7.
19. Xu XL, Singh HP, Wang L, Qi DL, Poulos BK, Abramson DH, et al. Rb suppresses human cone-precursor-derived retinoblastoma tumours. Nature. 2014;514(7522):385–8.
20. Rootman DB, Gonzalez E, Mallipatna A, Vandenhoven C, Hampton L, Dimaras H, et al. Hand-held high-resolution spectral domain optical coherence tomography in retinoblastoma: clinical and morphologic considerations. Br J Ophthalmol. 2013;97(1):59–65.
21. Soliman SE, VandenHoven C, MacKeen LD, Heon E, Gallie BL. Optical coherence tomography-guided decisions in retinoblastoma management. Ophthalmology. 2017;124(6):859–72.
22. Dimaras H, Khetan V, Halliday W, Orlic M, Prigoda NL, Piovesan B, et al. Loss of RB1 induces non-proliferative retinoma: increasing genomic instability correlates with progression to retinoblastoma. Hum Mol Genet. 2008;17(10):1363–72.
23. Ellsworth RM. The practical management of retinoblastoma. Trans Am Ophthalmol Soc. 1969;67:462–534.
24. Murphree AL. Intraocular retinoblastoma: the case for a new group classification. Ophthalmol Clin N Am. 2005;18:41–53.
25. Shields CL, Mashayekhi A, Au AK, Czyz C, Leahey A, Meadows AT, et al. The international classification of retinoblastoma predicts chemoreduction success. Ophthalmology. 2006;113(12):2276–80.
26. Edge S, Byrd DR, Compton CC, Fritz AG, Greene FL, Trotti A. AJCC cancer staging manual. 7th ed. New York: Springer; 2010. p. 648.
27. Rushlow D, Piovesan B, Zhang K, Prigoda-Lee NL, Marchong MN, Clark RD, et al. Detection of mosaic RB1 mutations in families with retinoblastoma. Hum Mutat. 2009;30(5):842–51.
28. Lohmann D, Gallie BL. Retinoblastoma. In: Pagon RA, Ardinger HH, Wallace SE, Amemiya A, Bean LGH, Bird TD, Fong C-T, Mefford HC, Smith RJH, Stephens K, editors. GeneReviews™. Seattle: University of Washington; 2015.
29. Soliman SE, Dimaras H, Khetan V, Gardiner JA, Chan HS, Heon E, et al. Prenatal versus postnatal screening for familial retinoblastoma. Ophthalmology. 2016;123(12):2610–7.
30. Zhang K, Vandezande K, Chen N, Sutherland J, Gallie BL, editors. RB1 splice variants and mutations detected by reverse transcriptase-polymerase chain reaction (RT-PCR) #2528. In: 94th American Association for Cancer Research Meeting; 2003.
31. Greger V, Debus N, Lohmann D, Hopping W, Passarge E, Horsthemke B. Frequency and parental origin of hypermethylated RB1 alleles in retinoblastoma. Hum Genet. 1994;94(5):491–6.
32. Dehainault C, Garancher A, Castera L, Cassoux N, Aerts I, Doz F, et al. The survival gene MED4 explains low penetrance retinoblastoma in patients with large RB1 deletion. Hum Mol Genet. 2014;23(19):5243–50.
33. Klutz M, Brockmann D, Lohmann DR. A parent-of-origin effect in two families with retinoblastoma is associated with a distinct splice mutation in the RB1 gene. Am J Hum Genet. 2002;71(1):174–9.
34. Schuler A, Weber S, Neuhauser M, Jurklies C, Lehnert T, Heimann H, et al. Age at diagnosis of isolated unilateral retinoblastoma does not distinguish patients with and without a constitutional RB1 gene mutation but is influenced by a parent-of-origin effect. Eur J Cancer. 2005;41(5):735–40.
35. Eloy P, Dehainault C, Sefta M, Aerts I, Doz F, Cassoux N, et al. A parent-of-origin effect impacts the phenotype in low penetrance retinoblastoma families segregating the c.1981C>T/p.Arg661Trp mutation of RB1. PLoS Genet. 2016;12(2):e1005888.
36. Kanber D, Berulava T, Ammerpohl O, Mitter D, Richter J, Siebert R, et al. The human retinoblastoma gene is imprinted. PLoS Genet. 2009;5(12):e1000790.
37. Skalet AH, Gombos DS, Gallie BL, Kim JW, Shields CL, Marr BP, et al. Screening children at risk for retinoblastoma: consensus report from the american association of ophthalmic oncologists and pathologists. Ophthalmology. 2018;125(3):453–8.
38. MacCarthy A, Bayne AM, Brownbill PA, Bunch KJ, Diggens NL, Draper GJ, et al. Second and subsequent tumours among 1927 retinoblastoma patients diagnosed in Britain 1951-2004. Br J Cancer. 2013;108(12):2455–63.

39. Villani A, Shore A, Wasserman JD, Stephens D, Kim RH, Druker H, et al. Biochemical and imaging surveillance in germline TP53 mutation carriers with Li-Fraumeni syndrome: 11 year follow-up of a prospective observational study. Lancet Oncol. 2016;17(9):1295–305.
40. Soliman SE, ElManhaly M, Dimaras H. Knowledge of genetics in familial retinoblastoma. Ophthalmic Genet. 2016;38(3):226–32.
41. Soliman SE, Ulster A, MacDonald H, VandenHoven C, Toi A, Heon E, et al. Psychosocial determinants for treatment decisions in familial retinoblastoma. Ophthalmic Genet. 2017;38(4):392–4.
42. Soliman SE, VandenHoven C, MacKeen LD, Gallie BL. Vision and visual potential for perifoveal retinoblastoma after optical coherence tomographic guided sequential laser photocoagulation. Br J Opthalmol. 2018;103(6):753–60.
43. Lo YM, Corbetta N, Chamberlain PF, Rai V, Sargent IL, Redman CW, et al. Presence of fetal DNA in maternal plasma and serum. Lancet. 1997;350(9076):485–7.
44. Langlois S, Brock JA, Genetics C. Current status in non-invasive prenatal detection of Down syndrome, trisomy 18, and trisomy 13 using cell-free DNA in maternal plasma. J Obstet Gynaecol Can. 2013;35(2):177–81.
45. Zhang J, Benavente CA, McEvoy J, Flores-Otero J, Ding L, Chen X, et al. A novel retinoblastoma therapy from genomic and epigenetic analyses. Nature. 2012;481(7381):329–34.
46. Pritchard EM, Dyer MA, Guy RK. Progress in small molecule therapeutics for the treatment of retinoblastoma. Mini Rev Med Chem. 2016;16(6):430–54.

Changing Trends in Retinoblastoma Management and What Is in Store for the Future

3

Jesse L. Berry

Key Points

- Retinoblastoma is the most common intraocular tumor in childhood
- The management of this tumor has changed significantly over the past several years including advances in local delivery of chemotherapy with intravitreal injection now done via safety enhanced techniques
- Seeding regression is nearly 100% with intravitreal chemotherapy however toxicity has been reported and the mechanisms and risk-factors have not yet been elucidated
- Advances have also been made in the use of hand-held Optical Coherence Tomography for diagnosis and monitoring
- The high-resolution imaging provided by OCT enables enhanced detection of tumors, including those that are "invisible' on fundoscopy.
- Optical coherence tomography has demonstrated the potential to detect recurrences masked by retinal scars
- Imaging of small tumors may help us better understand the cell of origin for retinoblastoma
- Retinoblastoma is known to have a genetic underpinning secondary to a mutation in the RB1 tumor-suppressor gene; nonetheless the genetic, genomic and epigenetic changes at the level of the tumor have not been readily assessed or correlated with clinical features or prognosis due to the inability to biopsy this tumor. This is a broad area for future research.

3.1 Retinoblastoma

Retinoblastoma (Rb) is the most common intraocular cancer of childhood with an incidence of 1 in 15,000 live births or about 12 per million children ages 0–4 years [1, 2]. Retinoblastoma accounts for 2% of all childhood cancers and approximately 8% percent of cancer in the first 4 years of life [3]. Worldwide there are 9000 new cases annually with the greatest number of cases seen in Asia and Africa where the birth rate is higher [4]. However the rate per live birth remains the same and no significant gender or racial predilection for the development of Rb has been described [5]. Maternal nutrition [6], HPV infection [7, 8], and advanced paternal age [9] have been suggested as predisposing etiologies but have not been definitively confirmed. Worldwide, the survival of children with retinoblastoma has improved [10] however disparities in the treatment and survival of children with this ocular cancer remain [11–16]. The treatment of retinoblastoma continues to evolve with a focus on

J. L. Berry (✉)
The Vision Center, Children's Hospital Los Angeles, Los Angeles, CA, USA

Department of Ophthalmology, USC Roski Eye Institute, Keck School of Medicine of the University of Southern California, Los Angeles, CA, USA
e-mail: Jesse.berry@med.usc.edu

V. Khetan (ed.), *Intraocular Tumors*, https://doi.org/10.1007/978-981-15-0395-5_3

more localized therapies to spare systemic toxicity. Nonetheless, there remains a critical need for personalized therapies. Retinoblastoma was one of the first cancers with a known genetic underpinning due to a mutation in the *RB1* retinoblastoma tumor suppressor gene (RB1) [17, 18], and has provided enormous insights into cancer biology; however, because this tumor cannot be safely biopsied, we still know very little about the genetic, genomic and epigenetic changes in this tumor that may affect treatment and prognosis for eye salvage [19]. This chapter will discuss the diagnosis, staging, and current treatment paradigms for retinoblastoma as well as discuss the future of this disease.

3.2 Diagnosis and Staging

The most common presenting sign of retinoblastoma is leukocoria, or loss of the red reflex, followed by strabismus [20]. Because retinoblastoma is rare, and screening requires a dilated, or low-light examination for loss of the normal red reflex, retinoblastoma remains undiagnosed until the cancer is quite advanced. Sometimes the tumor progresses to that point that it undergoes massive intratumoral necrosis and the child presents with significant ocular and periocular inflammation mimicking endophthalmitis or preseptal/orbital cellulitis [21].

Any child with leukocoria, strabismus or periocular inflammation should undergo a dilated fundus examination by an ophthalmologist followed by an examination under anesthesia (EUA) for any concern for retinoblastoma. The differential diagnosis of retinoblastoma includes other causes of leukocoria, such as Coats, persistent fetal vasculature (PFV), retinal astrocytic hamartoma, retinopathy of prematurity (ROP), familial exudative vitreoretinopathy (FEVR), retinal detachment, endophthalmitis, toxocariasis, toxoplasmosis, (old) vitreous hemorrhage and cataract [22].

On clinical examination, classically, retinoblastoma demonstrates single or multiple creamy white nodular retinal-based masses with prominent intralesional blood vessels. There are three primary clinical patterns of retinoblastoma growth: endophytic, exophytic and rarely diffuse infiltrating wherein a distinct mass is not seen. Endophytic growth occurs when the tumor grows from the retina into the vitreous cavity and is frequently associated with vitreous seeding, wherein small pieces of the tumor break off and proliferate in the vitreous compartment [23]. Exophytic growth occurs when the tumor expands in the subretinal space causing exudative retinal detachments and subretinal seeding. This growth pattern is more likely to demonstrate invasion to the choroid, a known risk factor for orbital relapse and metastatic disease [23]. Advanced tumors generally demonstrate a combination of these growth patterns. Pathognomonic features of retinoblastoma include intralesional calcium and tumor seeding, in the vitreous and subretinal spaces. This can occur either at diagnosis or in association with a tumor recurrence. More information on diagnosis can be found in Chap. 1.

3.3 Imaging Modalities for Retinoblastoma

Imaging modalities can be critical in the diagnosis of retinoblastoma. The most commonly used modality is b-scan ultrasonography which frequently demonstrates a dome-shaped retinal mass with diffuse intralesional calcium [24]. Calcium can often be most clearly seen on Computed Tomography (CT) scans, however it is not recommended that this modality be used if there is a suspicion for retinoblastoma given exposure to radiation in a child with a possible cancer predisposition syndrome [25, 26].

Magnetic resonance imaging (MRI) is the preferred imaging modality for most clinicians and recommended at initial staging. On *T1* imaging, retinoblastoma is slightly hyperintense (bright) to the vitreous. The tumor demonstrates moderate to marked enhancement. On gadolinium-enhanced *T1* weighted images, finely dispersed areas of low signal intensity correspond to areas of calcification. On T2 weighted imaging, the tumor is classically dark compared with the vitreous. The partially calcified areas may appear as hypointense foci [27]. Aside from its diagnostic value, MRI is performed with three main goals: (1) determine whether there is optic nerve extension, which is often better seen on fat-suppressed imaging [28] (2) extraocular/orbital extension, and (3) trilateral or tetralateral retinoblastoma. Trilateral retinoblastoma refers to a concomitant primitive midline neuroectodermal tumor (PNET) in the pineal region or the suprasellar cistern. Trilateral disease is found in 1.2–6.7% of patients with retinoblastoma and can be found at diagnosis or during/after treatment of the ocular disease [29]. Tetralateral (or quadrilateral) retinoblastoma is defined as the present of intraocular retinoblastoma and tumor in both suprasellar and pineal regions. MRI is often used as continued screening for these CNS tumors up to the age of 3 years (5 years in some centers). Post-enucleation enhancement in the orbit and the cut end of the optic nerve has been described on MRI and can be seen in these screening evaluations. Without a mass or clinical signs of orbital recurrence, this should be considered a benign finding [30]. Fluorescein angiography (FA) can also be critical in the diagnosis of retinoblastoma, particularly when Coat's disease is also being considered on the differential. Classically, FA demonstrates changes in the caliber of both small and large caliber vessels, with intratumoral retinal leakage and neo-vascularization of the iris [31]. General information on the imaging modalities available for choroidal tumors can be found in Chap. 4.

Finally, in the last several years, the advent of hand-held Optical Coherence Tomography (OCT), which allows for acquisition of images from an anesthetized, supine patient, has brought OCT into the realm of pediatric ocular oncology. The application of OCT has become critical for the management of retinoblastoma including detecting normal retinal anatomy underneath tumors, monitoring treatment response, identification of very small 'invisible' tumors, as well as early retinoblastoma recurrences [32–41]. As shown in Fig. 3.1, small retinoblastoma tumors appear as a smooth round, grey homogenous lesion involving the outer retina; there is 'tenting' of the overlying inner retinal layers. Larger tumors demonstrate posterior shadowing artifacts as well as more extensive involvement of the inner retinal layers [37]. It is difficult to distinguish retinoblastoma from benign retinocytomas on OCT, however, longitudinal perspective showing stability of the lesion can aid the clinician in making appropriate management decisions [42]. Use of OCT helps define other associated features such as subretinal fluid, intraretinal fluid, or intra-tumoral calcifications which may be difficult to assess when significant structural distortions from the tumor obscure the normal adjacent retina. For example, the ability to identify a fovea that has not been damaged by direct tumor involvement and/or associated fluid suggests that the future vision in the eye may be intact and thus the eye may merit salvaging therapy. Imaging of the vitreous with OCT imaging can also be valuable in clinical decision making. Even in the era of intravitreal injections of chemotherapy, vitreous seeding is the main cause of tumor relapse and requires more aggressive management. Clinically, vitreous seeds may be difficult to detect if they present as very fine dust type-seeds scattered just anterior to the retina. While difficult to detect on fundoscopy, these are well visualized with OCT [43]. As shown in Fig. 3.2, OCT can be used to image vitreous seeding of various morphologies including large spherical, hollow seeds, with posterior shadowing on the retina [44].

As smaller and smaller tumors are imaged, OCT may also help us understand the cell of origin for retinoblastoma, which remains unclear. An early description of small tumors on OCT described lesions "centered in the inner nuclear layer (INL)" that appeared to "consume" the middle layer while "sparing of the outer retinal layer" [36]. This led the authors of that paper to conclude that the cell responsible for retinoblastoma originated from the INL. However, the smallest lesions imaged to date appear to involve mostly the outer nuclear layer (ONL) and outer plexiform layer (OPL) with some extension into the INL. This supports the hypothesis that retinoblastoma shares a cellular lineage with the photoreceptors [40]. This is further supported by the characteristic finding of the normal outer plexiform and inner retinal layers "draping" over the outer retinal tumor [45]. Involvement of inner

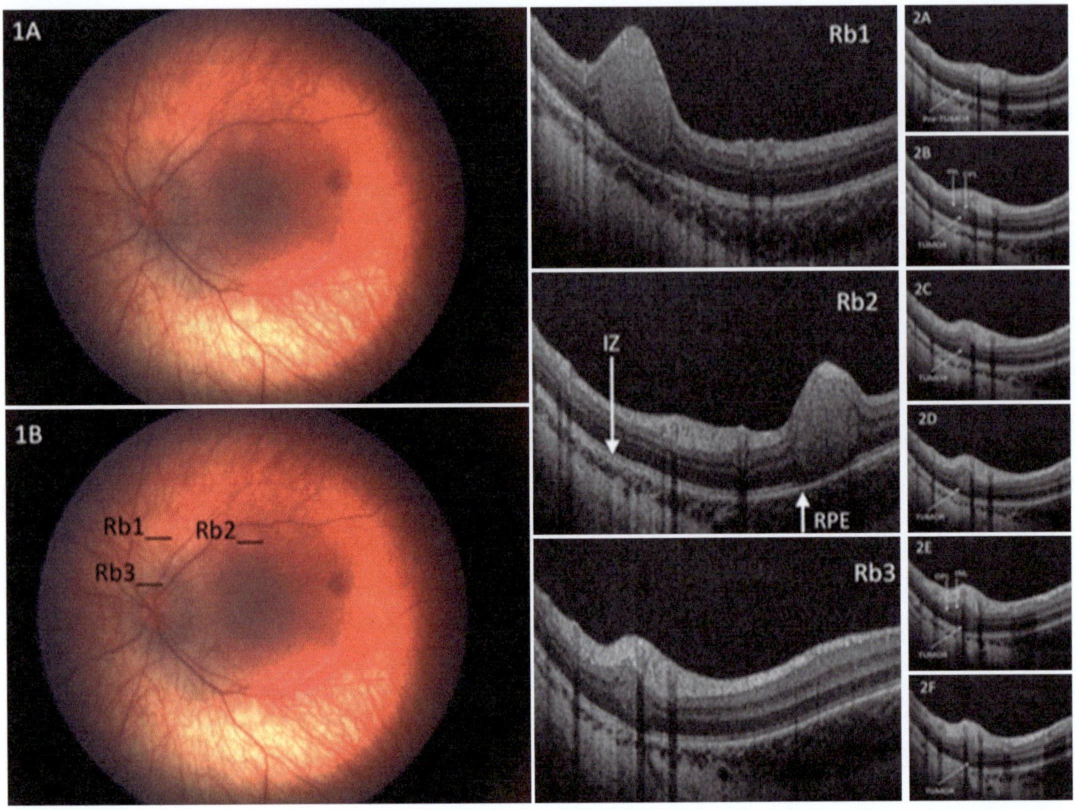

Fig. 3.1 OCT features of small retinoblastoma. (1A) Color fundus photograph of the left eye demonstrates 3 retinoblastoma tumors. (1B) Color fundus photograph of the left eye demonstrates 3 retinoblastoma tumors, marked by the arrows. The smallest tumor, barely visible on fundoscopy, lies just superior to the optic nerve. Rb1-3: Spectral-domain OCT of the three tumors shows homogenous dome shaped masses with overlying inner retinal draping. Tumor #3 is located in the outer retina involving the outer nuclear and possibly the outer plexiform layer. The inner nuclear (INL) and inner plexiform layer (IPL) drape over the tumor. There is also an outer retinal abnormality in all tumors affecting the external limiting membrane (ELM), inner segment-outer segment junction (ISOS), ellipsoid zone (EZ), and interdigitation zone (IZ). There is shadowing on OCT from the retinal vessels overlying the tumor which are also seen clinically. (2A–F) Optical Coherence Tomography (OCT) montage of images through the smallest lesion moving from the superior aspect towards the optic nerve. (2A) The lateral aspect of the larger tumor is seen peripherally. (2B) Most superior aspect of lesion. The inner nuclear layer (INL), outer nuclear layer (ONL) and outer plexiform layer (OPL) are shown in (2B, 2E) with the OPL and INL seen draping over the edges of the small tumor (Adapted from Berry et al. [40]. Reproduced with permission)

retinal structures may be from migration of malignant cells towards the inner retina and blood supply or general tumor expansion from the ONL. Imaging of small retinoblastoma tumors that primarily involve the outer nuclear layer is consistent with in vivo studies that suggest that the retinoblastoma cells of origin are the cone precursor cells. These cells are exquisitely sensitive to loss of a functional retinoblastoma protein [46, 47].

3.4 Grouping & Staging

Since the advent of the chemotherapy era in the late 1990s intraocular retinoblastoma has been classified according to the International Intraocular Retinoblastoma Classification (IIRC) described by Murphree [48]. The classification scheme separates intraocular retinoblastoma into five groups (A–E) based on size, location and presence of fluid, seeding and other clinical

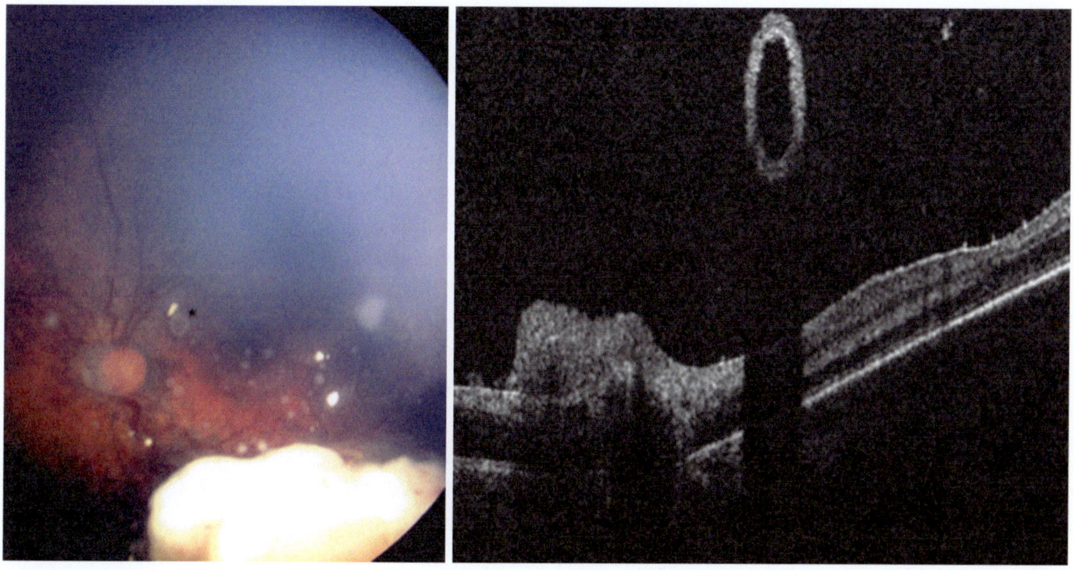

Fig. 3.2 Imaging of a spherical Seed in retinoblastoma. The clinical applications of handheld Optical Coherence Tomography (OCT) imaging (Bioptigen, USA) for retinoblastoma continue to evolve and include characterization of small tumors, tumor recurrences, evaluation of seeding and retinal anatomy. OCT done at staging examination of the left eye in a 13-month old child diagnosed with bilateral retinoblastoma (Group C right eye, Group D left eye) demonstrated normal foveal architecture, preretinal dusting of small hyper-reflective seeds and a hollow reflective cystic structure floating above the retina, with shadowing posteriorly, which correlated clinically with a large translucent spherical seed in the vitreous cavity (asterisk) (Adapted Berry et al. [44]. Reproduced with permission)

features. IIRC Group A eyes can generally be treated with local therapy only (laser therapy), with each classification progressively advancing until Group E, which is an eye functionally destroyed by tumor and according to the classification should be considered for salvage therapy only in very rare situations such as bilateral Group E eyes. Group A is associated with the greatest likelihood and Group E the least likelihood of ocular salvage based on chemoreduction protocols [49–52]. Recently however this has been supplanted with the AJCC 8th edition classification for retinoblastoma which includes a 4th factor to the TNM staging, H, for heredity and is the first cancer in the AJCC to have such a staging. This new staging classification is discussed in more detail in Chap. 1.

At most centers, staging consists of clinical examination and MRI (see imaging) however bone marrow aspiration or lumbar puncture may also be performed in patients if there is concern regarding the extent of disease such as extraocular extension, cerebrospinal fluid (CSF) or bone marrow metastases. This is not done routinely if the disease is confined to the globe.

3.5 Treatment

In the early 1900s the only successful treatment for retinoblastoma was enucleation. This treatment is still used today for advanced disease or recurrent tumors poorly responsive to other therapies, particularly in the setting of poor visual prognosis. However, given that 40% of new retinoblastoma cases involve both eyes this treatment modality was devastating for many children and thus attempts at globe salvage were undertaken.

3.6 EBRT

Historically external beam radiotherapy (EBRT) was a mainstay of treatment for many years however it is now rarely used except in certain salvage situations. Increased risk of orbital bony hypoplasia, which was very difficult to remedy cosmetically, and worse, second primary tumors, particularly in patients younger than 12 months of age, led clinicians to seek alternative therapies [53]. Even without EBRT, patients with heritable retinoblastoma are at an increased risk of many other types of second primary cancers throughout life including bony and soft tissue sarcomas and melanoma [10, 53–72].

Retinoblastoma survivors with a familial germline mutation are at slightly higher risk of a second primary tumor compared with those with a de novo germline mutation, in particular melanoma [69]. For germline patients, the risk of developing a second primary malignancy outside of the eye is approximately 30% at 40 years after the initial diagnosis [65, 67]. Unfortunately, patients at risk for a second non-ocular tumor are at risk of third and fourth tumors with increasing mortality regardless of EBRT exposure [73, 74].

EBRT has remained in the treatment arsenal for vitreous seeding, a common cause of relapse after systemic or intra-arterial chemotherapy [75]. However, a new treatment modality that involves intravitreal injection of chemotherapy has largely made this obsolete (see below). Recalcitrant retinal recurrences (particularly in an only remaining eye) may also still be treated with EBRT.

3.7 Systemic Chemoreduction

As an alternative to EBRT, Gallie, Murphree and several other ocular oncologists pioneered the use of chemotherapy in the 1990s [76, 77]. It has since become the backbone of treatment for retinoblastoma.

Systemic chemotherapy given for retinoblastoma is generally described as chemoreduction as the goal of chemotherapy administration is to shrink the tumor so that focal consolidative therapy (e.g. laser and/or cryotherapy) may be effective [78]. Focal consolidative therapy is directly destructive to tumor cells; it may also be used to augment penetration of chemotherapy into the eye [79]. Since the early 1990s, systemic 3-drug chemotherapy, along with local consolidation therapy, is a common and well documented therapy for globe salvage for patients with retinoblastoma [80].

Various regimens are used for systemic therapy, most typically carboplatin, vincristine, and etoposide with 3–6 cycles being given based on the extent of disease. Success rates for advanced Group D eyes are reported at approximately 50% with chemoreduction and local consolidation [51, 52]. At Children's Hospital Los Angeles, the chemoreduction protocol consists of intravenous carboplatin 390 mg/m^2 (13 mg/kg for children <36 months) × 2 days, etoposide 150 mg/m^2 (5 mg/kg for <36 months) × 2 days, and vincristine 1.5 mg/m^2 (0.05 mg/kg for <36 months) × 1 day, for 6 cycles every 28 days (i.e. CEV). Infants less than 6 months of age at diagnosis receive a modified dosing regimen with a 50% decrease in all agents for the first cycle [81]. Children with Group B eyes (less advanced) are treated with three initial cycles [82]. The therapy is augmented with local consolidation therapy, which includes diode or argon laser therapy (532 nm or 810 nm laser), and/or cryotherapy often used for larger lesions anterior to the equator.

While generally safe and well tolerated, systemic toxicity is known to occur. This leads to dangerous cytopenias, peripheral neuropathies [83], hearing loss [84] and rarely secondary leukemias [85–88]. Because of this, localized methods of chemotherapeutic delivery were touted to increase chemotherapeutic efficacy and minimize systemic toxicity. The main focus of this has been intra-arterial delivery of chemotherapy directly to the eye via the ophthalmic artery.

3.8 Intra-arterial Chemotherapy

Local methods of intra-arterial delivery of chemotherapeutic agents were pioneered by Suzuki and Kaneko in Japan [89] and Abramson and Gobin in the United States [79, 90–94]. Abramson and colleagues modified the Japanese protocol wherein, under general anesthesia, a cannula is introduced through the femoral artery and advanced to but not through the os of the ophthalmic artery. Fluoroscopy is used to confirm the position of the catheter before the chemotherapy is infused into the artery, approximately over 30 min [79]. Typically the initial agent of choice is melphalan although carboplatin, and/or topotecan can also be used. Initial doses are melphalan 0.4 mg/kg (with a maximum starting dose of 5 mg), carboplatin 50 mg and topotecan 0.2–4 mg [95].

This technique has been termed super selective ophthalmic artery chemotherapy or ophthalmic artery chemosurgery. Using Melphalan, Abramson and colleagues reported eye salvage rates superior to systemic chemoreduction, especially when used as primary versus second-line therapy for recurrent disease [95]. Group D eyes treated with intra-arterial chemotherapy have been reported with salvage rates ranging from 36% to 100% [96], with several large series of showing a rate between 78% and 100% [97–104]. Prospectively evaluated success rates for advanced Group D eyes have been reported as 100% when this is used as primary therapy [104]; however this has not been repeatable at all centers. A randomized clinical trial has been recommended to determine the efficacy and safety of this approach, as well as to determine the optimum chemotherapeutic agent. The Children's Oncology Group recently closed a trial of intra-arterial chemotherapy for patients with unilateral Group D disease, however results have not yet been reported.

Side effects, mostly vascular in nature, have also been described including ciliary flush, sectoral occlusive choroidopathy, and concerns exist about potential for stroke with this method of delivery [105–107]. There is also a learning curve with this technique with higher rates of vascular complications reported early on [108]. The total dose of whole body radiation given with multiple fluoroscopies also remains undefined. A more concerning trend, however, is that with greater success in salvage more advanced eyes are being treated with local chemotherapy only, this there may be an increased risk of both metastatic disease and orbital recurrences. A meta-analysis by Yousef et al. of intra-arterial chemotherapy for retinoblastoma found multiple reports of metastatic disease, while others have found equal, but relatively higher rates of metastatic disease and orbital relapse regardless of whether salvage therapy is attempted [109–114]. In general, as long as enucleation is reserved for the most advanced eyes, attempts at salvage therapy with enucleation for persistent or recurrent disease appear to be safe [115]. No therapy, including primary enucleation with adjuvant systemic chemotherapy, has been shown to completely eliminate the risk for metastatic disease. Thankfully, this remains a relatively rare event following a diagnosis of retinoblastoma confined to the intraocular space, regardless of treatment modality.

3.9 Intravitreal Chemotherapy

Seeding is one of the main indications for secondary enucleation in eyes that undergo attempted salvage therapy. Prior to 2012 recurrent seeding after chemotherapy was treated with EBRT, or if visual potential was poor, it may prompt enucleation in order to spare the child from radiation. This paradigm shifted dramatically in 2012 when Francis Munier introduced his safety-enhanced technique for intravitreal injection of chemotherapy which included a paracentesis with extraction of aqueous humor to lower the intraocular pressure prior to injection [116, 117]. This was not the first time that attempts had been made at injection of medication, chemotherapy or vectors had been made into the vitreous in retinoblastoma eyes [118, 119]. In fact, it was first described in 1962 by Ericson and Rosengren but reports of extraocular spread limited its use [120]. With the addition of the safety measures proposed by Munier, which were intended to lower the intraocular pressure and thus prevent reflux of intraocular fluid, intravitreal injection of melphalan has since been found to be safe when considering the risk of extraocular spread, and highly effective in eradicating vitreous seeding [89, 116, 117, 121–136]. As with any new therapy, the ideal dose of melphalan is not yet known and ranges widely from 8 to 50 μg with an equal range of number and interval of injection, although the average range is 20–30 μg given weekly until there is clearance of seeds [123, 124, 132]. Success rates are near 100% in eradicating vitreous seeds, and globe salvage even in advanced eyes is on par with previous studies using EBRT to control seeding [135, 137], however both anterior and posterior toxicity, loss of ERG function in doses over 30 μg and acute hemorrhagic retinopathy with devastating consequences have been reported (Fig. 3.3) [127, 134, 138, 139]. The mechanism of toxicity for the hemorrhagic retinopathy has been hypothesized to involve induction of a posterior vitreous detachment followed by retrohyaloidal injection of the medication causing toxicity secondary to concentration against the retina [134]. This however will require further research to better elucidate the mechanism for this acute toxicity. Nonetheless, the overall efficacy and relative safety of intraocular injection of chemotherapy have led to recent reports of use intracamerally for anterior segment seeding but the long term safety and outcomes of this are not yet known [140].

Given the new treatment paradigm for seeding, a new classification has been proposed, describing three patterns of vitreous seeding, based on their clinical morphology, which have prognostic significance [141]. These patterns include "dust," (type 1) which are small fine granules or vitreous haze, "spheres," (type 2) which are spherical vitreous opacities, which may have a translucent or opaque center, and "clouds," (type 3) which are dense, sheet-like collections of vitreous opacities. Seeds can occur in any of four vitreous compartments: retrohyaloidal, vitreous, subretinal, or anterior chamber. The seed classification has been shown to predict the number and overall dose of intravitreal melphalan injections required for local control [137, 142]. A retrospective study with a cohort of 28 patients found that at a mean dose of 25–30 μg, eyes with dust required three injections, eyes with spheres required four injections and eyes with clouds required the most number of injections (median 6) although some eyes responded to only one injection in all classification. Cloud type seeds also required the highest cumulative dose of melphalan [137]. These findings were similar to a larger study by Francis et al. that demonstrated dust type seeding required fewer injections and a lower overall dose than spheres and both lower than clouds for complete regression [142]. (Fig. 3.4) These studies found that the spherical seed class was the most likely to demonstrate recurrence and thus took the longest for complete clinical clearance (Fig. 3.5). This finding is supported by recent histopathologic correlation which found that spherical seeds can be composed of either non-necrotic viable retinoblastoma cells or an outer rim of active cells with a necrotic center however both types actively disperse viable cells which make them most likely to recur. This research also found that the cloud-type seed may take the longest to clear clinically but is mostly composed of macrophages and non-viable necrotic seeds and thus may not actually require more injections than the other seed classes [143].

3.10 Adjuvant Systemic Chemotherapy for High-Risk Histopathologic Features

There is no clear consensus on whether or not patients with high-risk pathologic features (such as massive choroidal invasive, post-laminar optic nerve invasion, and scleral invasion) should receive post enucleation adjuvant chemotherapy. A meta-analysis by Kim suggests that the risk with isolated post laminar involvement is 16% and with concomitant massive choroidal invasion the risk increases to nearly 33% and thus adjuvant chemotherapy is recommended and given at most centers [144]. Despite the lack of consensus on these features, there is general acceptance that optic-nerve invasion with involvement of the resection margin or bulky extra-scleral spread are highly predictive for extraocular relapse; in these scenarios, post-enucleation adjuvant systemic chemotherapy is indicated [145–147].

3.11 Orbital Relapse and Metastatic Disease

Orbital relapse occurs in about 4% of patients after primary enucleation, most within 12 months [148]. These patients are at increased risk for

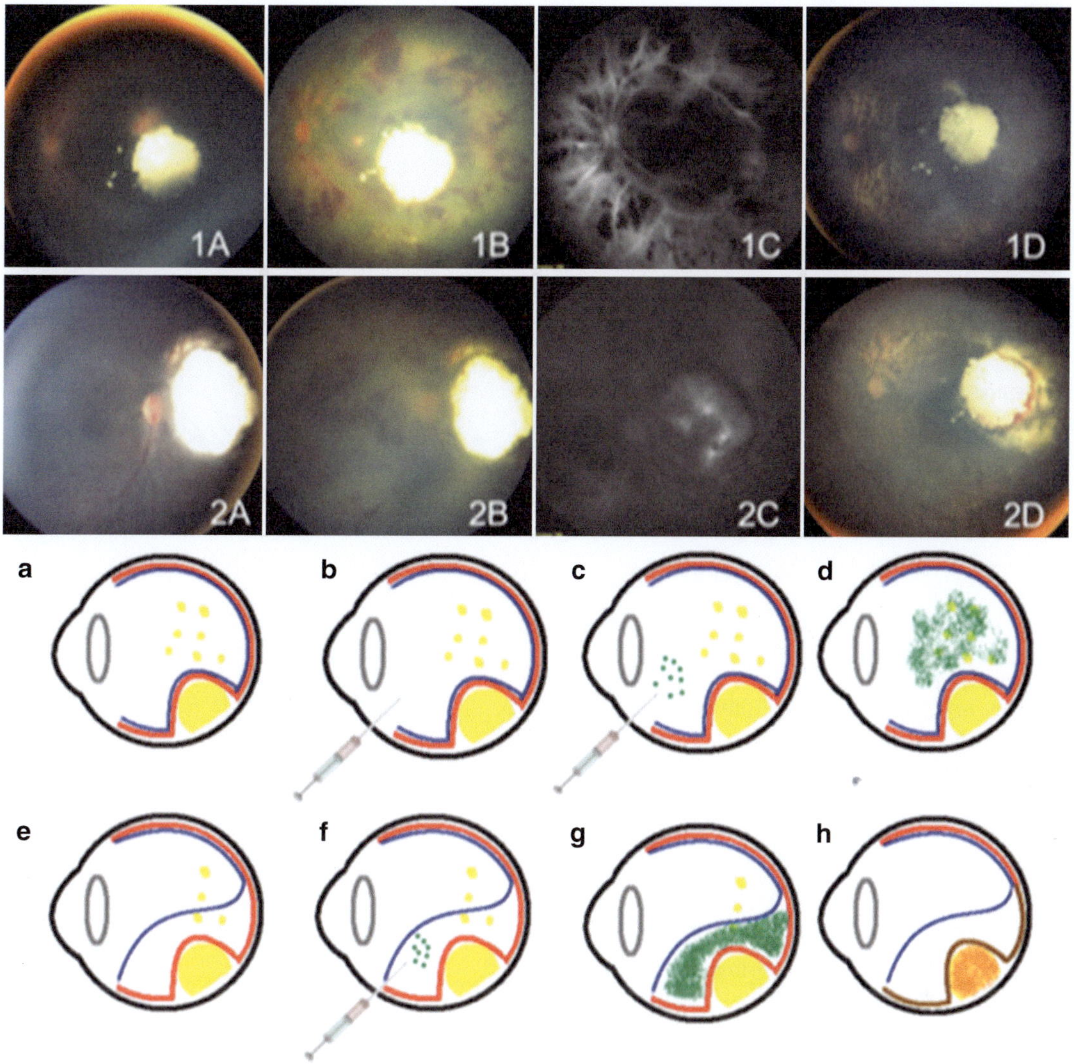

Fig. 3.3 Intravitreal melphalan toxicity. (1A, 2A) Fundus photographs of the left eye from patient 1 and right eye from patient 2 revealing partially treated retinoblastoma with associated vitreous seeding located in the macula and nasal to the optic disc respectively. (1B, 2B) Fundus photographs from patient 1 and patient 2, respectively, revealing diffuse retinal edema with associated intra and preretinal hemorrhages. (1C, 2C) Mid-phase fluorescein angiography of the left eye from patient 1 and the right eye from patient 2, respectively, revealing areas of blockage corresponding to the areas of retinal hemorrhage and intraocular tumor, with vascular sheathing. (1D, 2D) Fundus photographs at follow-up of the patient 1 and patient 2, respectively revealing diffuse chorioretinal atrophy in the posterior pole with a demarcation between the normal and atrophic retina. (**a**) Schematic rendition of an eye with retinoblastoma and associated vitreous seeding. The blue line represents the hyaloid face; the red line represents the retina and the yellow mass represents the tumor. (**b–d**) shows injection of melphalan (green) into the vitreous cavity via the pars plana. (**e**) represents a localized posterior hyaloid detachment over the tumor. (**f**, **g**) Injection of melphalan into the subhyaloid space due to the presence of a partial detachment. (**h**) Treated retinoblastoma (orange) with retinal atrophy (brown line) and resolution of vitreous seeding. (Adapted from Aziz et al. [134]. Reproduced with permission)

metastatic disease. Treatment for orbital recurrence (confined to the orbit) is systemic high-dose multi-agent chemotherapy as well as orbital radiotherapy. Patients with disseminated metastatic disease such as bone-marrow involvement receive high-dose 3–4 agent chemotherapy,

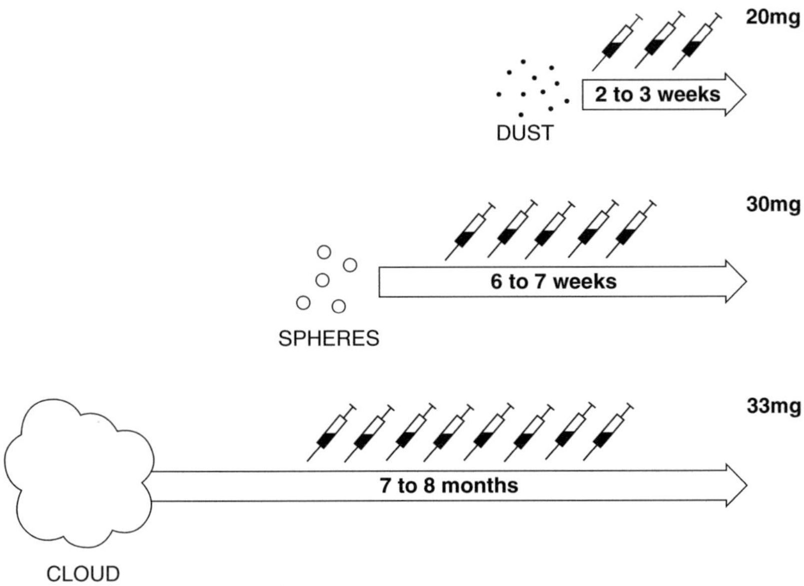

Fig. 3.4 Seeding classification and treatment response. Illustration summarizing vitreous seed classification and response to intravitreal melphalan: number of injections received, time to response, and median dose of melphalan per injection. (Adapted from Francis et al. [142]. Reproduced with permission)

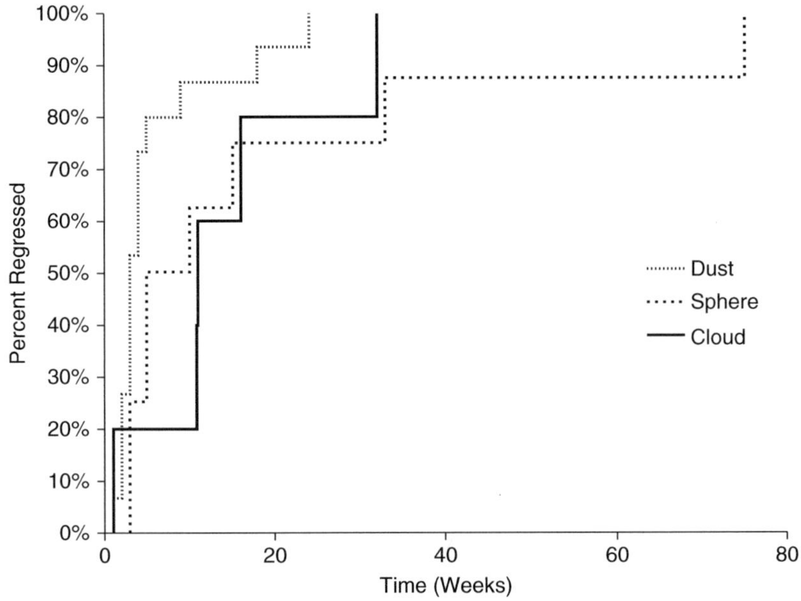

Fig. 3.5 Kaplan-Meier curves for seed regression based on classification. Median time to seed regression was 3 weeks for dust (range 1–24 weeks), 8 weeks for spheres (range 5–75) and 11 weeks for clouds (range 1–32 weeks) which was significant ($p = 0.07$). There was 100% seeding regression was seen in all classes of seed. Spheres were the most likely to recur and thus have the widest range from time to regression. (Adapted from Berry et al. [137]. Reproduced with permission)

bone marrow transplantation, and may also receive intrathecal radiotherapy [148].

Metastatic disease, while rare in the developed world, had remained largely fatal until recent trials of intensive multimodal therapy (including high-dose multi-agent chemotherapy and radiotherapy to bulky sites) with autologous hematopoietic stem cell rescue have shown success with reported 5-year event-free survival >60% [149–155].

3.12 Genetic Disease and Personalized Medicine for Retinoblastoma

Retinoblastoma is a known genetic disease. Tumorigenesis is initiated by a mutation in the *RB1* gene on chromosome 13q, which was the first tumor suppressor gene to be discovered [18, 156–161]. The inheritance pattern of retinoblastoma was instrumental in the discovery of the RB tumor suppressor gene [162]. Based on clinical genetics, there are three forms of Retinoblastoma: familial (10%), sporadic heritable (30%) in which a new mutation in the suppressor gene is present in all/many cells of the body, and non-heritable (60%) wherein both mutations in the *RB1* gene occur as somatic events in the tumor. Due to familial cases of retinoblastoma, it was known that retinoblastoma harbored a genetic underpinning. However, the genetic locus for this tumor was only elucidated in the past few decades. In 1971, Knudson first described the "two-hit hypothesis" suggesting that the RB gene requires mutations in both active gene copies in order for a child to manifest retinoblastoma [162]. The hypothesis suggested that in heritable cases a germline mutation was present in all (or most) cells of the body, and that a second somatic mutation was needed for tumor formation. Germline cases represent approximately 40% of retinoblastoma cases [163]. These patients tend to have bilateral and multifocal tumors and have a significantly increased risk for secondary tumors including pinealoblastoma (PNET). Their future offspring have a 45% chance of developing retinoblastoma (due to penetrance, it Is not 50%) [164].

In the non-heritable cases, both mutations in the *RB1* gene occur as somatic events, thereby explaining why somatic disease was always unilateral, unifocal and often seen in older children. Additionally, it did not predispose to second primary cancers. Approximately 15% of unilateral cases are found to have germline mutations [163, 165]. Some children may present with unilateral disease but subsequently progress asynchronously to bilateral involvement. Thus, serum genetic testing to determine whether the initial mutation is germline is critical to the management of these patients and families. It is recommended that children have genetic testing, particularly in the setting of unilateral disease regardless of age at presentation [166]. Further information on the genetics of retinoblastoma and testing for these mutations can be found in Chap. 2

Investigating the tumor suppressor pathway regulated by *RB1* has provided unprecedented insights into the genetic mechanisms of tumorigenesis, not only for retinoblastoma but also for virtually all human cancers. Despite this, we have not been able to leverage the growing field of cancer genomics for retinoblastoma patients which has dramatically impacted the care of breast, lung and prostate cancer patients [167–175]. This is primarily because we cannot safely biopsy this tumor and thus cannot correlate the genetic and epigenetic changes at the level of the tumor with clinical outcomes. Thus, since the 1990s the only real change in the management of retinoblastoma has been a focus on more localized delivery of chemotherapy to the eye with no role for tumor-derived genetic factors in the initial management of this disease. Preliminary research has, however, suggested that there are factors that predispose to increased tumor anaplasia, which correlates with a poor prognosis [176, 177]. Further studies have shown tumor-derived cell-free-DNA (cfDNA) is present in the aqueous humor of advanced retinoblastoma eyes. This cfDNA can be reliably collected, amplified and even evaluated for chromosomal alterations (e.g. small regions of gains and losses) [19]. It is also known from studies on tumor tissue, that chromosomal copy number alteration (gains and losses of partial sections of chromosomes) is a common secondary genomic change that allows for tumor progression [178, 179]. Interestingly, the tumor-derived cfDNA in the aqueous mimics the changes at the level of the tumor suggesting that the aqueous can be used as a liquid biopsy, or 'surrogate biopsy' for retinoblastoma (Fig. 3.6). This allows for the unique opportunity to evaluate these chromosomal changes in the tumor DNA found in the aqueous (e.g. before an eye has been enucleated) so that they can be associated with clinical tumor features, response to therapy and prognosis. Given that a paracentesis is now routinely performed before each injection of intravitreal melphalan (see intravitreal chemotherapy) and no cases of extraocular spread have been reported [180], it appears that a paracentesis is safe to perform in eyes with retinoblastoma even during active therapy. This method of isolating cfDNA from the aqueous has been termed the 'surrogate liquid tumor biopsy' and is the first time that retinoblastoma tumor-derived DNA has been isolated without enucleation from eyes undergoing

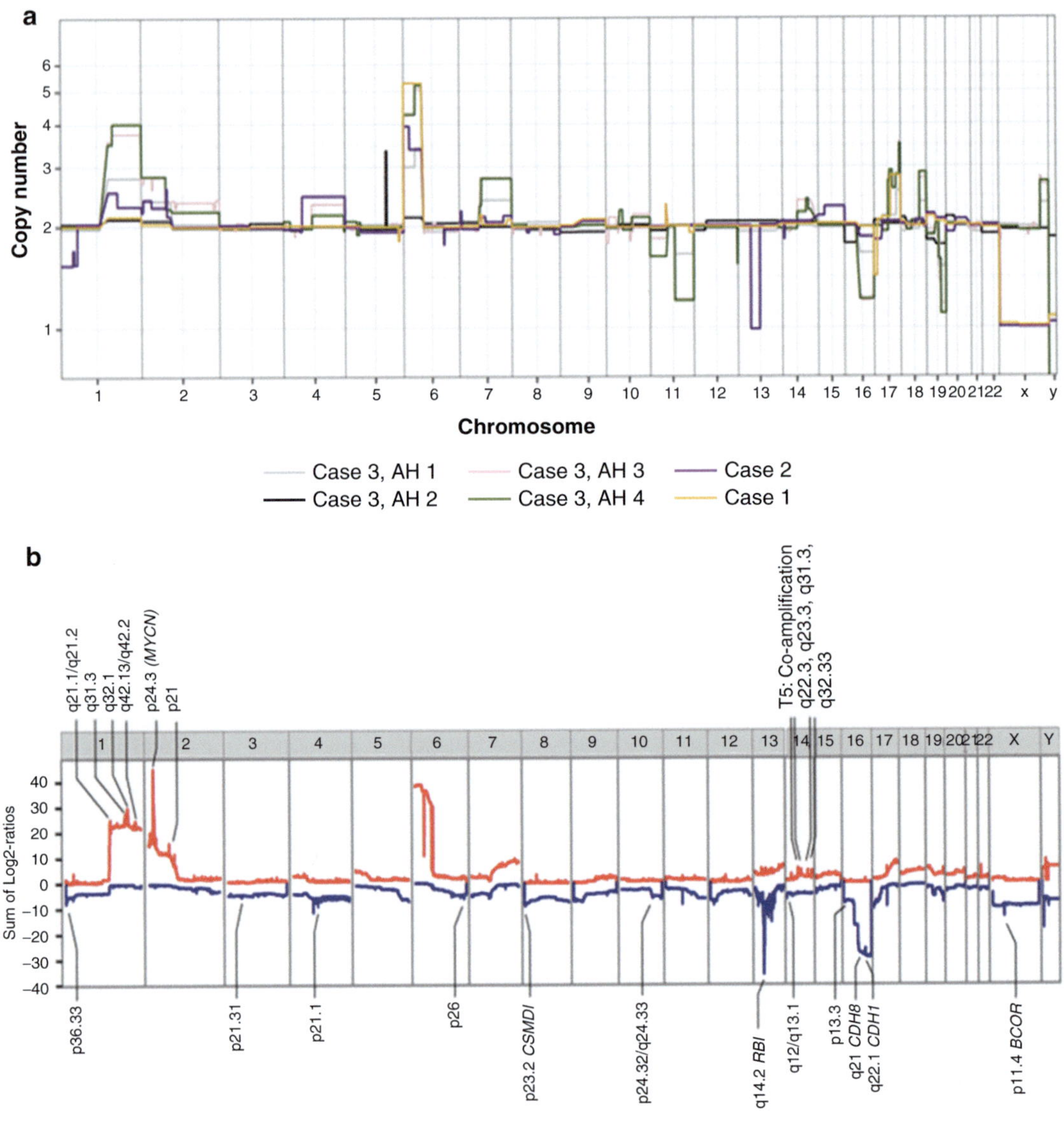

Fig. 3.6 Chromosomal copy number variation profiles from the aqueous humor and tumor composites. Chromosomal copy number variations (CNV) in single samples from the aqueous humor compared to Summative tumor CNV by Kooi et al., CNV from aqueous cfDNAs from 3 patients (**a**) compared to a summation of CNV profiles from 71 retinoblastoma tumor tissue samples from Kooi et al. [178]. (**b**) Show a very similar pattern of chromosomal gains and losses typical for retinoblastoma. (Adapted from Kooi et al. [178] and Berry et al. [19]. Reproduced with permission)

salvage therapy [19]. While this research is early, it may finally allow for identification of the *RB1* mutation in (nearly) all patients without enucleation and finally allow for genotypic-phenotypic correlation and important prognostic information. Evaluation of the aqueous humor during treatment for eyes with retinoblastoma has allowed for identification of a possible biomarker that portends a poor prognosis for globe salvage with therapy. In this study the authors found that identification of an increased copy number on a segment of chromosome 6p (termed gain of 6p) was associated with a 10× increased risk of the eye requiring enucleation after failed attempts at eye salvage [181]. Genes on 6p (*DEK, E2F*) are known to play a role in retinoblastoma tumorigenesis but the exact mechanism of 6p gain, or even the single gene player, is not yet known [182]. It will be important to obtain aqueous humor at diagnosis from eyes undergoing salvage and to evaluate the outcomes of these children prospectively before fully elucidating the prognostic impact of this potential biomarker. While there have been great strides in the diagnosis, imaging, staging and the local delivery of chemotherapy to augment globe salvage for these patients, there has been a complete lack of targeted therapies. The 'surrogate liquid tumor biopsy' may finally allow for the development of personalized medical therapy for retinoblastoma patients. Thus, we are entering into an exciting landscape for the management of this disease.

Acknowledgments Dr. Berry has grant support from the National Cancer Institute of the National Institute of Health Award Number K08CA232344, The Robert E. and May R. Wright Foundation, The Knights Templar Eye Foundation, the American Cancer Society #IRG-16-181-57, Hyundai Hope on Wheels and the Childhood Eye Cancer Trust.

Disclosure Statement The authors have no financial disclosures or conflicts of interests to disclose regarding the materials presented herein.

References

1. Broaddus E, Topham A, Singh AD. Incidence of retinoblastoma in the USA: 1975-2004. Br J Ophthalmol. 2009;93(1):21–3.
2. Seregard S, Lundell G, Svedberg H, Kivela T. Incidence of retinoblastoma from 1958 to 1998 in Northern Europe: advantages of birth cohort analysis. Ophthalmology. 2004;111(6):1228–32.
3. Steliarova-Foucher E, Colombet M, Ries LAG, Moreno F, Dolya A, Bray F, et al. International incidence of childhood cancer, 2001-10: a population-based registry study. Lancet Oncol. 2017;18(6):719–31.
4. Kivela T. The epidemiological challenge of the most frequent eye cancer: retinoblastoma, an issue of birth and death. Br J Ophthalmol. 2009;93(9):1129–31.
5. Dimaras H, Kimani K, Dimba EA, Gronsdahl P, White A, Chan HS, et al. Retinoblastoma. Lancet. 2012;379(9824):1436–46.
6. Lombardi C, Ganguly A, Bunin GR, Azary S, Alfonso V, Ritz B, et al. Maternal diet during pregnancy and unilateral retinoblastoma. Cancer Causes Control. 2015;26(3):387–97.
7. Anand B, Ramesh C, Appaji L, Kumari BS, Shenoy AM, Nanjundappa, et al. Prevalence of high-risk human papillomavirus genotypes in retinoblastoma. Br J Ophthalmol. 2011;95(7):1014–8.
8. Shetty OA, Naresh KN, Banavali SD, Shet T, Joshi R, Qureshi S, et al. Evidence for the presence of high risk human papillomavirus in retinoblastoma tissue from nonfamilial retinoblastoma in developing countries. Pediatr Blood Cancer. 2012;58(2):185–90.
9. Mills MB, Hudgins L, Balise RR, Abramson DH, Kleinerman RA. Mutation risk associated with paternal and maternal age in a cohort of retinoblastoma survivors. Hum Genet. 2012;131(7):1115–22.
10. Tamboli D, Topham A, Singh N, Singh AD. Retinoblastoma: a SEER dataset evaluation for treatment patterns, survival, and second malignant neoplasms. Am J Ophthalmol. 2015;160(5):953–8.
11. Gichigo EN, Kariuki-Wanyoike MM, Kimani K, Nentwich MM. Retinoblastoma in Kenya: survival and prognostic factors. Ophthalmologe. 2015;112(3):255–60.
12. Waddell KM, Kagame K, Ndamira A, Twinamasiko A, Picton SV, Simmons IG, et al. Clinical features and survival among children with retinoblastoma in Uganda. Br J Ophthalmol. 2015;99(3):387–90.
13. Waddell KM, Kagame K, Ndamira A, Twinamasiko A, Picton SV, Simmons IG, et al. Improving survival of retinoblastoma in Uganda. Br J Ophthalmol. 2015;99(7):937–42.
14. Chawla B, Hasan F, Azad R, Seth R, Upadhyay AD, Pathy S, et al. Clinical presentation and survival of retinoblastoma in Indian children. Br J Ophthalmol. 2016;100(2):172–8.
15. Li SY, Chen SC, Tsai CF, Sheu SM, Yeh JJ, Tsai CB. Incidence and survival of retinoblastoma in Taiwan: a nationwide population-based study 1998-2011. Br J Ophthalmol. 2016;100(6):839–42.
16. Temming P, Arendt M, Viehmann A, Eisele L, Le Guin CH, Schundeln MM, et al. How eye-preserving therapy affects long-term overall survival in heritable retinoblastoma survivors. J Clin Oncol. 2016;34(26):3183–8.
17. Benedict WF, Murphree AL, Banerjee A, Spina CA, Sparkes MC, Sparkes RS. Patient with 13 chromosome deletion: evidence that the retinoblastoma gene is a recessive cancer gene. Science. 1983;219(4587):973–5.
18. Dryja TP, Friend S, Weinberg RA. Genetic sequences that predispose to retinoblastoma and osteosarcoma. Symp Fundam Cancer Res. 1986;39:115–9.
19. Berry JL, Xu L, Murphree AL, Krishnan S, Stachelek K, Zolfaghari E, et al. Potential of aqueous humor as a surrogate tumor biopsy for retinoblastoma. JAMA Ophthalmol. 2017;135(11):1221–30.
20. Abramson DH, Beaverson K, Sangani P, Vora RA, Lee TC, Hochberg HM, et al. Screening for retinoblastoma: presenting signs as prognosticators of patient and ocular survival. Pediatrics. 2003;112(6 Pt 1):1248–55.
21. Foster BS, Mukai S. Intraocular retinoblastoma presenting as ocular and orbital inflammation. Int Ophthalmol Clin. 1996;36(1):153–60.

22. Maki JL, Marr BP, Abramson DH. Diagnosis of retinoblastoma: how good are referring physicians? Ophthalmic Genet. 2009;30(4):199–205.
23. Nawaiseh I, Al-Hussaini M, Alhamwi A, Meyar M, Sultan I, Alrawashdeh K, et al. The impact of growth patterns of retinoblastoma (endophytic, exophytic, and mixed patterns). Turk Patoloji Derg. 2015;31(1):45–50.
24. Novotny A, Krasny J. Diagnosis of retinoblastoma using ultrasound. Cas Lek Cesk. 1990;129(12):364–5.
25. Kaufman LM, Mafee MF, Song CD. Retinoblastoma and simulating lesions. Role of CT, MR imaging and use of Gd-DTPA contrast enhancement. Radiol Clin N Am. 1998;36(6):1101–17.
26. Danziger A, Price HI. CT findings in retinoblastoma. AJR Am J Roentgenol. 1979;133(4):695–7.
27. Razek AA, Elkhamary S. MRI of retinoblastoma. Br J Radiol. 2011;84(1005):775–84.
28. Ainbinder DJ, Haik BG, Frei DF, Gupta KL, Mafee MF. Gadolinium enhancement: improved MRI detection of retinoblastoma extension into the optic nerve. Neuroradiology. 1996;38(8):778–81.
29. de Jong MC, Kors WA, de Graaf P, Castelijns JA, Moll AC, Kivela T. The incidence of trilateral retinoblastoma: a systematic review and meta-analysis. Am J Ophthalmol. 2015;160(6):1116–26 e5.
30. Kim JW, Madi I, Lee R, Zolfaghari E, Jubran R, Lee TC, et al. Clinical significance of optic nerve enhancement on magnetic resonance imaging in enucleated retinoblastoma patients. Ophthalmol Retina. 2017;1(5):369–74.
31. Kim JW, Ngai LK, Sadda S, Murakami Y, Lee DK, Murphree AL. Retcam fluorescein angiography findings in eyes with advanced retinoblastoma. Br J Ophthalmol. 2014;98(12):1666–71.
32. Shields CL, Mashayekhi A, Luo CK, Materin MA, Shields JA. Optical coherence tomography in children: analysis of 44 eyes with intraocular tumors and simulating conditions. J Pediatr Ophthalmol Strabismus. 2004;41(6):338–44.
33. Shields CL, Materin MA, Shields JA. Review of optical coherence tomography for intraocular tumors. Curr Opin Ophthalmol. 2005;16(3):141–54.
34. Sony P, Garg SP. Optical coherence tomography in children with retinoblastoma. J Pediatr Ophthalmol Strabismus. 2005;42(3):134.
35. Yousef YA, Shroff M, Halliday W, Gallie BL, Heon E. Detection of optic nerve disease in retinoblastoma by use of spectral domain optical coherence tomography. J AAPOS. 2012;16(5):481–3.
36. Rootman DB, Gonzalez E, Mallipatna A, Vandenhoven C, Hampton L, Dimaras H, et al. Hand-held high-resolution spectral domain optical coherence tomography in retinoblastoma: clinical and morphologic considerations. Br J Ophthalmol. 2013;97(1):59–65.
37. Cao C, Markovitz M, Ferenczy S, Shields CL. Hand-held spectral-domain optical coherence tomography of small macular retinoblastoma in infants before and after chemotherapy. J Pediatr Ophthalmol Strabismus. 2014;51(4):230–4.
38. Pierro L, De Francesco S, Hadjistilianou D, Casalino G, Fusco F, Sergenti J, et al. Spectral-domain optical coherence tomography appearance of a posterior pole retinoma. J Pediatr Ophthalmol Strabismus. 2014;51(5):320.
39. Hasanreisoglu M, Dolz-Marco R, Ferenczy SR, Shields JA, Shields CL. Spectral domain optical coherence tomography reveals hidden fovea beneath extensive vitreous seeding from retinoblastoma. Retina. 2015;35(7):1486–7.
40. Berry JL, Cobrinik D, Kim JW. Detection and intraretinal localization of an 'invisible' retinoblastoma using optical coherence tomography. Ocul Oncol Pathol. 2016;2(3):148–52.
41. Park K, Sioufi K, Shields CL. Clinically invisible retinoblastoma recurrence in an infant. Retin Cases Brief Rep. 2017;13(2):108–10.
42. Malhotra PP, Bhushan B, Mitra A, Sen A. Spectral-domain optical coherence tomography and fundus autofluorescence features in a case of typical retinocytoma. Eur J Ophthalmol. 2015;25(6):e123–6.
43. Seider MI, Grewal DS, Mruthyunjaya P. Portable optical coherence tomography detection or confirmation of ophthalmoscopically invisible or indeterminate active retinoblastoma. Ophthalmic Surg Lasers Imaging Retina. 2016;47(10):965–8.
44. Berry JL, Anulao K, Kim JW. Optical coherence tomography imaging of a large spherical seed in retinoblastoma. Ophthalmology. 2017;124(8):1208.
45. Saktanasate J, Vongkulsiri S, Khoo CT. Invisible retinoblastoma. JAMA Ophthalmol. 2015;133(7):e151123.
46. Xu XL, Singh HP, Wang L, Qi DL, Poulos BK, Abramson DH, et al. Rb suppresses human cone-precursor-derived retinoblastoma tumours. Nature. 2014;514(7522):385–8.
47. Xu XL, Fang Y, Lee TC, Forrest D, Gregory-Evans C, Almeida D, et al. Retinoblastoma has properties of a cone precursor tumor and depends upon cone-specific MDM2 signaling. Cell. 2009;137(6):1018–31.
48. Linn Murphree A. Intraocular retinoblastoma: the case for a new group classification. Ophthalmol Clin N Am. 2005;18(1):41–53.
49. Kaliki S, Shields CL, Rojanaporn D, Al-Dahmash S, McLaughlin JP, Shields JA, et al. High-risk retinoblastoma based on international classification of retinoblastoma: analysis of 519 enucleated eyes. Ophthalmology. 2013;120(5):997–1003.
50. Shields CL, Shields JA. Basic understanding of current classification and management of retinoblastoma. Curr Opin Ophthalmol. 2006;17(3):228–34.
51. Shields CL, Mashayekhi A, Au AK, Czyz C, Leahey A, Meadows AT, et al. The international classification of Retinoblastoma predicts chemoreduction success. Ophthalmology. 2006;113(12):2276–80.
52. Berry JL, Jubran R, Kim JW, Wong K, Bababeygy SR, Almarzouki H, et al. Long-term outcomes of

Group D eyes in bilateral retinoblastoma patients treated with chemoreduction and low-dose IMRT salvage. Pediatr Blood Cancer. 2013;60(4):688–93.
53. Abramson DH, Frank CM. Second nonocular tumors in survivors of bilateral retinoblastoma: a possible age effect on radiation-related risk. Ophthalmology. 1998;105(4):573–9.
54. Abramson DH, Ronner HJ, Ellsworth RM. Second tumors in nonirradiated bilateral retinoblastoma. Am J Ophthalmol. 1979;87(5):624–7.
55. Abramson DH, Ellsworth RM, Kitchin FD, Tung G. Second nonocular tumors in retinoblastoma survivors. Are they radiation-induced? Ophthalmology. 1984;91(11):1351–5.
56. Eng C, Li FP, Abramson DH, Ellsworth RM, Wong FL, Goldman MB, et al. Mortality from second tumors among long-term survivors of retinoblastoma. J Natl Cancer Inst. 1993;85(14):1121–8.
57. Moll AC, Imhof SM, Bouter LM, Kuik DJ, Den Otter W, Bezemer PD, et al. Second primary tumors in patients with hereditary retinoblastoma: a register-based follow-up study, 1945-1994. Int J Cancer. 1996;67(4):515–9.
58. Li FP, Abramson DH, Tarone RE, Kleinerman RA, Fraumeni JF Jr, Boice JD Jr. Hereditary retinoblastoma, lipoma, and second primary cancers. J Natl Cancer Inst. 1997;89(1):83–4.
59. Moll AC, Imhof SM, Bouter LM, Tan KE. Second primary tumors in patients with retinoblastoma. A review of the literature. Ophthalmic Genet. 1997;18(1):27–34.
60. Rubin CZ, Rosenfield NS, Abramson SJ, Abramson DH, Dunkel IJ. The location and appearance of second malignancies in patients with bilateral retinoblastoma. Sarcoma. 1997;1(2):89–93.
61. Dunkel IJ, Gerald WL, Rosenfield NS, Strong EW, Abramson DH, Ghavimi F. Outcome of patients with a history of bilateral retinoblastoma treated for a second malignancy: the memorial sloan-kettering experience. Med Pediatr Oncol. 1998;30(1):59–62.
62. Hasegawa T, Matsuno Y, Niki T, Hirohashi S, Shimoda T, Takayama J, et al. Second primary rhabdomyosarcomas in patients with bilateral retinoblastoma: a clinicopathologic and immunohistochemical study. Am J Surg Pathol. 1998;22(11):1351–60.
63. Abramson DH. Second nonocular cancers in retinoblastoma: a unified hypothesis. The Franceschetti Lecture. Ophthalmic Genet. 1999;20(3):193–204.
64. Schlienger P, Campana F, Vilcoq JR, Asselain B, Dendale R, Desjardins L, et al. Nonocular second primary tumors after retinoblastoma: retrospective study of 111 patients treated by electron beam radiotherapy with or without TEM. Am J Clin Oncol. 2004;27(4):411–9.
65. Marees T, Moll AC, Imhof SM, de Boer MR, Ringens PJ, van Leeuwen FE. Risk of second malignancies in survivors of retinoblastoma: more than 40 years of follow-up. J Natl Cancer I. 2008;100(24):1771–9.
66. Sheen V, Tucker MA, Abramson DH, Seddon JM, Kleinerman RA. Cancer screening practices of adult survivors of retinoblastoma at risk of second cancers. Cancer. 2008;113(2):434–41.
67. Balaguer J, Harto M, Serra I, Oltra S, HernAndez M, Castel V. Mortality from second tumors among long-term survivors of retinoblastoma: an 87 case series report. Pediatr Blood Cancer. 2009;53(5):811.
68. Woo KI, Harbour JW. Review of 676 second primary tumors in patients with retinoblastoma: association between age at onset and tumor type. Arch Ophthalmol. 2010;128(7):865–70.
69. Kleinerman RA, Yu CL, Little MP, Li Y, Abramson D, Seddon J, et al. Variation of second cancer risk by family history of retinoblastoma among long-term survivors. J Clin Oncol. 2012;30(9):950–7.
70. MacCarthy A, Bayne AM, Brownbill PA, Bunch KJ, Diggens NL, Draper GJ, et al. Second and subsequent tumours among 1927 retinoblastoma patients diagnosed in Britain 1951-2004. Br J Cancer. 2013;108(12):2455–63.
71. Rodjan F, Graaf P, Brisse HJ, Verbeke JI, Sanchez E, Galluzzi P, et al. Second cranio-facial malignancies in hereditary retinoblastoma survivors previously treated with radiation therapy: clinic and radiologic characteristics and survival outcomes. Eur J Cancer. 2013;49(8):1939–47.
72. Fujiwara T, Fujiwara M, Numoto K, Ogura K, Yoshida A, Yonemoto T, et al. Second primary osteosarcomas in patients with retinoblastoma. Jpn J Clin Oncol. 2015;45(12):1139–45.
73. Abramson DH, Melson MR, Dunkel IJ, Frank CM. Third (fourth and fifth) nonocular tumors in survivors of retinoblastoma. Ophthalmology. 2001;108(10):1868–76.
74. Melson MR, Dunkel IJ, Frank CM, Abramson DH. Third (fourth and fifth) nonocular tumors in survivors of retinoblastoma. Invest Ophthalmol Vis Sci. 2000;41(4):S469.
75. Kaneko A, Suzuki S. Eye-preservation treatment of retinoblastoma with vitreous seeding. Jpn J Clin Oncol. 2003;33(12):601–7.
76. Gallie BL, Budning A, DeBoer G, Thiessen JJ, Koren G, Verjee Z, et al. Chemotherapy with focal therapy can cure intraocular retinoblastoma without radiotherapy. Arch Ophthalmol. 1996;114(11):1321–8.
77. Murphree AL, Villablanca JG, Deegan WF, Sato JK, Malogolowkin M, Fisher A, et al. Chemotherapy plus local treatment in the management of intraocular retinoblastoma. Arch Ophthalmol. 1996;114(11):1348–56.
78. Shields JA, Shields CL, De Potter P. Photocoagulation of retinoblastoma. Int Ophthalmol Clin. 1993;33(3):95–9.
79. Abramson DH, Dunkel IJ, Brodie SE, Kim JW, Gobin YP. A phase I/II study of direct intraarterial (ophthalmic artery) chemotherapy with melphalan for intraocular retinoblastoma initial results. Ophthalmology. 2008;115(8):1398–404.
80. Shields CL, De Potter P, Himelstein BP, Shields JA, Meadows AT, Maris JM. Chemoreduction in the initial management of intraocular retinoblastoma. Arch Ophthalmol. 1996;114(11):1330–8.

81. Berry JL, Jubran R, Lee TC, Murphree AL, Lee D, Kim JW. Low-dose chemoreduction for infants diagnosed with retinoblastoma before 6 months of age. Ocul Oncol Pathol. 2015;1:103–10.
82. Zhu DBJL, Ediriwickrema L, Wong K, Lee TC, Murphree AL, Kim JW, Jubran R. Long-term outcomes of group b eyes in patients with retinoblastoma treated with short-course chemoreduction: experience from Children's Hospital Los Angeles/University of Southern California. Ocul Oncol Pathol. 2016;2:105–11.
83. Mora E, Smith EM, Donohoe C, Hertz DL. Vincristine-induced peripheral neuropathy in pediatric cancer patients. Am J Cancer Res. 2016;6(11):2416–30.
84. Jehanne M, Lumbroso-Le Rouic L, Savignoni A, Aerts I, Mercier G, Bours D, et al. Analysis of ototoxicity in young children receiving carboplatin in the context of conservative management of unilateral or bilateral retinoblastoma. Pediatr Blood Cancer. 2009;52(5):637–43.
85. Weintraub M, Revel-Vilk S, Charit M, Aker M, Pe'er J. Secondary acute myeloid leukemia after etoposide therapy for retinoblastoma. J Pediatr Hematol Oncol. 2007;29(9):646–8.
86. Gombos DS, Hungerford J, Abramson DH, Kingston J, Chantada G, Dunkel IJ, et al. Secondary acute myelogenous leukemia in patients with retinoblastoma: is chemotherapy a factor? Ophthalmology. 2007;114(7):1378–83.
87. Nishimura S, Sato T, Ueda H, Ueda K. Acute myeloblastic leukemia as a second malignancy in a patient with hereditary retinoblastoma. J Clin Oncol. 2001;19(21):4182–3.
88. Rizzuti AE, Dunkel IJ, Abramson DH. The adverse events of chemotherapy for retinoblastoma: what are they? Do we know? Arch Ophthalmol. 2008;126(6):862–5.
89. Suzuki S, Aihara Y, Fujiwara M, Sano S, Kaneko A. Intravitreal injection of melphalan for intraocular retinoblastoma. Jpn J Ophthalmol. 2015;59(3):164–72.
90. Klufas MA, Gobin YP, Marr B, Brodie SE, Dunkel IJ, Abramson DH. Intra-arterial chemotherapy as a treatment for intraocular retinoblastoma: alternatives to direct ophthalmic artery catheterization. AJNR Am J Neuroradiol. 2012;33(8):1608–14.
91. Abramson DH, Marr BP, Brodie SE, Dunkel I, Palioura S, Gobin YP. Ophthalmic artery chemosurgery for less advanced intraocular retinoblastoma: five year review. PLoS One. 2012;7(4):e34120.
92. Abramson DH, Dunkel IJ, Brodie SE, Marr B, Gobin YP. Superselective ophthalmic artery chemotherapy as primary treatment for retinoblastoma (chemosurgery). Ophthalmology. 2010;117(8):1623–9.
93. Abramson DH, Dunkel IJ, Brodie SE, Marr B, Gobin YP. Bilateral superselective ophthalmic artery chemotherapy for bilateral retinoblastoma: tandem therapy. Arch Ophthalmol. 2010;128(3):370–2.
94. Brodie SE, Pierre Gobin Y, Dunkel IJ, Kim JW, Abramson DH. Persistence of retinal function after selective ophthalmic artery chemotherapy infusion for retinoblastoma. Doc Ophthalmol. 2009;119(1):13–22.
95. Abramson DH, Daniels AB, Marr BP, Francis JH, Brodie SE, Dunkel IJ, et al. Intra-arterial chemotherapy (ophthalmic artery chemosurgery) for group D retinoblastoma. PLoS One. 2016;11(1):e0146582.
96. Chung CY, Medina CA, Aziz HA, Singh AD. Retinoblastoma: evidence for stage-based chemotherapy. Int Ophthalmol Clin. 2015;55(1):63–75.
97. MacCarthy A, Birch JM, Draper GJ, Hungerford JL, Kingston JE, Kroll ME, et al. Retinoblastoma: treatment and survival in Great Britain 1963 to 2002. Br J Ophthalmol. 2009;93(1):38–9.
98. Naseripour M, Nazari H, Bakhtiari P, Modarres-zadeh M, Vosough P, Ausari M. Retinoblastoma in Iran: outcomes in terms of patients' survival and globe survival. Br J Ophthalmol. 2009;93(1):28–32.
99. Dimaras H, Dimba EA, Gallie BL. Challenging the global retinoblastoma survival disparity through a collaborative research effort. Br J Ophthalmol. 2010;94(11):1415–6.
100. Naseripour M. Retinoblastoma survival disparity: the expanding horizon in developing countries. Saudi J Ophthalmol. 2012;26(2):157–61.
101. Al-Nawaiseh I, Jammal HM, Khader YS, Jaradat I, Barham R. Retinoblastoma in Jordan, 2003-2013: ocular survival and associated factors. Ophthalmic Epidemiol. 2014;21(6):406–11.
102. Moreno F, Sinaki B, Fandino A, Dussel V, Orellana L, Chantada G. A population-based study of retinoblastoma incidence and survival in Argentine children. Pediatr Blood Cancer. 2014;61(9):1610–5.
103. Shields CL, Manjandavida FP, Lally SE, Pieretti G, Arepalli SA, Caywood EH, et al. Intra-arterial chemotherapy for retinoblastoma in 70 eyes: outcomes based on the international classification of retinoblastoma. Ophthalmology. 2014;121(7):1453–60.
104. Munier FL, Mosimann P, Puccinelli F, Gaillard MC, Stathopoulos C, Houghton S, et al. First-line intra-arterial versus intravenous chemotherapy in unilateral sporadic group D retinoblastoma: evidence of better visual outcomes, ocular survival and shorter time to success with intra-arterial delivery from retrospective review of 20 years of treatment. Br J Ophthalmol. 2017;101(8):1086–93.
105. Abruzzo T, Patino M, Leach J, Rahme R, Geller J. Cerebral vasoconstriction triggered by sympathomimetic drugs during intra-atrerial chemotherapy. Pediatr Neurol. 2013;48(2):139–42.
106. Shields CL, Bianciotto CG, Jabbour P, Griffin GC, Ramasubramanian A, Rosenwasser R, et al. Intra-arterial chemotherapy for retinoblastoma: report No. 2, treatment complications. Arch Ophthalmol. 2011;129(11):1407–15.
107. Marr B, Gobin PY, Dunkel IJ, Brodie SE, Abramson DH. Spontaneously resolving periocular erythema

and ciliary madarosis following intra-arterial chemotherapy for retinoblastoma. Middle East Afr J Ophthalmol. 2010;17(3):207–9.
108. Dalvin LA, Ancona-Lezama D, Lucio-Alvarez JA, Masoomian B, Jabbour P, Shields CL. Primary intra-arterial chemotherapy for retinoblastoma in the intravitreal chemotherapy era: five years of experience. Ocul Oncol Pathol. 2019;5:139–46.
109. Mathew AA, Sachdev N, Staffieri SE, McKenzie JD, Elder JE. Superselective intra-arterial chemotherapy for advanced retinoblastoma complicated by metastatic disease. J AAPOS. 2015;19(1):72–4.
110. Yousef YA, Soliman SE, Astudillo PP, Durairaj P, Dimaras H, Chan HS, et al. Intra-arterial chemotherapy for retinoblastoma: a systematic review. JAMA Ophthalmol. 2016;134(5):584–91.
111. Gobin YP, Dunkel IJ, Marr BP, Brodie SE, Abramson DH. Intra-arterial chemotherapy for the management of retinoblastoma: four-year experience. Arch Ophthalmol. 2011;129(6):732–7.
112. Shields CL, Lally SE, Leahey AM, Jabbour PM, Caywood EH, Schwendeman R, et al. Targeted retinoblastoma management: when to use intravenous, intra-arterial, periocular, and intravitreal chemotherapy. Curr Opin Ophthalmol. 2014;25(5):374–85.
113. Yannuzzi NA, Francis JH, Abramson DH. Incidence of orbital recurrence after enucleation or ophthalmic artery chemosurgery for advanced intraocular retinoblastoma--reply. JAMA Ophthalmol. 2016;134(1):114–5.
114. Yannuzzi NA, Francis JH, Marr BP, Belinsky I, Dunkel IJ, Gobin YP, et al. Enucleation vs ophthalmic artery chemosurgery for advanced intraocular retinoblastoma: a retrospective analysis. JAMA Ophthalmol. 2015;133(9):1062–6.
115. Berry JL, Kogachi K, Aziz HA, McGovern K, Zolfaghari E, Murphree AL, et al. Risk of metastasis and orbital recurrence in advanced retinoblastoma eyes treated with systemic chemoreduction versus primary enucleation. Pediatr Blood Cancer. 2017;64(4):26270.
116. Munier FL, Gaillard MC, Balmer A, Soliman S, Podilsky G, Moulin AP, et al. Intravitreal chemotherapy for vitreous disease in retinoblastoma revisited: from prohibition to conditional indications. Br J Ophthalmol. 2012;96(8):1078–83.
117. Munier FL, Gaillard MC, Balmer A, Beck-Popovic M. Intravitreal chemotherapy for vitreous seeding in retinoblastoma: recent advances and perspectives. Saudi J Ophthalmol. 2013;27(3):147–50.
118. Ildefonso CJ, Kong L, Leen A, Chai SJ, Petrochelli V, Chintagumpala M, et al. Absence of systemic immune response to adenovectors after intraocular administration to children with retinoblastoma. Mol Ther. 2010;18(10):1885–90.
119. Chevez-Barrios P, Chintagumpala M, Mieler W, Paysse E, Boniuk M, Kozinetz C, et al. Response of retinoblastoma with vitreous tumor seeding to adenovirus-mediated delivery of thymidine kinase followed by ganciclovir. J Clin Oncol. 2005;23(31):7927–35.
120. Ericson LA, Rosengren BH. Tests of intravitreous chemotherapy in retinoblastoma. Acta Ophthalmol. 1962;40:121–2.
121. Seregard S, Kock E, af Trampe E. Intravitreal chemotherapy for recurrent retinoblastoma in an only eye. Br J Ophthalmol. 1995;79(2):194–5.
122. Kivela T, Eskelin S, Paloheimo M. Intravitreal methotrexate for retinoblastoma. Ophthalmology. 2011;118(8):1689.
123. Ghassemi F, Shields CL. Intravitreal melphalan for refractory or recurrent vitreous seeding from retinoblastoma. Arch Ophthalmol. 2012;130(10):1268–71.
124. Shields CL, Fulco EM, Arias JD, Alarcon C, Pellegrini M, Rishi P, et al. Retinoblastoma frontiers with intravenous, intra-arterial, periocular, and intravitreal chemotherapy. Eye (Lond). 2013;27(2):253–64.
125. Smith SJ, Smith BD. Evaluating the risk of extraocular tumour spread following intravitreal injection therapy for retinoblastoma: a systematic review. Br J Ophthalmol. 2013;97(10):1231–6.
126. Sun YB, Hui P, Punyara K, Bi MC, Li SH, Teng SY, et al. Intravitreal injection of melphalan in the treatment of retinoblastoma with vitreous cavity seeding. Chin Med J. 2013;126(8):1587.
127. Francis JH, Schaiquevich P, Buitrago E, Del Sole MJ, Zapata G, Croxatto JO, et al. Local and systemic toxicity of intravitreal melphalan for vitreous seeding in retinoblastoma: a preclinical and clinical study. Ophthalmology. 2014;121(9):1810–7.
128. Ghassemi F, Shields CL, Ghadimi H, Khodabandeh A, Roohipoor R. Combined intravitreal melphalan and topotecan for refractory or recurrent vitreous seeding from retinoblastoma. JAMA Ophthalmol. 2014;132(8):936–41.
129. Lawson BM, Saktanasate J, Say EA, Shields CL. Intravitreal chemotherapy provides control for massive vitreous seeding from retinoblastoma. J Pediatr Ophthalmol Strabismus. 2014;51:e92–4.
130. Smith SJ, Smith BD, Mohney BG. Ocular side effects following intravitreal injection therapy for retinoblastoma: a systematic review. Br J Ophthalmol. 2014;98(3):292–7.
131. Manjandavida FP, Shields CL. The role of intravitreal chemotherapy for retinoblastoma. Indian J Ophthalmol. 2015;63(2):141–5.
132. Tuncer S, Balci O, Tanyildiz B, Kebudi R, Shields CL. Intravitreal lower-dose (20 microg) melphalan for persistent or recurrent retinoblastoma vitreous seeds. Ophthalmic Surg Lasers Imaging Retina. 2015;46(9):942–8.
133. Francis JH, Marr BP, Brodie SE, Gobin P, Dunkel IJ, Abramson DH. Intravitreal melphalan as salvage therapy for refractory retinal and subretinal retinoblastoma. Retin Cases Brief Rep. 2016;10(4):357–60.
134. Aziz HA, Kim JW, Munier FL, Berry JL. Acute hemorrhagic retinopathy following intravitreal

melphalan injection for retinoblastoma: a report of two cases and technical modifications to enhance the prevention of retinal toxicity. Ocul Oncol Pathol. 2017;3(1):34–40.

135. Berry JL, Shah S, Bechtold M, Zolfaghari E, Jubran R, Kim JW. Long-term outcomes of Group D retinoblastoma eyes during the intravitreal melphalan era. Pediatr Blood Cancer. 2017;64:26696.
136. Kiratli H, Koc I, Varan A, Akyuz C. Intravitreal chemotherapy in the management of vitreous disease in retinoblastoma. Eur J Ophthalmol. 2017;27(4):423–7.
137. Berry JL, Bechtold M, Shah S, Zolfaghari E, Reid M, Jubran R, et al. Not all seeds are created equal: seed classification is predictive of outcomes in retinoblastoma. Ophthalmology. 2017;124(12):1817–25.
138. Francis JH, Marr BP, Brodie SE, Abramson DH. Anterior ocular toxicity of intravitreous melphalan for retinoblastoma. JAMA Ophthalmol. 2015;133(12):1459–63.
139. Francis JH, Brodie SE, Marr B, Zabor EC, Mondesire-Crump I, Abramson DH. Efficacy and toxicity of intravitreous chemotherapy for retinoblastoma: four-year experience. Ophthalmology. 2017;124(4):488–95.
140. Munier FL. Intracameral chemotherapy (melphalan) for aqueous seeding in retinoblastoma: bicameral injection technique and related toxicity in a pilot case study. Ocul Oncol Pathol. 2017;3:149–55.
141. Munier FL. Classification and management of seeds in retinoblastoma. Ellsworth Lecture Ghent August 24th 2013. Ophthalmic Genet. 2014;35(4):193–207.
142. Francis JH, Abramson DH, Gaillard MC, Marr BP, Beck-Popovic M, Munier FL. The classification of vitreous seeds in retinoblastoma and response to intravitreal melphalan. Ophthalmology. 2015;122(6):1173–9.
143. Amram AL, Rico G, Kim JW, Chintagumpala M, Herzog CE, Gombos DS, et al. Vitreous seeds in retinoblastoma: clinicopathologic classification and correlation. Ophthalmology. 2017;124(10):1540–7.
144. Kim JW. Retinoblastoma: evidence for postenucleation adjuvant chemotherapy. Int Ophthalmol Clin. 2015;55(1):77–96.
145. Magramm I, Abramson DH, Ellsworth RM. Optic nerve involvement in retinoblastoma. Ophthalmology. 1989;96(2):217–22.
146. Shields CL, Shields JA, Baez KA, Cater J, De Potter PV. Choroidal invasion of retinoblastoma: metastatic potential and clinical risk factors. Br J Ophthalmol. 1993;77(9):544–8.
147. Yasui N, Kawamoto H, Fujiwara M, Aihara Y, Ogawa C, Hosono A, et al. High-dose chemotherapy for high-risk retinoblastoma: clinical course and outcome of 14 cases in the National Cancer Center, Japan. Bone Marrow Transplant. 2015;50(2):221–4.
148. Kim JW, Kathpalia V, Dunkel IJ, Wong RK, Riedel E, Abramson DH. Orbital recurrence of retinoblastoma following enucleation. Br J Ophthalmol. 2009;93(4):463–7.
149. Kremens B, Wieland R, Reinhard H, Neubert D, Beck JD, Klingebiel T, et al. High-dose chemotherapy with autologous stem cell rescue in children with retinoblastoma. Bone Marrow Transplant. 2003;31(4):281–4.
150. Dunkel IJ, Chan HS, Jubran R, Chantada GL, Goldman S, Chintagumpala M, et al. High-dose chemotherapy with autologous hematopoietic stem cell rescue for stage 4B retinoblastoma. Pediatr Blood Cancer. 2010;55(1):149–52.
151. Dunkel IJ, Jubran RF, Gururangan S, Chantada GL, Finlay JL, Goldman S, et al. Trilateral retinoblastoma: potentially curable with intensive chemotherapy. Pediatr Blood Cancer. 2010;54(3):384–7.
152. Dunkel IJ, Khakoo Y, Kernan NA, Gershon T, Gilheeney S, Lyden DC, et al. Intensive multimodality therapy for patients with stage 4a metastatic retinoblastoma. Pediatr Blood Cancer. 2010;55(1):55–9.
153. Matsubara H, Makimoto A, Higa T, Kawamoto H, Sakiyama S, Hosono A, et al. A multidisciplinary treatment strategy that includes high-dose chemotherapy for metastatic retinoblastoma without CNS involvement. Bone Marrow Transplant. 2005;35(8):763–6.
154. Lee SH, Yoo KH, Sung KW, Kim JY, Cho EJ, Koo HH, et al. Tandem high-dose chemotherapy and autologous stem cell rescue in children with bilateral advanced retinoblastoma. Bone Marrow Transplant. 2008;42(6):385–91.
155. Girnius S, Seldin DC, Skinner M, Finn KT, Quillen K, Doros G, et al. Hepatic response after high-dose melphalan and stem cell transplantation in patients with AL amyloidosis associated liver disease. Haematologica. 2009;94(7):1029–32.
156. Friend SH, Bernards R, Rogelj S, Weinberg RA, Rapaport JM, Albert DM, et al. A human DNA segment with properties of the gene that predisposes to retinoblastoma and osteosarcoma. Nature. 1986;323(6089):643–6.
157. Tien HF, Chuang SM, Chen MS, Lee FY, Hou PK. Cytogenetic evidence of multifocal origin of a unilateral retinoblastoma. A help in genetic counseling. Cancer Genet Cytogenet. 1989;42(2):203–8.
158. Lee SY, Jeon DG, Lee JS, Hwang CS, Huh K, Lee TW, et al. Deletion of Rb1 gene in late osteosarcoma from survivor of unilateral retinoblastoma--a case report. J Korean Med Sci. 1996;11(1):94–8.
159. Kim JW, Lee CG, Han SM, Kim KS, Kim JO, Lee JM, et al. Loss of heterozygosity of the retinoblastoma and p53 genes in primary cervical carcinomas with human papillomavirus infection. Gynecol Oncol. 1997;67(2):215–21.
160. Fung YK, Murphree AL, T'Ang A, Qian J, Hinrichs SH, Benedict WF. Structural evidence for the authenticity of the human retinoblastoma gene. Science. 1987;236(4809):1657–61.
161. Benedict WF, Fung YK, Murphree AL. The gene responsible for the development of retinoblastoma and osteosarcoma. Cancer. 1988;62(8 Suppl):1691–4.

162. Knudson AG Jr. Mutation and cancer: statistical study of retinoblastoma. Proc Natl Acad Sci U S A. 1971;68(4):820–3.
163. American Academy of P, Section on O, American Association for Pediatric O, Strabismus, American Academy of O, American Association of Certified O. Red reflex examination in neonates, infants, and children. Pediatrics. 2008;122(6):1401–4.
164. Abramson DH, Schefler AC. Update on retinoblastoma. Retina. 2004;24(6):828–48.
165. Ayari-Jeridi H, Moran K, Chebbi A, Bouguila H, Abbes I, Charradi K, et al. Mutation spectrum of RB1 gene in unilateral retinoblastoma cases from Tunisia and correlations with clinical features. PLoS One. 2015;10(1):e0116615.
166. Berry JL, Lewis L, Zolfaghari E, Green S, Le BHA, Lee TC, et al. Suprasellar arachnoid cyst presenting with bobble-head doll movements: a report of 3 cases. Neurol India. 2018;51(3):407–9.
167. Tang G, Paik S, Baehner FL, Liu Q, Jeong JH, Kim SR, et al. Prognostic impact of the 21-gene recurrence score (RS) on disease-free and overall survival of node-positive, ER-positive breast cancer patients (pts) treated with adjuvant chemotherapy: results from NSABP B-28. J Clin Oncol. 2012;30(27_suppl):1.
168. Torres-Torres B, Soberino J, Rios S, Gonzalez Rivas CS, Ruiz Vozmediano J, Castillo L, et al. The prognostic value of detection methylation level panel of gene in DNA circulating after and before treatment in patients with breast cancer. J Clin Oncol. 2012;30(30_suppl):67.
169. Tian S, Wang C, Chang HH, Sun J. Identification of prognostic genes and gene sets for early-stage non-small cell lung cancer using bi-level selection methods. Sci Rep. 2017;7:46164.
170. Peretti U, Ferrara R, Pilotto S, Kinspergher S, Caccese M, Santo A, et al. ALK gene copy number gains in non-small-cell lung cancer: prognostic impact and clinico-pathological correlations. Respir Res. 2016;17(1):105.
171. Lopes GL, Vattimo EF, Castro Junior G. Identifying activating mutations in the EGFR gene: prognostic and therapeutic implications in non-small cell lung cancer. J Bras Pneumol. 2015;41(4):365–75.
172. Tao KY, Li XX, Xu WZ, Wang Y, Zhu SM, Xie HX, et al. Prognostic role of apoptosis-related gene functional variants in advanced non-small-cell lung cancer patients treated with first-line platinum-based chemotherapy. Onco Targets Ther. 2015;8:147–55.
173. Hauke RJ Jr, Sissung TM, Figg WD. Discussing the predictive, prognostic, and therapeutic value of germline DNA-repair gene mutations in metastatic prostate cancer patients. Cancer Biol Ther. 2017;18(8):545–6.
174. Berg KD. The prognostic and predictive value of TMPRSS2-ERG gene fusion and ERG protein expression in prostate cancer biopsies. Dan Med J. 2016;63:12.
175. Kulda V, Topolcan O, Kucera R, Kripnerova M, Srbecka K, Hora M, et al. Prognostic significance of TMPRSS2-ERG fusion gene in prostate cancer. Anticancer Res. 2016;36(9):4787–93.
176. Mendoza PR, Specht CS, Hubbard GB, Wells JR, Lynn MJ, Zhang Q, et al. Histopathologic grading of anaplasia in retinoblastoma. Am J Ophthalmol. 2015;159(4):764–76.
177. Mendoza PR, Geisert EE, Ziesel AC, Specht CS, Hubbard GB, Wells JR, et al. Gene expression profiling of retinoblastoma and retinocytoma. Invest Ophthalmol Vis Sci. 2015;56:3444.
178. Kooi IE, Mol BM, Massink MP, Ameziane N, Meijers-Heijboer H, Dommering CJ, et al. Somatic genomic alterations in retinoblastoma beyond RB1 are rare and limited to copy number changes. Sci Rep. 2016;6:25264.
179. Kooi IE, Mol BM, Massink MP, de Jong MC, de Graaf P, van der Valk P, et al. A meta-analysis of retinoblastoma copy numbers refines the list of possible driver genes involved in tumor progression. PLoS One. 2016;11(4):e0153323.
180. Francis JH, Abramson DH, Ji X, Shields CL, Teixeira LF, Schefler AC, et al. Risk of extraocular extension in eyes with retinoblastoma receiving intravitreous chemotherapy. JAMA Ophthalmol. 2017;135(12):1426–9.
181. Berry JL, Xu L, Kooi I, Murphree AL, Prabakar RK, Reid M, et al. Genomic cfDNA analysis of aqueous humor in retinoblastoma predicts eye salvage: the surrogate tumor biopsy for retinoblastoma. Mol Cancer Res. 2018;16(11):1701–12.
182. Corson TW, Gallie BL. One hit, two hits, three hits, more? Genomic changes in the development of retinoblastoma. Genes Chromosomes Cancer. 2007;46(7):617–34.

Imaging of Intraocular Tumours

4

David Sia, Rana'a T. Al Jamal,
and Mandeep S. Sagoo

4.1 Color Photography

In the digital revolution, most film cameras have now been replaced by digital technology. The advantages of digital imaging are many, producing high resolution images with relatively inexpensive digital single lens reflex (DSLR) cameras, without the need for processing film or slides, hence giving an instant image [1]. Several devices are available with different ways of taking the image. This varies from ocular piece attachment, where a camera is attached to the eyepieces of the slit-lamp, to a beam attachment, where the camera is located to the optical beam path via a module (most slit lamp cameras), and finally instruments where the camera is integrated into the slit-lamp. In the latter type of machine, a beam splitter and camera are built into a single unit, requiring the camera to be connected to a computer.

D. Sia
Ocular Oncology Service, Moorfields Eye Hospital, London, UK

Retinoblastoma Service, Royal London Hospital, London, UK

R. T. Al Jamal
Ocular Oncology Service, Moorfields Eye Hospital, London, UK

M. S. Sagoo (✉)
Ocular Oncology Service, Moorfields Eye Hospital, London, UK

UCL Institute of Ophthalmology, London, UK
e-mail: Mandeep.sagoo@nhs.net

In ocular oncology, anterior segment color photography allows a good view of the anterior segment components. This is very helpful in documenting conjunctival lesions, iris tumours and pseudotumours, and the anterior chamber angle can be photographed with a gonioscopic lens. Slit-lamp colour photography is able to produce faithful colour reproduction of the tissues being photographed and has the advantage of slit-lamp magnification and utility of the slit-beam to highlight contours or to use diffuse illumination (Fig. 4.1).

Fundus photography is commonly used method for documenting fundus and intraocular pathology. The first device was introduced by Zeiss and Nordensen in 1926. It provided a 20° fundus image. Later, the field of view expanded to 30–45° which became the standard for the traditional fundus camera [2]. Fundus photography usually requires pupil dilation, multiple 45° images are captured, and then stitched together using computer software to create a panoramic view. Fluorescein angiography (FFA) or indocyanine green (ICG) can also be captured with these techniques.

Optomap ultra-widefield imaging (Optos PLC, Dunfermline, UK) was founded in 1992 by Douglas Anderson after the late detection of his child's retinal detachment. Optomap is a digital ultra-widefield (UWF) retinal imaging system (Scanning Laser Ophthalmoscope) with two low-powered laser wavelengths, green 532 nm and red 633 nm, that scan the fundus simultaneously. The green laser images the layers from the sensory

V. Khetan (ed.), *Intraocular Tumors*, https://doi.org/10.1007/978-981-15-0395-5_4

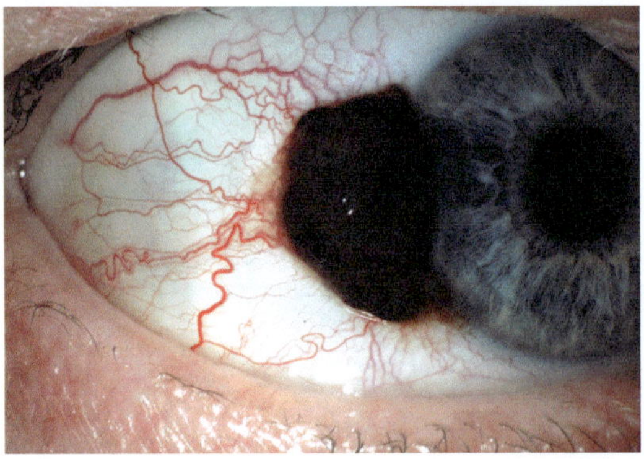

Fig. 4.1 Slit-lamp colour photograph showing a conjunctival melanoma at the temporal limbal area of the right eye

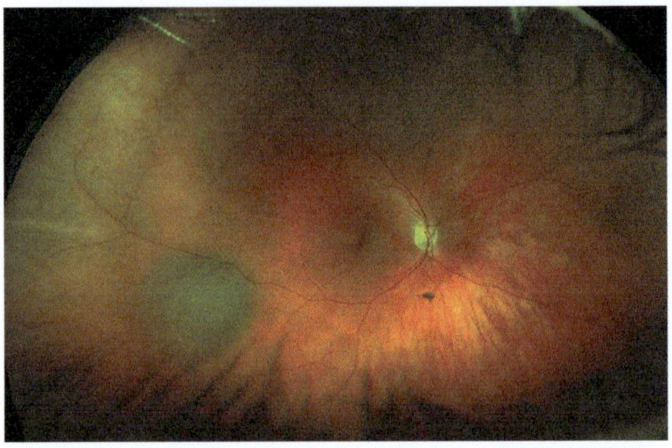

Fig. 4.2 Optomap ultra-widefield imaging (Optos PLC, Dunfermline, UK) of the right fundus showing a choroidal naevus in the inferotemporal mid-peripheral location

retina to the retinal pigment epithelium (RPE), whereas the red laser scans the deeper structures from the RPE to the choroid. In contrast to the simple illuminating effects of white light used in conventional ophthalmoscopy techniques, the Optomap allows review of retinal structures in their individual laser separations. The Optomap provides an ultra-widefield, non-mydriatic, 82% view (200°) of the retina, with a resolution of 14 μm, and higher resolution at 100°, of 11 μm, in single image capture, taking less than 1 s, while with traditional methods, only 10–15% of the retina is captured in one single shot.

UWF autofluorescence captures of the retina using autofluorescence and a green laser (532 nm). Colour imaging and autofluorescence can be carried out in one workflow and allows a brighter view of the macula than with a blue laser. It also allows FFA and ICG angiography [2]. In the evaluation of melanocytic fundus lesions, Shields et al. identified 5 risk factors that predict differentiating small choroidal melanomas from nevi [3]. Reznicek et al., studied the role of wide-field imaging and autofluorescence for evaluating of the criteria established by Shields. The mean fundus autofluorescence intensity of melanomas was significantly lower than the autofluorescence of choroidal nevi, which may help in differentiating between lesions [4]. Disadvantages of this camera system include false colours giving rise to erroneous pigmentation in amelanotic lesions, peripheral distortion, and eyelid and eyelash artefacts (Figs. 4.2 and 4.3).

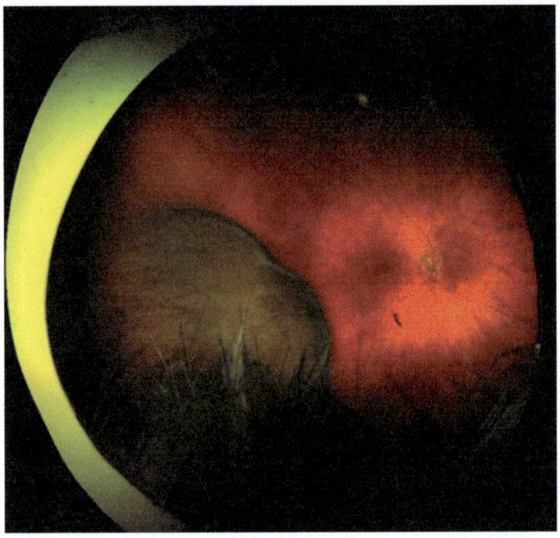

Fig. 4.3 Optomap ultra-widefield imaging (Optos PLC, Dunfermline, UK) of the same patient in Fig. 4.2, taken 3 years later, showing malignant transformation into choroidal melanoma

In paediatric ocular oncology, retinoblastoma specialists use an integrated fundus camera, the RetCam (Clarity Medical Systems, Pleasanton, California, USA) to document and monitor fundus tumours undergoing treatment during examinations under anaesthesia in the supine patient. This is used for screening neonates for retinopathy of prematurity as well as in other paediatric retinal diseases. Retinoblastoma, a childhood intraocular tumor accounts for 11% of all childhood cancers [5, 6]. This camera allows color fundus photos to be taken using a fiber optic light cable with a range of lenses that can image

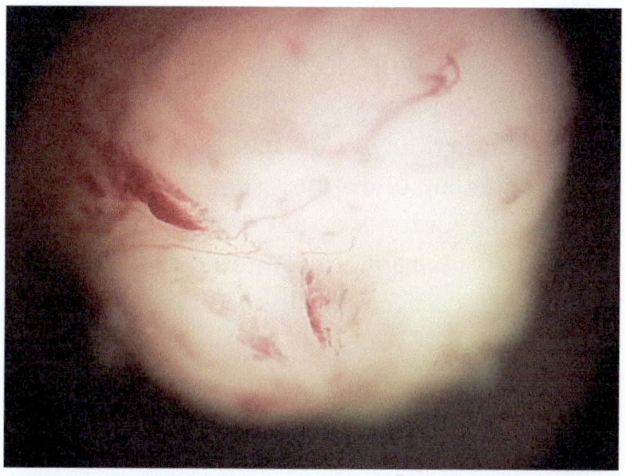

Fig. 4.4 RetCam (Clarity Medical Systems, Pleasanton, CA) image of the fundus in a paediatric patient demonstrating a retinoblastoma lesion (Group D, IRCB classification)

30–130° of the retina, and with appropriate filters can also take fluorescein angiograms. A handheld lens and light source unit is placed on the cornea with a viscoelastic gel coupling agent. It is possible to take anterior segment photos as well, but not with a slit beam source. It requires clear media making it more suited to use in infants and children rather than in adults [7]. Documentation with the RetCam is especially useful in the follow up of retinoblastoma patients, aiding careful comparison to judge therapeutic success (Fig. 4.4).

4.2 Fundus Fluorescein Angiography (FFA)

Sodium fluorescein is a fluorescent dye, of which 80% is protein bound and 20% is free in the plasma [8, 9]. It is the free form that is responsible for the emission of fluorescent light [9]. Due to these properties, fluorescein behaves like a micromolecule that diffuses easily from fenestrated blood vessels or any breakdown of endothelial tight junctions. It diffuses quickly into tissues but is also quickly washed out. When excited by blue light (460–490 nm), this dye fluoresces in the green-red visible light spectrum (520–630 nm) [10]. The fluorescent spectrum within visible light is blocked by retinal pigment epithelium (RPE) and therefore gives limited information on the choroidal circulation except on the choriocapillaris during the first 40–60 s of angiography [9].

Angiographic features of intraocular tumours depend on tumour pigmentation, depth of location within the choroid, intrinsic vascularity and associated secondary changes of the overlying retina.

For choroidal naevi, a small naevus confined to the outer choroid without involvement of overlying choriocapillaris may demonstrate a granular or normal appearing angiogram. A larger lesion that encroaches on the choriocapillaris as well as a highly pigmented lesion will appear more hypofluorescent [11]. Less-pigmented lesions and larger lesions with increased intrinsic vascularity may appear more hyperfluorescent [11]. Associated secondary changes of the overlying retina may give rise to patterns of hyperfluorescense (subretinal neovascular membrane (SRNVM), drusen and RPE atrophy, RPE detachment) or hypofluorescence (RPE clumping, RPE fibrous metaplasia (with late staining)) [11]. The diagnostic utility of FFA in choroidal naevi is often employed to differentiate subretinal fluid associated with a choroidal naevi arising from a SRVNM or from RPE failure.

Similarly, a small choroidal melanoma with normal overlying RPE may show no appreciable abnormality on angiography [11]. A large melanoma with overlying RPE disruption will show mottled hyperfluorescence in the arterial phase from filling of tumour vessels, and diffuse staining of the lesion and its overlying subretinal fluid in the late phases [11]. A larger amelanotic melanoma, particularly one that has broken through Bruch's membrane, might show more clearly the characteristic double circulation during the later arterial or early venous phase due to simultaneous filing of the choroidal and retinal vasculature [11, 12].

In choroidal metastasis, there is general hypofluorescence of the lesion in the arterial and early venous phases with pinpoint foci of hyperfluorescence appearing over the tumour beginning in the late venous phase (usually later than with choroidal haemangioma or melanoma), and increasing in intensity and extent with leakage of dye into overlying exudative retinal detachment [11].

In retinal capillary haemangiomas, there is rapid tumour filling via a dilated feeder vessel and visibility of fine intrinsic tumour vasculature in the arterial phase and late hyperfluorescence, often with leakage of dye into the vitreous [13]. FFA is particularly helpful in differentiating the feeder and drainage vessels to guide laser ablation of the tumor.

FFA in circumscribed choroidal haemangiomas generally adds little diagnostic information [13, 14]. Typically there is early filling of the tumour vessels before filling of the retinal vessels and diffuse late staining of the mass (Fig. 4.5) [13, 15].

In retinal arteriovenous malformation, FFA demonstrates the abnormal arteriovenous connection and presence or absence of intervening

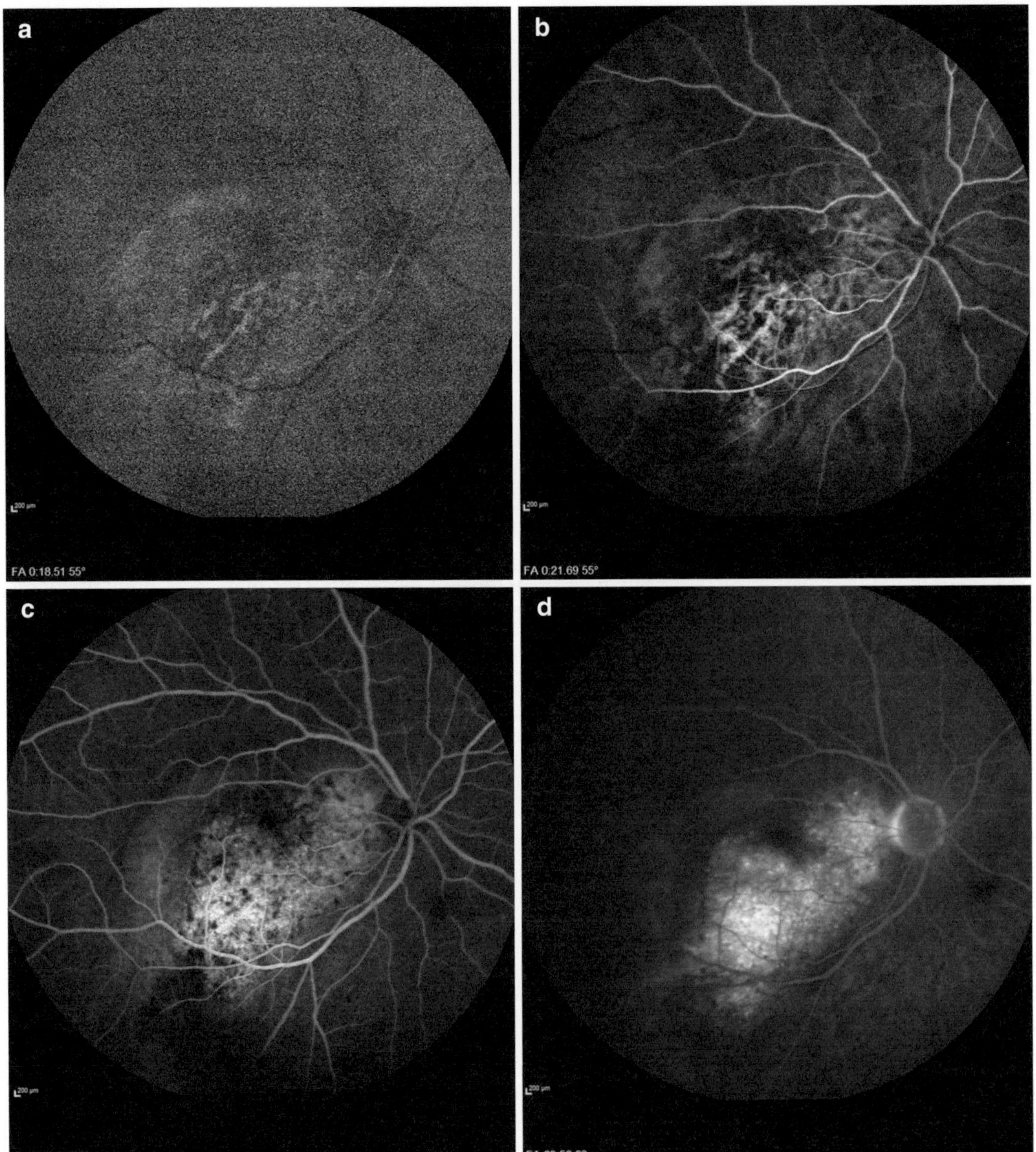

Fig. 4.5 Fundus fluorescein angiography of a circumscribed choroidal haemangioma showing early filling of the tumour vessels before filling of the retinal vessels (**a**) and progressive staining and leakage of the mass throughout the later stages (**b–d**)

capillaries [11, 16]. FFA in retinal cavernous haemangioma has a pathognomonic filling pattern, the tumour remains hypofluorescent throughout the arterial and early venous phases. In the late venous phase, the upper half of the saccular aneurysms begin to fill and appear as fluorescent caps. This is due to staining of supernatant plasma overlying sedimented blood cells [16]. There is usually no demonstrable leakage on angiography in both retinal arteriovenous malformations and retinal cavernous haemangiomas [11, 16].

FFA can be useful in the initial diagnosis of vasoproliferative tumours, in helping to differentiate it from peripheral exudative haemorrhagic chorioretinopathy by demonstrating the vascular supply of these lesions that show rapid filling in the early phase with diffuse leakage in the late phases [16, 17]. In contrast to retinal capillary haemangiomas, retinal feeder vessels are only mildly dilated in vasoproliferative tumours [13]. Due to the peripheral location, ultra-wide-field angiography is usually required to image these lesions.

4.3 Indocyanine Green Angiography (ICGA)

Indocyanine green (ICG) is a tricarbocyanine dye that is more protein bound compared to sodium fluorescein (98% vs 80%), and therefore diffuses out of fenestrated vasculature much slower than sodium flourescein [8, 18]. ICG maximally absorbs infrared light at 805 nm and maximally fluoresces at 835 nm wavelength. At these near-infrared wavelengths, penetration through ocular pigment and media opacities is much more efficient compared to shorter wavelengths of visible light used in fluorescein angiography (FA) [18]. These two properties make ICGA a more effective method at imaging the choroidal vasculature compared to FA.

ICGA is particularly useful in the differentiation of amelanotic choroidal tumours, such as amelanotic choroidal melanoma, choroidal haemangioma and metastasis.

Choroidal haemangiomas have the most consistent and characteristic ICG pattern amongst intraocular tumours (Fig. 4.6). In the early stages of the study (10–20 s), a network of small-caliber lacy vessels is seen rapidly fluorescing in a web configuration that completely obscures the normal choroidal pattern (Fig. 4.6a) [14, 19]. These vessels are distinctly different from those seen with choroidal melanomas and choroidal metastases [20]. Often, the fluorescence originates at the periphery of the lesion in a wreath pattern and spreads to the center of the tumour within seconds. By about 1 min, choroidal haemangiomas completely fill with dye and the tumour reaches maximal fluorescence (Fig. 4.6c). This maximal brightness at 1 min is brighter than any other intraocular tumour, and is very suggestive of the diagnosis [20]. In mid-phase (6–10 min), the hyperfluorescence usually begins to wane and in the very late phases (>30 min), the tumour becomes hypofluorescent relative to the surrounding choroid, a phenomenon known as 'wash-out' (Fig 4.6d) [19]. This phenomenon is due to the low-resistance, high-flow properties of the vascular tumour that causes a more rapid clearance of dye from the tumour compared to the normal surrounding choroid and is uniquely seen in choroidal haemangiomas [19, 20].

A choroidal naevus and a choroidal melanoma can show overlapping ICGA features, and have variable ICG fluorescent patterns depending on the degree of tumour pigmentation, tumour thickness and tumour vascularity. In general, more pigmented as well as minimally elevated lesions are less fluorescent. Whereas, amelanotic and thicker lesions are more fluorescent [20]. The speed of fluorescence is much slower compared to a choroidal haemangioma, and usually begins at about 1–2 min and reaches maximal fluorescence at about 18 min [14]. The intensity compared to the surrounding choroid is generally hypofluorescent [14]. The intrinsic tumour vasculature of choroidal naevi often resemble normal choroidal vessels in caliber, configuration and branching pattern but differ in being brighter and lacking small-caliber twig vessels [20]. On the other hand, intrinsic tumour vasculature in choroidal melanomas are identified early in the study (<20 s) as variable caliber, randomly branching vessels with small twig vessels arising

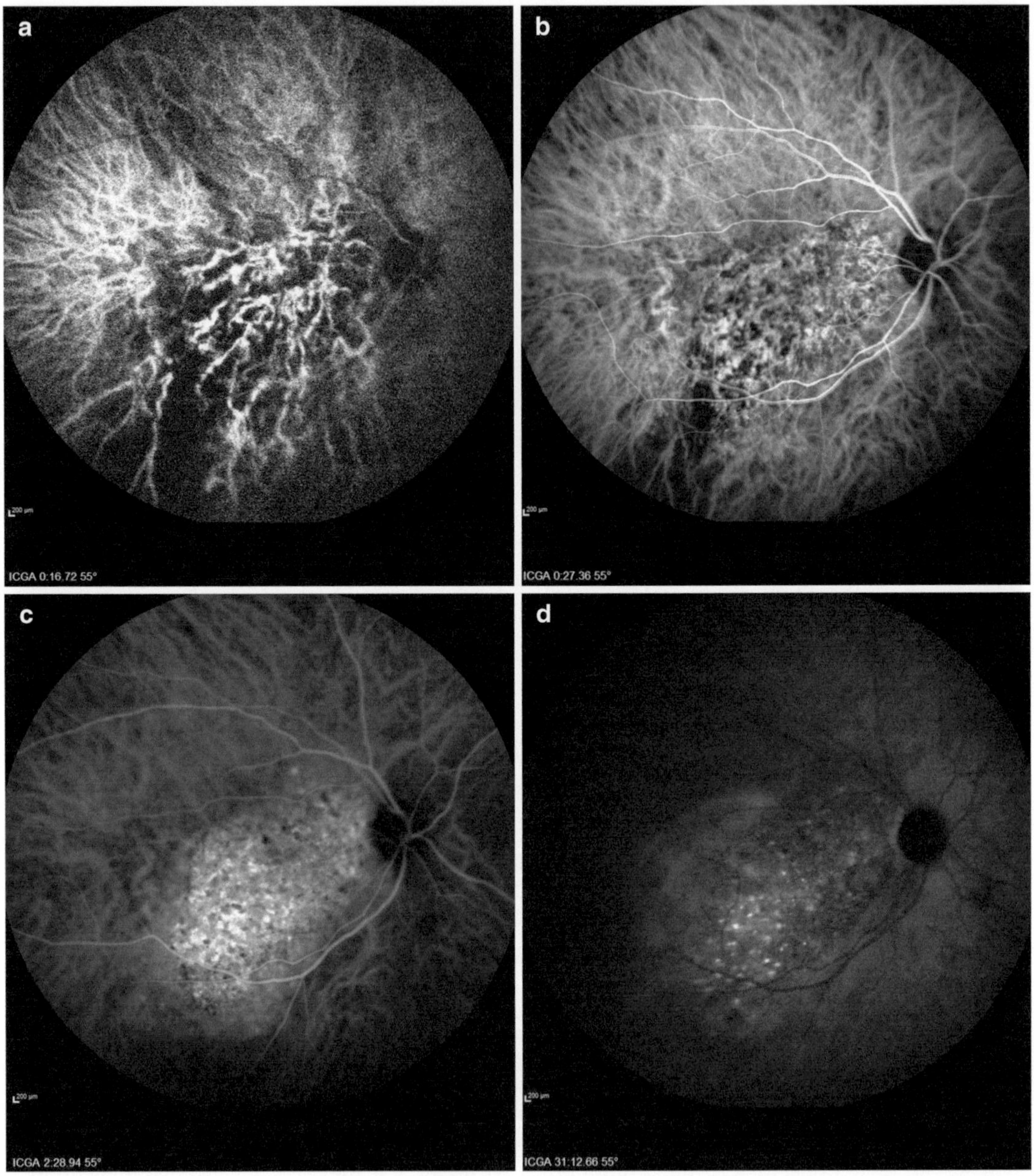

Fig. 4.6 Indocyanine green angiography of a circumscribed choroidal haemangioma showing characteristic early filling of lacy tumoural vessels (**a**), progressive filling of the tumour (**b**), maximal hyperfluorescence (**c**), and late 'washout' phenomenon (**d**)

from the main vessels [11]. The vessel walls show staining in the intermediate phase and leakage in the late phase (>30 min) [19]. They may also show abnormal features such as marked dilation, hairpin turns, corkscrew loops and random crisscrossing within the tumour [20]. Microvascular patterns of choroidal melanoma have been found to inform prognosis, with complex microcirculation patterns (parallel vessels with cross links, branching arcades, loops and networks) associated with poor prognosis [21].

In choroidal metastasis, there is a diffusely homogenous hypofluorescence compared to the surrounding choroid in the early frames (<1 min).

The normal perfusing choroidal pattern can often be faintly visualised underlying the lesion as if the tumour is acting as a relative filter. In the late frames (by 30 min), there may be persistent hypofluorescence, or late leakage into the overlying neurosensory detachment [20]. Intrinsic vessels are generally not observed because of the relative thinness of the tumour [19].

4.4 Fundus Autofluorescence (FAF)

Autofluorescence relies on the stimulated emission of light from naturally occuring fluorophores within human tissue. The main source of fundus autofluorescence is from lipofuscin, a product of degraded photoreceptor outer segments that accumulates within the RPE [22]. Intracellular lipofuscin accumulates with age and excessive lipofuscin accumulation within the RPE has been proposed as a marker of RPE disease and eventual photoreceptor degeneration [23, 24]. Other structures of the eye and their autofluorescence properties are listed in Table 4.1.

Choroidal tumours can secondarily affect the RPE. RPE hyperplasia, atrophy, fibrous and osseous metaplasia and drusen accumulation are associated with long-standing choroidal tumours, while intracellular lipofuscin accumulation is associated with more metabolically active tumours [22]. Lipofuscin accumulation appears as orange pigment when overlying pigmented choroidal tumours, but appears as brown pigment when overlying non-pigmented choroidal tumours [26].

Table 4.1 Fundus autofluorescence features of surrounding tissues related to intraocular tumours

Finding	Hyper-AF	Iso-AF	Hypo-AF
Orange/brown pigment (lipofuscin)	3+	–	–
Calcium	3+	–	–
Subretinal fluid	1+	–	–
Drusen	1+	–	–
Subretinal blood			
Fresh	–	–	3+
Old	1+	–	–
RPE hyperplasia	–	–	1+
RPE atrophy	–	–	2+
RPE fibrous metaplasia	–	–	2+

Adapted from Almeida et al. [25]

1+, mild; 2+, moderate; 3+, intense. *Hyper-AF* hyperautofluorescence, *hypo-AF* hypoautofluorescence, *NA* not applicable, *RPE* retinal pigment epithelium

Choroidal naevi and choroidal melanoma show only minimal intrinsic autofluorescence, with more pigmented lesions appearing more hypoautofluorescent and less pigmented lesions showing slight hyperautofluorescence. This is likely related to unmasking of deeper scleral autofluoresence [22, 27]. Extrinsic autofluorescence from secondary RPE changes are much more dramatic and informative. Choroidal naevi generally display extrinsic hypoautofluorescence from chronic RPE hyperplasia or atrophy, whereas choroidal melanoma generally show extrinsic hyperautofluorescence from lipofuscin accumulation and subretinal fluid [28]. Lipofuscin accumulation is particularly evident when the melanoma is small and active, and is less obvious with chronicity and tumour enlargement as the RPE degenerates with hyperplasia, atrophy, fibrous or osseous metaplasia [3]. Following treatment of choroidal melanoma, autofluorescence might increase due to increased lipofuscin, but eventually becomes hypoautofluorescent as lipofuscin fades from cell death [29, 30].

In choroidal metastasis, there is intrinsic hypoautofluorescence as the lesion blocks transmission of scleral autofluorescence [31]. Focal areas of lipofuscin (as brown pigmentation) may be seen overlying the lesion and these appear hyperautofluorescent [31, 32]. Following irradiation, there may be increased lipofuscin accumulation with confluent brown pigmentation over the lesion that appear intensely hyperautofluorescent [31]. Other areas of hyperautofluorescence associated with choroidal metastasis include the advancing tumour edge and subretinal fluid [31, 33].

Both circumscribed and diffuse choroidal haemangiomas have general intrinsic hypoautofluorescence or isoautofluorescence [34]. Extrinsic autofluorescence may be hyperautofluorescence from lipofuscin and subretinal fluid or hypoautofluorescence from RPE hyperplasia, metaplasia or atrophy. Following treatment, choroidal haemangiomas show increased intrinsic hypoautofluorescence and extrinsic hypoautofluorescence from further RPE hyperplasia or atrophy [34]. FAF is also useful in detecting prior resolved subretinal fluid and may show troughs of hypoautofluorescence from subtle RPE atrophy.

Choroidal osteomas show isoautofluorescence in the calcified portions where the RPE is intact, while decalcified portions show hypoautofluorescence due to RPE fibrous metaplasia or atrophy [35]. The periphery of the lesion have also been found to show hyperautofluorescence associated with granular hypoautofluorescent dots, which suggest an increased metabolic activity of the RPE along the margins of the tumour together with atrophic areas of RPE loss [36]. Associated overlying active CNV will appear hyperautofluorescent [35].

Intraocular lymphomas are divided into the uveal form and the retinovitreal form. Uveal lymphomas can be associated with overlying subretinal fluid which cause RPE irritation and multifocal dots of lipofuscin accumulation [25]. The retinovitreal form have a more diverse but distinctive FAF pattern. Yellow infiltrates seen ophthalmoscopically correspond to sub-RPE tumour infiltration and they appear weakly hyperautofluorescent possibly due to accumulation of lipofuscin within the tumour masses [37]. Brown clumps may develop overlying the subRPE yellow lesions, and these appear brightly hyperautofluorescent [37]. Yellow infiltrates may become confluent and spontaneously regress, leaving the RPE atrophic as a hypoautofluorescent area [37]. White infiltrates, on the other hand, are retinal infiltrates of tumour cells and these appear hypoautofluorescent due to blockage of underlying RPE autofluorescence [37].

Astrocytic hamartomas are classified into 3 types: Type 1 lesions are relatively flat, round or oval semitransparent, light-gray masses that are non-calcified. Type 2 lesions contain multiple calcified nodular areas with a mulberry-like appearance. Type 3 lesions contain features of both types 1 and 2, with a peripheral semitranslucent non-calcified rim and a calcified central portion [38]. Type 1 lesions have intrinsic hypoautofluorescence, as it partially blocks underlying RPE autofluorescence [39]. Type 2 lesions are brightly hyperautofluorescent from the calcification and type 3 lesions have a characteristic peripheral hypoautofluorescent rim, and a contrasting central bright hyperautofluorescent portion (Fig. 4.7) [39].

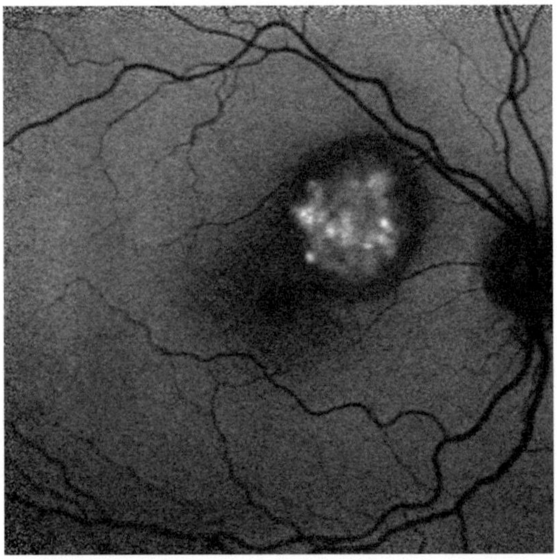

Fig. 4.7 Fundus autofluorescence of a type 3 astrocytic hamartoma showing characteristic peripheral hypoautofluorescent non-calcified rim and a contrasting central bright hyperautofluorescent calcified portion

4.4.1 Optical Coherence Tomography (OCT)

Optical coherence tomography (OCT) is a non-invasive diagnostic optical device, that was first introduced in early 1990s [40]. It is capable of providing cross-sectional view of both anterior and posterior segments. OCT is an important device in an ocular oncology practice and several types of OCTs are available: Anterior segment OCT (AS-OCT), ultra-high resolution OCT (UHR-OCT), spectral domain OCT (SD-OCT) and enhanced depth imaging OCT (EDI-OCT). These have varying resolution ranging from 1 to 25 μm. Spectral domain OCT has replaced time domain domain OCT because of higher speed and resolution [41]. It is commonly used in ocular oncology as it gives anatomic localization of tumors, and adds important features to the diag-

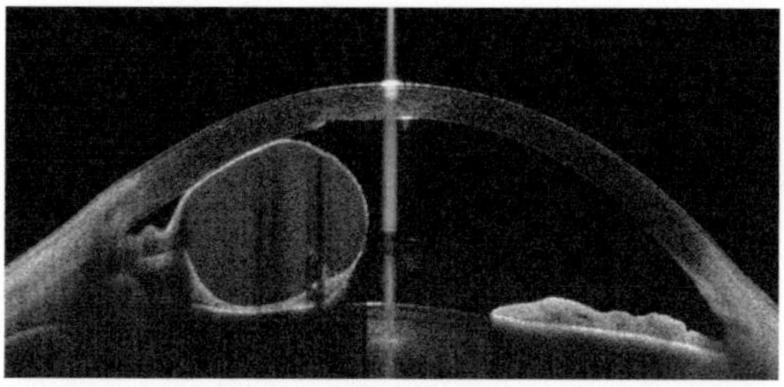

Fig. 4.8 Anterior segment optical coherence tomography showing a large iris stromal cyst with corneal apposition

nosis, treatment, follow up and response to treatment [42].

AS-OCT can be used for the diagnosis of ocular surface lesions. Some studies showed a good correlation with histopathology of the lesion [43, 44]. It is also used for imaging anterior segment tumours, mainly the iris (Fig. 4.8) [45], but ultrasound B scan or ultrasound biomicrosopy (UBM) remain the best methods to image anterior tumors, especially of the ciliary body with superior images to those on AS-OCT [43, 45].

Posterior segment OCT is helpful in identifying nevi from small choroidal melanomas, with a better view of subretinal fluid (SRF), and deeper layers of the choroid [46], especially when enhanced depth imaging (EDI-OCT) feature is used [41, 47]. Choroidal nevi appear as dome-shaped with overlying retinal pigment epithelium alterations, drusen, and even photoreceptor loss, while small melanoma shows moderately dome-shaped with overlying shallow SRF that often shows "shaggy" photoreceptors [42]. On the surface of choroidal naevi, chronic changes can lead to choroidal neovascularization and even outer retinal tabulation [48]. Choroidal metastases usually appear as a hyporeflective band in the deeper choroid causing enlargement of the suprachoroidal space, along with findings of intraretinal oedema and subretinal fluid [41, 49]. The anterior choroidal surface in choroidal metastasis often has a "lumpy, bumpy" appearance, as opposed to a "smooth" profile in choroidal melanomas [42]. In choroidal hemangiomas, there may be visible expansion of the affected small, medium, and large choroidal vessels in the macular or para-macular area [42, 50].

Medina et al. [49], studied amelanotic and melanotic choroidal naevus, choroidal melanoma, circumscribed choroidal haemangioma (CCH) and choroidal metastasis using EDI-OCT. They were able to identify the tumour distinctly from the surrounding normal choroid, suggesting that EDI-OCT may be used as a complementary technique to ultrasonography for measuring tumours less than 1 mm in height (Table 4.1).

Shields et al. described the appearance of choroidal lymphoma on EDI-OCT as the ocean surface with a "calm", flat infiltration of the choroid in a thin lesion; a "rippled" appearance in a thicker lesion; and undulating "seasick" appearance in a thick lesion [51]. In vitreoretinal lymphoma several distinct patterns on OCT are observed, including hyper-reflective subretinal infiltrates, hyper-reflective infiltration in inner retinal layers, retinal pigment epithelium undulation, clumps of vitreous cells and sub-RPE deposits. Of these, the hyper-reflective subretinal infiltrates have an appearance unique to vitreoretinal lymphoma, with features not seen in other diseases (Fig. 4.9) [52].

Choroidal osteoma appears as subtle horizontal hyper-reflective lines (bony lamellae), horizontal or vertical tubular channels (possible vessels), and an intrinsic sponge-like appearance within the choroid [42]. Retinal or retinal pigment epithelial changes overlying an osteoma, as well as choroidal neovascularization can also be observed [53].

Hand-held high-resolution SD-OCT is a useful device for children, mainly in retinoblastoma patients [54]. Tumours appear as thickened and disorganized outer retinal layers with posterior shadowing [49, 54] (Table 4.2).

4.5 Optical Coherence Tomography Angiography (OCT-A)

Optical coherence tomography angiography (OCT-A) is a novel, noninvasive modality that provides en-face retinal angiographic images

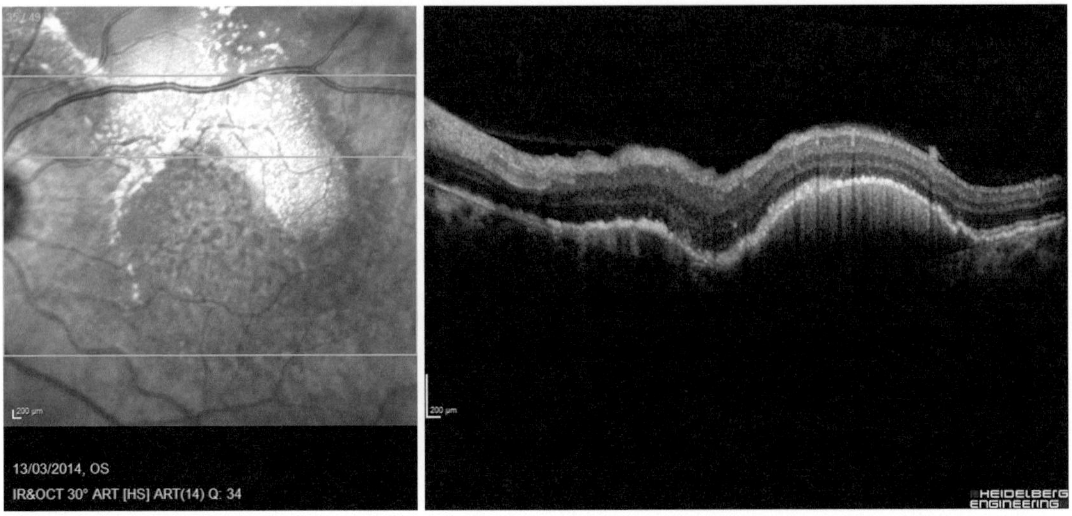

Fig. 4.9 Optical coherence tomography of the macula with vitreoretinal lymphoma showing hyper-reflective subretinal infiltrates and sub-retinal pigment epithelium deposits

Table 4.2 Enhanced depth-imaging OCT features of choroidal tumours

Clinical diagnosis	Choroidal reflectivity	Choroidal shadowing	Choriocapillaris visibility	Large vessel visibility	Inner sclera
Amelanotic naevus	Medium	–	+	+	+
Melanotic naevus	High	±	±	±	–
Melanoma	High	+	–	–	–
Haemangioma	Low to medium	+	±	–	–
Metastasis	Low	–	+	+	+

Adapted from Medina et al. [49]
+ detectable, – non-detectable, ± variably detectable

using the principle of split-spectrum amplitude decorrelation angiography [55, 56], providing an image of blood flow through vessels in different vascular layers. Preliminary studies have revealed interesting findings that suggest the possibility of differentiating choroidal melanoma from naevus using the OCT-A, but larger studies are needed to confirm these findings. Comparisons with the normal contralateral eye have shown that in choroidal naevi, there is no difference in the superficial foveal avascular zone (sFAZ), deep foveal avascular zone (dFAZ), superficial capillary vascular density (sCVD) or deep capillary vascular density (dCVD) [57]. However, suspicious choroidal naevi with three or more risk factors for transformation showed reduction in dCVD compared to contralateral eyes [57]. In treatment-naive choroidal melanomas, there was no difference in the sFAZ compared to the normal contralateral eye, however, dFAZ was enlarged, but only in macular choroidal melanomas [57, 58]. The sCVD is reduced only if subretinal fluid is present, and dCVD is reduced in all cases of choroidal melanoma regardless of subretinal fluid and tumour location, and the reduction is proportional to tumour thickness and diameter [57, 58]. Choroidal melanomas treated with plaque radiotherapy demonstrated significant enlargement of the foveal avascular zone and decreased capillary vascular density of both the superficial and deep plexuses, even in eyes with no clinical evidence of radiation maculopathy [59].

4.6 Summary

The ocular oncologist employs a range of imaging devices to diagnose, record and judge treatment response in tumours. As new devices appear, the ability to recognize patterns to make a final diagnosis becomes of ever increasing importance.

References

1. Peterson RC, Wolffsohn JS. The effect of digital image resolution and compression on anterior eye imaging. Br J Ophthalmol. 2005;89(7):828–30. https://doi.org/10.1136/bjo.2004.062240.
2. Shoughy SS, Arevalo JF, Kozak I. Update on wide- and ultra-widefield retinal imaging. Indian J Ophthalmol. 2015;63(7):575–81. https://doi.org/10.4103/0301-4738.167122.
3. Shields CL, Cater J, Shields JA, Singh AD, Santos MC, Carvalho C. Combination of clinical factors predictive of growth of small choroidal melanocytic tumors. Arch Ophthalmol. 2000;118(3):360–4.
4. Reznicek L, Stumpf C, Seidensticker F, Kampik A, Neubauer AS, Kernt M. Role of wide-field autofluorescence imaging and scanning laser ophthalmoscopy in differentiation of choroidal pigmented lesions. Int J Ophthalmol. 2014;7(4):697–703. https://doi.org/10.3980/j.issn.2222-3959.2014.04.21.
5. Sagong M, van Hemert J, Olmos de Koo LC, Barnett C, Sadda SR. Assessment of accuracy and precision of quantification of ultra-widefield images. Ophthalmology. 2015;122(4):864–6. https://doi.org/10.1016/j.ophtha.2014.11.016.
6. Wong JR, Tucker MA, Kleinerman RA, Devesa SS. Retinoblastoma incidence patterns in the US surveillance, epidemiology, and end results program. JAMA Ophthalmol. 2014;132(4):478–83. https://doi.org/10.1001/jamaophthalmol.2013.8001.
7. Kivela T. The epidemiological challenge of the most frequent eye cancer: retinoblastoma, an issue of birth and death. Br J Ophthalmol. 2009;93(9):1129–31. https://doi.org/10.1136/bjo.2008.150292.
8. Brubaker RF, Penniston JT, Grotte DA, Nagataki S. Measurement of fluorescein binding in human plasma using fluorescence polarization. Arch Ophthalmol. 1982;100(4):625–30.
9. Herbort CP. Fluorescein and indocyanine green angiography for uveitis. Middle East Afr J Ophthalmol. 2009;16(4):168–87. https://doi.org/10.4103/0974-9233.58419.
10. Ayyakkannu Manivannan AF. Instrumentation for fluorescein and indocyanine green angiography. In: Agrawal A, editor. Fundus fluorescein and indocyanine green angiography: a textbook and atlas. Thorofare: Slack; 2008.
11. Santosh Honavar MR, Shields CL, Shields JA. Intraocular tumours. In: Agrawal A, editor. Fundus fluorescein and indocyanine green angiography: a textbook and atlas. 1st ed. Thorofare: Slack; 2008.
12. Jerry A, Shields CLS. Posterior uveal melanoma: diagnostic approaches. In: Intraocular tumors: an atlas and textbook. 3rd ed. Philadelphia: LWW; 2016.
13. Heimann H, Jmor F, Damato B. Imaging of retinal and choroidal vascular tumours. Eye. 2013;27(2):208–16. https://doi.org/10.1038/eye.2012.251.
14. Schalenbourg A, Piguet B, Zografos L. Indocyanine green angiographic findings in choroidal hemangiomas: a study of 75 cases. Ophthalmologica. 2000;214(4):246–52. https://doi.org/10.1159/000027499.
15. Norton EW, Gutman F. Fluorescein angiography and hemangiomas of the choroid. Arch Ophthalmol. 1967;78(2):121–5.
16. Arun D, Singh PAR, Rennie IG. Retinal vascular tumors. In: Arun D, Singh BD, editors. Clinical ophthalmic oncology: retinal tumours. 2nd ed. Heidelberg: Springer; 2014. p. 17–344.
17. Tsui I, Jain A, Shah S, Schwartz SD, McCannel TA. Ultra widefield imaging of peripheral exudative hemorrhagic chorioretinopathy. Semin Ophthalmol. 2009;24(1):25–8. https://doi.org/10.1080/08820530802520178.
18. Hope-Ross MW. ICG dye: physical and pharmacologic properties. In: Lawrence A, Yannuzzi RWF, Slakter JS, editors. Indocyanine green angiography. 1st ed. St. Louis: Mosby; 1997. p. 46–9.
19. Shields CL, Shields JA, De Potter P. Patterns of indocyanine green videoangiography of choroidal tumours. Br J Ophthalmol. 1995;79(3):237–45.
20. Shields CL. Chapter 21: clinical evaluation of choroidal tumors. In: Yannuzzi, editor. Indocyanine green angiography. 1st ed. St. Louis: Mosby; 1997.
21. Mueller AJ, Freeman WR, Schaller UC, Kampik A, Folberg R. Complex microcirculation patterns detected by confocal indocyanine green angiography predict time to growth of small choroidal melanocytic tumors: MuSIC Report II. Ophthalmology. 2002;109(12):2207–14.
22. Shields CL, Bianciotto C, Pirondini C, Materin MA, Harmon SA, Shields JA. Autofluorescence of orange pigment overlying small choroidal melanoma. Retina. 2007;27(8):1107–11. https://doi.org/10.1097/IAE.0b013e31814934ef.
23. Dorey CK, Wu G, Ebenstein D, Garsd A, Weiter JJ. Cell loss in the aging retina. Relationship to lipofuscin accumulation and macular degeneration. Invest Ophthalmol Vis Sci. 1989;30(8):1691–9.
24. Delori FC, Fleckner MR, Goger DG, Weiter JJ, Dorey CK. Autofluorescence distribution associated with drusen in age-related macular degeneration. Invest Ophthalmol Vis Sci. 2000;41(2):496–504.
25. Almeida A, Kaliki S, Shields CL. Autofluorescence of intraocular tumours. Curr Opin Ophthalmol. 2013;24(3):222–32. https://doi.org/10.1097/ICU.0b013e32835f8ba1.

26. Shields JA, Rodrigues MM, Sarin LK, Tasman WS, Annesley WH Jr. Lipofuscin pigment over benign and malignant choroidal tumors. Trans Sect Ophthalmol Am Acad Ophthalmol Otolaryngol. 1976;81(5):871–81.
27. Shields CL, Pirondini C, Bianciotto C, Materin MA, Harmon SA, Shields JA. Autofluorescence of choroidal nevus in 64 cases. Retina. 2008;28(8):1035–43. https://doi.org/10.1097/IAE.0b013e318181b94b.
28. Spaide R. Autofluorescence from the outer retina and subretinal space: hypothesis and review. Retina. 2008;28(1):5–35. https://doi.org/10.1097/IAE.0b013e318158eca4.
29. Gunduz K, Pulido JS, Bakri SJ, Amselem L, Petit-Fond E, Link T. Fundus autofluorescence of choroidal melanocytic lesions and the effect of treatment. Trans Am Ophthalmol Soc. 2007;105:172–8.
30. Hashmi F, Rojanaporn D, Kaliki S, Shields CL. Orange pigment sediment overlying small choroidal melanoma. Arch Ophthalmol. 2012;130(7):937–9. https://doi.org/10.1001/archophthalmol.2011.1907.
31. Ishida T, Ohno-Matsui K, Kaneko Y, Tobita H, Hayashi K, Shimada N, et al. Autofluorescence of metastatic choroidal tumor. Int Ophthalmol. 2009;29(4):309–13. https://doi.org/10.1007/s10792-008-9234-2.
32. Collet LC, Pulido JS, Gunduz K, Diago T, McCannel C, Blodi C, et al. Fundus autofluorescence in choroidal metastatic lesions: a pilot study. Retina. 2008;28(9):1251–6. https://doi.org/10.1097/IAE.0b013e318188c7d0.
33. Natesh S, Chin KJ, Finger PT. Choroidal metastases fundus autofluorescence imaging: correlation to clinical, OCT, and fluorescein angiographic findings. Ophthalmic Surg Lasers Imaging. 2010;41(4):406–12. https://doi.org/10.3928/15428877-20100426-03.
34. Ramasubramanian A, Shields CL, Harmon SA, Shields JA. Autofluorescence of choroidal hemangioma in 34 consecutive eyes. Retina. 2010;30(1):16–22. https://doi.org/10.1097/IAE.0b013e3181bceedb.
35. Navajas EV, Costa RA, Calucci D, Hammoudi DS, Simpson ER, Altomare F. Multimodal fundus imaging in choroidal osteoma. Am J Ophthalmol. 2012;153(5):890–5. https://doi.org/10.1016/j.ajo.2011.10.025.
36. Ascaso FJ, Villen L. Fundus autofluorescence imaging findings in choroidal osteoma. Retina. 2011;31(5):1004–5. https://doi.org/10.1097/IAE.0b013e31820d37a6.
37. Ishida T, Ohno-Matsui K, Kaneko Y, Tobita H, Shimada N, Takase H, et al. Fundus autofluorescence patterns in eyes with primary intraocular lymphoma. Retina. 2010;30(1):23–32. https://doi.org/10.1097/IAE.0b013e3181b408a2.
38. Nyboer JH, Robertson DM, Gomez MR. Retinal lesions in tuberous sclerosis. Arch Ophthalmol. 1976;94(8):1277–80.
39. Mennel S, Meyer CH, Eggarter F, Peter S. Autofluorescence and angiographic findings of retinal astrocytic hamartomas in tuberous sclerosis. Ophthalmologica. 2005;219(6):350–6. https://doi.org/10.1159/000088377.
40. Huang D, Swanson EA, Lin CP, Schuman JS, Stinson WG, Chang W, et al. Optical coherence tomography. Science. 1991;254(5035):1178–81.
41. Torres VL, Brugnoni N, Kaiser PK, Singh AD. Optical coherence tomography enhanced depth imaging of choroidal tumors. Am J Ophthalmol. 2011;151(4):586–93. https://doi.org/10.1016/j.ajo.2010.09.028.
42. Shields CL, Manalac J, Das C, Saktanasate J, Shields JA. Review of spectral domain enhanced depth imaging optical coherence tomography of tumors of the choroid. Indian J Ophthalmol. 2015;63(2):117–21. https://doi.org/10.4103/0301-4738.154377.
43. Bianciotto C, Shields CL, Guzman JM, Romanelli-Gobbi M, Mazzuca D Jr, Green WR, et al. Assessment of anterior segment tumors with ultrasound biomicroscopy versus anterior segment optical coherence tomography in 200 cases. Ophthalmology. 2011;118(7):1297–302. https://doi.org/10.1016/j.ophtha.2010.11.011.
44. Shields CL, Belinsky I, Romanelli-Gobbi M, Guzman JM, Mazzuca D Jr, Green WR, et al. Anterior segment optical coherence tomography of conjunctival nevus. Ophthalmology. 2011;118(5):915–9. https://doi.org/10.1016/j.ophtha.2010.09.016.
45. Bakri SJ, Singh AD, Lowder CY, Chalita MR, Li Y, Izatt JA, et al. Imaging of iris lesions with high-speed optical coherence tomography. Ophthalmic Surg Lasers Imaging. 2007;38(1):27–34.
46. Sayanagi K, Pelayes DE, Kaiser PK, Singh AD. 3D Spectral domain optical coherence tomography findings in choroidal tumors. Eur J Ophthalmol. 2011;21(3):271–5. https://doi.org/10.5301/EJO.2010.5848.
47. Cennamo G, Romano MR, Breve MA, Velotti N, Reibaldi M, de Crecchio G, et al. Evaluation of choroidal tumors with optical coherence tomography: enhanced depth imaging and OCT-angiography features. Eye. 2017;31(6):906–15. https://doi.org/10.1038/eye.2017.14.
48. Papastefanou VP, Nogueira V, Hay G, Andrews RM, Harris M, Cohen VM, et al. Choroidal naevi complicated by choroidal neovascular membrane and outer retinal tubulation. Br J Ophthalmol. 2013;97(8):1014–9. https://doi.org/10.1136/bjophthalmol-2013-303234.
49. Medina CA, Plesec T, Singh AD. Optical coherence tomography imaging of ocular and periocular tumours. Br J Ophthalmol. 2014;98(Suppl 2):ii40–6. https://doi.org/10.1136/bjophthalmol-2013-304299.
50. Shields CL, Honavar SG, Shields JA, Cater J, Demirci H. Circumscribed choroidal hemangioma: clinical manifestations and factors predictive of visual outcome in 200 consecutive cases. Ophthalmology. 2001;108(12):2237–48.
51. Shields CL, Arepalli S, Pellegrini M, Mashayekhi A, Shields JA. Choroidal lymphoma shows calm,

rippled, or undulating topography on enhanced depth imaging optical coherence tomography in 14 eyes. Retina. 2014;34(7):1347–53. https://doi.org/10.1097/IAE.0000000000000145.
52. Barry RJ, Tasiopoulou A, Murray PI, Patel PJ, Sagoo MS, Denniston AK, et al. Characteristic optical coherence tomography findings in patients with primary vitreoretinal lymphoma: a novel aid to early diagnosis. Br J Ophthalmol. 2018;102(10):1362–6. https://doi.org/10.1136/bjophthalmol-2017-311612.
53. Papastefanou VP, Pefkianaki M, Al Harby L, Arora AK, Cohen VM, Andrews RM, et al. Intravitreal bevacizumab monotherapy for choroidal neovascularisation secondary to choroidal osteoma. Eye. 2016;30(6):843–9. https://doi.org/10.1038/eye.2016.50.
54. Rootman DB, Gonzalez E, Mallipatna A, Vandenhoven C, Hampton L, Dimaras H, et al. Hand-held high-resolution spectral domain optical coherence tomography in retinoblastoma: clinical and morphologic considerations. Br J Ophthalmol. 2013;97(1):59–65. https://doi.org/10.1136/bjophthalmol-2012-302133.
55. Jia Y, Bailey ST, Hwang TS, McClintic SM, Gao SS, Pennesi ME, et al. Quantitative optical coherence tomography angiography of vascular abnormalities in the living human eye. Proc Natl Acad Sci U S A. 2015;112(18):E2395–402. https://doi.org/10.1073/pnas.1500185112.
56. Spaide RF, Klancnik JM Jr, Cooney MJ. Retinal vascular layers imaged by fluorescein angiography and optical coherence tomography angiography. JAMA Ophthalmol. 2015;133(1):45–50. https://doi.org/10.1001/jamaophthalmol.2014.3616.
57. Valverde-Megias A, Say EA, Ferenczy SR, Shields CL. Differential macular features on optical coherence tomography angiography in eyes with choroidal nevus and melanoma. Retina. 2017;37(4):731–40. https://doi.org/10.1097/IAE.0000000000001233.
58. Li Y, Say EA, Ferenczy S, Agni M, Shields CL. Altered parafoveal microvasculature in treatment-naive choroidal melanoma eyes detected by optical coherence tomography angiography. Retina. 2017;37(1):32–40. https://doi.org/10.1097/IAE.0000000000001242.
59. Shields CL, Say EA, Samara WA, Khoo CT, Mashayekhi A, Shields JA. Optical coherence tomography angiography of the macula after plaque radiotherapy of choroidal melanoma: comparison of irradiated versus nonirradiated eyes in 65 patients. Retina. 2016;36(8):1493–505. https://doi.org/10.1097/IAE.0000000000001021.

Ultrasound Examination in Intraocular Tumours

5

Marie Restori and Mandeep S. Sagoo

5.1 B-Mode Ultrasound

A transducer emits ultrasonic pulses and echoes received by the same transducer are recorded as electrical signals and displayed on a screen as brightness modulated spots. Strong echoes are displayed as bright spots and weak echoes as dim spots [1, 2]. The transducer is moved in a straight line (Fig. 5.1) or rocked through an angle and the echoes are plotted on the display, their positions on the screen based on an assumed average speed of sound in the tissue of 1550 m/s. This B-Scan represents a cross sectional image of the eye and orbit. Most dedicated eye scanners use a mechanically rocked single transducer to produce trapezoidal shaped (sector) B-Scans. The transducer is usually housed in a column of oil or water within a plastic case, the outer front surface of which forms the probe footprint for contact to the eye or eyelid. Typical frame rates are 24 B-Scans per second. Operators often scan on the open anaesthetised eye using a viscous gel couplant. Each line of echoes that comprises the B-Scan is known as an A-line. Some operators measure echo amplitude using an A-Scan (like an A-line but echoes plotted as spikes) in addition to B-Scan to help differentiate pathology. Good grey-scale on the B-scan enables a wide range of echo amplitudes to be displayed as different shades of grey and so A-scan measurements can be unnecessary. A maximum amplitude echo is recorded when the sound pulses strike tissues perpendicularly. This can be achieved by either moving the probe or asking the patient to move the eye or a combination of both.

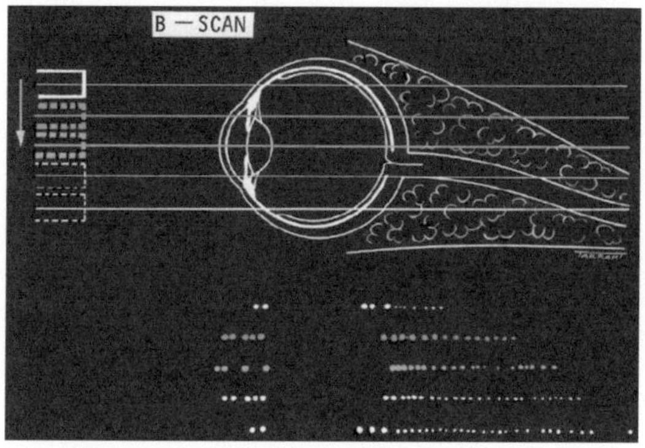

Fig. 5.1 B-scan technique

Solid state array probes are comprised of numerous transducers which are electronically fired in sequence to simulate a single moving transducer to produce either a trapezoidal shaped

M. Restori
Ultrasound Department, Moorfields Eye Hospital, London, UK
e-mail: m.restori@nhs.net

M. S. Sagoo (✉)
Ocular Oncology Service, Moorfields Eye Hospital, London, UK

Retinoblastoma Service, Royal London Hospital, London, UK

NIHR Biomedical Research Centre for Ophthalmology at Moorfields Eye Hospital and UCL Institute of Ophthalmology, London, UK
e-mail: Mandeep.sagoo@nhs.net

V. Khetan (ed.), *Intraocular Tumors*, https://doi.org/10.1007/978-981-15-0395-5_5

(sector) or rectangular shaped (linear) image. Scanners that use array probes assume a system velocity of 1540 m/s. Much higher frame rates are achievable with array probes, typically using 42 B-Scans per second and working through closed eyelids. Sector arrays have a smaller footprint, give a wider-angle view and are useful for imaging the equatorial globe. Disadvantages are poor anterior globe view and decreasing lateral resolution with depth. Linear arrays have a larger footprint, poorer equatorial view but image the anterior structures well and the lateral resolution is constant with depth. Higher frequencies enable shorter pulses which give better axial resolution but these frequencies are preferentially absorbed. A compromise between axial resolution and penetration of sound is required. Most images shown herein were taken at 14 MHz. The probe is moved across the eye to produce a whole series of B-Scan images which the operator can visualise as a virtual 3D image in seconds.[1]

5.1.1 Tumour Appearances on B-mode

Tumours are seen as a group of echoes attached to the coats of the eye in a domed, 'collar-stud' or sessile overall shape (Figs. 5.2, 5.3, 5.4, 5.5, 5.6, and 5.7) [1]. The anterior surface of a tumour may be smooth or irregular. Internal echo amplitudes may be uniform or varied.

Malignant melanomas, tend to be domed or 'collar-stud' in shape and are generally of mixed, medium and low, internal echogenicity (Fig. 5.2) [3]. 'Choroidal excavation' (Fig. 5.2a)—replacement of normal stronger choroidal echoes by lower amplitude tumour echoes—is often detected. Choroidal haemangiomas show uniform, high or medium, echo amplitude (Fig. 5.3a, b). Calcifications, seen as very high amplitude echoes, are detected in osteoma (Fig. 5.3c) and retinoblastoma (Fig. 5.8). Calcifications, even micro-calcifications, cause shadowing (Figs. 5.3c and 5.8). Extra-scleral spread of tumours (Figs. 5.5 and 5.7) into fat is recognised by the contrast in brightness between the lower echogenicity of the tumour and that of normal fat.

Measurements are taken of the lesion base in two orthogonal meridians and the maximum tumour elevation. Repeat measurements at regular intervals can be used to assess growth or regression.

5.2 Ultra High Frequency B-scanners (Ultrasound Biomicroscope-UBM)

If only the anterior globe structures are of interest then higher frequency transducers (30 MHz, 50 MHz, 60 MHz or even 100 MHz) can be used. Such high frequency probes are difficult to deploy as an array and therefore, UBMs tend to have a single transducer mechanically rocked. As sound attenuation is problematic at these frequencies, probes need to couple to the open anesthetised eye. Manufacturers have devised innovative, disposable coupling techniques for these scanners. UBMs are useful for examining for example, very small ciliary body tumours. If the anterior structures are not optically opaque then anterior segment optical coherence tomography is preferable.

5.3 Imaging of Movements

At frame rates of 24 B-Scans per second and higher, any movements of the eye and contained pathology are seen clearly in real time. Haemorrhage can be seen to swirl following eye deviations whereas most of the internal echoes within a solid lesion are static. Blood flowing in tumour vessels can be visible on the real-time B-Scans but this requires the patient's eye and the probe to be static. Whether blood flow is visible in this way is determined by the B-Scan frame rate and the velocity of the blood flow during systole[2] and system sensitivity.

[1] Examination times should be kept as short as possible to minimise exposure times. Also the power outputs settings on scanners should be set as low a practical and ideally should have an MI setting ~0.2 or less.

[2] Nyquist theorem.

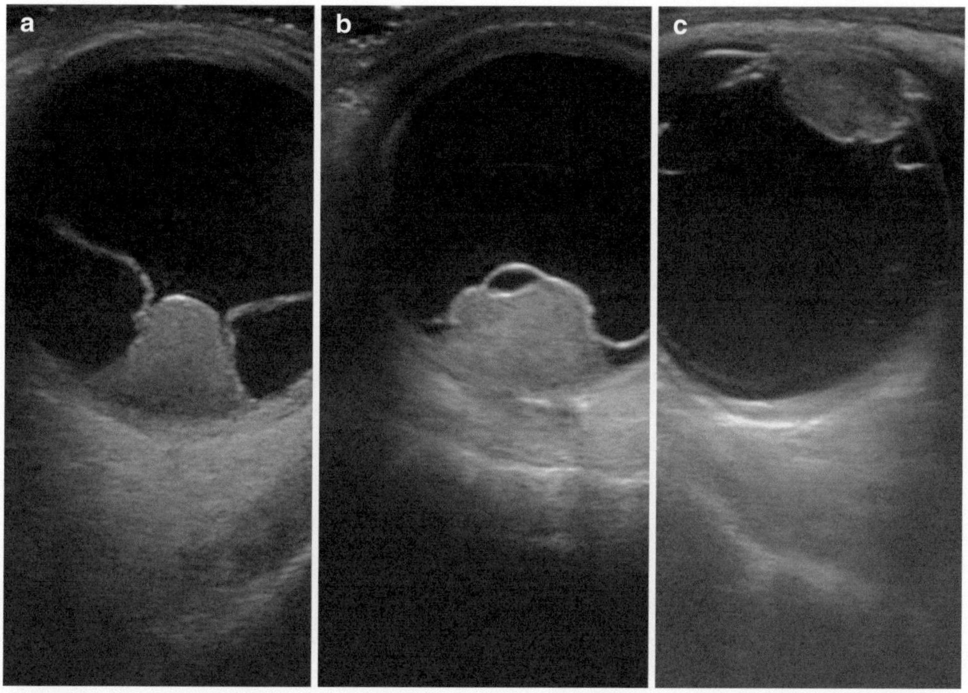

Fig. 5.2 B-Scans malignant melanoma: medium and low internal echogenicity: retinal detachment. (**a**) Posterior 'collar-stud'. (**b**) Bi-lobed posterior 'collar-stud'. (**c**) Ciliary body lesion

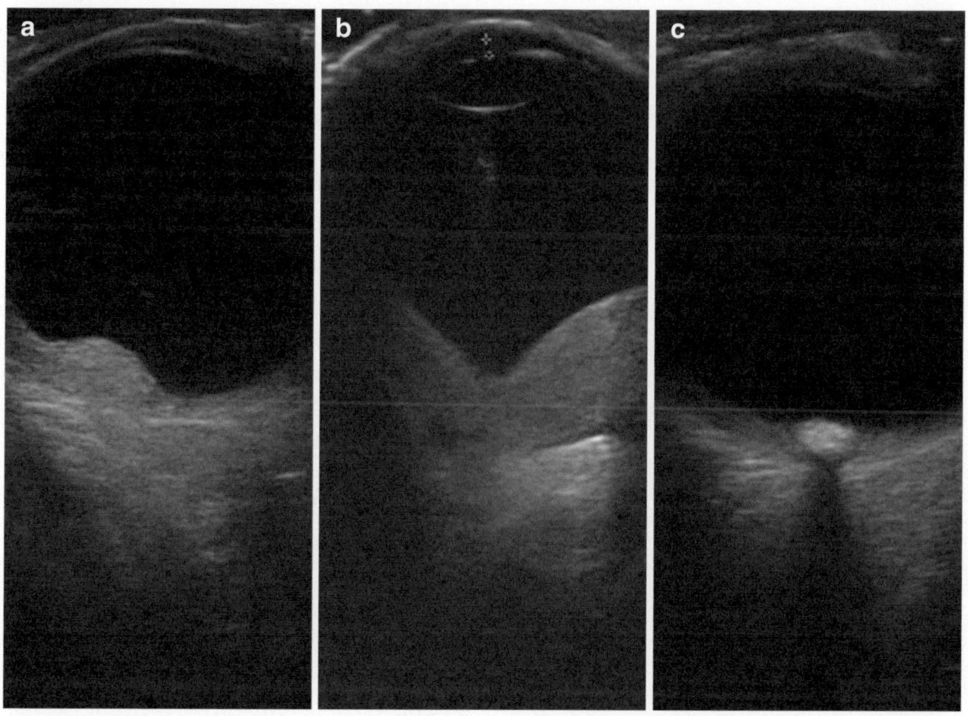

Fig. 5.3 B-Scans. (**a**) Choroidal haemangioma: uniform high internal echogenicity. (**b**) Choroidal haemangioma: uniform medium internal echogenicity: closed funnel retinal detachment; shallow anterior chamber; Sturge-Weber syndrome. (**c**) Choroidal osteoma: high internal echogenicity shadowing from calcification

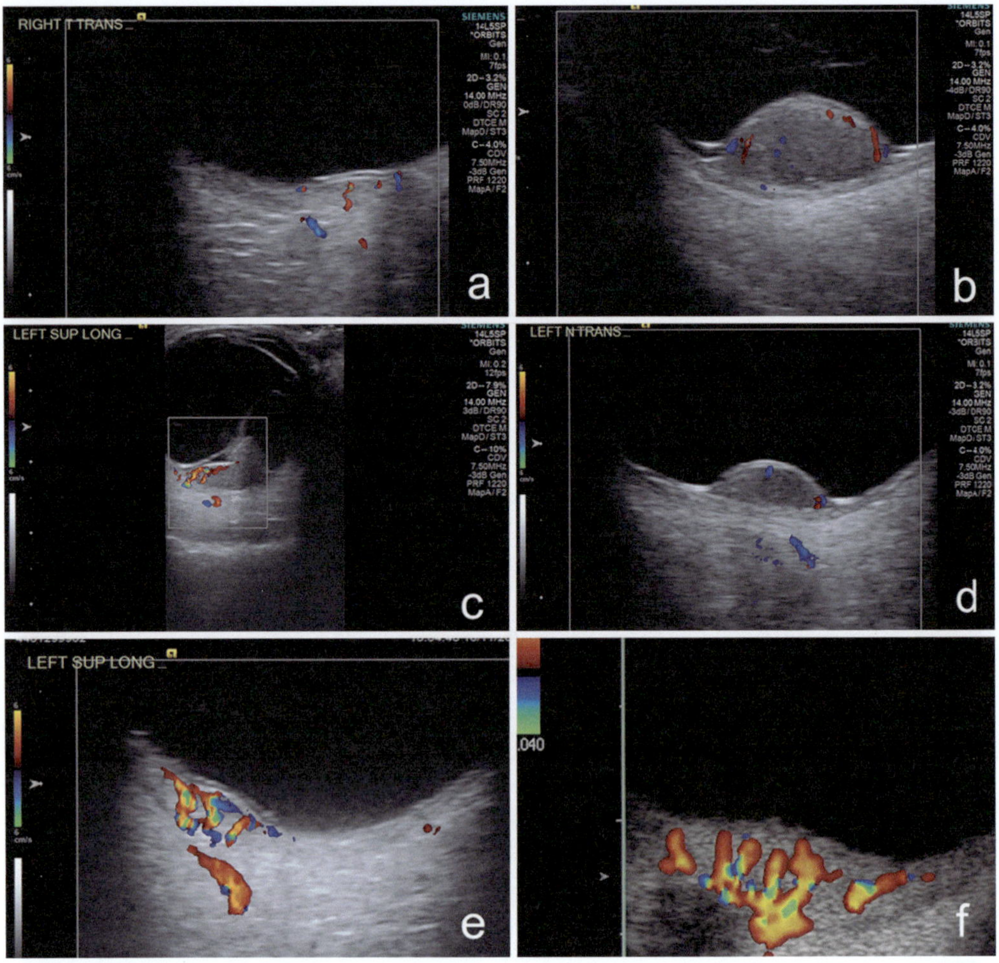

Fig. 5.4 Colour flow maps showing internal blood vessels; (**a**–**d**) malignant melanoma. (**e**, **f**) Choroidal haemangioma

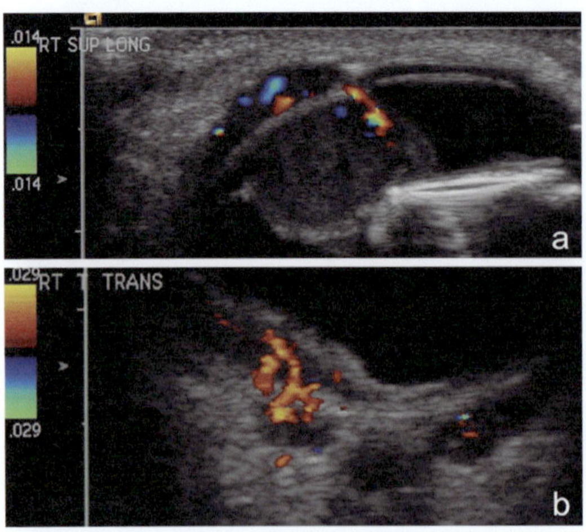

Fig. 5.5 Colour flow maps: zoomed images: intra-ocular lymphoma. (**a**) Iris lesion with anterior spread. (**b**) Posterior sessile lesion with spread into orbital fat pad

Following measurements and movement examination operators may wish to perform blood flow studies.

5.4 Colour Flow Mapping and Spectral Doppler Techniques

Colour Flow Mapping is a technique to image blood flow in colour and is available on array scanners. A window of variable size is positioned on a region of interest on the B-Scan. The patient's eye and the probe should be static to detect small displacements in echo positions over short time intervals. Any displacements detected are con-

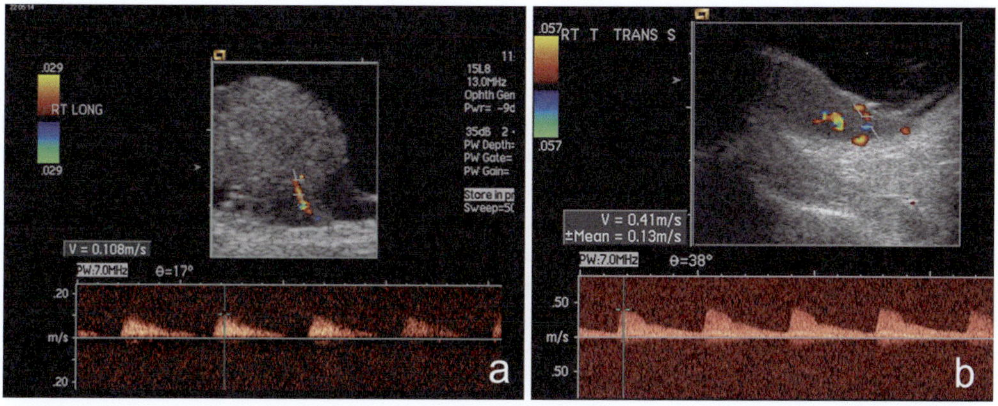

Fig. 5.6 Colour flow maps with spectrogram. (**a**) Malignant melanoma: systolic velocity of internal flow 11 cm/s. (**b**) Choroidal haemangioma: systolic velocity of internal flow 41 cm/s

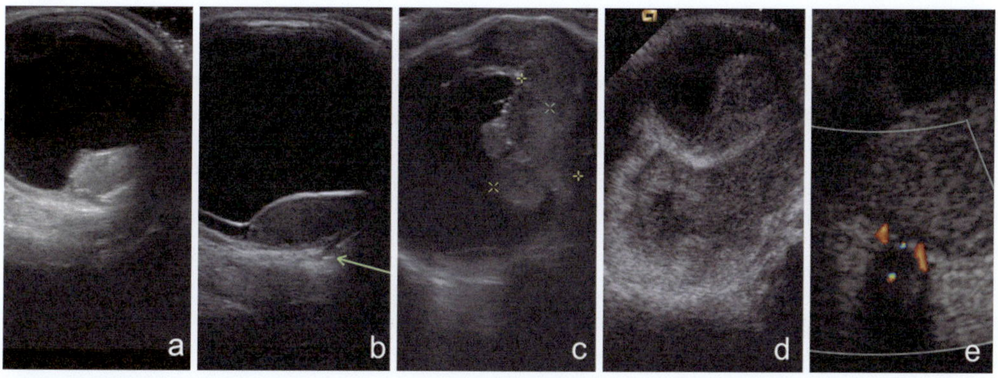

Fig. 5.7 Malignant melanoma. (**a**, **b**) Small extra-scleral spread (arrow). (**c**) Massive anterior extra-ocular spread: cursors mark intra-ocular portion of lesion. (**d**) Massive posterior extra-ocular spread filling entire orbital cavity. (**e**) Spread into the optic nerve sheath detected on colour flow map (arrow)

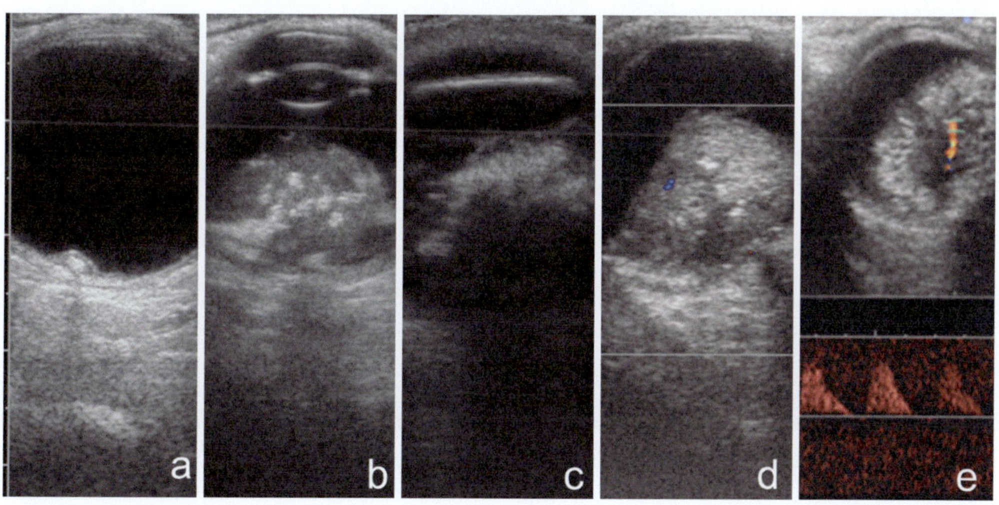

Fig. 5.8 Retinoblastoma (**a-d**) showing varying degrees of calcification and consequent shadowing. (**e**) Velocity of blood flow in retinoblastoma of 13 cm/s

verted to velocities and plotted in real time onto the B-Scan in colour. Any inadvertent movements of the patient's eye or the probe is seen as a burst of colour on the screen. Arteries are seen as colour flashes at the heart rate and veins as a continuous colour. Convention in all body parts is to show flow towards the probe in red and away from the probe in blue. If the velocity scale is set too low the colours wrap around and the directional information is lost. Colour flow maps showing blood flow in tumours are shown in Figs. 5.4, 5.5, 5.6, 5.7, and 5.8. A gate (seen as two horizontal white lines on image) is placed on the imaged blood vessel and an angle correction made by aligning a marker along the vessel. A graph of blood flow velocity against time, known as a spectrogram or spectrograph (Figs. 5.6, 5.7, and 5.8) is plotted. Arterial traces on the Spectrogram repeat with each heart beat whereas veins show no fluctuation in velocity on the display. The spectrogram is a quantitative technique which allows measurement of the maximum systolic velocity. Usually a tumour depth of 2 mm is required to measure accurate velocities.

Most melanomas have a maximum systolic velocity around 11 cm/s (range 5–30 cm/s). The higher velocities in this range are only seen in aggressively growing lesions. Choroidal haemangiomas appear highly vascular on colour flow mapping (Fig. 5.4e, f) and systolic velocity within most are around 20 cm/s. (range 15–50 cm/s). Similarly, higher velocities in this range are only seen in actively growing lesions. Posterior mucosa associated lymphoid tissue (MALT) lymphomas appear sessile, the base of the tumours is much larger than the elevation. Although lesions are often very shallow they frequently spread into the orbit. Internal echogenicity is mixed, medium and low. Blood flow is easy to detect within both the intra-ocular and orbital portions of posterior lymphoma (Fig. 5.5b).

Metastatic tumours vary in appearance considerably, sometimes reflecting the appearance of the primary. The appearance can change rapidly.

Shallowly elevated echolucent dilated vortex veins (Fig. 5.9a), may mimic a small lesion but can be observed to flatten on compression. Eccentric disciform or peripheral exudative

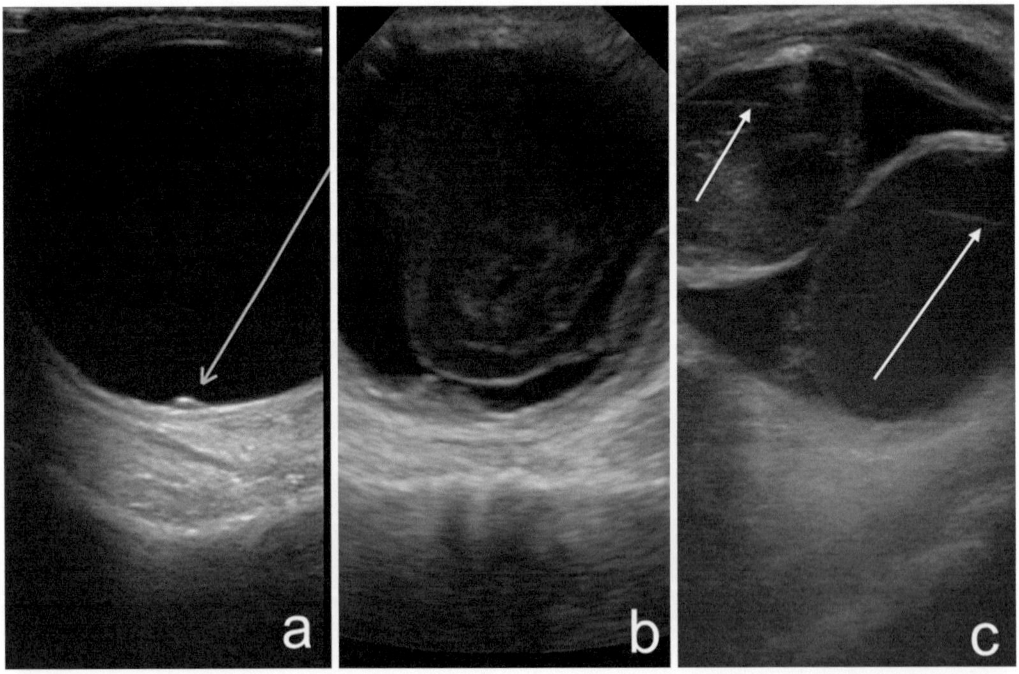

Fig. 5.9 (**a**) Echolucent dilated vortex vein: flattens on compression. (**b**) Posterior vitreous detachment with dense intra gel haemorrhage: disciform lesion (peripheral exudative haemorrhagic chorioretinopathy) with areas of sub-retinal haemorrhage. (**c**) Supra-choroidal haemorrhage; attachment to vortex ampullae of vortex vein seen as a straight lines (arrows)

haemorrhagic chorioretinopathy with associated subretinal haemorrhage (Fig. 5.9b) may mimic a metastatic deposit. Supra-choroidal haemorrhage (Fig. 5.9c) with active bleeding can be confusing but will be seen to reduce in size on follow up.

5.5 Standardized A Scans

A-scans can be used once the B scan determines the site and topography of the tumour [4, 5]. These are able to give information on reflectivity and attenuation of the ultrasound waves by internal structures. However, good grey-scale B-Mode with high frame rates to echo amplitudes of pathology to be assessed, enable dynamic studies of pathology and blood flow movement to be imaged on the B-Scan. B-Mode images as described here are comprised of numerous A-Scan data lines but presented in a different format. Although, some workers place stress on the exact echo amplitude as measured on an A-scan line, this may reflect the use of scanners with poorer grey scale facility.

With experience of diagnostic B-Scans the need to access the raw A-scan data becomes unnecessary. Echo amplitude is highly dependent on angle of incidence of incoming sound pulses. Probe movement and good B-Mode grey-scale enable relevant echo amplitude data to be quickly assessed. Colour flow mapping and spectral Doppler can be used instead on suitable B mode scanners to provide additional data in tumours studies.

5.6 Conclusions

Ultrasound techniques are an essential part of ocular oncology, particularly as most intraocular tumours do not undergo diagnostic biopsy. B-scan with colour flow mapping is very useful in refining the differential diagnosis.

References

1. Coleman DJ, Abramson DH, Jack RL, Franzen LA. Ultrasonic diagnosis of tumors of the choroid. Arch Ophthalmol. 1974;91(5):344–54.
2. ter Haar G. Is modern diagnostic ultrasound safe? Rad Mag. 2016;42(492):23–4.
3. Sobottka B, Schlote T, Krumpaszky HG, Kreissig I. Choroidal metastases and choroidal melanomas: comparison of ultrasonographic findings. Br J Ophthalmol. 1998;82(2):159–61.
4. Ossoinig KC. Standardized echography: basic principles, clinical applications, and results. Int Ophthalmol Clin. 1979;19(4):127–210.
5. Ossoinig KC, Byrne SF, Weyer NJ. Standardized echography. Part II: performance of standardized echography by the technician. Int Ophthalmol Clin. 1979;19(4):283–5.

Uveal Melanoma: Diagnosis, Classification and Management

6

Ronel Veksler and Ido Didi Fabian

6.1 Introduction

Uveal melanoma (UM) is the most common primary intraocular malignancy in adults, yet a relatively rare cancer. Among all melanoma cases, approximately 5% arise from the ocular and adnexal structures [1]. Of these, the majority are uveal in origin. There are approximately 1400 newly diagnosed cases in the US and 500 in the UK each year. Incidence of UM varies by various factors. UM mainly affects light-skinned individuals, though it can occur less frequently in dark-skinned. In the US, the incidence is approximately 5 per million population, but higher in non-Hispanic whites with approximately 6 new cases per million population per year. In Hispanics, incidence is 1.7 per million and in blacks <0.5 per million population [2–4]. In Europe, incidence increases with latitude, with approximately 2 cases per million in Mediterranean countries, up to 6 per million in central European countries and >8 per million population in Scandinavia [5]. UM is rare in Asians. The malignancy affects males and females at a similar rate, with a slight predominance among males. The mean age of diagnosis is approximately 60 years; however, the peak range is in the eighth decade of life [3, 6].

R. Veksler · I. D. Fabian (✉)
Ocular Oncology Service, Goldschleger Eye Institute, Sheba Medical Center, Tel-Aviv University, Tel Aviv, Israel
e-mail: didi@didifabian.com

UM arises from melanocytes in the choroid, ciliary body, referred together as posterior UM, or iris. Approximately 95% of the cases are posterior UM, with the vast majority involving the choroid, and the remaining 5% are iris melanomas. Risk factors associated with UM include fair skin, light eyes and northern European ancestry. The development of UM is considered to be a sporadic event, although several syndromes are known to be associated with higher risk to develop the eye cancer, including ocular melanocytosis, dysplastic nevus and BAP1 cancer predisposition syndrome [7–9]. There is currently no definite evidence linking UV light with UM. Choroidal nevus, which is found in approximately 5% of the general population [10], rarely transforms into melanoma (1/9000) [11]. However, the presence of typical clinical features, including the presence lipofuscin, tumor >2 mm in elevation, proximity to the optic disc, presence of subretinal fluid and symptoms, are associated with increased risk for tumor growth and transformation into UM [12].

The most common presenting symptom in patients with UM is blurred vision, followed by photopsia, floaters, visual field defects and less common symptoms. In approximately 1/3 of UM patients, tumors are incidentally found on routine eye examination (i.e. asymptomatic) [13]. Patients with Iris melanoma often present with complaints of iris color changes. Clinical diagnosis of UM requires the expertise of an ocular oncologist. In most cases, the diagnosis is

V. Khetan (ed.), *Intraocular Tumors*, https://doi.org/10.1007/978-981-15-0395-5_6

established following clinical examination, in which a pigmented dome-shaped mass is observed. Ultrasound (US) examination, both A- and B-mode, is a critical tool in the diagnosis and evaluation of UM, demonstrating an elevated intraocular lesion (B-scan) with low-medium internal reflectivity (A-scan). Additional imaging tools, among others, include optical coherence tomography (OCT), with enhanced depth imaging (EDI), and fluorescein angiography (FA). Suspicious iris or choroidal nevi may require serial fundus photographs to demonstrate tumor growth (i.e. malignant transformation). Tumor biopsy by various techniques is rarely used for diagnosis, but commonly performed for prognostication [14].

The American Joint Committee on Cancer (AJCC), which uses the universal tumor (T), node (N), and metastasis (M) (TNM) staging, divides UM into anterior (i.e. iris) and posterior (i.e. ciliary body and choroidal) systems, which differ anatomically and prognostically. On analysis, higher AJCC stage was found to correlate with an increased risk of metastatic spread and death [15].

Various treatment modalities are available today for UM. Historically, enucleation was the only treatment option, still used today as the primary modality, mainly for large tumors. Most cases nowadays, however, are treated conservatively by means of radiotherapy, mainly plaque brachytherapy or proton-beam radiotherapy [16]. Several laser-based techniques, used for other ophthalmic indications, were also tested for UM, including laser photocoagulation and photodynamic therapy, showing variable results [17].

This chapter will discuss the diagnosis, classification and management options for UM.

6.2 Diagnosis

The history for UM or any suspicious intraocular tumor should include questions about the past general medical history, family history of cancer as well as history of any type of malignancy with the individual, past ocular problems and interventions, systemic and ocular use of medication, and current visual symptoms. In a review by Damato et al. of 2384 UM patients in the UK [13], nearly 40% had blurred vision, 9% photopsia, 7% floaters, 6% visual field loss, 3% visible tumor, 2% pain, and 2% metamorphopsia. Interestingly, 30% of patients reported no symptoms.

In contrast to most systemic malignancies, UM diagnosis is based on clinical examination, rather than tissue-biopsy. The reasons are, one, to avoid intraocular biopsy-related complications, and two, because in the vast majority of cases, clinically-based diagnosis is sufficiently accurate. In the Collaborative Ocular Melanoma Study (COMS), the largest prospective multicenter trial in the field of ocular oncology, 413 cases clinically diagnosed with UM were examined also by means of histopathology (following enucleation) [18]. Of these, 411 (99.5%) were confirmed to be UM. The definite diagnosis, treatment and monitoring of UM should be done by an expert in the field of ocular oncology. Clinical examination is based primarily on biomicroscopy and indirect ophthalmoscopy. Most cases of posterior UM demonstrate a pigmented mass with overlying retinal detachment (Fig. 6.1). Iris melanoma, the rarest form of uveal melanoma, usually appears in the inferior part of the iris, with presenting symptoms include iritis, glaucoma, hyphema and sector cataract [19]. Secondary glaucoma can result either because of compression of the anterior-chamber angle,

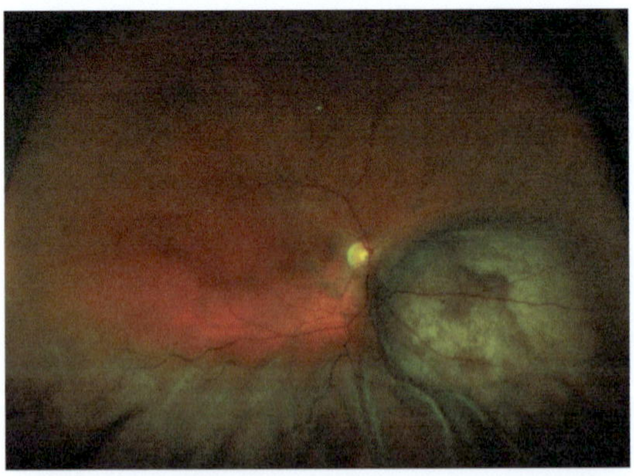

Fig. 6.1 A color photo of a right eye juxtapapillary choroidal melanoma on the nasal side of the optic disc. Note the inferior retinal detachment

Table 6.1 Common pseudomelanomas [20–22]

Choroidal pseudomelanoma	Ciliary body pseudomelanoma	Iris pseudomelanoma
Choroidal nevus	Iris cyst arising from the pigment epithelium	Iris cyst
Peripheral exudative hemorrhagic chorioretinopathy	Medulloepithelioma	Iris nevus
Congenital hypertrophy of the retinal pigment epithelium	Leiomyoma	Essential iris atrophy
Hemorrhagic detachment of the retina or pigment epithelium	Age-related hyperplasia of the non-pigmented ciliary epithelium (Fuchs adenoma)	Foreign body
Circumscribed choroidal hemangioma	Adenocarcinoma	Peripheral anterior synechia
Age-related macular degeneration	Adenoma	Secondary metastasis

tumor invasion of the angle or blockage of the trabecular meshwork due to infiltration of either tumor cells or macrophages. The tumor color is brown in most cases but can also be amelanotic. Ophthalmoscopy may reveal intrinsic tumor vessels, sentinel episcleral vessels, anterior segment pigment dispersion, synechiae, corectopia and ectropion uvea.

Several conditions can simulate UM (Table 6.1). However, clinical examination in addition to ancillary tests are usually sufficient to make a diagnosis. Ancillary tests commonly used include color fundus photography, US, OCT, FA, indocyanine green (ICG) angiography, and fundus autofluorescence, used as needed, tailored per patient. The most important auxiliary test is the US, with both A- and B-modes. The most important feature of the A-mode is the internal reflectivity, which typically shows low-medium spikes in case of UM. Although not a pathognomonic feature, however, it greatly assists in differentiating UM from other benign (e.g. choroidal hemangioma) and malignant (e.g. choroidal metastasis) tumors. In B-mode, the choroidal tumor appears as a dome-shaped or mushroom-shaped mass (Fig. 6.2). Using B-mode (and independently A-mode), tumor dimensions can be measured, including base diameter and height, and internal vascularity, using a Doppler probe, can also be evaluated. In addition, a choroidal excavation and orbital shadowing may be observed, as well as areas of extraocular extension. Ciliary body melanoma may remain asymptomatic and unrecognized for a long period of time, before symptoms develop due to dislocation of the lens (which causes astigmatism), cataract, elevated intraocular pressure or iris root detachment (Fig. 6.3). Dilated episcleral blood vessels (sentinel vessels) can also be noticed. Ultrasound biomicroscopy (UBM) is especially valuable in the detection and follow-up of ciliary body melanomas, specifically small ones (<4 mm in elevation), which are harder to detect using

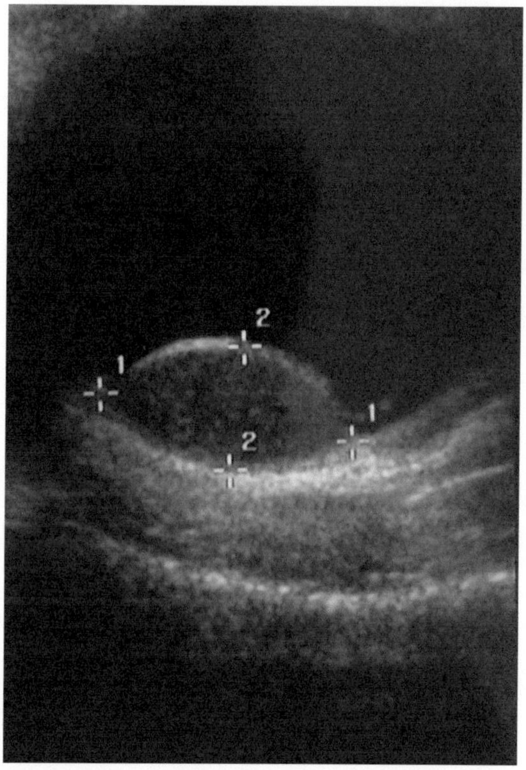

Fig. 6.2 Dome-shape choroidal mass as demonstrated by B-mode ultrasonography

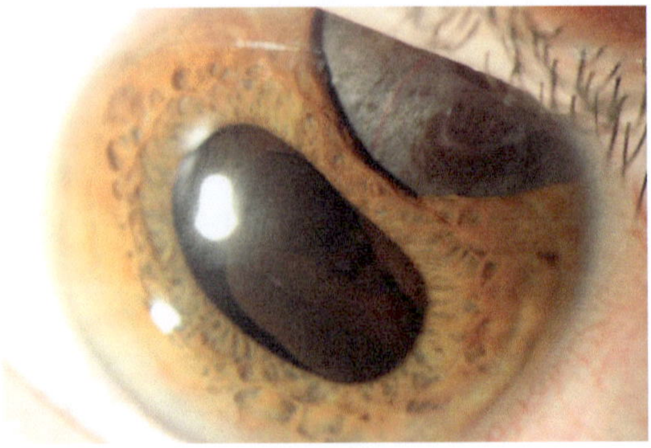

Fig. 6.3 A color photo of a large ciliary body melanoma that have detached the iris root and can be seen also through the pupil

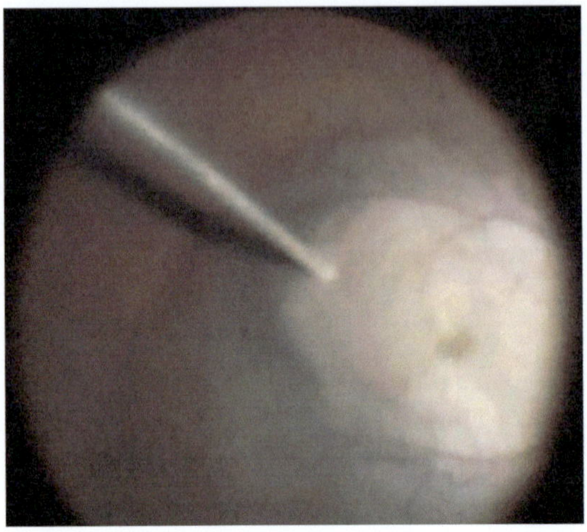

Fig. 6.4 A right eye Transvitreal biopsy of a posterior amelanotic choroidal melanoma using a 25G needle. Histopathological analysis confirmed the diagnosis of a melanoma and demonstrated monosomy 3, a prognostic factor known to be associated with higher chances to develop distant metastasis

other methods and allows differentiation from a cyst as well evaluation of extension of the tumor [23]. The output of US examination not only assists in establishing the correct diagnosis, but also guides treatment (enucleation vs. conservative, and radiotherapy planning) and is a very powerful tool in monitoring cases following primary treatment. OCT is a useful non-invasive tool to detect overlying subretinal fluid as well as changes in the retina and sub-retinal layers. With enhanced depth imaging EDI-OCT, it is possible to evaluate also deeper structures such as the choroid and sclera. Using EDI-OCT, Shields et al. were able to characterize small choroidal melanoma and differ the malignant lesions from benign choroidal nevi [24]. Features of choroidal melanoma included increased tumor thickness, subretinal fluid, subretinal lipofuscin deposition, and retinal irregularities. OCT is also a useful imaging tool in monitoring post-radiotherapy complications, such as macular edema. FA and ICG are not commonly used for the initial diagnosis of UM. However, in certain cases these modalities are found useful, for example, in demonstrating early filling of a choroidal hemangioma, differentiating it from an amelanotic melanoma. FA features of UM include intra-tumor as well as choroidal circulation ("double circulation"). Angiography tests are also useful in detecting neovascularization of the disc or retina post-radiotherapy [24].

Biopsy is rarely performed to establish the diagnosis of UM. However, in certain cases it is a useful tool to differentiate between tumor types. Tumor biopsy can be performed by various ways, depending on tumor site (iris, ciliary body or choroid), size, equipment and expertise. Sampling can be done by use of a fine needle aspiration biopsy (i.e. cytology), incisional or excisional tumor biopsy (i.e. pathology). A ciliary body mass can be reached via transscleral route, whereas a post-equatorial choroidal tumor by a transvitreal approach (using a needle (Fig. 6.4), or vitrectomy). Tissue is often used for prognostic evaluation as well and biopsy yield is considered to be very high [25].

At times, differentiating a choroidal nevus from an early melanoma can be challenging (Fig. 6.5). Radiotherapy, the most common treatment modality used for UM, may result with complications such as retinopathy, papillopathy, maculopathy, neovascularization, secondary glaucoma and need for secondary enucleation [26], hence treatment should be used only in cases of definite tumor growth or highly suspected tumors. Shields et al. analyzed 2514 consecutive cases of choroidal nevi, investigating predictive features for growth into melanoma [12]. Tumor growth was observed in 9% and 13% of eyes after 5 and 10 years, respectively. Factors found to be predictive of growth included tumor thickness greater than 2 mm, subretinal fluid,

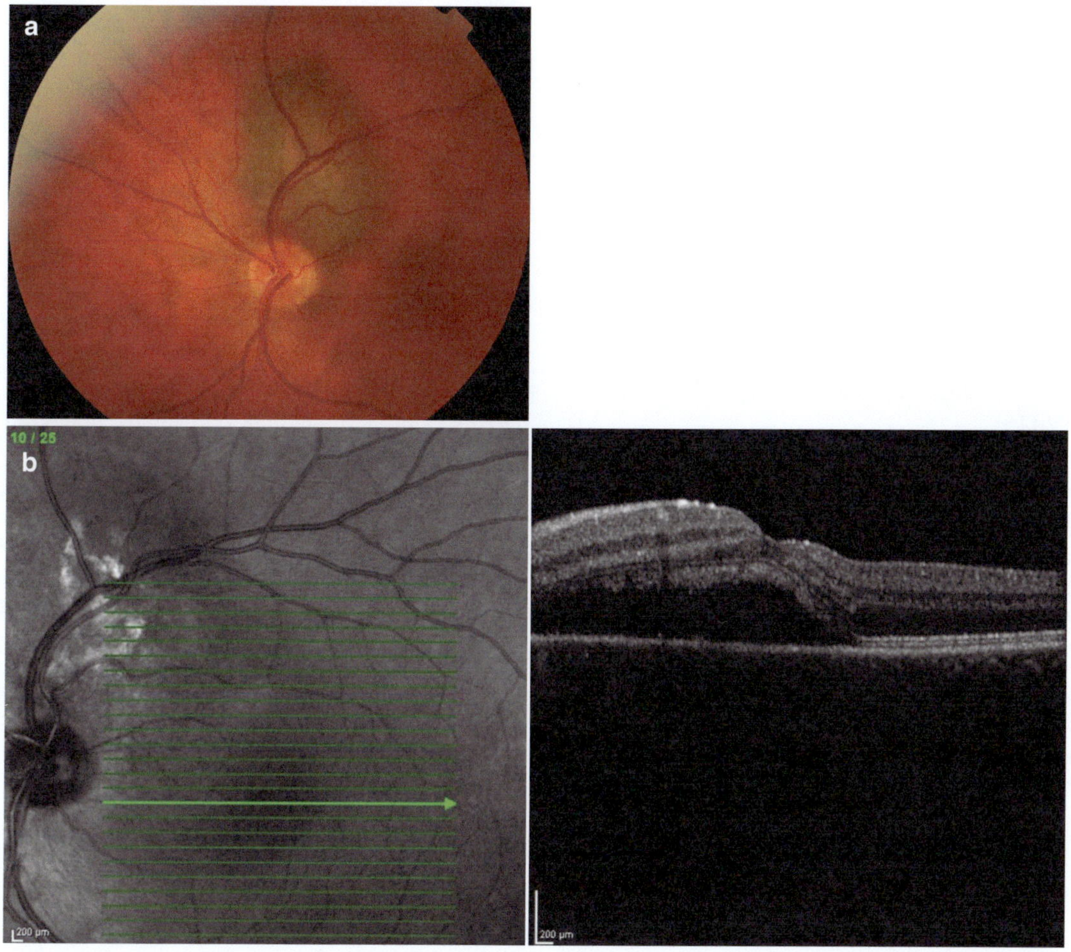

Fig. 6.5 A right eye juxtapapillary choroidal A color photo of a left eye juxtapapillary suspicious choroidal lesion (**a**). Risk factors for growth included presence of symptoms, proximity to the optic disc, orange pigment and subretinal fluid, also seen on optical coherence tomography (OCT; **b**)

presence of symptoms, orange pigment, tumor margin within 3 mm of the optic disc, ultrasonographic hollowness, and halo absence. A useful mnemonic to recall these risk factors is "To find small ocular melanoma using helpful hints", representing thickness, fluid, symptoms, orange pigment, margin, ultrasonographic hollowness, and halo absence.

6.3 Classification

UMs are routinely classified according to tumor dimensions, although different studies used different size definitions. According to the COMS, small tumors are 1.5–3.0 mm in height and 5.0–16.0 mm in diameter, medium tumors are 3.1–8.0 mm in height and ≤16.0 mm in diameter and large tumors are >8.0 mm in height and >16.0 mm in base diameter [27]. The COMS have specified tumor size as the strongest indicator for metastasis and metastatic death [28]. Ten-year survival rates for UM have been published as 81% for small melanomas, 60% for medium melanomas, and 35% for large UMs [29].

The AJCC classification of posterior UM is based on tumor dimensions (base diameter and tumor height), ciliary body involvement and extraocular extension (T category) [15]. Staging, which combines T categorization with lymph node involvement (N) and distant metastasis (M), is used for prognostic estimation. Shields et al.

investigated the clinical features and prognosis of posterior UM based on the seventh edition AJCC staging system. Of the 7731 patients enrolled, after therapy, Kaplan-Meier estimates of metastasis at 1, 5, 10, and 20 years were <1%, 5%, 12%, and 20% for stage I; 2%, 17%, 29%, and 44% for stage II; 6%, 44%, 61%, and 73% for stage III, and 100% by 1 year for stage IV. Kaplan-Meier estimates of death at 1, 5, 10, and 20 years were <1%, 3%, 6%, and 8% for stage I; <1%, 9%, 15%, and 24% for stage II; 3%, 27%, 39%, and 53% for stage III, and 100% by 1 year for stage IV [15].

AJCC classification of iris melanoma is based on tumor size in the iris, existence of secondary glaucoma, extension into the ciliary body, choroid and sclera, as well as extraocular extension [30]. Mostly due to the visibility of iris tumors, 75% of patients are diagnosed with T1 tumors, 19% with T2, <1% with T3 and 5% with T4. Secondary metastasis is more common when secondary glaucoma exists, with a hazard ratio (HR) of 4.51, when the tumor is categorized as T2 (vs. T1, HR 4.09) and when the tumor category is T4 (vs. T1, HR 30.8). Melanoma-related death risk increases with age, T2 category (vs. T1, HR 8.07) and T4 category (vs. T1, HR 20.3).

With genetic analysis taking a more central part in prognostication in oncology in general, and ocular oncology in specific, cytogenetic studies enable classification of UM based on molecular properties of the tumor. This topic will be further discussed in the UM genetics chapter.

6.4 Management

UM is potentially a deadly metastatic cancer that can spread hematogenously primarily to the liver, but also to the lung, bone, and skin [31]. Once metastasis occurs, survival is estimated at 9 months [32]. As mentioned, a major risk factor for distant spread is the tumor size at presentation. It is therefore important to detect a choroidal tumor as early as possible and begin treatment. While a watchful waiting approach is not warranted in case of a definite UM, it may be employed in selected cases of small suspicious nevi, if close monitoring can be guaranteed. However, once tumor has shown evidence of growth, intervention to reach tumor control should be practiced.

Historically, enucleation (i.e. eye removal) was the only treatment modality available for UM. In enucleation surgery, the whole eye is removed, while the extraocular muscles and other orbital tissues remain intact. In advance cases of large extraocular extension, enucleation may not suffice, and exenteration (i.e. removal of the content of the globe) should be practiced. In the 1970's, Zimmerman and colleagues noted an increase in the rate of metastasis and death following enucleation [33]. The authors hypothesized (known as the "Zimmerman hypothesis") that a rise in intraocular pressure at the time of cutting of the optic nerve causes systemic dissemination of tumor cells. Consequently, various enucleation-enhanced techniques were introduced in an attempt to reduce this risk. However, further investigations suggested that metastases are dispatched to the systemic circulation early in the course of disease, regardless of the primary surgery, likely at or before presentation and treatment. Today, enucleation is reserved for large UM, cases associated with a circumferential drainage angle component ("ring melanoma"), melanoma encircling the optic disc, melanoma with large extraocular extension and as a secondary treatment modality after failure of conservative measures [34].

Plaque radiotherapy or brachytherapy for UM was first explored by Stallard in England in the 1940's [35]. The first used applicator was radioactive cobalt 60, followed by iridium 192, ruthenium 106, Iodine 125 and palladium 103. The COMS' medium-sized UM arm demonstrated no significant difference in mortality rate between conservatively treated patients (by means of a iodine 125 applicator) and patients undergoing primary enucleation [36]. Consequently, plaque brachytherapy became the mainstay treatment for medium-sized UM, whereas enucleation was generally abandoned as a primary modality for this indication. The most commonly used applicator today is iodine 125, mainly in north America, and ruthenium 106 in Europe. The

COMS included only selected cases of choroidal melanoma, excluding cases of extraocular extension, juxtapapillary tumors, ciliary body and iris melanomas. Further investigations, however, on these UM subtypes, found plaque brachytherapy to be very useful in reaching tumor control, establishing the treatment modality as the main option for most UM cases [37–39] Using ruthenium 106 plaques for iris melanoma in 19 consecutive cases, Agraval and colleagues reported a 100% tumor control and eye retention rate after a mean follow-up of over 5 years [40]. Fernandes et al. reported similar results using iodine 125 plaques for iris melanoma [41]. Sagoo et al. reported their results in treating juxtapapillary choroidal melanoma with plaque brachytherapy [42]. Tumor control was found in 14% and 21% after 5 and 10 years, respectively. They also found on analysis that eyes treated with adjuvant transpupillary thermotherapy (TTT) had lower chances of recurrence. Krema and colleagues used iodine 125 plaques for ciliary body melanomas in 42 patients [43]. After a median follow-up time of 43 months, tumor control was reported to be 98%. Shields et al. used plaque brachytherapy for large posterior UM (≥8 mm in thickness) and found it to be useful, reaching tumor control after 10 years of follow-up in 87% of cases.

Proton beam radiotherapy for UM was first described in Boston in 1980 by Gragoudas and colleagues [44]. Since its introduction, it became an important conservative therapeutic alternative for this indication, used by many centers across the world [45–47]. It utilizes a beam of protons to irradiate a tissue with the dose deposited over a narrow depth range. As it is delivered from an external device (subtype of external beam radiotherapy), rather than positioned on the eye wall, like radioactive plaque surgery, it may cause side effects in extraocular structures, such as the eyelids, lacrimal gland, and the tear ducts. Damato et al. reported the results of a total of 349 UM patients (all choroidal melanoma) [47]. The 5-year actuarial rates were 3.5% for local tumor recurrence and 9.4% for enucleation. Papakostas and colleagues have also used this modality for large UM [48]. Inclusion criteria included tumors with a height of 10 mm or greater or a longest linear diameter greater than 16 mm or a height greater than 8 mm when the optic nerve was involved. Ten years following primary treatment, 70% of eyes were retained and tumor control was achieved in 88% of eyes.

Complications of radiotherapy, whether plaque or proton beam radiotherapy, include radiation retinopathy, papillopathy, maculopathy, cataract, neovascularization, secondary glaucoma and phthisis bulbi. Sagoo et al. investigated 650 cases of juxtapapillary choroidal melanoma treated by means of plaque radiotherapy [26]. After 10 years of follow-up nonproliferative retinopathy was present in 75% of eyes, proliferative retinopathy in 32%, maculopathy in 65%, papillopathy in 77%, cataract in 80%, neovascular glaucoma in 22%, vitreous hemorrhage in 42%, and secondary enucleation was performed in 26% of eyes. In addition, a final visual acuity of 20/200 or worse was measured in 77% eyes. Damato and colleagues reported a final visual acuity of 20/200 or better after 8 years of follow-up in 42% of UM patients treated with proton beam radiotherapy [47]. Using 4-monthly intervals of intravitreal injections of bevacizumab to UM patients that underwent plaque brachytherapy, Shah et al. showed that macular edema and radiation maculopathy were reduced and visual acuity improved [49]. Yet, the long-term impact of intravitreal injections of anti-vascular endothelial growth factors for this indication remains to be proven.

Focal laser therapy for small UM was explored in the 1970's and on with variable results. Xenon-arc and argon laser were used in various centers in an attempt to reach tumor control while preserving vision [50, 51]. Oosterhuis and colleagues subsequently introduced TTT, a diode laser that can penetrate deeper into the melanoma [52]. The technique was adopted by several centers as a primary treatment modality for small UM, but some have questioned its efficacy in terms of local tumor control and specifically the risk of iatrogenic extraocular spread [53]. TTT is also used in conjunction to plaque brachytherapy to achieve better tumor control. Photodynamic therapy (PDT) using various photosensitizers was also tested for small UM, in both pigmented and non-pigmented choroidal tumors [54, 55]. Fabian et al. used PDT with verteporfin for small pigmented posterior-pole choroidal melanoma, with encouraging results, achieving 80% tumor control rate after 15 months of follow-up, elimination of sub-retinal and significant improvement of visual acuity [17]. Further investigation however, on a larger cohort and for a longer period, were less encouraging, showing that this modality was useful only in 60% of eyes, and according to Kaplan-Meier estimates, 51% of eyes after 3 years [56].

External tumor resection is another, yet not commonly used treatment modality for posterior UM. It allows pathological confirmation and genetic analysis while preserving the globe. However, because of the surgical complexity and length and since it is considered useful only for selected cases, only a handful of centers offer this treatment. Another approach used by several clinicians is to resect the tumor using a vitrectomy technique (i.e. internal approach). However, this too hasn't gained much popularity among experts in the field. A common approach to treat iris melanoma is by tumor resection, although plaque brachytherapy is used currently for this indication in most centers. Interestingly, it was found that after a very long follow-up time of over 30 years, late solitary extraocular recurrence from previously resected iris melanoma may occur [27].

Future management of UM is likely to rely on the use of multimodality imaging techniques, focus on early tumor detection and treatment by means of focal therapy, which will result with a high tumor control rate and improved side effect profile.

References

1. Chang AE, Karnell LH, Menck HR. The National Cancer Data Base report on cutaneous and noncutaneous melanoma: a summary of 84,836 cases from the past decade. The American College of Surgeons Commission on Cancer and the American Cancer Society. Cancer. 1998;83:1664–78.
2. Hu D-N, Yu G-P, McCormick SA, Schneider S, Finger PT. Population-based incidence of uveal melanoma in various races and ethnic groups. Am J Ophthalmol. 2005;140:612.e1–8.
3. Singh AD, Turell ME, Topham AK. Uveal melanoma: trends in incidence, treatment, and survival. Ophthalmology. 2011;118:1881–5.
4. Egan KM, Seddon JM, Glynn RJ, Gragoudas ES, Albert DM. Epidemiologic aspects of uveal melanoma. Surv Ophthalmol. 1988;32:239–51.
5. Virgili G, et al. Incidence of uveal melanoma in Europe. Ophthalmology. 2007;114:2309–2315.e2.
6. McLaughlin CC, et al. Incidence of noncutaneous melanomas in the U.S. Cancer. 2005;103:1000–7.
7. Harbour JW, et al. Frequent mutation of BAP1 in metastasizing uveal melanomas. Science. 2010;330:1410–3.
8. Shields CL, et al. Association of ocular and oculodermal melanocytosis with the rate of uveal melanoma metastasis: analysis of 7872 consecutive eyes. JAMA Ophthalmol. 2013;131:993–1003.
9. Gallagher RP, et al. Risk factors for ocular melanoma: Western Canada Melanoma Study. J Natl Cancer Inst. 1985;74:775–8.
10. Chien JL, Sioufi K, Surakiatchanukul T, Shields JA, Shields CL. Choroidal nevus: a review of prevalence, features, genetics, risks, and outcomes. Curr Opin Ophthalmol. 2017;28:228–37.
11. Singh AD, Kalyani P, Topham A. Estimating the risk of malignant transformation of a choroidal nevus. Ophthalmology. 2005;112:1784–9.
12. Shields CL, et al. Choroidal nevus transformation into melanoma. Arch Ophthalmol. 2009;127:981.
13. Damato EM, Damato BE. Detection and time to treatment of uveal melanoma in the United Kingdom: an evaluation of 2384 patients. Ophthalmology. 2012;119:1582–9.
14. Finn AP, Materin MA, Mruthyunjaya P. Choroidal tumor biopsy. Retina. 2018;38:S79–87.
15. Shields CL, et al. American joint committee on cancer classification of uveal melanoma (anatomic stage) predicts prognosis in 7731 patients. Ophthalmology. 2015;122:1180–6.
16. Shields JA, Shields CL. Management of posterior uveal melanoma: past, present, and future: the 2014 Charles L. Schepens lecture. Ophthalmology. 2015;122:414–28.
17. Fabian ID, et al. Primary photodynamic therapy with verteporfin for small pigmented posterior pole choroidal melanoma. Eye. 2017;31:519–28.
18. Accuracy of diagnosis of choroidal melanomas in the Collaborative Ocular Melanoma Study. COMS report no. 1. Arch Ophthalmol. 1990; 108:1268–1273.
19. Khan S. Clinical and pathologic characteristics of biopsy-proven iris melanoma. Arch Ophthalmol. 2012;130:57.

20. Shields JA, Eagle RC, Ferguson K, Shields CL. Tumors of the nonpigmented epithelium of the ciliary body. Retina. 2015;35:957–65.
21. Shields JA, Sanborn GE, Augsburger JJ. The differential diagnosis of malignant melanoma of the iris. A clinical study of 200 patients. Ophthalmology. 1983;90:716–20.
22. Shields JA, Mashayekhi A, Ra S, Shields CL. Pseudomelanomas of the posterior uveal tract: the 2006 Taylor R. Smith Lecture. Retina. 2005;25:767–71.
23. Bianciotto C, et al. Assessment of anterior segment tumors with ultrasound biomicroscopy versus anterior segment optical coherence tomography in 200 cases. Ophthalmology. 2011;118:1297–302.
24. Shields CL, Kaliki S, Rojanaporn D, Ferenczy SR, Shields JA. Enhanced depth imaging optical coherence tomography of small choroidal melanoma: comparison with choroidal nevus. Arch Ophthalmol. 2012;130:850–6.
25. Shields CL, et al. Chromosome 3 analysis of uveal melanoma using fine-needle aspiration biopsy at the time of plaque radiotherapy in 140 consecutive cases. Arch Ophthalmol. 2007;125:1017.
26. Sagoo MS, et al. Plaque radiotherapy for juxtapapillary choroidal melanoma. JAMA Ophthalmol. 2014;132:697.
27. Margo CE. The collaborative ocular melanoma study: an overview. Cancer Control. 2004;11:304–9.
28. McLean IW, Foster WD, Zimmerman LE, Martin DG. Inferred natural history of uveal melanoma. Invest Ophthalmol Vis Sci. 1980;19:760–70.
29. McLean IW, Foster WD, Zimmerman LE, Martin DG. Inferred natural history of uveal melanoma. Invest Ophthalmol Vis Sci. 1980;19:760–70.
30. Shields CL, et al. Iris melanoma outcomes based on the American joint committee on cancer classification (eighth edition) in 432 patients. Ophthalmology. 2018;125:913–23.
31. Zakka KA, Foos RY, Omphroy CA, Straatsma BR. Malignant melanoma. Analysis of an autopsy population. Ophthalmology. 1980;87:549–56.
32. Kath R, et al. Prognosis and treatment of disseminated uveal melanoma. Cancer. 1993;72:2219–23.
33. Zimmerman LE, McLean IW, Foster WD. Does enucleation of the eye containing a malignant melanoma prevent or accelerate the dissemination of tumour cells. Br J Ophthalmol. 1978;62:420–5.
34. Fabian ID, et al. Secondary enucleations for uveal melanoma: a 7-year retrospective analysis. Am J Ophthalmol. 2015;160:1104–1110.e1.
35. Stallard HB. Radiotherapy for malignant melanoma of the choroid. Br J Ophthalmol. 1966;50:147–55.
36. Collaborative Ocular Melanoma Study Group. The COMS randomized trial of iodine 125 brachytherapy for choroidal melanoma: V. Twelve-year mortality rates and prognostic factors: COMS report No. 28. Arch Ophthalmol. 2006;124:1684–93.
37. Gündüz K, Shields CL, Shields JA, Cater J, Brady L. Plaque radiotherapy for management of ciliary body and choroidal melanoma with extraocular extension. Am J Ophthalmol. 2000;130:97–102.
38. Shields CL, et al. Iris melanoma management with iodine-125 plaque radiotherapy in 144 patients: impact of melanoma-related glaucoma on outcomes. Ophthalmology. 2013;120:55–61.
39. Sagoo MS, et al. Plaque radiotherapy for juxtapapillary choroidal melanoma overhanging the optic disc in 141 consecutive patients. Arch Ophthalmol. 2008;126:1515–22.
40. Agraval U, et al. Use of ruthenium-106 brachytherapy for iris melanoma: the Scottish experience. Br J Ophthalmol. 2018;102:74–8.
41. Fernandes BF, et al. Management of iris melanomas with 125Iodine plaque radiotherapy. Am J Ophthalmol. 2010;149:70–76.e2.
42. Sagoo MS, et al. Plaque radiotherapy for juxtapapillary choroidal melanoma. Ophthalmology. 2011;118:402–7.
43. Krema H, et al. Management of ciliary body melanoma with iodine-125 plaque brachytherapy. Can J Ophthalmol. 2009;44:395–400.
44. Gragoudas ES, et al. Proton beam irradiation. An alternative to enucleation for intraocular melanomas. Ophthalmology. 1980;87:571–81.
45. Zografos L, et al. Rapport sur le traitement conservateur des mélanomes de l'uvée a la clinique ophtalmologique universitaire de Lausanne*. Klin Monatsbl Augenheilkd. 1988;192:572–8.
46. Dendale R, et al. Proton beam radiotherapy for uveal melanoma: results of Curie Institut–Orsay Proton Therapy Center (ICPO). Int J Radiat Oncol. 2006;65:780–7.
47. Damato B, Kacperek A, Chopra M, Campbell IR, Errington RD. Proton beam radiotherapy of choroidal melanoma: the Liverpool-Clatterbridge experience. Int J Radiat Oncol Biol Phys. 2005;62:1405–11.
48. Papakostas TD, Lane AM, Morrison M, Gragoudas ES, Kim IK. Long-term outcomes after proton beam irradiation in patients with large choroidal melanomas. JAMA Ophthalmol. 2017;135:1191.
49. Shah SU, et al. Intravitreal bevacizumab at 4-month intervals for prevention of macular edema after plaque radiotherapy of uveal melanoma. Ophthalmology. 2014;121:269–75.
50. Shields JA, Glazer LC, Mieler WF, Shields CL, Gottlieb MS. Comparison of xenon arc and argon laser photocoagulation in the treatment of choroidal melanomas. Am J Ophthalmol. 1990;109:647–55.
51. Meyer-Schwickerath G, Vogel M. Treatment of malignant melanomas of the choroid by photocoagulation. Trans Ophthalmol Soc U K. 1977;97:416–20.

52. Oosterhuis JA, Journée-de Korver HG, Kakebeeke-Kemme HM, Bleeker JC. Transpupillary thermotherapy in choroidal melanomas. Arch Ophthalmol. 1995;113:315–21.
53. Singh AD, Kivelä T, Seregard S, Robertson D, Bena JF. Primary transpupillary thermotherapy of 'small'; choroidal melanoma: is it safe? Br J Ophthalmol. 2008;92:727–8.
54. Jmor F, Hussain RN, Damato BE, Heimann H. Photodynamic therapy as initial treatment for small choroidal melanomas. Photodiagn Photodyn Ther. 2017;20:175–81.
55. Rundle P. Treatment of posterior uveal melanoma with multi-dose photodynamic therapy. Br J Ophthalmol. 2014;98:494–7.
56. Fabian ID, et al. Primary photodynamic therapy with verteporfin for pigmented posterior pole cT1a choroidal melanoma: a 3-year retrospective analysis. Br J Ophthalmol. 2018;102(12):1705–10. https://doi.org/10.1136/bjophthalmol-2017-311747.

7 Genetics of Uveal Melanoma

Helen Kalirai, Alexander Iu. Tsygankov, Sophie Thornton, Svetlana V. Saakyan, and Sarah E. Coupland

7.1 Introduction

Uveal melanoma (UM) is the most common primary intraocular tumor in adults [1], arising in the three main structures of the uveal tract: the choroid, the ciliary body and less frequently in the iris. Unlike tumors occurring in the choroid or ciliary body, those found in the iris are generally associated with a good prognosis [2, 3]. About half of all patients with choroidal or ciliary body UM, in contrast, develop hematogenous dissemination mainly to the liver. In the last 10 years, we have seen the introduction of molecular genetic testing/techniques into routine clinical practice for the stratification of UM patients according to their risk of developing metastatic disease; aiding subsequent clinical management [4–6]. Despite this, once metastatic disease has developed, there is little in the way of effective treatment (reviewed in [7–9]). Recent, innovative high-resolution and detailed genetic analyses are increasing our understanding of the molecular biology of UM not only to further enhance prognostication and patient management but also in the development of targeted therapies to improve survival.

H. Kalirai · S. Thornton
Molecular and Clinical Cancer Medicine, Institute of Translational Medicine, University of Liverpool, Liverpool, UK
e-mail: h.kalirai@liverpool.ac.uk; sophie.thornton@liverpool.ac.uk

A. I. Tsygankov
Department of Ocular Oncology and Radiology, Moscow Helmholtz Research Institute of Eye Diseases, Moscow, Russian Federation

S. V. Saakyan
Department of Ocular Oncology and Radiology, Moscow Helmholtz Research Institute of Eye Diseases, Moscow, Russian Federation

Department of Eye Diseases, Moscow Helmholtz Research Institute of Eye Diseases, Moscow, Russian Federation

S. E. Coupland (✉)
Molecular and Clinical Cancer Medicine, Royal Liverpool and Broadgreen University, Hospital NHS Trust, University of Liverpool, Liverpool, UK
e-mail: s.e.coupland@liverpool.ac.uk

7.2 Uveal Melanoma Prognosis

7.2.1 Chromosomal Changes

Specific chromosomal changes of prognostic value are commonly found in UM cells. Loss of one copy of chromosome 3 (monosomy 3; M3) and polysomy 8q (8qG) are strongly associated with the development of metastatic disease, reportedly resulting in an intermediate metastatic risk when occurring in isolation and a high metastatic risk when both occur together, with a 70–80% reduction in the 5 year survival rate [8–10]. In contrast, the gain of the short arm of chromosome 6 (polysomy 6p) is often found in choroidal melanoma with disomy 3 (D3) and has been associated with a good prognosis [11–13].

V. Khetan (ed.), *Intraocular Tumors*, https://doi.org/10.1007/978-981-15-0395-5_7

Cases in which polysomy 6p occurs together with M3 or 8qG have, however, also been reported suggesting a more complex classification and evolution of copy number variation (CNV) in UM [11, 14–17]. In a recent comprehensive molecular analysis of UM by The Cancer Genome Atlas (TCGA), four groups were described based on somatic CNV ordered by increasing chromosomal instability [13]. The four groups could be further defined by the mutation status of three key genes *EIF1AX*, *SF3B1* and *BAP1* as described later in this chapter. In addition to chromosomal alterations, both M3 and 8qG are associated with the following clinical and histological features; large tumor size, ciliary body involvement, epithelioid cell morphology, high mitotic count and Periodic Acid Schiff (PAS)-positive closed loops [18, 19]. Using data from patients treated at the Liverpool Ocular Oncology Centre, an interactive web based tool, Liverpool Uveal Melanoma Prognosticator Online (LUMPO), has been developed which combines clinical, histopathological and chromosome 3 status of the tumor to produce a personalized survival curve for each patient [20]; this is used for patient management and screening frequency. External validation of the LUMPO tool in a cohort of patients treated at the University of California San Francisco confirmed the utility of the interpolation of such datasets to predict UM specific mortality [21]. In support of this, another web-based prognostic tool "Prediction of Risk of Metastasis in Uveal Melanoma (PRiMeUM)" was recently described [22]. This tool provides an individualized prediction of metastatic risk within 48 months following treatment using clinical and tumor characteristics and the copy number status of chromosomes 1p, 3, 6 and 8 when known. The continued refinement and external validation of these metastatic risk models is necessary as our understanding of the involvement of other genetic alterations increases and as tests to detect these changes are introduced into routine clinical practice. In this regard, version III of LUMPO, which includes chromosome 8q data, is currently undergoing internal validation; examples of a patient with a low metastatic risk and a high metastatic risk UM are shown in Fig. 7.1.

To assess chromosomal CNV a variety of molecular genetic methods are routinely used by molecular pathology laboratories. These include; fluorescence in situ hybridization (FISH), microsatellite analysis (MSA), multiplex ligation dependent probe amplification (MLPA), comparative genomic hybridization (CGH) and single nucleotide polymorphism (SNP) analysis (reviewed in [23]). Not only do the sensitivities of these techniques to detect chromosomal CNV differ but also their requirement for differing amounts and quality of input DNA, which may influence their utility for small biopsy and formalin fixed paraffin embedded specimens. In addition, MSA requires a matched blood sample from the patient [24]. Of importance for prognostic testing is the ability of the chosen technique to provide reliable results in samples taken following radiotherapy. This has recently been demonstrated for both MLPA and MSA when testing biopsy samples taken following completion of proton beam radiotherapy [25].

7.3 Gene Expression Profiling

Gene expression profiling (GEP) has been used by several groups to stratify UM patients according to their metastatic risk and to gain further insight into the pathogenesis of the disease [26–28]. Using microarray techniques, differences in gene expression patterns between low metastatic risk D3 UM and high metastatic risk M3 UM could be demonstrated. Data generated by Onken et al. [26] have since been used to develop a commercially available assay, DecisionDx UM, (Castle Biosciences, Friendswood, Texas, USA) that examines 12 differentially expressed target genes and classifies tumours as either Class 1 (low risk) or Class 2 (high risk) [6]. Class 1 choroidal melanomas are reported to resemble normal uveal melanocytes and melanocytic low-grade tumors, whereas class 2 tumors have a more de-differentiated profile that resembles primitive neural/ectodermal stem cells, which

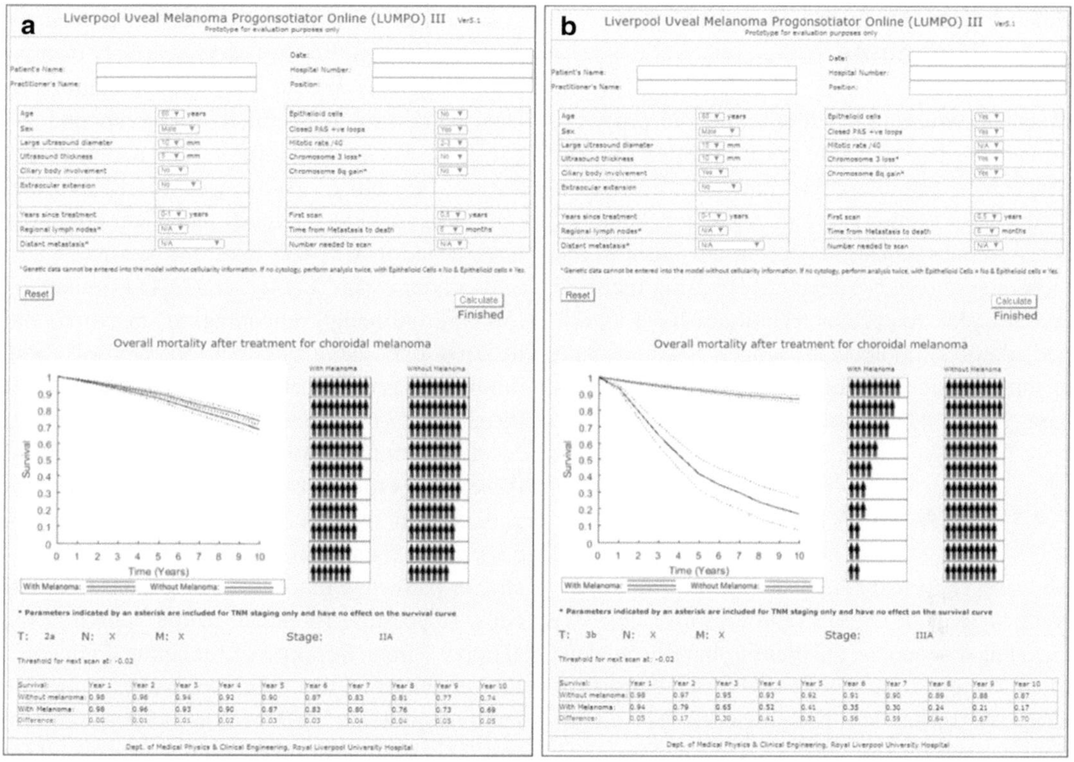

Fig. 7.1 Representative images of LUMPO III output showing a 68 year old male with (**a**) a low metastatic risk UM and (**b**) a high metastatic risk UM

may contribute to their metastatic potential [29]. Similar to the refinements made to classifications based on chromosomal CNV, GEP classifications have recently been expanded to include an additional category (class 1B) for tumors with intermediate metastatic risk [30]. Class 1B tumors that gave rise to metastatic disease, could be identified by their expression of PRAME mRNA (preferentially expressed antigen in melanoma) [31]. The 5-year actuarial rate of metastasis was 0% for Class 1 (PRAME-), 38% for Class 1 (PRAME+), and 71% for Class 2 tumors. Median metastasis-free survival for Class 1 (PRAME+) patients was 88 months, compared to 32 months for Class 2 patients.

The DecisionDx®-UM test uses RNA extracted from a variety of specimen types including fine needle aspiration biopsy (FNAB), FFPE specimens, or resected tumor and the metastatic risk classification provided is not further imputed using clinical or histological features of the tumor. Whether RNA-based GEP or DNA-based analysis of chromosomal CNV is more accurate in predicting UM metastatic risk remains controversial and is dependent on the sensitivity of the method used to determine chromosomal CNV, in particular M3. In a Collaborative Ocular Oncology Group Report it was suggested that GEP provides more reliable predictions for metastasis-free survival compared to multi-SNP analysis [32]. However, it should be noted that the median follow-up time in this prospective study was only 17.4 months. In addition, GEP was compared only with respect to chromosome 3 status as a measure of metastatic risk, but not with a predictive model that includes genetic, clinical and histopathological features of the tumor.

7.4 Genetic Mutations in Uveal Melanoma

Despite progress in the development of prognostic models, UM that take an unexpected clinical course have been described and it is clear, that a binary classification into high and low risk tumors is an oversimplification. Recent advances in the molecular characterisation of UM using multiple and complex molecular techniques have identified additional molecular changes that contribute to the development and progression of this disease [13, 33–42]; these are discussed below.

7.4.1 GNAQ/GNA11

Mutually exclusive mutations in *GNAQ* (chromosome 9q21.2) or *GNA11* (chromosome 19p13.3) encoding α subunits of G proteins have been identified in approximately 86–89% of all primary UM [39, 40, 43, 44]. The *GNAQ*/*GNA11* alterations described so far are missense mutations (i.e., single amino acid substitutions) occurring most commonly in codon 209 (exon 5) and less frequently in codon 183 (exon 4) of both genes. The occurrence of *GNAQ*/*GNA11* mutations in benign uveal nevi (including melanocytomas) [39, 43, 45, 46] and the majority of UM, independent of prognosis, suggests that they are an initiating event in tumor development. Detection of *GNAQ*/*GNA11* mutations, whilst not of prognostic value, can be used to classify melanoma metastases with unclear primary tumors and may be of use as biomarkers of tumour spread. For example, *GNAQ/GNA11* mutations in circulating cell-free DNA were detected in the plasma of 9/22 UM patients with metastasis [47]. Similar results were achieved by Saakyan S.V. et al. in the Moscow ocular oncology lab (unpublished data).

The altered *GNAQ/GNA11* gene product suppresses the intrinsic guanosine triphosphatase (GTPase) activity, which normally inactivates the α subunit of the G protein. This results in an increased activation of downstream signaling pathways, such as MAPK and PKC, influencing proliferation, differentiation and apoptosis [48]. MAPK activation depends on Ras. RasGRP3, a guanine exchange factor for Ras, was recently shown to be significantly and selectively overexpressed in response to *GNAQ/11* mutations in UM, suggesting its potential as a therapeutic target [49]. Using the information about downstream signaling pathways, MAPK, PI3K (phosphoinositide 3-kinase) and PKC inhibitors were tested in UM cell lines and xenograft animal models with *GNAQ* or *GNA11* mutations [50–55]. Although encouraging in vitro and in vivo data demonstrating efficacy of these inhibitors has driven clinical trials of these agents in patients with metastatic UM, the initial data from these human studies show little success of these agents to improve overall survival for UM patients with metastatic disease (reviewed in [56, 57]). One explanation for this is that other downstream pathways modulate the response of UM cells. A possible candidate in this regard is the "Hippo Tumor Suppressor Signaling Pathway". Key enzymes of this signaling pathway include the oncoproteins *YAP* (yes-associated protein) and *TAZ* (transcriptional coactivator with PDZ-binding motif), which regulate the activity of transcription factors. Studies demonstrate that *GNAQ*/*GNA11* mutations promote tumorigenesis by activating the YAP oncoprotein independently of the Hippo tumor suppressor signaling pathway [58, 59]. Because of the potential for multiple signaling pathways to be activated downstream of GNAQ/GNA11 studies have focused on the identification of upstream effectors that could be targeted therapeutically. Recently, the small GTPase ARF6 was identified as such an effector of oncogenic GNAQ signaling to induce multiple downstream signalling pathways including PLC/PKC, Rho/Rac and YAP, as well as β-catenin signalling [60]. Inhibition of ARF6 with a small-molecule inhibitor reduced UM cell proliferation and tumorigenesis in a mouse model [60].

7.4.2 BAP1

Biallelic inactivation of the *BRCA1*-associated protein 1 (*BAP1*; Chromosome 3p21) gene due to chromosome 3 loss and the presence of a *BAP1* mutation on the remaining copy, is associated with an increased risk of metastasis in patients with UM [35, 61–63]. BAP1 is a nuclear-localised deubiquitylase (DUB) belonging to the ubiquitin carboxy-terminal hydrolase (UCH) family of DUBs [64]. It has multiple functions, including involvement in DNA damage responses, chromatin remodelling, cell differentiation and proliferation [65]. In in vitro studies of UM cell lines, knockdown of *BAP1* led to dedifferentiation of UM cells and the acquisition of stem cell like characteristics [66].

The identification of somatic *BAP1* gene mutations in ~85% of all metastatic primary UM supports its role as a tumor suppressor in this disease [13, 35]. *BAP1* inactivating mutations occur along the entire length of the gene and are associated with a loss of nuclear expression of the BAP1 protein (nBAP1) [67], with data supporting the use of BAP1 immunohistochemistry to evaluate metastatic risk [67–70]. It is of interest, however, that not all metastatic UM have *BAP1* mutations or loss of nBAP1 protein [68, 71, 72] (Fig. 7.2). Moreover, nBAP1-positive/M3 UM were shown to be associated with prolonged survival compared to nBAP1-negative/M3 UM [73].

Treating the loss of a tumor suppressor therapeutically is much more difficult than inhibiting an oncogene. One approach is "synthetic lethality"; for example, *BAP1* loss may result in the activation of alternative signalling pathways, which in turn can be targeted by drugs. According to this principle, histone deacetylase inhibitors (HDACi) were identified as a possible class of drugs for *BAP1*-mutated UM. Preliminary results of in vitro and in vivo HDACi-treated UM cells indicate an effect of these agents to slow tumor growth and increase the expression of genes associated with differentiated melanocytes [74].

In addition to somatic mutations, truncating germline mutations of the *BAP1* gene have been demonstrated in families predisposed to the development of a variety of malignant tumors [75–77]. These include amongst others UM, renal cell carcinoma, mesothelioma and cutaneous melanoma. In a recent study examining families with two or more family members diagnosed with UM, which has an incidence of around 1% of all UM, germline *BAP1* mutations were identified in 19–22% of the families tested [78]. Of interest in the families without *BAP1* mutations were distinct family histories and high rates of prostate cancer in first- and second-degree relatives, suggesting the presence of other cancer predisposition genes. It is important therefore, that family histories for patients with UM are collected; current evidence indicates that genetic testing and counselling should be recommended for families with first or second degree relatives who have developed two or more of the tumours commonly associated with the *BAP1* predisposition syndrome (reviewed in [79, 80]).

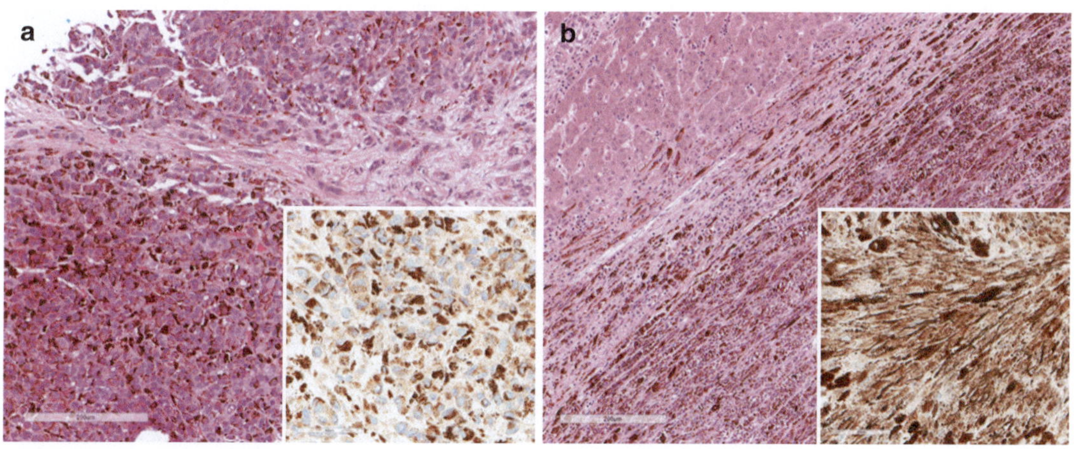

Fig. 7.2 BAP1 protein expression in metastatic uveal melanoma to the liver. H&E images of two cases of liver metastases with high power inserts showing (**a**) BAP1 negative uveal melanoma cells and (**b**) BAP1 positive uveal melanoma cells

7.4.3 SF3B1

Harbour et al. [36] first described mutations in codon 625 of the splice factor 3B subunit 1 gene (*SF3B1*) in UM with a favorable prognosis. Further studies confirmed this mutational hotspot together with codon 666 [81, 82] in 9–24% of all UM [34, 37, 42, 82]. *SF3B1* is a component of a spliceosome whose role is to transform precursor mRNA into mature mRNA by separating the introns. Although the exact function in UM is unclear, *SF3B1* mutations are reportedly associated with alternative mRNA splicing at the 3 'end of genes [82]. Although originally associated with a good prognosis, data now demonstrate that *SF3B1* mutations identify a subset of D3 tumors with late-onset metastases [42]. In support of this, Griewank et al. [71] detected an *SF3B1* mutation in codon 625 in one of 26 metastases. Recently mutations in another splice factor *SRSF2* have been described predominantly in D3-UM, which similar to *SF3B1* mutations can alter translation initiation [13].

7.4.4 EIF1AX

Mutations in the amino terminal region of eukaryotic translational initiation factor 1A gene on chromosome X (*EIF1AX*) have been reported in 13–19% of ciliary body and choroidal UM [13, 34, 37] and 42% of iris melanomas [44]. *EIF1AX* mutations are associated with good prognosis D3 [13, 34, 37, 61] and Class 1 tumors [33] and are generally mutually exclusive to the presence of *SF3B1* or *BAP1* mutations. The functional significance of *EIF1AX* mutations in UM remains unclear, however a recent study suggests that aberrant translational regulation occurs in *EIF1AX* mutant cells possibly leading to their positive clonal selection [83].

7.4.5 Additional Molecular Changes

Alongside the genetic alterations commonly associated with UM development and metastasis, a number of less frequent alterations have been described that are also likely to have prognostic and/or functional implications for UM progression. A gain-of-function mutation in *PLCB4* (chromosome 20p12.3) was detected in 1 out of 56 UM sequenced [84]. PLCB4 is a downstream target of GNAQ/GNA11 suggesting that this is an alternative way of activating this signaling pathway. Similarly, a recurrent mutation in *CYSLTR2* in 4 of 9 UM samples that lacked mutations in *GNAQ/GNA11* was reported [85]. CYSLTR2 is a G-coupled protein receptor that activates the Gα subunits, again acting as an alternative means of activating downstream signaling pathways. In support of this *GNAQ*, *GNA11*, *PLCB4* and *CYSLTR2* mutations are found in a mutually exclusive pattern. Royer-Bertrand *et al* also report five somatic mutations identified in more than one of 33 UM samples examined; *TP53BP1*, *CSMD1*, *TTC28*, *DLK2*, and *KTN1* [38]; the biological significance of these is not yet clear. Other genetic changes of relevance to metastatic progression include the amplification of *DDEF1* [86] and *PTP4A3* [87] on chromosome 8q.

It is not only genetic but also epigenetic alterations that regulate gene expression, thereby playing an important role in carcinogenesis. Epigenetic changes that silence tumor suppressor genes (TSG) or activate oncogenes include DNA methylation and changes in the expression levels of both small and long non-coding RNAs (lncRNA). Six small non coding microRNAs (let-7b, miR-199a, miR-199a*, miR-143, miR-193b and miR-652) were found to differentiate class 1 and class 2 UM [88]. Another study identified 30 miRNAs that were differentially expressed between UM that had metastasised and those that had not [89]. Other studies examining individual miRNAs describe the upregulation of miR-367, miR-149, miR-134 and miR-20a in UM tissues and cell lines, promoting proliferation and migration [90–92]. Conversely, miR-34a [93], miR-137 [94] and miR-32 [95] expression levels are reported to be downregulated in UM samples and cell lines.

Long non-coding RNAs are non-protein coding transcripts longer than 200 nucleotides. In recent years, the importance of these molecules to regulate gene expression has been increasingly recognized. Unlike miRNAs, lncRNAs display complex secondary and tertiary structures allowing them to bind to key regulatory proteins, RNA and DNA; regulating processes such as transcription, tumorigenesis and metastasis. Of particular note in UM, the knockdown of *RHPN1 antisense RNA 1* (*RHPN1-AS1*) a 2030-bp transcript on chromosome 8q24, inhibited cell proliferation and migration both in vitro and in vivo [96]. In addition, the lncRNAs *LINC00152* (*CYTOR*) and *BANCR*, are reported at higher abundance in poor prognosis as compared with good prognosis UM [13].

Abnormal promoter hyper-methylation of CpG islands has been shown to play an important role in the inactivation of TSG in cancer. In UM, promoter methylation of the TSG *RAS association domain family 1* (*RASSF1*), located on chromosome 3p21.3, was associated with an increased risk of metastatic disease [97]. In the recent analysis of samples by TCGA four DNA methylation clusters were identified. Within these clusters D3-UM possessed distinct DNA methylation patterns dependent upon whether they had an *EIF1AX* or *SF3B1/SRFR2* mutation; M3/BAP1-aberrant UM showed a single profile associated predominantly with low levels of methylation [13].

Genome wide association studies (GWAS) are large scale genetic analyses aimed at identifying common variants associated with a specific disease. In UM, the first reported GWAS study identified a susceptibility locus at 5p15.33 in or around the *CLPTM1L* locus. Further work is now necessary to determine the significance of these findings for UM oncogenesis [98].

7.5 Future Challenges for Molecular Genetics of Uveal Melanoma

Our knowledge and understanding of the molecular pathology of UM has improved dramatically over the last 20 years. This has been made possible not only due to advances in molecular techniques, but also by the availability of well-characterised and clinically annotated tumor samples from patients consenting to scientific research. Nevertheless, the data presented above show the complexities of these analyses and the current gaps in our understanding of how they contribute to UM progression and metastasis. This is further highlighted by atypical UM that do not fit the current prognostic classifications and thus require additional evaluation.

In order to improve the molecular classification of tumors both for prognostic and therapeutic purposes, custom designed genetic panels are being developed for clinical use; with the ultimate goal to be able to turn molecular knowledge into targeted therapeutic approaches stratified according to the genetic profile of each individual patient. In this regard, genetic testing is currently performed on primary UM samples due to a lack of availability of metastatic tissue. In order to use this information in the treatment of individual patients with metastatic disease, we must assume that few genetic differences exist between the primary and the metastatic UM. Whilst this may be the case, our current understanding of the molecular landscape of UM metastases in the liver is limited, with only few studies examining (a) infiltrating immune cells [99] (b) chromosomal aberrations [72, 100, 101], (c) mutations [71, 102] and (d) GEP [103]. In order to better understand the UM metastases, international multicentre research groups have been formed that focus their research on these tumors (e.g. UMCure2020, http://www.umcure2020.org/en/).

References

1. Damato BE, Coupland SE. Differences in uveal melanomas between men and women from the British Isles. Eye (Lond). 2012;26(2):292–9.
2. Khan S, Finger PT, Yu GP, Razzaq L, Jager MJ, de Keizer RJ, et al. Clinical and pathologic characteristics of biopsy-proven iris melanoma: a multicenter international study. Arch Ophthalmol. 2012;130(1):57–64.
3. Krishna Y, Kalirai H, Thornton S, Damato BE, Heimann H, Coupland SE. Genetic findings in treatment-naive and proton-beam-radiated iris melanomas. Br J Ophthalmol. 2016;100(7):1012–6.
4. Caines R, Eleuteri A, Kalirai H, Fisher AC, Heimann H, Damato BE, et al. Cluster analysis of multiplex ligation-dependent probe amplification data in choroidal melanoma. Mol Vis. 2015;21:1–11.

5. Coupland SE, Lake SL, Zeschnigk M, Damato BE. Molecular pathology of uveal melanoma. Eye (Lond). 2013;27(2):230–42.
6. Harbour JW. A prognostic test to predict the risk of metastasis in uveal melanoma based on a 15-gene expression profile. Methods Mol Biol. 2014;1102:427–40.
7. Carvajal RD. Update on the treatment of uveal melanoma. Clin Adv Hematol Oncol. 2016;14(10):768–70.
8. Carvajal RD, Schwartz GK, Tezel T, Marr B, Francis JH, Nathan PD. Metastatic disease from uveal melanoma: treatment options and future prospects. Br J Ophthalmol. 2017;101(1):38–44.
9. Woodman SE. Metastatic uveal melanoma: biology and emerging treatments. Cancer J. 2012;18(2):148–52.
10. Carvajal RD, Yavuzyigitoglu S, Drabarek W, Smit KN, van Poppelen N, Koopmans AE, et al. Update on the treatment of uveal melanoma. Clin Adv Hematol Oncol. 2016;14(10):768–70.
11. Damato B, Dopierala JA, Coupland SE. Genotypic profiling of 452 choroidal melanomas with multiplex ligation-dependent probe amplification. Clin Cancer Res. 2010;16(24):6083–92.
12. Ehlers JP, Worley L, Onken MD, Harbour JW. Integrative genomic analysis of aneuploidy in uveal melanoma. Clin Cancer Res. 2008;14(1):115–22.
13. Robertson AG, Shih J, Yau C, Gibb EA, Oba J, Mungall KL, et al. Integrative analysis identifies four molecular and clinical subsets in uveal melanoma. Cancer Cell. 2017;32(2):204–20.e15.
14. de Lange MJ, van Pelt SI, Versluis M, Jordanova ES, Kroes WG, Ruivenkamp C, et al. Heterogeneity revealed by integrated genomic analysis uncovers a molecular switch in malignant uveal melanoma. Oncotarget. 2015;6(35):37824–35.
15. Ehlers JP, Harbour JW. Molecular pathobiology of uveal melanoma. Int Ophthalmol Clin. 2006;46(1):167–80.
16. Kilic E, van Gils W, Lodder E, Beverloo HB, van Til ME, Mooy CM, et al. Clinical and cytogenetic analyses in uveal melanoma. Invest Ophthalmol Vis Sci. 2006;47(9):3703–7.
17. Singh N, Singh AD, Hide W. Inferring an evolutionary tree of uveal melanoma from genomic copy number aberrations. Invest Ophthalmol Vis Sci. 2015;56(11):6801–9.
18. Damato B, Eleuteri A, Taktak AF, Coupland SE. Estimating prognosis for survival after treatment of choroidal melanoma. Prog Retin Eye Res. 2011;30(5):285–95.
19. Dogrusoz M, Bagger M, van Duinen SG, Kroes WG, Ruivenkamp CA, Bohringer S, et al. The prognostic value of AJCC staging in uveal melanoma is enhanced by adding chromosome 3 and 8q status. Invest Ophthalmol Vis Sci. 2017;58(2):833–42.
20. Eleuteri A, Damato B, Coupland SE, Taktak A. Enhancing survival prognostication in patients with choroidal melanoma by integrating pathologic, clinical and genetic predictors of metastasis. Int J Biomed Eng Technol. 2012;8(1):18–35.
21. DeParis SW, Taktak A, Eleuteri A, Enanoria W, Heimann H, Coupland SE, et al. External validation of the liverpool uveal melanoma prognosticator online. Invest Ophthalmol Vis Sci. 2016;57(14):6116–22.
22. Vaquero-Garcia J, Lalonde E, Ewens KG, Ebrahimzadeh J, Richard-Yutz J, Shields CL, et al. PRiMeUM: a model for predicting risk of metastasis in uveal melanoma. Invest Ophthalmol Vis Sci. 2017;58(10):4096–105.
23. Coupland SE, Damato BE. Molecular analysis of uveal melanoma. Ophthalmology. 2013;120(7):e50.
24. Tschentscher F, Prescher G, Zeschnigk M, Horsthemke B, Lohmann DR. Identification of chromosomes 3, 6, and 8 aberrations in uveal melanoma by microsatellite analysis in comparison to comparative genomic hybridization. Cancer Genet Cytogenet. 2000;122(1):13–7.
25. Hussain RN, Kalirai H, Groenewald C, Kacperek A, Errington RD, Coupland SE, et al. Prognostic biopsy of choroidal melanoma after proton beam radiation therapy. Ophthalmology. 2016;123(10):2264–5.
26. Onken MD, Worley LA, Ehlers JP, Harbour JW. Gene expression profiling in uveal melanoma reveals two molecular classes and predicts metastatic death. Cancer Res. 2004;64(20):7205–9.
27. Tschentscher F, Husing J, Holter T, Kruse E, Dresen IG, Jockel KH, et al. Tumor classification based on gene expression profiling shows that uveal melanomas with and without monosomy 3 represent two distinct entities. Cancer Res. 2003;63(10):2578–84.
28. Zuidervaart W, van der Velden PA, Hurks MH, van Nieuwpoort FA, Out-Luiting CJ, Singh AD, et al. Gene expression profiling identifies tumour markers potentially playing a role in uveal melanoma development. Br J Cancer. 2003;89(10):1914–9.
29. Chang SH, Worley LA, Onken MD, Harbour JW. Prognostic biomarkers in uveal melanoma: evidence for a stem cell-like phenotype associated with metastasis. Melanoma Res. 2008;18(3):191–200.
30. Field MG, Harbour JW. Recent developments in prognostic and predictive testing in uveal melanoma. Curr Opin Ophthalmol. 2014;25(3):234–9.
31. Field MG, Durante MA, Decatur CL, Tarlan B, Oelschlager KM, Stone JF, et al. Epigenetic reprogramming and aberrant expression of PRAME are associated with increased metastatic risk in Class 1 and Class 2 uveal melanomas. Oncotarget. 2016;7(37):59209–19.
32. Onken MD, Worley LA, Char DH, Augsburger JJ, Correa ZM, Nudleman E, et al. Collaborative Ocular Oncology Group report number 1: prospective validation of a multi-gene prognostic assay in uveal melanoma. Ophthalmology. 2012;119(8):1596–603.
33. Decatur CL, Ong E, Garg N, Anbunathan H, Bowcock AM, Field MG, et al. Driver mutations in uveal melanoma: associations with gene expression

profile and patient outcomes. JAMA Ophthalmol. 2016;134(7):728–33.
34. Dono M, Angelini G, Cecconi M, Amaro A, Esposito AI, Mirisola V, et al. Mutation frequencies of GNAQ, GNA11, BAP1, SF3B1, EIF1AX and TERT in uveal melanoma: detection of an activating mutation in the TERT gene promoter in a single case of uveal melanoma. Br J Cancer. 2014;110(4):1058–65.
35. Harbour JW, Onken MD, Roberson ED, Duan S, Cao L, Worley LA, et al. Frequent mutation of BAP1 in metastasizing uveal melanomas. Science. 2010;330(6009):1410–3.
36. Harbour JW, Roberson ED, Anbunathan H, Onken MD, Worley LA, Bowcock AM. Recurrent mutations at codon 625 of the splicing factor SF3B1 in uveal melanoma. Nat Genet. 2013;45(2):133–5.
37. Martin M, Masshofer L, Temming P, Rahmann S, Metz C, Bornfeld N, et al. Exome sequencing identifies recurrent somatic mutations in EIF1AX and SF3B1 in uveal melanoma with disomy 3. Nat Genet. 2013;45(8):933–6.
38. Royer-Bertrand B, Torsello M, Rimoldi D, El Zaoui I, Cisarova K, Pescini-Gobert R, et al. Comprehensive genetic landscape of uveal melanoma by whole-genome sequencing. Am J Hum Genet. 2016;99(5):1190–8.
39. Van Raamsdonk CD, Bezrookove V, Green G, Bauer J, Gaugler L, O'Brien JM, et al. Frequent somatic mutations of GNAQ in uveal melanoma and blue naevi. Nature. 2009;457(7229):599–602.
40. Van Raamsdonk CD, Griewank KG, Crosby MB, Garrido MC, Vemula S, Wiesner T, et al. Mutations in GNA11 in uveal melanoma. N Engl J Med. 2010;363(23):2191–9.
41. Yavuzyigitoglu S, Drabarek W, Smit KN, van Poppelen N, Koopmans AE, Vaarwater J, et al. Correlation of gene mutation status with copy number profile in uveal melanoma. Ophthalmology. 2017;124(4):573–5.
42. Yavuzyigitoglu S, Koopmans AE, Verdijk RM, Vaarwater J, Eussen B, van Bodegom A, et al. Uveal melanomas with SF3B1 mutations: a distinct subclass associated with late-onset metastases. Ophthalmology. 2016;123(5):1118–28.
43. Onken MD, Worley LA, Long MD, Duan S, Council ML, Bowcock AM, et al. Oncogenic mutations in GNAQ occur early in uveal melanoma. Invest Ophthalmol Vis Sci. 2008;49(12):5230–4.
44. Scholz SL, Moller I, Reis H, Susskind D, van de Nes JAP, Leonardelli S, et al. Frequent GNAQ, GNA11, and EIF1AX mutations in iris melanoma. Invest Ophthalmol Vis Sci. 2017;58(9):3464–70.
45. Mudhar HS, Doherty R, Salawu A, Sisley K, Rennie IG. Immunohistochemical and molecular pathology of ocular uveal melanocytoma: evidence for somatic GNAQ mutations. Br J Ophthalmol. 2013;97(7):924–8.
46. Vader MJC, Madigan MC, Versluis M, Suleiman HM, Gezgin G, Gruis NA, et al. GNAQ and GNA11 mutations and downstream YAP activation in choroidal nevi. Br J Cancer. 2017;117(6):884–7.
47. Metz CH, Scheulen M, Bornfeld N, Lohmann D, Zeschnigk M. Ultradeep sequencing detects GNAQ and GNA11 mutations in cell-free DNA from plasma of patients with uveal melanoma. Cancer Med. 2013;2(2):208–15.
48. Shoushtari AN, Carvajal RD. GNAQ and GNA11 mutations in uveal melanoma. Melanoma Res. 2014;24(6):525–34.
49. Chen X, Wu Q, Depeille P, Chen P, Thornton S, Kalirai H, et al. RasGRP3 mediates MAPK pathway activation in GNAQ mutant uveal melanoma. Cancer Cell. 2017;31(5):685–96.e6.
50. Ambrosini G, Pratilas CA, Qin LX, Tadi M, Surriga O, Carvajal RD, et al. Identification of unique MEK-dependent genes in GNAQ mutant uveal melanoma involved in cell growth, tumor cell invasion, and MEK resistance. Clin Cancer Res. 2012;18(13):3552–61.
51. Amirouchene-Angelozzi N, Frisch-Dit-Leitz E, Carita G, Dahmani A, Raymondie C, Liot G, et al. The mTOR inhibitor Everolimus synergizes with the PI3K inhibitor GDC0941 to enhance anti-tumor efficacy in uveal melanoma. Oncotarget. 2016;7(17):23633–46.
52. Chen X, Wu Q, Tan L, Porter D, Jager MJ, Emery C, et al. Combined PKC and MEK inhibition in uveal melanoma with GNAQ and GNA11 mutations. Oncogene. 2014;33(39):4724–34.
53. Ho AL, Musi E, Ambrosini G, Nair JS, Deraje Vasudeva S, de Stanchina E, et al. Impact of combined mTOR and MEK inhibition in uveal melanoma is driven by tumor genotype. PLoS One. 2012;7(7):e40439.
54. Khalili JS, Yu X, Wang J, Hayes BC, Davies MA, Lizee G, et al. Combination small molecule MEK and PI3K inhibition enhances uveal melanoma cell death in a mutant GNAQ- and GNA11-dependent manner. Clin Cancer Res. 2012;18(16):4345–55.
55. Musi E, Ambrosini G, de Stanchina E, Schwartz GK. The phosphoinositide 3-kinase alpha selective inhibitor BYL719 enhances the effect of the protein kinase C inhibitor AEB071 in GNAQ/GNA11-mutant uveal melanoma cells. Mol Cancer Ther. 2014;13(5):1044–53.
56. Komatsubara KM, Manson DK, Carvajal RD. Selumetinib for the treatment of metastatic uveal melanoma: past and future perspectives. Future Oncol. 2016;12(11):1331–44.
57. Luke JJ, Triozzi PL, McKenna KC, Van Meir EG, Gershenwald JE, Bastian BC, et al. Biology of advanced uveal melanoma and next steps for clinical therapeutics. Pigment Cell Melanoma Res. 2015;28(2):135–47.
58. Feng X, Degese MS, Iglesias-Bartolome R, Vaque JP, Molinolo AA, Rodrigues M, et al. Hippo-independent activation of YAP by the GNAQ uveal melanoma oncogene through a trio-regulated

rho GTPase signaling circuitry. Cancer Cell. 2014;25(6):831–45.
59. Yu FX, Luo J, Mo JS, Liu G, Kim YC, Meng Z, et al. Mutant Gq/11 promote uveal melanoma tumorigenesis by activating YAP. Cancer Cell. 2014;25(6):822–30.
60. Yoo JH, Shi DS, Grossmann AH, Sorensen LK, Tong Z, Mleynek TM, et al. ARF6 is an actionable node that orchestrates oncogenic GNAQ signaling in uveal melanoma. Cancer Cell. 2016;29(6):889–904.
61. Ewens KG, Kanetsky PA, Richards-Yutz J, Purrazzella J, Shields CL, Ganguly T, et al. Chromosome 3 status combined with BAP1 and EIF1AX mutation profiles are associated with metastasis in uveal melanoma. Invest Ophthalmol Vis Sci. 2014;55(8):5160–7.
62. van Essen TH, van Pelt SI, Versluis M, Bronkhorst IH, van Duinen SG, Marinkovic M, et al. Prognostic parameters in uveal melanoma and their association with BAP1 expression. Br J Ophthalmol. 2014;98(12):1738–43.
63. Yavuzyigitoglu S, Mensink HW, Smit KN, Vaarwater J, Verdijk RM, Beverloo B, et al. Metastatic disease in polyploid uveal melanoma patients is associated with BAP1 mutations. Invest Ophthalmol Vis Sci. 2016;57(4):2232–9.
64. Jensen DE, Rauscher FJ 3rd. BAP1, a candidate tumor suppressor protein that interacts with BRCA1. Ann N Y Acad Sci. 1999;886:191–4.
65. Carbone M, Yang H, Pass HI, Krausz T, Testa JR, Gaudino G. BAP1 and cancer. Nat Rev Cancer. 2013;13(3):153–9.
66. Matatall KA, Agapova OA, Onken MD, Worley LA, Bowcock AM, Harbour JW. BAP1 deficiency causes loss of melanocytic cell identity in uveal melanoma. BMC Cancer. 2013;13:371.
67. Koopmans AE, Verdijk RM, Brouwer RW, van den Bosch TP, van den Berg MM, Vaarwater J, et al. Clinical significance of immunohistochemistry for detection of BAP1 mutations in uveal melanoma. Mod Pathol. 2014;27(10):1321–30.
68. Kalirai H, Dodson A, Faqir S, Damato BE, Coupland SE. Lack of BAP1 protein expression in uveal melanoma is associated with increased metastatic risk and has utility in routine prognostic testing. Br J Cancer. 2014;111(7):1373–80.
69. Shah AA, Bourne TD, Murali R. BAP1 protein loss by immunohistochemistry: a potentially useful tool for prognostic prediction in patients with uveal melanoma. Pathology. 2013;45(7):651–6.
70. Szalai E, Wells JR, Ward L, Grossniklaus HE. Uveal melanoma nuclear BRCA1-associated protein-1 immunoreactivity is an indicator of metastasis. Ophthalmology. 2018;125(2):203–9. https://doi.org/10.1016/j.ophtha.2017.07.018.
71. Griewank KG, van de Nes J, Schilling B, Moll I, Sucker A, Kakavand H, et al. Genetic and clinicopathologic analysis of metastatic uveal melanoma. Mod Pathol. 2014;27(2):175–83.
72. McCarthy C, Kalirai H, Lake SL, Dodson A, Damato BE, Coupland SE. Insights into genetic alterations of liver metastases from uveal melanoma. Pigment Cell Melanoma Res. 2016;29(1):60–7.
73. Farquhar N, Thornton S, Coupland S, Coulson J, Sacco J, Krishna Y, et al. Patterns of BAP1 protein expression provide insights into prognostic significance and the biology of uveal melanoma. J Pathol Clin Res. 2017;4(1):26–38.
74. Landreville S, Agapova OA, Matatall KA, Kneass ZT, Onken MD, Lee RS, et al. Histone deacetylase inhibitors induce growth arrest and differentiation in uveal melanoma. Clin Cancer Res. 2012;18(2):408–16.
75. Abdel-Rahman MH, Pilarski R, Cebulla CM, Massengill JB, Christopher BN, Boru G, et al. Germline BAP1 mutation predisposes to uveal melanoma, lung adenocarcinoma, meningioma, and other cancers. J Med Genet. 2011;48(12):856–9.
76. Haugh AM, Njauw CN, Bubley JA, Verzi AE, Zhang B, Kudalkar E, et al. Genotypic and phenotypic features of BAP1 cancer syndrome: a report of 8 new families and review of cases in the literature. JAMA Dermatol. 2017;153(10):999–1006.
77. Testa JR, Cheung M, Pei J, Below JE, Tan Y, Sementino E, et al. Germline BAP1 mutations predispose to malignant mesothelioma. Nat Genet. 2011;43(10):1022–5.
78. Rai K, Pilarski R, Boru G, Rehman M, Saqr AH, Massengill JB, et al. Germline BAP1 alterations in familial uveal melanoma. Genes Chromosomes Cancer. 2017;56(2):168–74.
79. Pilarski R, Cebulla CM, Massengill JB, Rai K, Rich T, Strong L, et al. Expanding the clinical phenotype of hereditary BAP1 cancer predisposition syndrome, reporting three new cases. Genes Chromosomes Cancer. 2014;53(2):177–82.
80. Rai K, Pilarski R, Cebulla CM, Abdel-Rahman MH. Comprehensive review of BAP1 tumor predisposition syndrome with report of two new cases. Clin Genet. 2016;89(3):285–94.
81. Alsafadi S, Houy A, Battistella A, Popova T, Wassef M, Henry E, et al. Cancer-associated SF3B1 mutations affect alternative splicing by promoting alternative branchpoint usage. Nat Commun. 2016;7:10615.
82. Furney SJ, Pedersen M, Gentien D, Dumont AG, Rapinat A, Desjardins L, et al. SF3B1 mutations are associated with alternative splicing in uveal melanoma. Cancer Discov. 2013;3(10):1122–9.
83. Johnson CP, Kim IK, Esmaeli B, Amin-Mansour A, Treacy DJ, Carter SL, et al. Systematic genomic and translational efficiency studies of uveal melanoma. PLoS One. 2017;12(6):e0178189.
84. Johansson P, Aoude LG, Wadt K, Glasson WJ, Warrier SK, Hewitt AW, et al. Deep sequencing of uveal melanoma identifies a recurrent mutation in PLCB4. Oncotarget. 2016;7(4):4624–31.
85. Moore AR, Ceraudo E, Sher JJ, Guan Y, Shoushtari AN, Chang MT, et al. Recurrent activating mutations

of G-protein-coupled receptor CYSLTR2 in uveal melanoma. Nat Genet. 2016;48(6):675–80.
86. Ehlers JP, Worley L, Onken MD, Harbour JW. DDEF1 is located in an amplified region of chromosome 8q and is overexpressed in uveal melanoma. Clin Cancer Res. 2005;11(10):3609–13.
87. Laurent C, Valet F, Planque N, Silveri L, Maacha S, Anezo O, et al. High PTP4A3 phosphatase expression correlates with metastatic risk in uveal melanoma patients. Cancer Res. 2011;71(3):666–74.
88. Worley LA, Long MD, Onken MD, Harbour JW. Micro-RNAs associated with metastasis in uveal melanoma identified by multiplexed microarray profiling. Melanoma Res. 2008;18(3):184–90.
89. Radhakrishnan A, Badhrinarayanan N, Biswas J, Krishnakumar S. Analysis of chromosomal aberration (1, 3, and 8) and association of microRNAs in uveal melanoma. Mol Vis. 2009;15:2146–54.
90. Ling JW, Lu PR, Zhang YB, Jiang S, Zhang ZC. miR-367 promotes uveal melanoma cell proliferation and migration by regulating PTEN. Genet Mol Res. 2017;16:3. https://doi.org/10.4238/gmr16039067.
91. Venkatesan N, Kanwar J, Deepa PR, Khetan V, Crowley TM, Raguraman R, et al. Clinicopathological association of delineated miRNAs in uveal melanoma with monosomy 3/disomy 3 chromosomal aberrations. PLoS One. 2016;11(1):e0146128.
92. Zhou J, Jiang J, Wang S, Xia X. Oncogenic role of microRNA20a in human uveal melanoma. Mol Med Rep. 2016;14(2):1560–6.
93. Yan D, Zhou X, Chen X, Hu DN, Dong XD, Wang J, et al. MicroRNA-34a inhibits uveal melanoma cell proliferation and migration through downregulation of c-Met. Invest Ophthalmol Vis Sci. 2009;50(4):1559–65.
94. Chen X, Wang J, Shen H, Lu J, Li C, Hu DN, et al. Epigenetics, microRNAs, and carcinogenesis: functional role of microRNA-137 in uveal melanoma. Invest Ophthalmol Vis Sci. 2011;52(3):1193–9.
95. Ma YB, Song DW, Nie RH, Mu GY, Yoo JH, Shi DS, et al. MicroRNA-32 functions as a tumor suppressor and directly targets EZH2 in uveal melanoma. Genet Mol Res. 2016;15(2):889–904.
96. Lu L, Yu X, Zhang L, Ding X, Pan H, Wen X, et al. The long non-coding RNA RHPN1-AS1 promotes uveal melanoma progression. Int J Mol Sci. 2017;18(1):pii: E226. https://doi.org/10.3390/ijms18010226.
97. Maat W, van der Velden PA, Out-Luiting C, Plug M, Dirks-Mulder A, Jager MJ, et al. Epigenetic inactivation of RASSF1a in uveal melanoma. Invest Ophthalmol Vis Sci. 2007;48(2):486–90.
98. Mobuchon L, Battistella A, Bardel C, Scelo G, Renoud A, Houy A, et al. A GWAS in uveal melanoma identifies risk polymorphisms in the CLPTM1L locus. NPJ Genom Med. 2017;2:pii: 5. https://doi.org/10.1038/s41525-017-0008-5.
99. Krishna Y, McCarthy C, Kalirai H, Coupland SE. Inflammatory cell infiltrates in advanced metastatic uveal melanoma. Hum Pathol. 2017;66:159–66.
100. Singh AD, Tubbs R, Biscotti C, Schoenfield L, Trizzoi P. Chromosomal 3 and 8 status within hepatic metastasis of uveal melanoma. Arch Pathol Lab Med. 2009;133(8):1223–7.
101. Trolet J, Hupe P, Huon I, Lebigot I, Decraene C, Delattre O, et al. Genomic profiling and identification of high-risk uveal melanoma by array CGH analysis of primary tumors and liver metastases. Invest Ophthalmol Vis Sci. 2009;50(6):2572–80.
102. Luscan A, Just PA, Briand A, Burin des Roziers C, Goussard P, Nitschke P, et al. Uveal melanoma hepatic metastases mutation spectrum analysis using targeted next-generation sequencing of 400 cancer genes. Br J Ophthalmol. 2015;99(4):437–9.
103. Meir T, Dror R, Yu X, Qian J, Simon I, Pe'er J, et al. Molecular characteristics of liver metastases from uveal melanoma. Invest Ophthalmol Vis Sci. 2007;48(11):4890–6.

Choroidal Melanoma: Clinical Trials and What Have We Learned from Them

8

Sidharth Puri and Aparna Ramasubramanian

The last decade has seen a paradigm shift in oncology care, especially with respect to clinical trial design. This has ensured quick translation of biological knowledge to clinical practice [1]. Uveal melanoma is the most common primary intraocular tumor with an estimated annual incidence between 4.3 and 8.6 cases per one million in the Western world [2]. The current management and understanding of choroidal melanoma have benefitted greatly from well conducted research and clinical trials. In this chapter, we will review the impact of clinical trials and how they have influenced the current management of choroidal melanoma.

8.1 Risk Factors

Several risk factors have been implicated with uveal melanomas, most notably host factors [3, 4].

Weis and Shah (2005) conducted a meta-analysis of patients with uveal melanoma and ultraviolet light exposure looking at 133 published reports and suggested welding as a risk factor [3]. Their meta-analysis yielded inconsistent results associating ultraviolet light with development of uveal melanoma. It has been suggested that chronic occupational sunlight exposure non-significantly increases the risk of uveal melanoma.

Another meta-analysis by Weis and Shah (2006) showed strong evidence associating the host susceptibility factors of iris color, skin color, and ability to tan with uveal melanoma [4].

8.2 Pathogenesis

Uveal melanomas have been characterized by numerous genetic mutations. While cutaneous melanomas are associated with mutations in BRAF, uveal melanomas are associated with somatic mutations in GNAQ and GNA11. GNAQ and GNA11 are genes that code for the α-subunit of G proteins that act with G protein coupled receptors [5]. Uveal melanoma samples had 83% rate of mutations in GNAQ/GNA11 [6–8]. These mutations result in a persistently active Gα-subunit.

Activation of Gα results in upregulation of MAPK, PI3K-Akt-mTOR, and Hippo pathways [5]. These downstream pathways are associated with cell proliferation regulation and have been implicated in uveal melanomas.

Additional genes have been found to affect uveal melanoma. BAP1 is a nuclear deubiquitinase on chromosome 3p that acts as a tumor suppressor [5]. Mutations in BAP1 inactivate the gene and have been found in primary uveal melanomas (47%) and metastatic melanomas (84%). SF3B1 is a gene that encodes splicing factor 3B

S. Puri · A. Ramasubramanian (✉)
Kentucky Lions Eye Center, University of Louisville, Louisville, KY, USA
e-mail: aparna.ramasubramanian@louisville.edu

V. Khetan (ed.), *Intraocular Tumors*, https://doi.org/10.1007/978-981-15-0395-5_8

subunit1. Mutations in this gene have been associated with improved prognosis and features of younger age, fewer undifferentiated cells, and disomy 3. EIF1AX mutations are associated with disomy 3 and are less frequently associated with metastases. Immune checkpoint inhibitors have shown efficacy in many tumors, including cutaneous melanoma, and further research could lead to better treatment for metastatic uveal melanoma involving the mutations described.

8.3 Collaborative Ocular Melanoma Study

The Collaborative Ocular Melanoma Study (COMS) was a National Eye Institute funded study that commenced in 1985. The COMS predominantly consisted of 2 multicenter clinical trials to compare treatment outcomes in medium and large choroidal melanoma and also to assess the natural history in small choroidal melanoma. The findings of the COMS are detailed as follows:

- *Small Choroidal Melanoma*—Diameter of 5–16 mm and 1.5–2.4 mm height. These patients were enrolled in a clinical registry and monitored.
- *Medium Choroidal Melanoma*—Diameter ≤16 mm and 2.5–10 mm height. These patients were randomized to either enucleation or Plaque brachytherapy with Iodine-125.
- *Large Choroidal Melanoma*—Diameter >16 mm and >10 mm apical height. Patients with large choroidal melanoma were randomized to external beam radiation (20 Gy) after enucleation or enucleation alone.

8.3.1 Main Results

- *Small Choroidal Melanoma*—204 patients were enrolled in the registry and median follow up was 92 months. 75% patients were treated and 6 deaths were reported due to metastatic melanoma.
- *Medium Choroidal Melanoma*—Total 1317 patients were enrolled. There was no statistically significant difference in mortality between the enucleation and the brachytherapy group.
- *Large Choroidal Melanoma*—Total 1003 patients were enrolled in this trial. Patients that received pre-enucleation radiation did not show a statistically significant 5-year mortality benefit. In this study the 5-year mortality related mortality was 27%.

8.3.2 Additional Information Obtained from COMS by Report Numbers

1. *Report # 1—Accuracy of Diagnosis*—The Collaborative Ocular Melanoma Study misdiagnosis rate was 0.48%, emphasizing that the challenge in choroidal melanoma is optimizing treatment and not determining correct diagnosis [9].
2. *Report # 2—Enucleation Complication*—The COMS included 981 eyes that were enucleated and there were no perioperative deaths and no accidental ruptures of the globe [10]. Unanticipated extrascleral extension was found in 1.5% and overall complication rate was 2.8%.
3. *Report # 3—Trial for an uncommon disease*—This report discussed the formulation and conduct of trials for an uncommon disease like choroidal melanoma [11]. The COMS recruited very good number in spite of being a rare condition.
4. *Report # 4—Mortality for small melanoma*—Of the 204 patients followed with small melanoma, 6 deaths were reported by the clinical center as due to metastatic melanoma [12]. The Kaplan-Meier estimate of 5-year all-cause mortality was 6.0%.
5. *Report # 5—Small Melanoma Growth Predictors*—Of all small choroidal melanomas that were subjected to observation, 21% demonstrated growth at 2 years and at 5 years 31% had documented growth [13]. As per

the COMS report, factors significantly associated with growth were greater initial tumor thickness and diameter, presence of orange pigment, absence of drusen, and absence of areas of retinal pigment epithelial changes adjacent to the tumor.

6. *Report # 6—Histopathologic characteristics*—In choroidal melanomas, the most common cell type was mixed cell (86%) followed by spindle cell (9%) and epitheloid cell (5%) [14]. Overall, 81.1% on histopathological examination showed local invasion, scleral invasion was present in 55.7% of eyes, and extrascleral extension was visible in 8.2%.
7. *Report # 7—Sociodemographic and Clinical Predictors of Participation*—The variables that were significantly predictive of enrollment were older age, residence in the same state as the trial, larger tumor basal diameter, and worse initial visual acuity in the study eye [15]. This report is useful not only for uveal melanoma but also understanding patient willingness to enroll in any clinical trial.
8. *Report # 8—Clear cell differentiation*—Two patients on histopathology showed clear cell features and the cytoplasm contained scattered glycogen granules, premelanosomes, and melanosomes [16]. These can be misdiagnosed as metastatic clear cell carcinoma to the choroid.
9. *Report # 9—External Validity Large Tumors*—Eligible patients who enrolled in the trial were similar to eligible patients who did not enroll with respect to most factors considered and hence the results of the COMS large melanoma study can be generalized to all patients [17].
10. *Report # 10—Mortality in large choroidal melanoma*—There was no survival difference attributable to pre-enucleation radiation of large choroidal melanoma [18].
11. *Report # 11—Complications of treatment of large choroidal melanoma*—Complications were infrequent (early pain and later poor prosthetic mobility being most common) during the 5-year period following enucleation surgery [19]. There was no indication that pre-enucleation radiation had resulted in more serious complications.
12. *Report # 12—Ultrasound characteristics in the COMS study* [20].
13. *Report # 13—Ultrasonography consistency*—The COMS Echography Center demonstrated that its grading protocol is consistent over time [21].
14. *Report # 14—Cause Specific Mortality Coding*—As in all clinical trials, accurate reporting of cause-specific mortality in patients is difficult. In the COMS study also death certificates underestimated the proportion of deaths due to metastatic choroidal melanoma [22].
15. *Report # 15—Metastatic Status at the time of death*—There were 1003 patients that were enrolled in the large melanoma subgroup and of these 457 patients died during the study monitoring with an estimated median survival (from time of enrollment) of 7.4 years [23]. Of all the deaths 62% (269 patients) had histopathologically confirmed melanoma metastasis at the time of death, and an additional 215 (92 patients) had suspected based on imaging and tests but without pathological confirmation. Multiple sites of metastasis was identified in 87% of patients. The most common site of metastasis as liver (93%) followed by lung (24%), and bone (16%).
16. *Report # 16—Visual acuity after brachytherapy for medium tumors*—Vision loss is one of the most common side effect from brachytherapy and after 3 years of treatment 43% of patients had vision of 20/200 or worse and 49% of eyes had lost 6 or more lines of visual acuity from the pretreatment level [24]. The predictors of poor vision included history of diabetes, thicker tumors, tumors close to or beneath the FAZ, tumor-associated retinal detachment, or tumors that were not dome shaped [24].
17. *Report # 17—External Validity Medium Tumors*—This report was conceived to document that the enrolled patients in the trial depicted the patients in routine clinical practice that are treated with brachytherapy [25].

18. *Report # 18—Mortality Rates in Medium Tumors*—In the medium size tumor group, after a follow up of 12 years the mortality was same in the enucleation group and the brachytherapy group. The five-year rates of melanoma related death were 11% and 9% following enucleation and brachytherapy [26].
19. *Report # 19—Predictors of treatment failure after Brachytherapy*—Of the 638 patients that were followed after brachytherapy, 11% were enucleated and 9% had documented treatment failure [27]. The most common risk factors for treatment failure were older age, greater tumor thickness and proximity of the tumor to the foveal avascular zone. Treatment failure accounted for most enucleation in the first 3 years of life and after 3 years the most common cause was ocular pain.
20. *Report # 20—Time trends in tumor size*—This COMS report analyzed the management trends over 10 years and found that the more recent tumors are smaller in size and enucleation is employed less for tumors with less than 15 mm basal diameter. Enucleation is reserved more for larger tumors greater than 15 mm [28].
21. *Report # 21—Comparison of clinical and histopathological measurements*—The clinical measurement was less than the histopathological measurement by more than 2 mm in 32 eyes (5%), which occurred more frequently when the tumor was within 2 mm of the optic disc [29]. The echographic and histopathological measurements of apical height agreed within ±2 mm in 579 eyes (90%). This report indicated that the ultrasonographic measurements are accurate for brachytherapy planning.
22. *Report # 22—Fellow eye changes after treatment*—There was no evidence that fellow eyes of patients whose affected eye was treated with pre-enucleation radiation or with brachytherapy were at greater risk of loss of vision or new ophthalmic diagnoses than eyes of patients treated with enucleation alone [30].
23. *Report # 23—Screening for metastasis*—COMS patients were screened annually for metastasis and new cancers using liver function test (alkaline phosphatase, AST, ALT, or bilirubin) [31]. Elevated findings (1.5–2 times upper limit of normal) prompted a diagnostic or imaging test to confirm or rule out cancer recurrence. Use of liver function test has high specificity (92%) and predictive values (46%) but low sensitivity (15%).
24. *Report # 24—Mortality at 10 years in the large choroidal melanoma study*—On longer follow up of the large melanoma group it was confirmed that pre-enucleation radiation did not confer any survival advantage. Ten year all-cause mortality was 61% for the enucleation only group and the pre-enucleation radiation group. Melanoma related death was also not difference in the two arms (45% in the pre-enucleation radiation arm and 40% in the enucleation alone arm) [32].
25. *Report # 25—Second Primary Cancer*—The most common second primary cancer was prostate (23%) followed by breast (17%). Prior radiation did not increase the occurrence of second cancer. Excluding basal or squamous cell skin cancer, the 5 year rate of a second primary cancer was 7.7% [33]. Routine medical surveillance is warranted, especially for those with a history of smoking.
26. *Report # 26—Metastatic Characteristics*—Patients with choroidal melanoma had a metastasis rate of 25% at 5 years and 34% at 10 years. [34] Most common metastatic site was liver (89%). Survival after metastasis was poor with a death rate of 80% at 1 year and 92% at 2 years.
27. *Report # 27—Cataract after Brachytherapy*—By 5 years, 83% of study eyes were reported to have a cataract and 12% had undergone cataract surgery in the study eye [35]. As expected the rates of cataract surgery increased with the radiation dosage to the lens. Eighteen percentage of eyes that received higher than 24 Gy radiation required cataract surgery. Only 4% of eyes that received less than 12 Gy underwent cataract surgery. The median visual acuity improved from 20/125 before cataract to

20/50 after cataract surgery. The most common cause of lack of visual improvement after cataract surgery was presence of radiation retinopathy.

28. *Report # 28—Long term mortality after brachytherapy*—Mortality rates were not different in the brachytherapy arm (43%) versus the enucleation arm (41%) [36]. The primary predictors of time to death were older age and larger maximum basal tumor diameter.

8.3.3 Quality of Life Reports from the COMS

The COMS report studied the difference in quality of life between the plaque brachytherapy group and the enucleation group. Until 2 years the brachytherapy group reported better visual function (peripheral vision for driving) and that difference was negated by 3–5 years [37]. The COMS study did document that patients who underwent plaque brachytherapy noted more symptoms of anxiety compared to the enucleation group.

8.4 Treatment

From enucleation to more conservative, globe-saving methods, the management and treatment of choroidal melanomas have evolved over recent decades. For moderately sized tumors, the COMS demonstrated that enucleation versus plaque brachytherapy resulted in similar outcomes for patients [26]. In addition to these techniques, other modalities include transpupillary thermotherapy (TTT), proton beam radiotherapy, photocoagulation therapy and internal resection.

8.4.1 Transpupillary Thermotherapy

Mashayekhi et al. (2015) investigated the outcomes of primary TTT upon choroidal melanomas [38]. At 10-year follow up, there was a 42% chance of tumor recurrence in patients who underwent primary TTT. Tumor recurrence was associated with several high-risk features, including ocular symptoms (decreased visual acuity), presence of subretinal fluid, tumor thickness, elevation of residual tumor scar after treatment, and proximity of tumor to optic disc. It was noted that a higher number of high risk tumor features was associated with greater recurrence, e.g. 3–5 factors at 35% risk and 6–7 factors at 55% risk. Further, additional TTT after recurrence still resulted in a 50% probability of tumor recurrence.

When used in conjunction with plaque radiotherapy, TTT may prove useful. In particular for juxtapapillary melanomas, plaque radiotherapy with TTT demonstrated a slight but nonsignificant improvement in local tumor control and reduced metastatic rates [39].

8.4.2 Proton Beam Radiotherapy

Proton beam radiotherapy has emerged as an alternative, globe-salvaging treatment for choroidal melanoma. Dendale et al. (2005) observed that 5-year overall survival and metastasis-free survival were 79% and 80.6%, respectively [40]. Risk factors for local tumor recurrence were increased tumor diameter and greater macular area receiving more than 30 CGE (cobalt Gray equivalent). The 5-year enucleation for complications rate was 7.7%. Those at risk for enucleation were associated with tumor thickness and lens volume receiving at least 30 CGE.

8.4.3 Transscleral Resection

Transscleral resection (TSR) can serve as a possible surgical treatment for uveal melanomas [41]. TSR was first reported in the 1960s by Stallard and Muller and may be an appropriate surgical treatment for patients ineligible for plaque brachytherapy, proton beam irradiation, or for those wishing to retain their eye. For TSR, 5- and 10-year recurrence rates have been reported at 24% and 32%, respectively. Local recurrence was associated with large tumor base diameter greater than 16 mm, absence of adjuvant plaque brachytherapy, and retinal detachment. Metastasis rates following TSR at 5- and 10-year were 28% and 44%, respectively. While TSR may also carry a heightened risk of metastasis at 5- and 10-years (28%, and 44% respectively), possible pre-operative proton beam radiotherapy may aid in improving recurrence and survival [41].

8.4.4 Minimizing Radiation Retinopathy

Radiotherapy for choroidal melanoma has been associated with increased retinal ischemic drive and VEGF production [42]. Radiation maculopathy is a serious complication of radiotherapy. OCT-evident macular edema may be detected as early as 4 months after radiotherapy. Prophylactic intravitreal bevacuzimab injections were found to reduce the radiation-related macular edema. In a study by Shah et al. (2014), bevacuzimab injection at time of plaque removal and every 4 months thereafter for two years was associated with a significant reduction in radiation-related macular edema and improved visual outcomes [42].

8.4.5 Fine Needle Aspiration Biopsy for Cytogenetics

Fine needle aspiration biopsy (FNAB) can aid in the diagnosis and prognosis of uveal melanomas [43]. Singh et al. (2016) investigated the utility of FNAB of uveal melanoma with 25 gauge needle. FNAB was found to have a 92% positive diagnostic and 84% prognostic yield. The study demonstrated the safety and efficacy of FNAB in establishing the diagnosis and prognosis of uveal melanomas.

8.5 Cytogenetics

Cytogenetic analysis has allowed for a greater understanding of uveal melanoma prognosis. Immunotherapies are currently under investigation to guide specific treatment of uveal melanomas.

8.5.1 Chromosome 3

The most significant chromosomal abnormality associated with uveal melanomas is a full or partial loss of chromosome 3 (monosomy 3) [44]. Monosomy 3 demonstrates the strongest association with metastasis and decreased survival. Other chromosomal abnormalities associated with uveal melanomas are chromosome 1p, 6q, 8q.

8.5.2 Gene Profile Assay

The COOG (Collaborative Ocular Oncology Group) multicenter study established the superiority of gene expression profile (GEP) classification in determining uveal melanoma prognosis. GEP signaling and molecular signatures of RNA expression have helped categorize uveal melanoma (UM) into class 1 (low metastatic risk) and class 2 (high metastatic risk) [45]. The 15 gene incorporated assay utilizes PCR to quantify mRNA of key genes obtained from enucleation sample or fine needle aspiration biopsy samples. The COOG study demonstrated that the GEP assay successfully classified 97.2% of cases. The GEP was class 1 in 62% and class 2 38.1% of cases. At mean 18 month follow up, metastasis was detected in 1% of class 1 cases and 26% of class 2 cases.

Further, the only significant factor that enhanced the accuracy of the GEP classification was found to be largest basal tumor diameter (LBD). The 5-year metastasis-free survival estimates were [46]

- Class 1, basal diameter <12 mm—97%
- Class 1, basal diameter ≥12 mm—90%
- Class 2, basal diameter <12 mm—90%
- Class 2, basal diameter ≥12 mm—30%

The response to treatment also varied based on the gene profile. Class 1 UM tumors tend to regress more rapidly than class 2 tumors in the first 6 months after plaque radiotherapy. Class 1A and 1B tumors regress at similar rates after plaque radiotherapy [47].

8.5.3 Newer Markers

Several new markers have been investigated for determining uveal melanoma prognosis.

The cancer-testis antigen PRAME (preferentially expressed antigen of melanoma) has been found to be expressed in several malignancies, including uveal melanoma [48]. PRAME was found to be expressed in 45% of primary uveal melanomas and both PRAME and HLA class 1 were expressed in 50% of uveal metastases. PRAME-specific T cells can target PRAME positive uveal melanomas. Through PRAME T cell receptor (TCR) gene therapy, T cell-directed immunotherapy may serve as a novel and effective means by which to target uveal melanomas.

In addition to GEP and PRAME, five particular genes have been found to also be associated with uveal melanoma: GNAQ, GNA11, BAP1, SF3B1, and EIF1AX. BAP1 was associated with higher risk of metastasis and poor prognostic factors (class 2 and older age) [49]. EIF1AX and SF3B1 were associated with better prognosis factors (EIF1AX with class 1 GEP and SF3B1 with younger age). GNAQ and GNA11 were not associated with prognosis. By further understanding the relationships between specific mutations and uveal melanoma prognosis, targeted therapies may be developed to improve patient outcomes.

8.6 Metastatic Melanoma

8.6.1 Prognosis

The Helsinki University Hospital Working Formulation was developed for staging uveal melanoma [50]. Three prognostic variables for metastasis were used to establish this model: performance index (patient overall health), largest diameter of the largest metastasis, and serum alkaline phosphatase (evaluation of hepatic function). The model divides newly diagnosed metastatic uveal melanoma into 3 prognostic stages with a predicted median overall survival of either >12 months (IVa), <12 to 6 months (IVb), or <6 months (IVc). The work by Kivelä et al. (2016) validated the Working Formulation as a reliable tool to categorize prognosis of metastatic uveal melanoma.

8.6.2 Adjuvant Therapy for High Risk Patients

Uveal melanomas typically have demonstrated resistance to adjuvant chemotherapy [51]. Systemic adjuvant use of dacarbazine, an intravenous alkylating agent, for uveal melanoma did not demonstrate any improvement in survival outcomes. Adjuvant interferon has not been shown to improve overall survival. Several novel cytotoxic, immunomodulatory, and targeted compounds are being investigated in the metastatic setting, alone and in combinations, which may be applicable to the adjuvant setting. Also several immune check point agents are currently being investigated.

8.6.3 Treatment

The evolution of our understanding of uveal melanoma tumorigenesis has created increased possibilities for targeted therapies. There have been numerous recent and ongoing investigations into specific systemic therapies for uveal melanoma.

Targeted therapies have investigated particular genes on chromosome 3, in particular BAP1 [52, 53]. BAP1 is located on chromosome 3p21.1 and is a tumor suppressor gene that encodes histone H2A ubiquitin hydrolase. Mutations resulting in loss of function or silencing of BAP1 have been implicated in class 2 uveal melanoma and poor survival. Currently, there has been increased interest into histone deactylase (HDAC) inhibitors to target the downstream effects of absent BAP1 in uveal melanoma.

As referred to prior, GNAQ and GNA11 somatic mutations have been implicated in uveal melanoma [52]. In the presence of these mutations, the MAPK (mitogen-activated protein kinase) pathway is upregulated in uveal melanoma tumors and liver metastases. Protein kinase C (PKC) plays a critical role in this pathway and has served as a therapy target. PKC inhibitors, such as AEB071 or AHT956, have shown increased apoptosis and tumor reduction in uveal melanoma cell lines with GNAQ or GNA11 mutations. In a phase II multicenter trial, PKC inhibitor selumetinib demonstrated successful tumor shrinking and survival compared to chemotherapy. Further work to target the MAPK pathway may reveal not only enhanced ways to control uveal melanoma, but also insight into the complex pathways that promote tumorigenesis.

Uveal melanoma upregulation of IGF-1 receptor (IGF-1R) may also serve as a targeted therapy modality [52]. IGF-1 signaling can induce cell migration and invasion. The liver has been demonstrated to produce IGF-1 and may promote an environment conducive to high rates of metastasis. Current studies into IGF-IR inhibitors, such as cyclolignan picropodophyllin, has shown in human UM-derived cell lines to reduce tumor cell proliferation, invasion, and migration. Research into cixutumamab, a monoclonal antibody against IGF-IR, has shown merit in its reduction of UM cell migration.

While anti-VEGF therapies have developed an expanded role in ophthalmology, their role in targeting angiogenesis in the tumors remains critical. Currently, bevacizumab with temozolaomide (phase II) and ranibiuzimab with proton beam irradiation (phase I) are currently under investigation [52]. Sunitinib is also a potential therapy, with inhibition of VEGF, platelet-derived growth factor receptor (PDGFR), c-KIT, FMS-like tyrosine kinase 3 (FLT-3) and RET.

Further work into immunotherapy has provided additional insight into treatment of uveal melanoma. Ipilimumab is a CTLA4 inhibitor that has gained greater attention recently for its role in targeting uveal melanomas [52]. The GEM1 study suggested an improved disease control rate and survival rate with use of ipilimumab monotherapy.

Nivolumab and pembrolizumab are monoclonal antibodies against PD-1, a co-inhibitor receptor that decreases anti-tumor activity of T cells [52]. Currently there are phase II trials investigating the role of pembrolizumab in patients with metastatic uveal melanoma.

These numerous, novel systemic targeted therapies highlight the advances in our understanding of uveal tumor biology.

The management and treatment of uveal melanomas is evolving rapidly. Improved diagnostic and prognostic measures, such as gene expression assays, can aid in early detection of uveal melanoma and improve survival outcomes. Novel therapeutic strategies through targeted therapy can help ophthalmologists effectively counsel and provide appropriate treatment to improve morbidity and mortality. Extensive clinical trials will continue to help shape the way in which we understand and treat uveal melanomas over decades to come.

Acknowledgements No financial interest associated with manuscript

- "This work was supported in part by an unrestricted institutional grant from Research to Prevent Blindness, NY, NY."

References

1. Sargent DJ, Korn EL. Decade in review—clinical trials: shifting paradigms in cancer clinical trial design. Nat Rev Clin Oncol. 2014;11:625–6.
2. McLaughlin CC, Wu XC, Jemal A, et al. Incidence of noncutaneous melanomas in the U.S. Cancer. 2005;103(5):1000–7.
3. Shah CP, Weis E, Lajous M, et al. Intermittent and chronic ultraviolet light exposure and uveal melanoma: a meta-analysis. Ophthalmology. 2005;112(9):1599–607.
4. Weis E, Shah CP, Lajous M, et al. The association between host susceptibility factors and uveal melanoma: a meta-analysis. Arch Ophthalmol. 2006;124(1):54–60.
5. Krantz BA, Dave N, Komatsubara KM, Marr BP, Carvajal RD. Uveal melanoma: epidemiology, etiology, and treatment of primary disease. Clin Ophthalmol. 2017;11:279–89.
6. Van Raamsdonk CD, Bezrookove V, Green G, et al. Frequent somatic mutations of GNAQ in uveal melanoma and blue naevi. Nature. 2009;457(7229):599–602.

7. Van Raamsdonk CD, Griewank KG, Crosby MB, et al. Mutations in GNA11 in uveal melanoma. N Engl J Med. 2010;363(23):2191–9.
8. Shoushtari AN, Carvajal RD. GNAQ and GNA11 mutations in uveal melanoma. Melanoma Res. 2014;24(6):525–34.
9. Collaborative Ocular Melanoma Study Group. Accuracy of diagnosis of choroidal melanomas in the Collaborative Ocular Melanoma Study. Arch Ophthalmol. 1990;108:1268–73.
10. Collaborative Ocular Melanoma Study Group. Complications of enucleation surgery. COMS report no. 2. In: Franklin RM, editor. Proceedings of the symposium on retina and vitreous, New Orleans Academy of Ophthalmology. New York: Kugler Publications; 1993. p. 181–90.
11. Collaborative Ocular Melanoma Study Group. Design and methods of a clinical trial for a rare condition: the collaborative ocular melanoma study. COMS report no. 3. Control Clin Trials. 1993;14:362–91.
12. Collaborative Ocular Melanoma Study Group. Mortality in patients with small choroidal melanoma. COMS report no. 4. Arch Ophthalmol. 1997;115:886–93.
13. Collaborative Ocular Melanoma Study Group. Factors predictive of growth and treatment of small choroidal melanoma. COMS report no. 5. Arch Ophthalmol. 1997;115:1537–44.
14. Collaborative Ocular Melanoma Study Group. Histopathologic characteristics of uveal melanomas in eyes enucleated from the Collaborative Ocular Melanoma Study. COMS report no. 6. Am J Ophthalmol. 1998;125:745–66.
15. Collaborative Ocular Melanoma Study Group. Sociodemographic and clinical predictors of participation in two randomized trials: findings from the Collaborative Ocular Melanoma Study. COMS report no. 7. Control Clin Trials. 2001;22:526–37.
16. Grossniklaus HE, Albert DM, Green WR, Conway BP, Hovland KR. Clear cell differentiation in choroidal melanoma. COMS report no. 8. Collaborative Ocular Melanoma Study Group. Arch Ophthalmol. 1997;115:894–8.
17. Collaborative Ocular Melanoma Study Group. The Collaborative Ocular Melanoma Study (COMS) randomized trial of pre-enucleation radiation of large choroidal melanoma. I: characteristics of patients enrolled and not enrolled. COMS report no. 9. Am J Ophthalmol. 1998;125:767–78.
18. Collaborative Ocular Melanoma Study Group. The Collaborative Ocular Melanoma Study (COMS) randomized trial of pre-enucleation radiation of large choroidal melanoma. II. Initial mortality findings. COMS report no. 10. Am J Ophthalmol. 1998;125:779–96.
19. Collaborative Ocular Melanoma Study Group. The Collaborative Ocular Melanoma Study (COMS) randomized trial of pre-enucleation radiation of large choroidal melanoma. III. Local complications and observations following enucleation. COMS Report No. 11. Am J Ophthalmol. 1998;126:362–72.
20. Collaborative Ocular Melanoma Study Group, et al. J Ophthalmic Nurs Technol. 1999;18(4):143–9, Part II, 18(5):219-232
21. Collaborative Ocular Melanoma Study Group. Consistency of observations from echograms made centrally in the Collaborative Ocular Melanoma Study. COMS report no. 13. Ophthalmic Epidemiol. 2002;9:11–27.
22. Collaborative Ocular Melanoma Study Group. Cause-specific mortality coding: methods in the Collaborative Ocular Melanoma Study. COMS report no. 14. Control Clin Trials. 2001;22:248–62.
23. Collaborative Ocular Melanoma Study Group. Assessment of metastatic disease status at death in 435 patients with large choroidal melanoma in the Collaborative Ocular Melanoma Study. COMS report no. 15. Arch Ophthalmol. 2001;119:670–6.
24. Collaborative Ocular Melanoma Study Group. Collaborative Ocular Melanoma Study (COMS) randomized trial of I-125 brachytherapy for medium choroidal melanoma. I. Visual acuity after 3 years. COMS report no. 16. Ophthalmology. 2001;108(2):348–66.
25. Collaborative Ocular Melanoma Study Group. The COMS randomized trial of iodine 125 brachytherapy for choroidal melanoma. II. Characteristics of patients enrolled and not enrolled. COMS report no. 17. Arch Ophthalmol. 2001;119:951–65.
26. Collaborative Ocular Melanoma Study Group. The COMS randomized trial of iodine 125 brachytherapy for choroidal melanoma. III. Initial mortality findings. COMS report no. 18. Arch Ophthalmol. 2001;119:969–82.
27. Collaborative Ocular Melanoma Study Group. The COMS randomized trial of iodine 125 brachytherapy for choroidal melanoma. Local treatment failure and enucleation in the first 5 years after brachytherapy. COMS report no. 19. Ophthalmology. 2002;198:2197–206.
28. Collaborative Ocular Melanoma Study Group. Trends in size and treatment of recently diagnosed choroidal melanoma, 1987-1997. Findings from patients evaluated at Collaborative Ocular Melanoma Study centers. COMS report no. 20. Arch Ophthalmol. 2003;121:1156–62.
29. Collaborative Ocular Melanoma Study Group. Comparison of clinical, echographic, and histologic measurements from eyes with medium-sized choroidal melanoma in the Collaborative Ocular Melanoma Study. COMS report no. 21. Arch Opthalmol. 2003;121:1163–71.
30. Collaborative Ocular Melanoma Study Group. Ten-year follow-up of fellow eyes of patients enrolled in Collaborative Ocular Melanoma Study (COMS) randomized trials. COMS report no. 22. Ophthalmology. 2004;111:996–76.
31. Diener-West M, Reynolds SM, Agugliaro DJ, Caldwell R, et al. Screening for metastasis from choroidal melanoma: experience of the Collaborative Ocular Melanoma Study. Collaborative Ocular

Melanoma Study report no. 23. Am J Clin Oncol. 2004;22:2438–44.
32. Collaborative Ocular Melanoma Study Group. The Collaborative Ocular Melanoma Study (COMS) randomized trial of pre-enucleation radiation of large choroidal melanoma. IV. Ten-year mortality findings and prognostic factors. COMS report no. 24. Am J Ophthalmol. 2004;138:936–51.
33. Collaborative Ocular Melanoma Study Group. Second primary cancers after enrollment in the COMS trials for treatment of choroidal melanoma. COMS report no. 25. Arch Ophthalmol. 2005;123:601–4.
34. Collaborative Ocular Melanoma Study Group. Development of metastatic disease after enrollment in the COMS trials for treatment of choroidal melanoma. Collaborative Ocular Melanoma Study Group report no. 26. Arch Ophthalmol. 2005;123:1639–43.
35. Collaborative Ocular Melanoma Study Group. Incidence of cataract and outcomes after cataract surgery in the first 5 years after 125I brachytherapy in the COMS. COMS report no. 27. Ophthalmology. 2007;114:1363.
36. Collaborative Ocular Melanoma Study Group. The COMS randomized trial of iodine 125 brachytherapy for choroidal melanoma. V. Twelve-year mortality rates and prognostic factors. COMS report no. 28. Arch Ophthalmol. 2006;124:1684–93.
37. Collaborative Ocular Melanoma Study -- Quality of Life Study Group. Quality of life after iodine 125 brachytherapy versus enucleation for choroidal melanoma: 5-year results from the Collaborative Ocular Melanoma Study prospective study. COMS-QOLS report no. 3. Arch Ophthalmol. 2006;124:226–38.
38. Mashayekhi A, Shields CL, Rishi P, et al. Primary transpupillary thermotherapy for choroidal melanoma in 391 cases: importance of risk factors in tumor control. Ophthalmology. 2015;122(3):600–9.
39. Sagoo MS, Shields CL, Mashayekhi A, et al. Plaque radiotherapy for juxtapapillary choroidal melanoma: tumor control in 650 consecutive cases. Ophthalmology. 2011;118(2):402–7.
40. Dendale R, Lumbroso-Le Rouic L, Noel G, et al. Proton beam radiotherapy for uveal melanoma: results of Curie Institut-Orsay proton therapy center (ICPO). Int J Radiat Oncol Biol Phys. 2006;65(3):780–7.
41. Bechrakis NE, Petousis V, Willerding G, et al. Ten-year results of transscleral resection of large uveal melanomas: local tumour control and metastatic rate. Br J Ophthalmol. 2010;94(4):460–6.
42. Shah SU, Shields CL, Bianciotto CG, et al. Intravitreal bevacizumab at 4-month intervals for prevention of macular edema after plaque radiotherapy of uveal melanoma. Ophthalmology. 2014;121(1):269–75.
43. Singh AD, Medina CA, Singh N, et al. Fine-needle aspiration biopsy of uveal melanoma: outcomes and complications. Br J Ophthalmol. 2016;100(4):456–62.
44. Damato B, Duke C, Coupland SE, et al. Cytogenetics of uveal melanoma: a 7-year clinical experience. Ophthalmology. 2007;114(10):1925–31. Epub 2007 Aug 27
45. Onken MD, Worley LA, Char DH, et al. Collaborative Ocular Oncology Group report number 1: prospective validation of a multi-gene prognostic assay in uveal melanoma. Ophthalmology. 2012;119(8):1596–603.
46. Walter SD, Chao DL, Feuer W, et al. Prognostic implications of tumor diameter in association with gene expression profile for uveal melanoma. JAMA Ophthalmol. 2016;134:734–40.
47. Mruthyunjaya P, Seider MI, Stinnett S, Schefler A, Ocular Oncology Study Consortium. Association between tumor regression rate and gene expression profile after iodine 125 plaque radiotherapy for uveal melanoma. Ophthalmology. 2017;124:1532–9.
48. Gezgin G, Luk SJ, Cao J, et al. PRAME as a potential target for immunotherapy in metastatic uveal melanoma. JAMA Ophthalmol. 2017;135(6):541–9.
49. Decatur CL, Ong E, Garg N, et al. Driver mutations in uveal melanoma: associations with gene expression profile and patient outcomes. JAMA Ophthalmol. 2016;134(7):728–33.
50. Kivelä TT, Piperno-Neumann S, Desjardins L, et al. Validation of a prognostic staging for metastatic uveal melanoma: a collaborative study of the European Ophthalmic Oncology Group. Am J Ophthalmol. 2016;168:217–26.
51. Triozzi PL, Singh AD. Adjuvant therapy of uveal melanoma: current status. Ocul Oncol Pathol. 2014;1:54–62.
52. Goh AY, Layton CJ. Evolving systemic targeted therapy strategies in uveal melanoma and implications for ophthalmic management: a review. Clin Exp Ophthalmol. 2016;44(6):509–19.
53. Buder K, Gesierich A, Gelbrich G, et al. Systemic treatment of metastatic uveal melanoma: review of literature and future perspectives. Cancer Med. 2013;2(5):674–86.

9 Pathology of Intraocular Tumors

Subramanian Krishnakumar

9.1 Intraocular Tumors

9.1.1 Introduction

Intraocular tumors are generally challenging to the general pathologist. The challenges are due to several reasons such as the less of ophthalmic pathology training in the undergraduate and postgraduate pathology curriculum, the need for the background knowledge of ophthalmology and finally the small sample size [1].

The intraocular components of the eye includes the iris tissue and ciliary body which are part of the anterior segment, and the posterior segment which comprises the vitreous fluid, vascular choroid, which is a continuation of the ciliary body, the multilayered retinal tissue in front of choroid and retinal pigment epithelium that is located between the retina and the choroid. These structures are involved in inflammation and also have the potential to develop both primary malignant tumors because of the genetic events/mutation/chromosomal aberrations and also secondarily invaded by malignant tumors that spread from outside the eye and metastasize from other organs. Structures such as sclera, the outer coat of the eye and optic disc/nerve can be involved by inflammation and tumors and may mimic intraocular tumors. Thus, diagnosing intraocular tumors has its own challenges.

The diagnosis of intraocular tumors needs the knowledge gained from various non-invasive techniques such as ultrasound bio microscopy, ultrasound, Optical Coherence Tomography (OCT) imaging, computed tomography (CAT) scan, magnetic resonance imaging (MRI) imaging and fundus photography. This supports the light microscopy observation and complemented by immunohistochemistry technique, molecular techniques such as Polymerase Chain reaction (PCR) for diagnosis of tuberculosis and PCR-Sequencing for identifying MYD88L265P and IgH gene clonal rearrangements for diagnosing primary intraocular large cell lymphoma [2].

The applications of molecular techniques like microarray based gene expression profiling in uveal melanoma [3], retinoblastoma [4] and studying chromosomal aberrations in uveal melanoma [5] helps in prognosticating the tumors. The newer digital pathology is sure to advance ophthalmic pathology by helping the ophthalmic pathologist to share the images with peers for second opinion and later could enable the application of machine learning in ophthalmic pathology [1].

S. Krishnakumar (✉)
Research Fellowship in Ophthalmic Pathology from Doheny Eye Institute, University of Southern California, Los Angeles, CA, USA

Larsen and Toubro Ocular Pathology Department-Vision Research Foundation, Sankara Nethralaya, Chennai, Tamil Nadu, India
e-mail: drkk@snmail.org

V. Khetan (ed.), *Intraocular Tumors*, https://doi.org/10.1007/978-981-15-0395-5_9

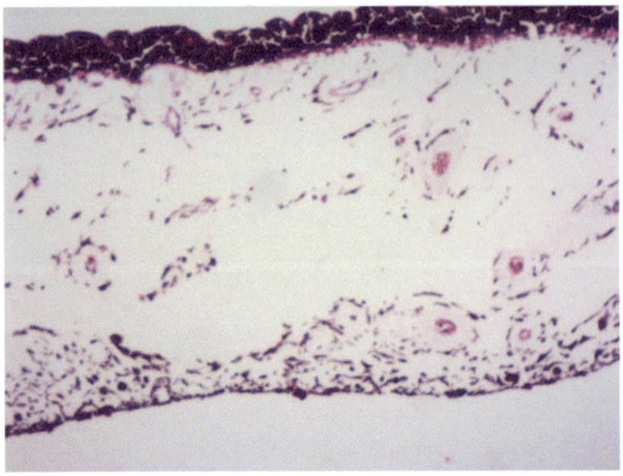

Fig. 9.1 Iris tissue showing the pigmented epithelium and the stroma

9.2 Iris

9.2.1 Background

The components of the iris tissue include pigment epithelium, non-pigment epithelium, blood vessels, smooth muscle fibers and the stroma composed of mesenchyme, immune cells, and blood vessels (Fig. 9.1) [6]. Iris tissue is involved in many disorders ranging from genetic diseases that have a structural defect [7] to inflammatory disorders [8] where iris is inflamed and presents as iris nodules [9]. In recent years, many high-throughput technologies like proteomics and sequencing are used to study the iris tissue which will help in understanding the biology, functions and diseases of iris tissue [10–12].

9.3 Iris Tumors

9.3.1 Introduction

Iris is involved in both primary and secondary tumors, where the clinical presentation is just an iris mass [13, 14]. It is also involved by secondary tumors extending from the adjacent tissues such as from the ciliary body, retina, and ocular surface and from the solid tumors from distant organs which metastasis to the iris. Iris tissue also involved in hematological malignancies [15].

9.3.2 Classification of the Iris Tumors Based on the Clinical Behaviour

9.3.2.1 Benign Tumors

- Iris nevus
- Iris melanocytoma
- Iris pigment epithelial adenoma
- Iris leiomyoma
- Iris leiomyoepithelioma
- Iris neurofibroma

9.3.2.2 Intermediate Grade Tumors

- Iris melanocytic tumors of uncertain malignant potential
- Epstein-Barr virus–associated smooth muscle tumor

9.3.2.3 Malignant Tumors

- Iris melanoma
- Iris pigment epithelial adenocarcinoma
- Rhabdomyosarcoma
- Ewing's sarcoma

9.3.2.4 Vascular Tumors

- Capillary/cavernous/racemose hemangioma

9.3.2.5 Hematological Tumors

- Lymphoma-primary/secondary
- Plasmacytoma

9.3.2.6 Metastatic Tumors of Iris

9.3.2.7 Secondary Iris Tumors Resulting from Extension of Local Tumors

9.3.3 Benign Primary Tumors of the Iris

9.3.3.1 Iris Nevus

Clinical Notes This arises from the melanocytes in the iris stroma. It presents as pigmented spot in the iris. Iris nevi can be either focal or diffuse. Focal iris nevus can be slightly elevated. Diffuse iris nevus can involve large component of the iris.

Histopathology Iris nevus is pigmented. Bleaching is necessary to study the cell morphology. The nevus is composed of both spindle cells and polygonal cells. The nevus cells have tiny nucleoli. Rarely, these nevus cells can have clear cytoplasm and form rosettes [16, 17]. There is no atypia in these nevus cells. The risk of melanoma transformation of iris nevi is less than 10% [18].

Histopathology Differential Diagnosis Iris nevus should be differentiated from iris melanoma. If there are clear cells, then balloon cell nevus [17, 19], xanthomathous infiltration [20] and metastatic renal cell tumor all come in the differential diagnosis [21].

Immunohistochemistry Melanocyte lineage markers such as Melan-A and SOX 10 will help to identify the nevus. However CD68 may be needed to identify xanthoma and when metastatic tumor is suspected a panel of immunohistochemical markers is needed as given in Table 9.1.

9.3.3.2 Iris Melanocytoma

Clinical Notes Iris melanocytoma presents as a black nodule in the iris. It can be localized or show a diffuse pattern. There could be pressure effect and invasion in to the adjacent structures [22, 23]. Iris melanocytomas may show spontaneous necrosis [24] and regress spontaneously [25]. Iris melanocytic lesions have a favorable outcome and malignant transformation is rare [25–29]

Histopathology Bleach preparation of the tumor shows oval to round cells with low nucleocytoplasmic ratio. There is a tiny nucleolus with no atypia or mitotic activity.

Histopathology Differential Diagnosis Iris Melanocytic Tumors of Uncertain Malignant Potential and Iris melanoma.

Immunohistochemistry and Genetic Study Immunohistochemistry has limitations except proliferative index Ki-67, which is low in melanocytoma. However, mutation studies on iris melanocytoma for mutations such as GNAQ, GNA11, and EIF1AX are absent.

9.3.3.3 Iris Pigment Epithelial Adenoma

Clinical Notes Iris Pigment Epithelial (IPE) adenoma is seen in adults and present as an iris nodule. Clinically it mimics melanoma. These tumors are located in the superficial portion of iris and do not invade the iris stroma [30].

Histopathology Bleached preparation is required. The tumor shows intensely pigmented epithelial cells which are arranged in tubular and cord like pattern with a cystic component that contain melanophages. Periodic acid–Schiff (PAS) stain shows deposition of basement membrane material around the tumor cells.

Table 9.1 A basic panel for immunohistochemical markers for metastatic tumors

	Site of the tumor					
Immunohistochemical markers	Breast	Colon	Lung	Prostate	Thyroid	Melanoma
Cytokeratin 7	+	±	+	±	+	–
Cytokeratin 20	±	+	±	±	–	–
GATA3	+	–	–	–	–	–
TTF1	–	–	+	–	+	–
CDX2	–	+	–	–	–	–
GCDFP-15	+	–	–	–	–	–
HMB45	–	–	–	–	–	+

The full immunohistochemical staining panel is outside the scope of this volume

Histopathology Differential Diagnosis IPE adenocarcinoma to be considered if mitotic activity and nuclear atypia is present [14, 30–33].

Immunohistochemistry Epithelial markers such as cytokeratin and epithelial membrane antigen (EMA) are positive.

9.3.3.4 Iris Leiomyoma

Clinical Notes This tumor is common in younger age group and in females. The tumor presents as a nodule in the iris. These tumors are usually not pigmented and are slow growing. The tumor could cause pressure effects on the adjacent tissues causing glaucoma and cataract [34–37].

Histopathology Iris leiomyoma is composed of spindle cells arranged in a fascicular pattern with oval nuclei and myxoid changes can be seen in the tumor. There is no atypia and no mitotic activity.

Histopathological Differential Diagnoses Spindle cell melanoma and Epstein-Barr virus (EBV) associated smooth muscle tumor of the iris.

Immunohistochemistry The tumor cells express smooth muscle actin (SMA), desmin and are negative for melanocyte markers such as SOX-10, Microphthalmia transcription factor (MITF), S-100 and HMB45 and negative for Epstein Barr virus associated RNA by insitu hybridization.

9.3.3.5 Iris Leiomyoepithelioma

Clinical Notes This tumor is pigmented and mimics melanocytoma. There is only one case report [38]. It is seen in younger age group and presents as a nodule.

Histopathology The tumor is composed of spindle and polygonal cells. The polygonal cells representing the epithelial origin and spindle cells show the smooth muscle differentiation and the polygonal cells may have a prominent nucleolus. There is no atypia and mitotic activity.

Histopathology Differential Diagnosis Melanocytoma and melanoma.

Immunohistochemistry The tumor cells are positive for smooth muscle actin (SMA), desmin, mesenchymal marker vimentin, epithelial marker-EMA and may be positive for melanocyte lineage markers such as SOX-10, MITF, S-100 and HMB45

9.3.3.6 Iris Neurofibroma

Clinical Notes The tumor presents as iris nodule. There is associated neurofibromatosis type 1.

Histopathology The tumor is composed of spindle cells with wavy nuclei and no nuclear atypia. The spindle cells are intermixed with collagen tissue and a few scattered mast cells are seen.

Histopathology Differential Diagnosis Leiomyoma and spindle cell nevus if there is no pigmentation [39]

Immunohistochemistry S-100, SOX- 10 proteins are moderately positive, as these proteins are also expressed in melanocytes correlation with light microscopy is required.

9.3.4 Intermediate Grade Tumors

9.3.4.1 Iris Melanocytic Tumors of Uncertain Malignant Potential

Clinical Notes These tumors present as a pigment nodule in the iris. This is a small subset of iris nevus which has BRCA1 associated protein 1 [BAP1] mutation and could transform to melanoma [40].

Histopathology This arises from the melanocytes in the iris stroma. The nevus cells are composed of spindle cells and epithelioid cells with minimal nuclear atypia or local invasion. These atypical nevus cells have prominent nucleoli.

Histopathology Differential Diagnosis Iris melanoma is an important differential diagnosis.

Immunohistochemistry There is loss of nuclear staining for BAP1 protein in the epithelioid cells.

9.3.4.2 Epstein-Barr Virus (EBV): Associated Smooth Muscle Tumor

Clinical Notes Epstein-Barr virus (EBV)–associated smooth muscle tumor is rare and presents as a solitary mass in the iris or systemically in other organs. These tumors are usually fleshy, vascularized and not pigmented. This tumor occurs in immune suppressed patients due to post-transplant medications and infection with human immunodeficiency virus [41].

Histopathology The tumor is cellular and composed of a mixture of predominantly spindle cells arranged in a fascicular pattern and small foci of epithelioid cells with prominent nucleoli. There could be minimal nuclear atypia and mitotic activity and this should not be mistaken for evidence of a sarcoma [42]. These tumors have favorable prognosis [41]. There is infiltration by lymphocytes and the prognosis and histopathology severity depends on the level of immunosupression.

Histopathological Differential Diagnosis Leiomyoma, amelanotic melanoma, leiomyosarcoma and metastatic spindle cell tumors.

Immunohistochemistry and Molecular Techniques The tumor cells are positive for SMA, desmin and negative for melanocyte markers such as SOX10, MITF, S-100 and HMB45. Epstein Barr virus associated RNA by in situ hybridization is positive in the tumor and confirms the diagnosis.

9.3.5 Malignant Tumors of the Iris

9.3.5.1 Iris Melanoma

Clinical Notes Iris melanoma presents as pigmented nodule in the iris.

Histopathology Bleached preparation of the tumor shows both spindle and epithelioid cells or one cell type. Iris melanomas behave aggressively and can invade the orbit [43] and metastasize [44]. Thus, iris melanomas can be classified in to class 1 and class 2 melanomas based on their biological behaviour similar to the choroidal melanomas based on gene expression profiling. Most of the iris melanomas show monosomy 3 [45, 46].

Histopathology Differential Diagnosis Iris melanocytic tumors of uncertain malignant potential.

9.3.5.2 Iris Pigment Epithelial Adenocarcinoma

Clinical Notes This is a pigmented tumor and presents as an iris nodule. The tumor mimics iris melanoma [47, 48].

Histopathology This tumor originates from the fully differentiated iris pigment epithelium. Bleach preparation shows a tumor composed of atypical pigment epithelial cells arranged in tubular and tubulo-acinar arrangement. These cells are oval to cuboidal with adequate cytoplasm. There is moderate high nucleo cytoplasmic ratio with prominent nucleoli. There is deposition of perioidic acid Schiff (PAS) positive basement membrane around the tumor cells. Scattered vascular channels are seen within the tumor. There could be local invasion into the adjacent structures.

Histopathological Differential Diagnosis Metastatic adenocarcinoma from the various solid organs such as breast, lung, kidney, esophagus etc. that could metastasize to the iris [49–53].

Immunohistochemistry These tumors are positive for S-100, vimentin, cytokeratin and negative for HMB45 and EMA.

9.3.5.3 Iris Rhabdomyosarcoma

Clinical Notes This tumor presents as a nodule in the iris. Only 3 cases have been reported [54–56]. These tumors are considered to be predominantly rhabdomyoblastic differentiation of the iris medulloepithelioma. These tumors could arise either from the mesenchymal cells in the iris stroma or from rhabdomyoblastic differentiation of the primitive medullary epithelial cells in iris [55].

Histopathology The histopathology is like rhabdomyosarcoma elsewhere. The tumor is cellular and composed of tumor cells which are oval cells with prominent nucleoli and spindle cells. Nuclear atypia and mitosis are seen.

Histopathological Differential Diagnosis Teratoid medulloepithelioma with a rhabdomyoblastic component to be ruled out with serial sections. Metastatic rhabdomyosarcoma to the iris should be ruled out with clinical information [57]. Malignant Rhabdoid Tumor both primary and metastatic to be ruled out with imaging studies on the kidney.

Immunohistochemistry Muscle markers such as desmin, actin and myogenin are positive and there is negative expression of the nuclear SMARCB1/INI1protein by immunohistochemistry in the rhabdoid tumor cells [58–60].

9.3.5.4 Ewing's Sarcoma of Iris

Clinical Notes Ewing's sarcoma is a primary bone tumor in childhood and can present as an iris mass [61].

Histopathology The tumor is cellular and there is diffuse infiltration of small round cells. The cells have minimal cytoplasm and contain glycogen which can be stained by PAS. The nucleus of the tumor cell has indentations and tiny nucleoli. The tumor is divided in to lobular arrangement by fibrous septa.

Histopathology Differential Diagnosis The round cells can morphologically mimic Retinoblastoma, acute lymphoblastic leukemia cells, and lymphoma cells. A diagnosis of primary Ewing's sarcoma should be made only after metastatic Ewing's tumor is excluded [62].

Immunohistochemistry and Molecular Tests Immunohistochemistry shows strong membranous CD99 positivity, and molecular testing for the fusion gene EWS-FLI1, caused by the t(11;22)(q24;q12) translocation, helps in diagnosis [63].

9.3.5.5 Vascular Tumors of Iris

Clinical Notes Vascular tumors in the iris have been reported. These tumors include capillary hemangioma, cavernous hemangioma, racemose hemangiomas and micro hemangiomatosis. Hemangiomas are noted at birth they can either regress or enlarge [64]. Capillary hemangiomas are rare. Racemose hemangiomas [arteriovenous malformation] are common [65]. Iris hemangiomas may be associated with choroidal hemangiomas [66].

Histopathology The tumor is composed of vascular spaces filled with blood, similar to cavernous hemangioma elsewhere.

9.3.6 Hematological Disorders of Iris

9.3.6.1 Iris Lymphoma

Clinical Notes Iris lymphomas present as iris nodules and thickening of iris. Iris lymphoma can be classified into 2 categories. In the first, iris lymphoma is a component of the extra nodal marginal zone B cell lymphoma or mucosa-associated lymphoid tissue (MALT) lymphoma. These lymphomas are usually low grade lymphomas [67, 68]. In the second, iris tissue is the primary presentation of non-Hodgkin's lymphomas such as Mantle cell lymphoma, T cell lymphoma and Anaplastic large cell lymphoma. Primary Mantle cell lymphoma has been reported in the iris. This lymphoma has aggressive behavior [68, 69]. T cell lymphoma and Anaplastic large cell lymphoma can invade the iris and present as iris nodules, and diffuse infiltration [70, 71].

Histopathology Diffuse infiltration with atypical lymphoid cells is seen. Plasma cells can be seen in malt lymphoma. Large cells with atypia can be seen in anaplastic large cell lymphoma.

Immunohistochemistry A panel of immunohistochemical markers for B cell, T cell, NK cell, CD 30, ALK, cyclin D1 is needed. A detailed description of lymphomas is beyond the scope of this chapter. Lymphomas are in detail discussed elsewhere.

9.3.6.2 Plasmacytoma of Iris

Clinical Notes Plasmacytoma in the iris could be part of multiple myeloma or isolated plasmacytoma of iris. It can present as an iris mass. Histopathology and immunohistochemistry are needed to establish the diagnosis [72]. Serum immunoelectrophoresis is needed to rule out monoclonal gammopathy.

Histopathology Diffuse infiltration with plasma cells is present. The plasma cells can have intranuclear inclusions.

Immunohistochemistry Kappa and lambda chains are needed to confirm the clonality of the plasma cells. In reactive plasma cell infiltrates both kappa and lambda chains will be positive and in monoclonal disease such as plasmacytoma only one of these chain is positive and helps to make the diagnosis.

9.3.6.3 Metastatic Tumors of Iris

Clinical Notes Metastatic tumors to iris are rare. Iris secondary deposits can present as a nodule or thickening of the iris. The patient could present with pain or hyphema. Tumors both from solid organs and lymphoreticular disorders can involve the iris. Iris involvement accounts for less than 10% of uveal metastases [73]. Solitary iris metastasis is rare [74, 75]. Clinicopathological correlation is important [53, 76].

Histopathology The tumors could be arranged in diffuse pattern composed of small round cells, or glandular pattern with atypia and areas of necrosis. A panel of Immunohistochemistry markers is needed to know the site of organ from which it has originated. This is discussed in Table 9.1.

9.3.6.4 Secondary Iris Tumors Resulting from Extension of Local Tumors

Clinical Notes Secondary iris tumors present either as pigmented or amelanotic, fleshy vascularized nodule. Ciliary body melanoma and medulloepithelioma can extend into the iris and mimic an iris tumor [77] (Fig. 9.2). Anteriorly situated retinoblastoma can invade the iris and can present as a nodules in the iris [78] (Fig. 9.3). Tumors from the ocular surface especially squa-

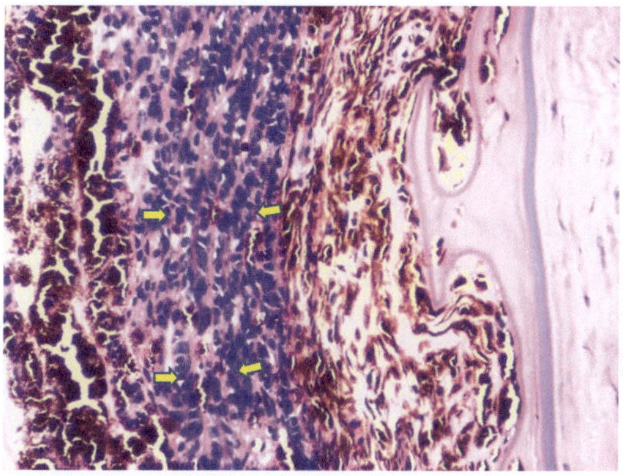

Fig. 9.2 Ciliary body teratoid medulloepithelioma tumor cells (arrows) invading the iris tissue. The tumor cells are seen arranged in a thin cord like pattern invading in to the iris stroma

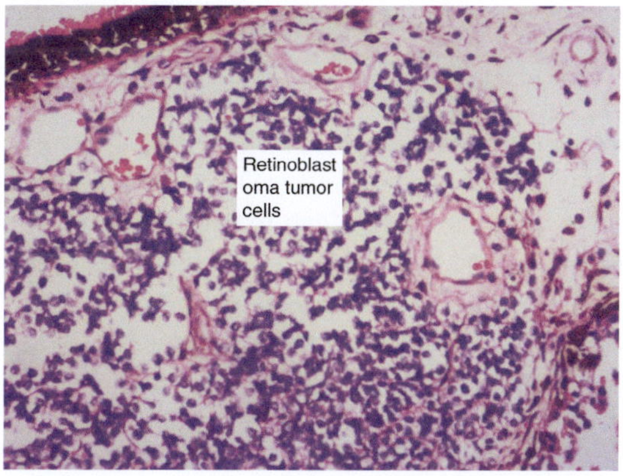

Fig. 9.3 Retinoblastoma tumor cells invading the iris tissue. The tumor cells are undifferentiated and arranged in a nodular pattern in the iris stroma. There are numerous blood vessels in the iris stroma

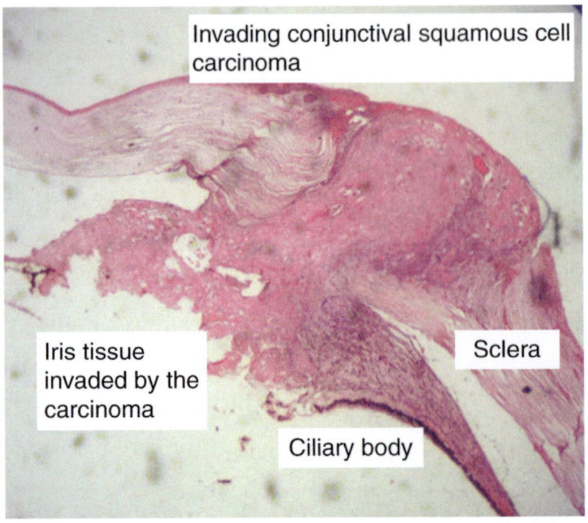

Fig. 9.4 Part of the enucleated sample shows the anterior segment. The pinkish stained tumor cells from the limbus and the conjunctiva are seen invading the corneal stroma and invading into the anterior chamber and invading the iris tissue and portions of the ciliary body

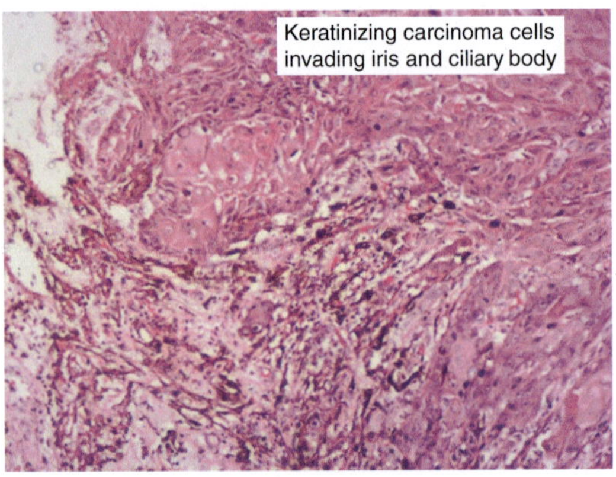

Fig. 9.5 Conjunctival Squamous cell carcinoma invading the iris tissue and portions of the ciliary body

mous cell carcinomas can extend in to the iris (Figs. 9.4 and 9.5) to simulate primary iris tumor [79]. Conjunctival carcinomas and melanomas can extend intraocularly and invade the iris [80–82].

9.4 Ciliary Body

9.4.1 Introduction

Ciliary body is continuation of the iris and an important component of the uveal tract. The components of ciliary body include the pigment epithelium which secretes the aqueous humor, non-pigmented epithelium which secretes the vitreous fluid, blood vessels and smooth muscle fibers which control the lens shape and the stroma composed of blood vessels, dendritic cells, macrophages, lymphocytes and mesenchymal cells (Fig. 9.6). Proteomics studies done on ciliary body has identified novel proteins that may help to understand diseases of the ciliary body [83, 84]. Ciliary body can be involved in both primary tumors and secondary tumors.

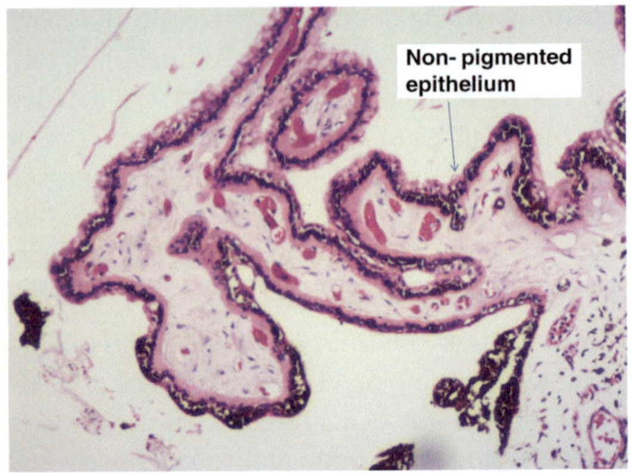

Fig. 9.6 Ciliary body with processes with pigmented and non pigmented epithelium

9.4.2 Tumors of the Ciliary Body

9.4.2.1 Classification of Ciliary Body Tumors Based on Their Clinical Behavior

Benign Primary Tumors

- Ciliary body Nevus
- Ciliary body melanocytoma
- Adenoma of the ciliary pigment epithelium
- Fuch's Adenoma of the ciliary non-pigment epithelium
- Adenoma of the ciliary non-pigment epithelium
- Ciliary body leiomyoma
- Ciliary body Schwannoma
- Glioneuroma
- Astrocytoma

Intermediate Grade Tumors

- Perivascular epithelioid cell tumor, also known as PEComa

Malignant Tumors of the Ciliary Body

- Ciliary body melanoma
- Ciliary adenocarcinoma from pigment epithelium
- Ciliary adenocarcinoma from non-pigment epithelium
- Leiomyosarcoma
- Medulloepithelioma

Hematological Tumors of Ciliary Body

- Lymphoma-primary/secondary

Miscellaneous Tumors

- Solitary fibrous tumor
- IgG4 Inflammatory tumor

Metastatic Tumors

Benign primary tumors of the ciliary body

9.4.2.2 Ciliary Body Nevus

Clinical Notes This is usually seen in adults and presents as ciliary body mass [85]. There could be pigmentation extending to the adjacent structures [86]. Clinically, it mimics melanocytoma and melanoma.

Histopathology The nevus is pigmented. Bleaching shows the nevus is composed of spindle cells with bland nuclei. There is no atypia or mitotic activity. The nevus could be seen extending to sclera and adjacent structures [86, 87]

Histopathology Differential Diagnosis Ciliary body melanocytoma/melanoma.

Immunohistochemistry Melanocyte lineage markers such as Melan-A and SOX 10 are positive.

9.4.2.3 Ciliary Body Melanocytoma

Clinical Notes This presents as a black nodule in the ciliary body and mimics melanoma. There could be pigmentation in the anterior chamber and adjacent sclera. Invasion into the anterior chamber is common. This must not be mistaken for melanoma with extension, ciliary body adenoma, and pigmented adenocarcinoma [88, 89].

Histopathology This arises from the melanocytes in the ciliary body stroma [88]. The tumor shows densely pigmented cells. Bleached preparation shows that there are 2 types of cells. Type 1 melanocytoma cells are polyhedral with a small round uniform with nucleus showing a low nucleo-cytoplasmic ratio. They have tiny nucleoli. Type 2 melanocytoma cells have a spindle cell appearance [90]. Melanocytomas undergo spontaneous necrosis and numerous pigment laden macrophages are seen in histopathology [91]. There could be extra ocular extension of the nevus [92]. Transformation to a melanoma is rare but has been reported [93].

Histopathological Differential Diagnosis Ciliary body melanoma.

Immunohistochemistry Ki 67 is very low in melanocytoma.

9.4.2.4 Adenoma of the Ciliary Pigmented Epithelium

Clinical Notes These tumors are rare and seen in middle age around 50 years. Clinically presents as multiple nodules in the ciliary body. There could be extension into the iris and anterior chamber.

Histopathology The tumor can be densely pigmented or partially pigmented. The tumor shows a varied pattern ranging from trabecular to pseudo glandular pattern containing cystic spaces that are filled with acid mucopolysaccharide. PAS positive basement membrane is seen around the tumor cells. Bleach preparation shows intermediate to large size oval round cells with small to prominent nucleoli. The tumors may show necrosis and mitotic activity is low. Invasion in to the adjacent structures is seen [94].

Histopathology Differential Diagnosis Adenomas of the non-pigmented ciliary epithelium, which can be pigmented due to reactive proliferation of the pigmented epithelium, melanocytoma and melanoma.

Immunohistochemistry These tumors are positive for vimentin, cytokeratin 18 and negative for melanocyte markers [95].

9.4.2.5 Ciliary Fuchs's Adenoma-from Non-pigmented Epithelium

Clinical Notes This presents as a ciliary body nodule and patients can have visual blurring due to pressure effects. It mimics ciliary body melanoma.

Histopathology There are duct like structures of the non-pigmented epithelium in the tumor. PAS positive eosinophilic basement membrane material surrounds the duct like structures. There is no atypia or mitotic activity [96].

9.4.2.6 Ciliary Adenoma of the Non-pigmented Epithelium

Clinical Notes These tumors rare and are reported in adults. These tumor presents as a ciliary body nodule. The tumor could be partially pigmented. The tumor nodule is usually well defined [97–101]. Clinically it mimics melanoma.

Histopathology The tumor shows a combination of solid, glandular and papillary areas in a myxoid background. The tumor cells are small size with oval to polygonal with tiny nucleoli. The tumor cells are surrounded by a PAS positive basement membrane like material. There is no necrosis, atypia and no mitotic activity. Smooth muscle differentiation [102] and areas of calcifications have been reported [103].

Histopathological Differential Diagnosis Important ones are the low-grade ciliary adenocarcinoma, epithelioid leiomyoma.

Immunohistochemistry These tumors are positive for vimentin, cytokeratin 18 and S-100. Melanocyte markers such as SOX-10, Melan-A and HMB45 are negative.

9.4.2.7 Primary Ciliary Body Leiomyoma

Clinical Notes This tumor is usually not pigmented and presents as a nodule. There are 2 types of this tumor based on the cell of origin. Mesodermal leiomyoma originates from the smooth muscle layer of vessel walls. Mesoectodermal leiomyoma arises from the ciliary muscle which is a neural crest derivative [104–109]. These tumors are associated with local eye complications because of the mass effect such as lens dislocation, glaucoma and retinal detachment [104–107, 110].

Histopathology These tumors are usually well circumscribed. Mesodermal leiomyoma is a cellular tumor and composed of bland spindle cells showing a fascicular pattern of arrangement. The spindle cells have elongated nuclei. There is no nuclear atypia. Mesoectodermal leiomyoma is a cellular tumor and composed of spindle cells that show a fascicular pattern with fibrillary cytoplasm with focal areas showing cystic degeneration [111]. The tumors stain for both smooth muscle marker and neural marker [112, 113].

Histopathological Differential Diagnosis Epithelioid variant of leiomyoma should not be mistaken for melanoma [114].

Immunohistochemistry Mesodermal leiomyoma tumor cells are positive for smooth muscle actin, vimentin and negative for melanocyte markers such as SOX-10, MITF, and Melan-A. Mesoectodermal leiomyoma positive for smooth muscle actin, vimentin and negative for melanocyte markers and S-100 known neural marker is positive in mesoectodermal leiomyoma.

9.4.2.8 Ciliary Body Schwannoma

Clinical Notes These tumors present as an amelanotic mass in the ciliary body [115]. These tumors arise from the posterior ciliary nerve. The tumors are slow growing and cause pressure effects to the local adjacent structures of the eye. It is important to rule out systemic disorders such as neurofibromatosis or Carney complex [115].

Histopathology The tumor is composed of spindle cells that are wavy and have bland nuclei and abundant eosinophilic cytoplasm. The tumor cells are arranged in a cellular pattern (Antoni A) with palisaded called verocay bodies and with a hypocellular myxoid component (Antoni B) (Figs. 9.7 and 9.8). The tumor could be pigmented or have a plexiform pattern [116–119].

Histopathology Differential Diagnosis Ciliary body spinde cell amelanotic melanoma.

Immunohistochemistry The tumors are positive for S-100 in the cytoplasm and nucleus of the tumor cells and vimentin and negative for melanocyte markers such as Melan-A and SOX-10.

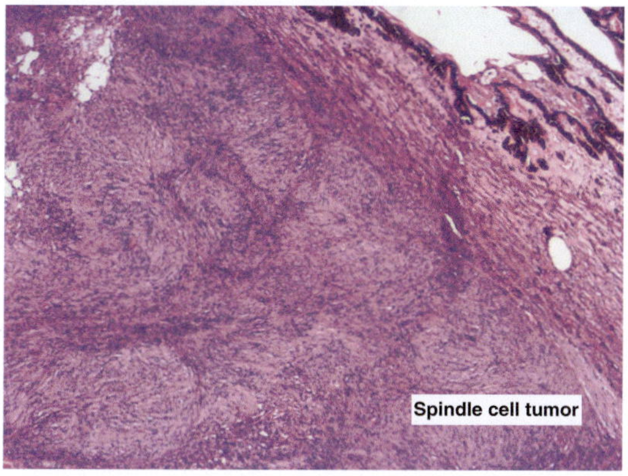

Fig. 9.7 Cilio choroid schwannoma showing spindle cells

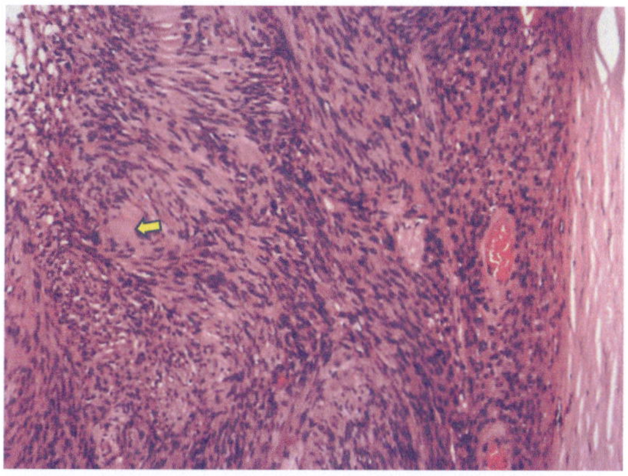

Fig. 9.8 Cilio choroid schwannoma showing a cellular tumor composed of spindle cells arranged in Antony A pattern showing verocay body formation (arrow)

9.4.2.9 Glioneuroma

Clinical Notes This arises in the ciliary body presenting as a fleshy mass in the anterior chamber angle. These tumors are classified under choristoma and contains both glial and neuronal elements [120, 121].

Histopathology The tumor has hypocellular appearance and made of wavy cells which show markers for glial tissue and axonal cells. There could be dysplastic rosettes and calcification. There is no atypia [122].

Histopathology Differential Diagnosis Serial sections are needed along with clinical information and imaging to rule out teratoid medulloepithelioma of the ciliary body.

Immunohistochemistry Glial fibrillary acidic protein (GFAP) is positive in the glial portion of the tumor and synapotophysin is positive in the neuronal portion of the tumor.

9.4.2.10 Astrocytoma

Clinical Notes Astrocytoma of the ciliary body is a benign tumor. It is thought to be a choristoma or metaplastic process from the normal ciliary epithelium [123–125].

Histopathology The tumor is composed of spindle cells in a fibrillary stroma. There could be minimal variation in nuclei size and shape.

Immunohistochemistry GFAP is positive in the spindle cells.

9.4.3 Borderline Malignant Tumor

9.4.3.1 Perivascular Epithelioid Cell Tumor/PEComa

Clinical Notes Perivascular epithelioid cell tumor, also known as PEComa is a mesenchymal neoplasm originating from perivascular myoid cells. It presents as a ciliary body tumor and mimics melanoma [126, 127].

Histopathology The tumor is cellular and has both spindle and epithelioid cells in perivascular arrangement. The cytoplasm appearance ranges from clear to granular. The tumors biologically behave in both benign and aggressive ways. Benign PEComas do not show atypia, however malignant PEComas show areas of necrosis, with nuclear atypia and mitotic activity [128] (Fig. 9.9).

Histopathology Differential Diagnosis Alveolar soft part sarcoma, (Figs. 9.10 and 9.11) amelanotic melanoma and metastatic tumors.

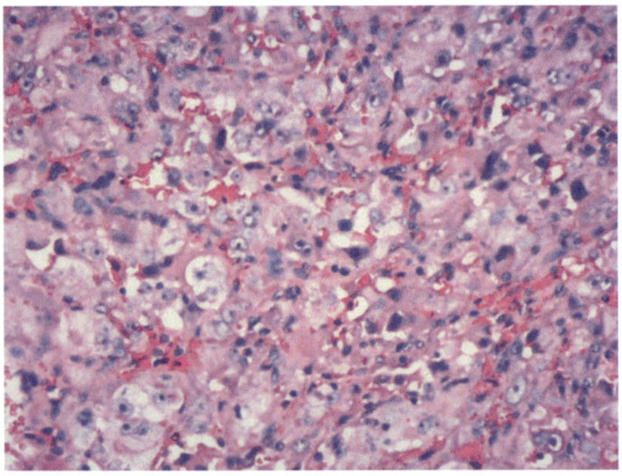

Fig. 9.9 PECOMA—the tumor is composed of cells arranged around the vessels and predominantly epithelioid cells and less of spindle cells are seen. The epithelioid cells have prominent nucleoli. There is nuclear atypia (representative histology from orbital biopsy)

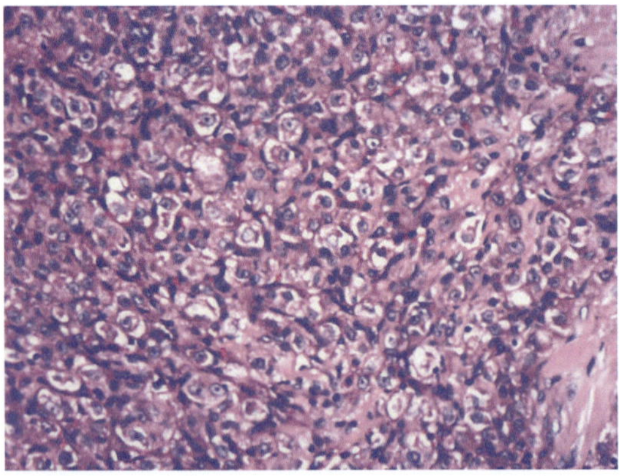

Fig. 9.10 Alveolar soft part sarcoma tumor showing nests of tumor cells separated by septa. The tumor cells are large epithelioid with prominent nucleoli. The cytoplasm shows vacuolation and granularity

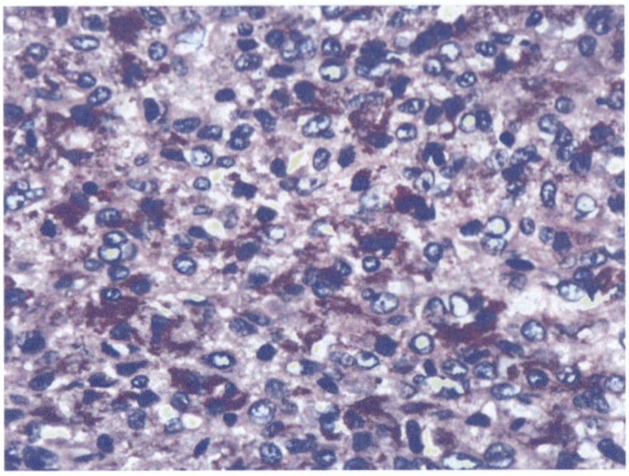

Fig. 9.11 PAS stain in alveolar soft part sarcoma showing PAS positive inclusions in the cytoplasm of the tumor cells

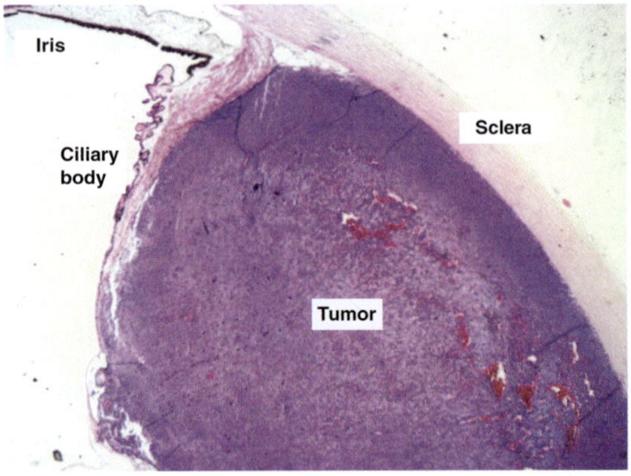

Fig. 9.12 Ciliary body tumor that is not pigmented

Immunohistochemistry PEComas express both muscle markers and melanocytic markers such as Melan-A, HMB 45. Cytokeratins are usually negative.

9.4.4 Malignant Tumors of the Ciliary Body

9.4.4.1 Ciliary Body Melanoma

Clinical Notes Ciliary body melanoma presents as a nodule (Fig. 9.12) or a diffuse mass involving both the ciliary body and the choroid [129] or involve the ciliary body in a circumscribed diffuse pattern known as ring melanoma. The prognosis is not good in ring melanoma [130].

Histopathology Bleaching is needed to study the cell morphology. The tumor is cellular and composed of spindle and epithelioid cells. Spindle cells are elongated cells with a spindle nucleus and tiny nucleoli. Epithelioid cells are round to polygonal cells with high nucleo-cytoplasmic ration and prominent nucleoli. Mitotic activity can be seen. If the tumor is composed of spindle cells it is called as spindle cell melanoma. If both the spindle and epithelioid cells it is called as mixed melanoma and only epithelioid cells it is called as epithelioid cell melanoma.

Histopathology Differential Diagnosis If the tumor is amelanotic ciliary body leiomyoma, epithelioid cell type leiomyoma, benign peripheral nerve sheath tumor and solitary fibrous tumor are to be ruled out.

Molecular Study Prognostication based on both chromosomal aberrations and gene expression profiling for class 1 and class 2 signature is applicable to ciliary body melanoma similar to choroidal melanoma [131].

9.4.4.2 Ciliary Adenocarcinoma Arising from the Pigmented Epithelium

Clinical Notes This is a rare tumor and presents as a nodule in the ciliary body with secondary cataract and glaucoma due to pressure effect of the adjacent structures [132, 133]. Clinical examination and imaging studies alone have limitations in the diagnosis and differentiation from melanoma.

Histopathology These tumors are pigmented and show infiltrative growth patterns into the ciliary body stroma and choroid. The tumor is composed of epithelial cells arranged in a cord and glandular pattern. PAS positive basement membrane material is seen around the tumor cells. The tumor cells have moderate nucleo cytoplasmic ration with a prominent nucleolus. Nuclear atypia is present [134, 135].

Histopathology Differential Diagnosis Pigmented adenoma arising from the ciliary epithelium and metastatic tumor in the ciliary body. Local stromal invasion, nuclear atypia and mitotic activity are the clue to differentiate it from pigmented adenoma.

Immunohistochemistry Markers for melanocyte origin such as SOX-10, MITF, S-100 are variably positive and the tumors cells are positive for EMA, pancytokeratin (AE1/AE3), cytokeratin 8/18 and cytokeratin 5/6.

9.4.4.3 Ciliary Adenocarcinoma Arising from the Non-pigmented Epithelium

Clinical Notes These are rare tumors and occur in both children and adults. They present as anterior chamber mass, non-pigmented and fleshy and vascularized or as an epibulbar mass. There could be hyphema with pressure effects on the adjacent structures [136].

Histopathologically The tumors can have patterns such as solid, papillary, and a special type of tumor known as pleomorphic adenocarcinoma. The solid tumor pattern shows the arrangement of the tumor cells in gland like patterns, surrounded by PAS positive material. The tumor cells have round to polygonal in shape with a high nucelo-cytoplasmic ratio with a prominent nucleolus. The papillary pattern shows the arrangement of the tumor cells in tubular and papillary patterns. There is mitosis and atypia and these tumors are graded from low grade to high grade [137, 138] based on the mitosis and invasiveness.

Pleomorphic adenocarcinoma of the non pigmented epithelium of the ciliary body is a variant of the tumor which is more aggressive and can spread locally and also have metastasis [136, 139].

Histopathology Differential Diagnosis Medulloepithelioma and retinoblastoma should be ruled out when it occurs in children. Metastatic tumors from breast, lung, and gastrointestinal tract carcinomas can show the papillary and glandular patterns [140, 141].

Immunohistochemistry Markers for melanocyte origin such as SOX-10, MITF, S-100 are negative and the tumors cells are positive for EMA and cytokeratins. Proliferative index Ki 67 is high in the tumor. A panel of markers to identify the source of metastatic tumor should be done (Table 9.1).

9.4.4.4 Primary Ciliary Leiomyosarcoma

Clinical Notes The tumor presents as a ciliary body mass with obstruction to the vision. These tumors are not pigmented [142, 143]. Important clinical differential diagnosis include amelanotic melanoma and medulloepithelioma.

Histopathology These tumors arise from the ciliary body stroma. The tumor is cellular and is composed of both polygonal cells and spindle cells. The polygonal cells have a hyperchromatic nuclei and eosinophilic cytoplasm. Nuclear atypia and mitotic activity are seen in the tumor cells.

Histopathology Differential Diagnosis Amelanoitc melanoma and teratoid medulloepithelioma with a sarcomatous component to be ruled out.

Immunohistochemistry Smooth muscle alpha actin, pan-actin HHF-35, and desmin is positive whereas immunohistochemistry for melanocytic markers, such as S-100, Melan-A, and HMB-45, are negative [142].

9.4.4.5 Medulloepithelioma

Clinical Notes This tumor originates from the non-pigmented ciliary epithelium, but can be partially pigmented [144]. It presents as a ciliary body mass and can extend into the iris and extrascleral extension can be seen (Figs. 9.13 and 9.14). These tumor are reported in children [145–148] and also in adults.

Histopathologically The tumor is heterogeneous and shows both solid and cystic portions. The tumor is composed of poorly differentiated neuroepithelial cells arranged in a spindle cell pattern (Fig. 9.15). The tumor may also show

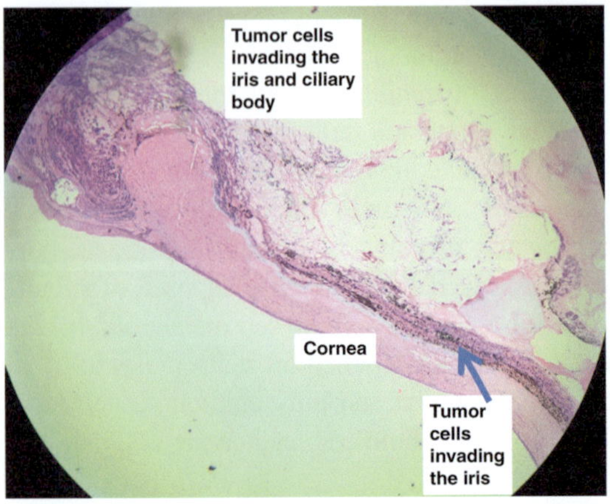

Fig. 9.13 Medulloepithelioma of the ciliary body with anterior segment extension

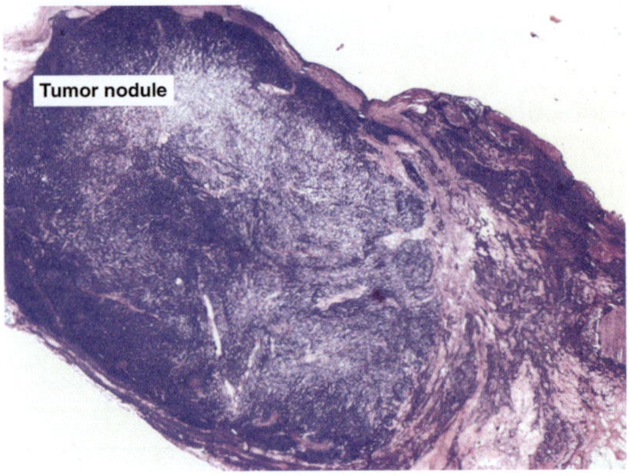

Fig. 9.14 Medulloepithelioma of the ciliary body with scleral and extrascleral extension

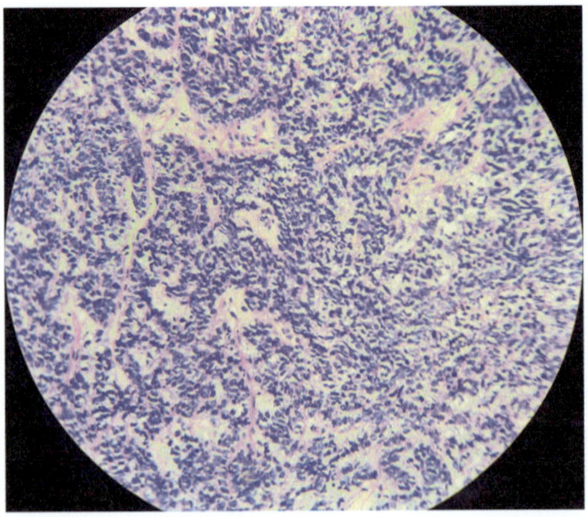

Fig. 9.15 Primitive spindle cells of the medulloepithelioma

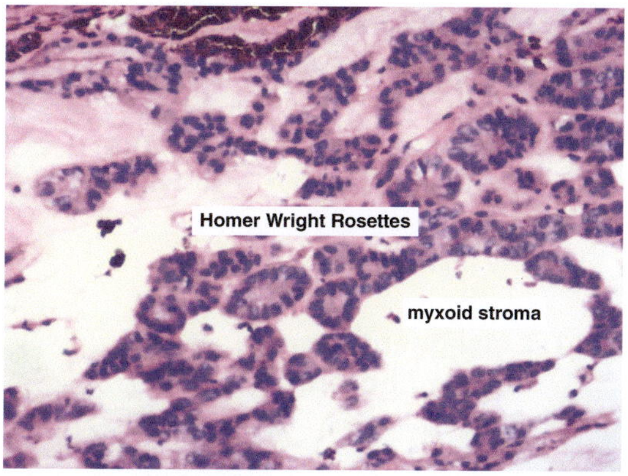

Fig. 9.16 Ciliary body medulloepithelioma tumor showing Homer-Wright rosettes with tumor cells arranged around a central neural material and in a myxoid stroma

duct and cord like pattern in a myxoid stroma. The tumor may show homer-wright rosettes (Fig. 9.16) and rarely Flexner-wintersteiner rosettes. These tumors are subtyped as teratoid medulloepithelioma when hyaline cartilage, rhabdomyoblasts and brain tissue is seen and non-tertaoid medulloepithelioma in absence of them [149]. Medulloepitheliomas spreads locally in the adjacent structures and also to distant site [150–152]. All medulloepitheliomas are potentially malignant tumors and graded as follows (adapted from [153])

Grade I medulloepithelioma (benign, no atypia, no mitosis, no spindle cell atypical component). Grade II medulloepithelioma, local invasion present [invasion into ciliary body iris]. (Pleomorphism, mitotic activity in both the rosettes, and presence of sarcomatous spindle cell component) and Grade III medulloepithelioma with extra scleral extension [153].

Histopathology Differential Diagnosis Anterior retinoblastoma with extension in to the iris and ciliary body has to be ruled out. Ciliary body adenomas, primary adenocarcinoma of the iris and ciliary body and metastatic neuroblastoma have also to be ruled out.

Special Stains and Immunohistochemistry Acid mucopolysaccharide stain such as colloidal iron stain and alcian blue stain are positive in the mucinous stroma in the tumor. Immunohistochemistry has limitations and mesenchymal markers such as vimentin may be positive in the spindle cells. The other markers such as neuron specific enolase, synaptophysin are not specific for medulloepithelioma. Pigmented medulloepithelioma may be positive for S 100 and HMB45 (Figs. 9.17 and 9.18).

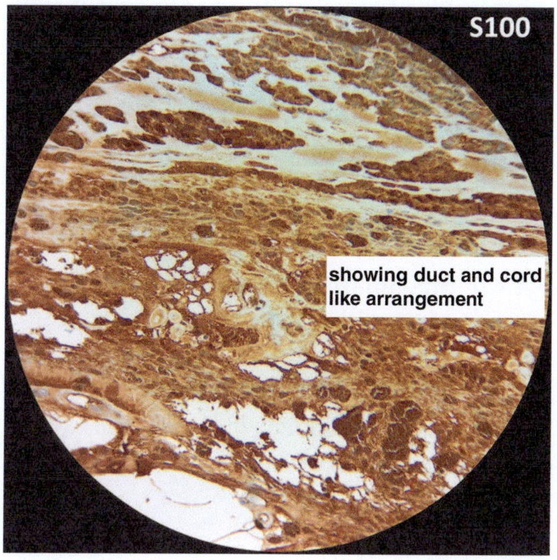

Fig. 9.17 Medulloepithelioma tumor cells showing duct and cord like arrangement positive for S-100 protein by Immunohistochemistry

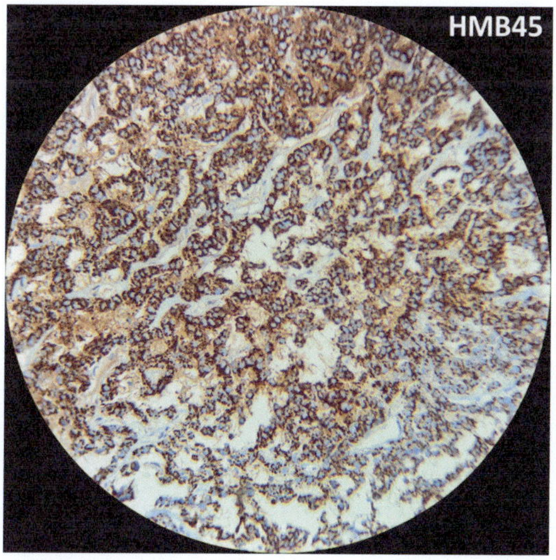

Fig. 9.18 Medulloepithelioma tumor cells showing duct and cord like arrangement positive for HMB45 protein by Immunohistochemistry

9.4.4.6 Hematological Disorders of Ciliary Body

Clinical Notes Ciliary body is involved by non-Hodgkin lymphomas (NHL), in two ways. In the first, there is primary lymphoma of the ciliary body in diffuse ring like pattern. This occur in both extra nodal marginal zone lymphoma-MALT type which is a low grade lymphoma [154] and also in both diffuse large cell B lymphoma which is a high grade lymphoma where there could be involvement of iris too [155] and in the rare aggressive Mantle cell lymphoma (MCL) [156]. A detailed description of lymphomas is beyond the scope of this chapter. Lymphomas are in detail discussed elsewhere.

9.4.4.7 Miscellaneous Tumors of the Ciliary Body

Solitary Fibrous Tumor of the Ciliary Body [157], and IgG4-related intraocular inflammation have been reported in the ciliary body [158] and oligodendrogliomas of the ciliary body [159].

9.5 Choroid

Choroid is highly vascular and is sandwiched between the retinal pigment epithelium and sclera. Choroid tissue contains melanocytes, blood vessels and nerves. The melanocytes in the choroid belong to two categories. First type of melanocyte does not respond to cytokines, growth factors and hormones unlike the second one which belongs to the nevus category which responds to all stimuli. Choroid, because of its rich vascular supply and pigmentation is home to primary tumors and secondary tumors from solid organs.

9.5.1 Classification of Choroidal Tumors Based on Clinical Behaviour

9.5.1.1 Benign Primary Tumors

- Choroidal melanocytoma
- Bilateral diffuse uveal melanocytic hyperplasia/bilateral diffuse uveal melanocytic proliferation (BDUMP)
- Choroidal leiomyoma
- Choroidal schwannoma
- Choroidal neurofibroma

9.5.1.2 Intermediate Grade Tumors

- Perivascular epithelioid cell tumor, also known as PEComa
- Solitary fibrous tumor

9.5.1.3 Malignant Tumors of the Choroid

- Choroidal melanoma

9.5.1.4 Vascular Tumors of Choroid

- Cavernous hemangioma

9.5.1.5 Hematological Tumors of the Choroid

- Primary choroidal lymphoma-part of MALT lymphoma
- Secondary lymphomatous infiltration
- Leukemic infiltration

9.5.1.6 Metastatic Tumors of Choroid

9.5.1.7 Secondary Choroidal Tumors Resulting from Extension from a Local Tumor

- Retinoblastoma
- RPE adenocarcinoma
- Conjunctival squamous cell carcinoma

9.5.1.8 Miscellaneous Tumors

- Choroidal osteoma

9.5.2 Benign Primary Tumors of the Choroid

9.5.2.1 Choroidal Melanocytoma

Clinical Notes Choroidal melanocytomas are rare. These tumors are heavily pigmented and they could mimic choroidal melanoma when it presents as a choroidal mass [89, 160, 161].

Histopathology Bleaching of the tumor is needed. The tumor is made of oval to polyhedral cells with a low nucleo cytoplasmic ratio, the nucleus is bland and a tiny nucleoli (Figs. 9.19 and 9.20). There is no atypia and mitotic activity. Melanocytomas undergo

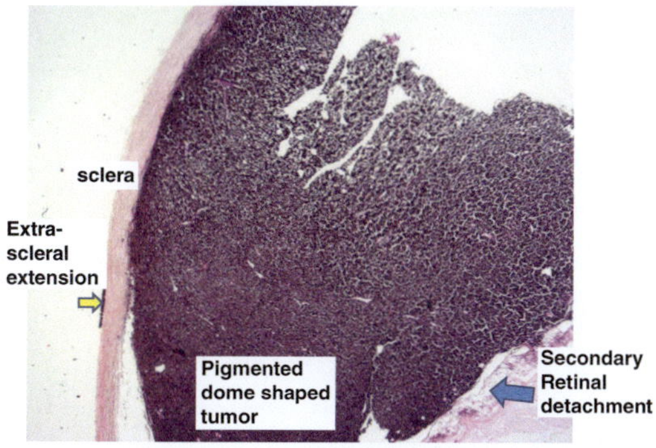

Fig. 9.19 Choroidal melanocytoma with extrascleral extension (arrow). The tumor is densely pigmented

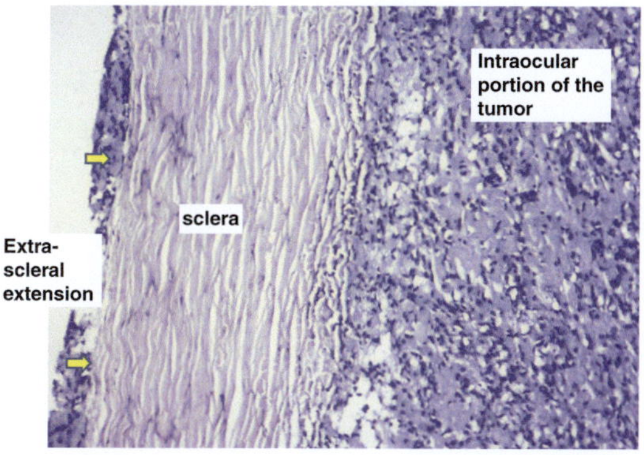

Fig. 9.20 Bleached preparation of the choroidal melanocytoma with extrascleral extension (arrow). The tumor cells are bland with bland nuclei

necrosis and attract numerous melanophages [162, 163]. Malignant transformation of melanocytoma to melanoma is rare, however has been reported. It is challenging to identify melanoma transformation in a necrotic melanocytoma [163]. However, serial sections are required not to miss foci of epithelioid cells or atypia. Melanocytomas may show extra scleral extension [164].

Histopathology Differential Diagnosis Chororidal melanoma mush be differentiated based on the cell type and nuclear atypia.

Molecular Studies Chromosomal abeerations such as Monosomy 3 is negative in melanocytoma.

9.5.2.2 Bilateral Diffuse Uveal Melanocytic Proliferation (BDUMP)

Clinical notes BDUMP (Bilateral diffuse uveal melanocytic proliferation) is a rare paraneoplastic eye manifestation of an underlying systemic tumors such as lymphomas. This can lead to visual loss. It presents as choroidal thickening [165, 166].

Histopathology Enucleated eye shows there is increased numbers of spindle cells which are mostly choroidal nevus type melanocytes. These melanocytes have bland nuclei. There is no atypia [167].

Differential Diagnosis Diffuse uveal melanoma, however the clinical context is different and chromosomal aberrations as reported in uveal melanoma are not there and absent GNAQ mutation.

9.5.2.3 Leiomyoma-Choroid

Clinical Notes Leiomyomas are smooth muscle tumors and they arise from the mesenchyme of the choroidal stroma. These tumors can lead to reduced vision and presents as an intraocular tumor.

Histopathology The tumor expands the choroid in a dome shaped mass situated in the choroid and there could be secondary retinal detachment. The tumor is cellular and composed of interlacing spindle cells. There is usually no atypia and the tumors are not pigmented [168–171].

Histopathology Differential Diagnosis Neurilemmoma, amelanotic melanoma and solitary fibrous tumor of the choroid.

Immunohistochemistry Leiomyoma cells are strongly positive for muscle markers especially smooth muscle actin (SMA), desmin, and h-caldesmon and negative for melanocyte markers. Solitary fibrous tumor is positive for nuclear STAT 6 protein.

9.5.3 Vascular Tumors of the Choroid

9.5.3.1 Hemangiomas

Clinical Notes Choroidal hemangiomas are benign vascular hamartomas without systemic associations. Lesions are usually solitary and unilateral. Intravenous fluorescein angiography, indocyanine green angiography, ultrasonography, optical coherence tomography are helpful ancillary tests for diagnosis of circumscribed choroidal hemangiomas [172].

Histopathology The vascular tumor shows features seen in cavernous hemangioma at other sites.

9.5.4 Intermediate Grade Malignant Tumors

9.5.4.1 Solitary Fibrous Tumor (SFT)/ Hemangiopericytoma

Clinical Notes This tumors is common in the orbit, however it can present as a choroidal mass [173]. There is reduced vision because of the secondary retinal detachment.

Histopathology The tumor originates from the choroid mesenchyme. The tumor is composed of both cellular and myxoid area. The cellular portion of the tumor is composed of spindle cells mixed with fibroblasts with thickened collagen (Fig. 9.20). Scattered branching blood vessels with a few inflammatory cells are seen within the tumor. These tumors range from benign to malignancy in their biological behavior. Aggressive tumors show necrosis, mitosis >4 per ten high power fields.

Histopathology Differential Diagnosis Monophasic synovial sarcoma, spindle cell melanoma and leiomyoma.

Immunohistochemistry and Molecular Study Solitary fibrous tumors and hemangiopericytoma (HPC) are part of the same tumor with NAB2-STAT 6 fusion gene. STAT6 immunohistochemistry reflects the fusion status. Immunohistochemistry for nuclear STAT6 protein expression is confirmative [173] (Figs. 9.21 and 9.22).

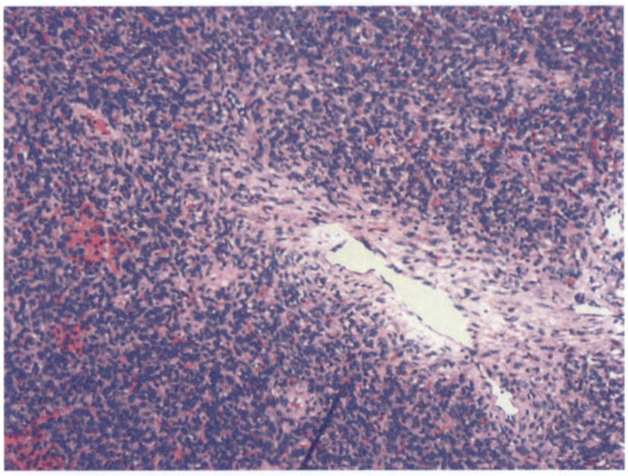

Fig. 9.21 Solitary fibrous tumor showing dilated sinusoidal channel with cellular tumor in a pattern less pattern (representative histology from orbital biopsy)

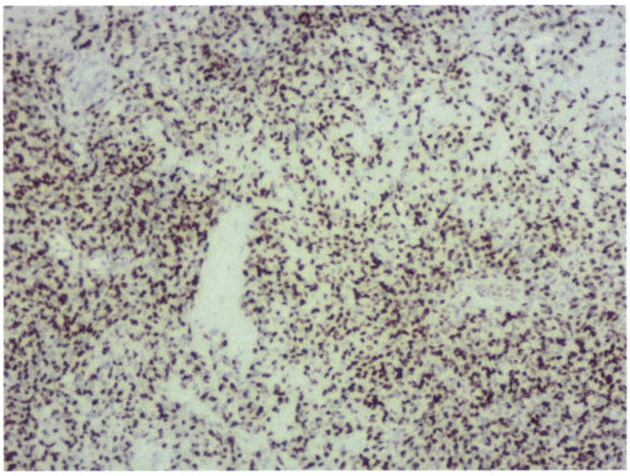

Fig. 9.22 Solitary fibrous tumor showing nuclear STAT6 protein positivity (representative histology from orbital biopsy)

9.5.4.2 Perivascular Epithelioid Cell Tumor, Also Known as PEComa

Clinical Notes These are rare tumors occurring in the eye. One case has been reported in the choroid [174].

Histopathology and Immunohistochemistry These tumors have been described under the ciliary body tumors.

Histopathology Differential Diagnosis Amelanotic melanoma and metastatic tumor.

9.5.5 Malignant Tumors of Choroid

9.5.5.1 Choroidal Melanoma

Clinical Notes Melanoma of choroid is common primary intraocular tumor in adults in US/Europe. It is less common in the Asian Indians [175]. The tumor can present as choroidal mass (Figs. 9.23 and 9.24) or as diffuse choroidal melanoma. Focal choroidal melanoma presents as a dome shape arises from the choroidal melanocytes. The enucleated eye ball shows the pigmented tumor having either a dome shaped or a mushroom shaped tumor depending on the break in bruch's membrane. Diagnosis of choroidal melanoma is based on fundus photography and MRI imaging. The tumor dimensions are measured from the height and base of the tumor. Based on the largest tumor diameter [LTD] the melanomas are classified in to small choroidal melanoma <10 mm in diameter, medium sized between 11 to 15 mm and large tumors >15 mm [176].

Histopathology Bleach preparation of the tumor to remove the melanin is necessary to study the cell morphology clearly. The tumor is cellular and has 2 types of cells. Spindle cells (A and B) and epithelioid cells. Spindle A cells have a nuclear groove and spindle B cells have tiny nucleoli (Figs. 9.25, 9.26, and 9.27). Epithelioid cells are large with oval to polygonal shape with a low nucleo-cytoplasmic ratio with the nucleus showing a vesicular chromatin and prominent nucleoli (Fig. 9.28). Spindle cell melanoma is predominantly made up of spindle cells and epithelioid cell melanomas are composed of epithelioid cells respectively. Mixed cell melanomas are composed of both spindle cells and epithelioid cells. Melanoma cells can have rhabdoid featured with intracytoplasmic inclusions and also show rhabdomyoblastic differentiation when they are extrascleral extension (Figs. 9.29 and 9.30).

Prognostic Parameters Ciliochoroidal melanoma and choroidal melanomas develop hematogenous metastasis to liver, lung and bone marrow. The biological behavior of uveal melanoma is based on many factors ranging from size of tumor and histopathological information. Large tumor volume, large tumor diameter [176] epithelioid cells, nuclear atypia, mitosis, presence of tumor infiltrating lymphocytes (Fig. 9.31),

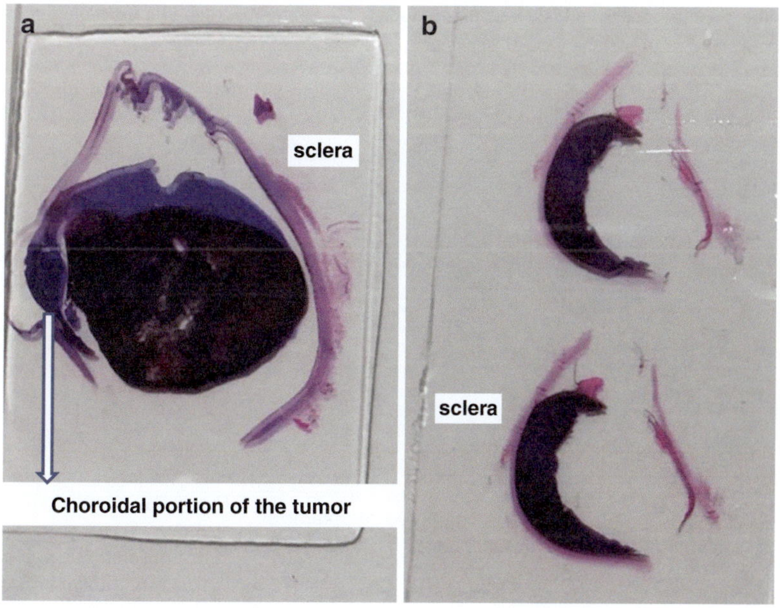

Fig. 9.23 Photomicrograph of the slides showing sections from enucleated eye ball showing choroidal melanoma tumors. (**a**) Shows a choroidal pigmented tumor which is large and broken the bruch's membrane and projecting into the vitreous. (**b**) Shows a pigmented choroidal tumor which is extending throughout the choroid on one side

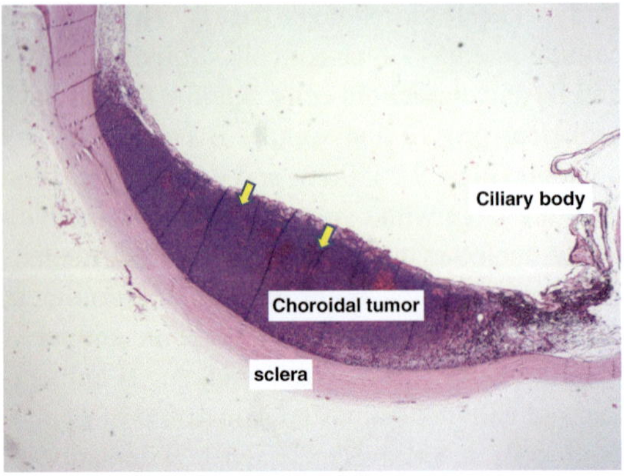

Fig. 9.24 Enucleated Eye ball showing a dome shaped tumor of the choroid-choroidal melanoma (arrow)

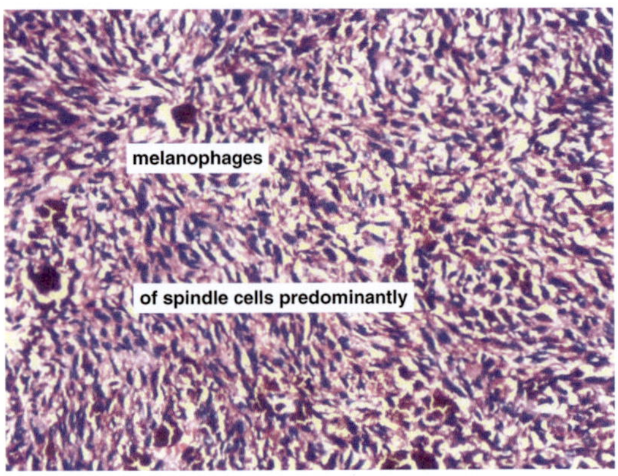

Fig. 9.25 Choroidal melanoma composed of spindle A cells predominantly with scattered melanophages

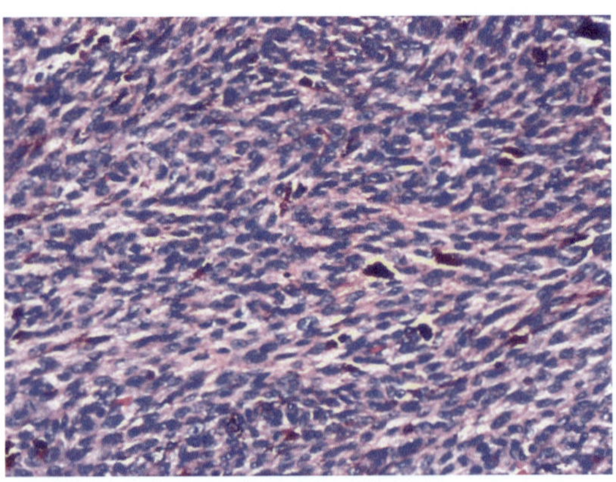

Fig. 9.26 Choroidal melanoma composed of spindle B cells predominantly with tiny nucleoli

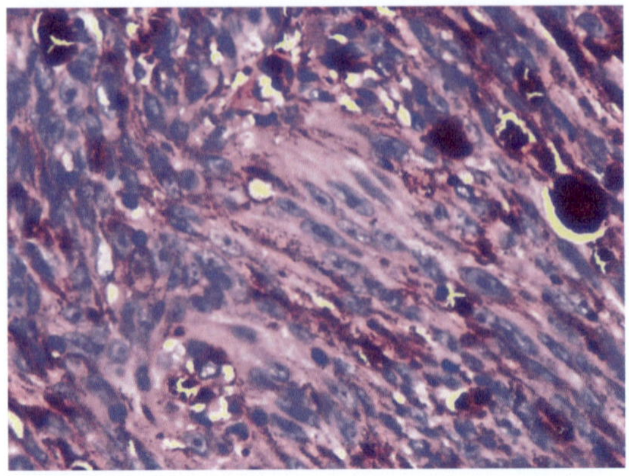

Fig. 9.27 Higher magnification of the tumor showing the spindle B cells in choroidal melanoma with tiny nucleoli

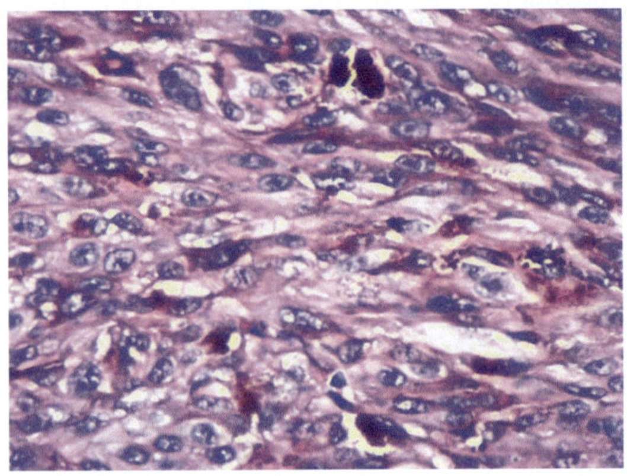

Fig. 9.28 Choroidal melanoma showing the epithelioid cells with prominent nucleoli

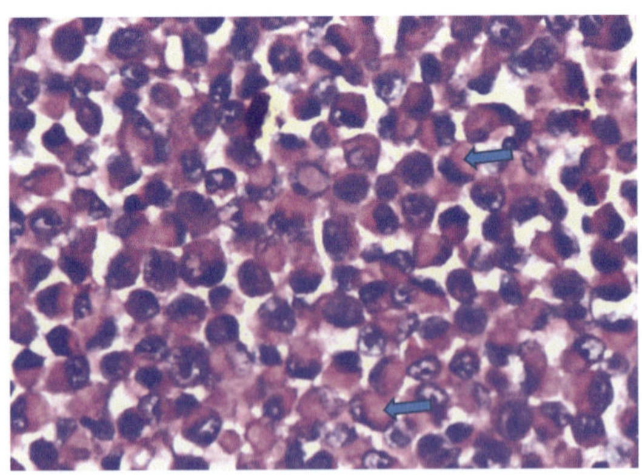

Fig. 9.29 Amelanotic epithelioid melanoma cells with rhabdoid features in choroidal tumor. The tumor cells show eosinophilic inclusions (shown by arrow) in the cytoplasm of the tumor cells and the nucleus of the tumor cell is pushed to the periphery

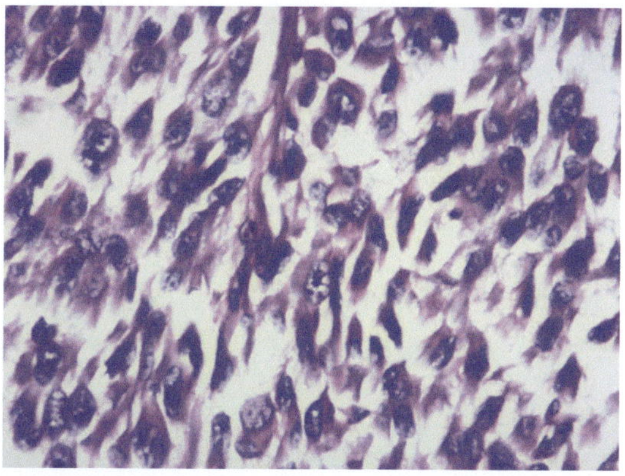

Fig. 9.30 Amelanotic choroidal melanoma cells with rhabdomyoblastic pattern

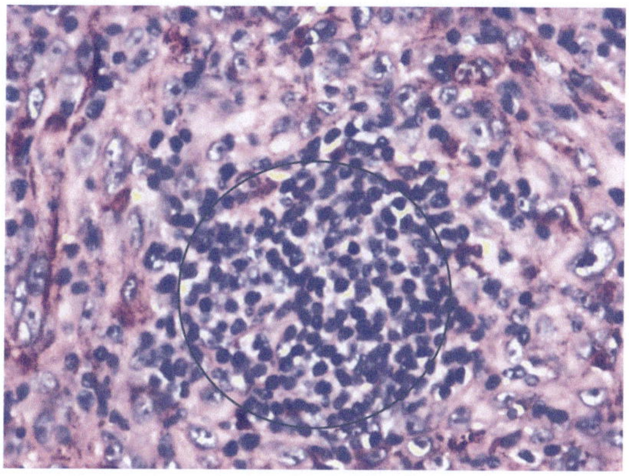

Fig. 9.31 Tumor infiltrating lymphocytes (marked by circle) amongst the choroid melanoma cells

and presence of extra vascular matrix patterns mostly loops and networks contribute to aggressive behavior of the melanoma [177, 178].

However, many of the histopathological parameters such as cell types [179]. Nucleolar grade assessment, tumor infiltrating lymphocytes, and vascular patterns have shown to have limitations and these may not be applicable when the ophthalmologist does FNAB for diagnosis and prognosticating the melanoma and manages the eye melanoma with local therapy without enucleation.

Molecular Testing Currently 2 molecular tests are available as standard of care in ocular oncology. One technique is based on gene expression profiling using microarray. The authors have identified a set of genes to predict risk of a patient's tumor spreading in 5 years [3, 180–183]. This test measures a list of up regulated and down regulated genes in uveal melanoma and the melanoma is classified in to class 1 (low risk) and class 2 (high risk tumor). Uveal melanoma patients with class 2 gene expression profile have a high risk for developing liver metastasis in next 5 years compared to uveal melanoma patients with class 1 gene expression in their tumor samples who have a less chance for developing liver metastasis. There are limitations in using gene expression profiling as the panel cannot differentiate between metastatic tumors to the choroid and class 2 melanoma from a Fine needle aspiration biopsy sample [184] and recently intratumoral heterogeneity in gene expression profile results has been reported in uveal melanomas [185].

The second technique relies on the use of chromosomal aberrations to prognosticate choroidal melanoma. Loss of chromosome 3 and gain of chromosome 8 are associated with liver metastasis. Chromosomal aberrations can be studied using FISH [186–190]. Intratumoral heterogeneity has also been reported in chromosomal aberrations too [191].

Histopathology Differential Diagnosis Choroidal melanocytoma, Leiomyoma, solitary fibrous tumor, neurilemmoma and metastatic tumor in the choroid if the tumor is amelanotic.

Immunohistochemistry It is usually not needed, however if the tumor is amelanotic then immunohistochemistry is needed. Choroidal melanoma is positive of Melanocyte markers such as Melan-1, SOX-10 and HMB45.

9.5.5.2 Choroidal Osteoma

Clinical Notes It is a choristoma and develops from the choroidal mesenchyme. It is usually bilateral [192].

Histopathology The tumor is seen in the middle portion of the choroid and surrounded by the choroidal mesenchyme. The tumor is composed of compact bone. There are marrow spaces that contain dilated thin-walled blood vessels and mesenchymal cells. These tumors grow very slowly [193, 194]. Occasional fast growth of the tumor has been reported [195]. The overlying retina shows thinning.

Histopathology Differential Diagnosis It has to be differentiated from the osseous metaplasia of the retinal pigment epithelium (RPE) in pthysicial eye.

9.5.5.3 Choroid Metastasis

Clinical Notes Choroidal vascularity makes it a favourable site for the hematogenous spread of tumors from other sites such as the breast, thyroid, lung, kidney, GI tract, cutaneous melanoma, or others [196]. Choroidal metastasis indicates poor prognosis [197, 198].

Breast and lung primary tumors are the common primary tumors that metastasize to the choroid [73].

Histopathology Rarely eye is enucleated for diagnosis of metastatic tumors of choroid. In the enucleated tumor there are tumor cells forming a papillary and glandular pattern and may contain mucin secreting cells (Fig. 9.32).

Histopathology Differential Diagnosis Amelanotic secondary tumor deposits in the choroid from primary tumor elsewhere may simulate chorodial melanoma. However, clinical information and immunohistochemistry for melanocyte markers helps to confirm the tumor is melanocyte origin. Choroidal deposits from cutaneous melanoma are rare but diagnosis is made with clinical information and imaging. With the availability of immunotherapy for skin melanoma, choroidal secondary deposits may be seen.

Immunohistochemistry Clinical information, imaging and a panel of immunohistochemistical markers are needed to identify the type of tumor [199]. Please refer to Table 9.1 for panel of markers. A detailed panel is beyond the scope of this book [200].

9.5.5.4 Secondary Choroidal Tumors Resulting from Extension from a Local Tumor

Choroid can be invaded by retinoblastoma tumor and also from intraocular invasion of ocular surface squamous cell carcinoma and rarely from the adenocarcinoma of retinal pigment epithelium. Intraocular extension of lacrimal gland adenocarcinoma may secondarily invade the choroid (Fig. 9.33). Intraocular extension of ocular surface carcinoma may mimic intraocular tumor or inflammation and the eviscerated or enucleated portion of the eye may show the tumor in the choroid. Presence of keratinizing atypical cells or keratin pearl formation by the tumor cells is diagnositic (Figs. 9.34 and 9.35).

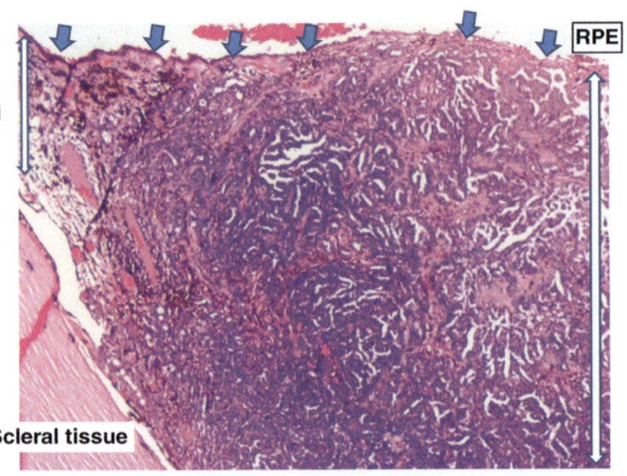

Fig. 9.32 Metastatic adenocarcinoma deposit in the choroid (marked by double arrowhead) underlying the retinal pigment epithelium (RPE) (shown by single arrow). The tumor cells show a papillary pattern

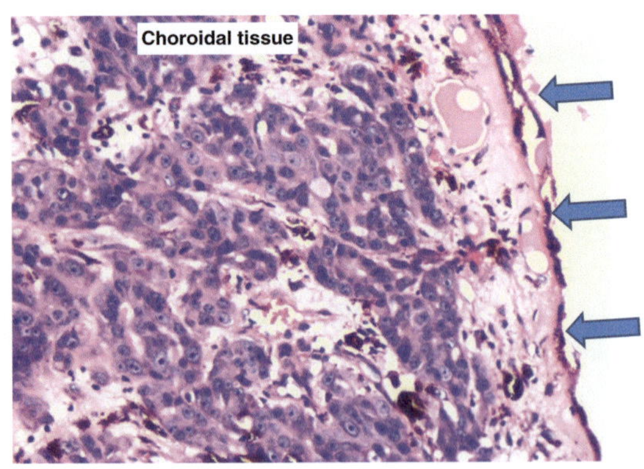

Fig. 9.33 Choroidal invasion of adenocarcinoma of the lacrimal gland. The tumor cells have invaded in the choroid and are arranged in glandular pattern with duct like structures are seen in the tumor. The retinal pigment epithelium is shown by arrow

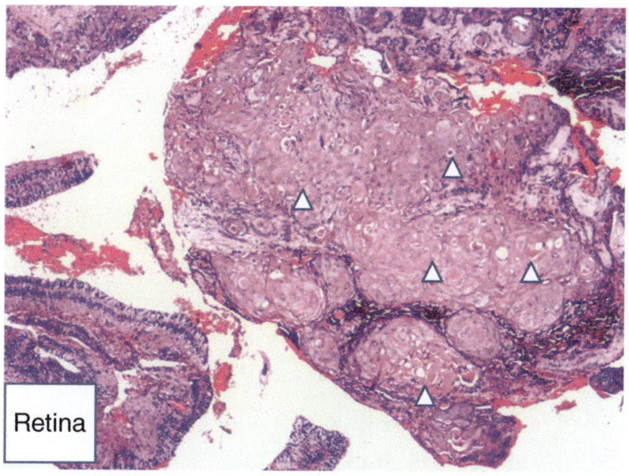

Fig. 9.34 Eviscerated portion of the intraocular contents showing local intraocular extension of conjunctival squamous cell carcinoma in to choroid (shown by triangle cartoon) with portions of the retina are seen

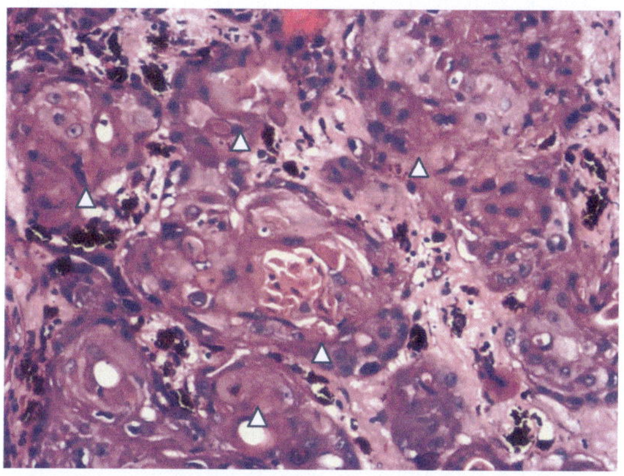

Fig. 9.35 Well differentiated keratinized conjunctival squamous cell carcinoma (shown by triangle cartoon) in the choroid (shown by triangle cartoon) in to choroid. Scattered choroidal melanocytes are seen

9.6 Tumors Arising from the Retina

Retina is a special multilayered neural tissue. Retina is prone not only to genetic diseases, retinal infections by virus, parasites and immune mediated disorders and metabolic disorders but also to tumors, both primary and secondary.

9.6.1 Benign Retinal Tumors

Retinal vascular tumors

- Retinal hemangioblastoma
- Cavernous hemangioma of the retina
- Retinal vasoproliferative tumor

9.6.2 Intermediate Grade Tumors

- Retinoma

9.6.2.1 Malignant Retinal Tumors

Primary

- Retinoblastoma
- Vitreo retinal lymphoma

Secondary

- Leukemic infiltration into retina
- Melanoma cells infiltrating retina
- Metastatic tumor cells in retina

9.6.2.2 Rare Intraocular Tumors-Possibly from Retina

- Primitive Neuroectodermal tumor/Ewing's sarcoma-retina
- Synovial Sarcoma
- Extra renal Rhabdoid tumor

9.6.3 Benign Tumors

9.6.3.1 Vascular Tumors of Retina

Retinal Hemangioblastoma

Clinical Notes Retinal capillary hemangioblastoma may be an isolated lesion within the retina or associated with von Hippel-Lindau (VHL) syndrome when there could be hemangioblastomas of the central nervous system [201]. Patient could have vision loss because of retinal detachment.

Histopathology The vascular tumors are seen in the retinal tissue that could show secondary detachment because of serous exudates. The vascular tumor is composed of numerous small capillaries, spindle cells and surrounded by foamy stromal cells. There is no atypia [202]. The stromal cells are the neoplastic cells and they are positive for CD133 [203].

Histopathological Differential Diagnosis Coat's disease, when there is more retinal and vitreous exudates.

Cavernous Hemangioma of the Retina

Clinical Notes Retinal cavernous hemangioma could lead to vision loss [204]. There could be associated Central nervous system hemangioma.

Histopathology The retinal tissue shows blood-filled sinusoidal spaces. There could be associated fibro glial proliferation within the inner retinal layers [205, 206]

Histopathological Differential Diagnosis Coat's disease, retinal hemangioblastoma.

Retinal Vasoproliferative Tumor (VPTRs)

Clinical Notes Retinal VPTR is rare vascular tumor also known as nodular and massive retinal gliosis. They could be unilateral with no associated systemic disorder or bilateral associated with retinitis pigmentosa, retinopathy of prematurity, and coats disease etc. [207].

Histopathology The vascular tumor arises from the retina and there is secondary retinal detachment. The vascular tumor takes a nodular shape that may be small or large one causing significant retinal detachment. There are secondary changes in the retinal pigment epithelium such as osseous metaplasia and exudates in the vitreous. The tumor predominantly shows spindle cell proliferation around the dilated thickened blood vessels of retina. The spindle cells are mostly astrocytes and glial cells. The thickened material around the blood vessels is PAS positive. There is no atypia and no mitosis.

Histopathological Differential Diagnosis Retinal hemangioblastoma, astrocytoma and oligodendroglioma.

Immunohistochemistry S 100 and GFAP are positive in the spindle cells. CD 34 is positive in the blood vessels. Ki 67 is low.

9.6.4 Intermediate Grade Tumors of the Retina

9.6.4.1 Retinoma

Clinical Notes Retinoma is the benign precursor to retinoblastoma. In most cases, it remains benign for the lifetime of the individual, rarely progressing to retinoblastoma [208].

Retinoma has three (3) characteristic clinical features: a grey, translucent mass in the retina; cottage cheese-like calcification; and a hyperplastic retinal epithelium/chorioretinal scar [209]. Vitreous seeds have also been observed associated with retinoma though rarely [210]. Retinoma has been observed clinically in 1.8% [209] to 3.2% [211] of retinoblastoma cases and by pathology in 15.6% [212] to 20.4% [213] of enucleated retinoblastoma specimens.

Histopathology Retinoma is histologically distinct from retinoblastoma. Retinoma displays abundant fleurettes, eosinophilic cytoplasm, foci of calcification and non-proliferative cells [212, 214] (Fig. 9.36).

Histopathology Differential Diagnosis Retinoma lacks the typical features of retinoblastoma (Homer Wright and Flexner-Wintersteiner rosettes, nuclear moulding, abundant mitoses and necrosis), and is often observed adjacent to retinoblastoma tumor in enucleated specimens [212].

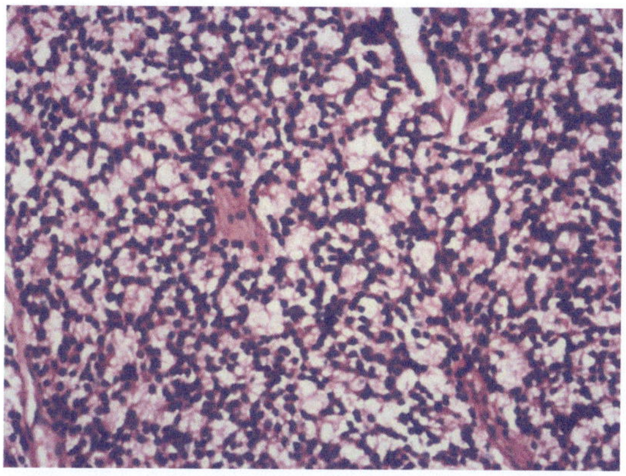

Fig. 9.36 Tumor lobule showing extensive fleurettes with no atypia, no mitosis and no necrosis. This pattern is seen in retinoma

Immunohistochemistry Proliferative index Ki 67 is low and p75NTR protein is expressed in retinoma and not in retinoblastoma.

9.6.5 Malignant Tumors of Retina

9.6.5.1 Retinoblastoma

Clinical Notes Retinoblastoma is a common intraocular tumor in children. More than 90% of the tumors are diagnosed before the age of 3. The clinical presentation varies from leukocoria/squint/proptosis. Mutations in retinoblastoma (RB1) gene, an important tumor suppressor gene, with subsequent loss of functional retinoblastoma protein have been attributed as one of the common events in development of several tumors and as a sole contributor to majority of germinal retinoblastoma tumors.

Genetics Based on the pattern of RB1 gene inactivation, retinoblastoma is classified as hereditary (germline) and non-hereditary form. The germ line form tends to present earlier and mostly bilateral in manifestation with multifocal tumors while the non-hereditary form is usually unilateral in manifestation with unifocal tumors [215]. Although, RB1 gene mutation is an initiating event, several secondary genetic lesions following the RB1 gene mutation is required for the tumorigenesis and progression. Copy number gains have been frequently identified on 1q, 2p, 6p and loss on 16q in most retinoblastoma samples. Recent studies [216] exploring the characterization of the genomic regions have thrown light on the identity of gains in several oncogenes and loss in tumor suppressors such as CDH11, DDX1, DEK, E2F3,KIF14, MDM4, MYCN and RBL2 which might play a role in RB progression. Recent reports suggest that approximately 2.7% of unilateral sporadic retinoblastoma tumors do not carry any mutation in the RB1 gene. These samples screened for other copy number gains revealed NMYC amplification. It is now widely accepted that NMYC amplification, albeit at low frequencies, can be an initiator in subset of RB tumors where a fully functional RB protein is detectable [217].

Histopathology The eye grossing of the enucleated retinoblastoma and sectioning is done according to the International Retinoblastoma Staging Working Group (IRSWG) guidelines (Fig. 9.37) [218]. In tumors which are enucleated prior chemotherapy, the enucleated globe on sectioning shows a basophilic tumor arising from the layers of retina with retina detached (Fig. 9.38).

The tumor is arranged in lobules around the central blood vessels. There are areas in the periphery of the tumor lobules showing necrotic/apoptotic zones (Figs. 9.39 and 9.40).

When the tumor is subjected to chemotherapy, the tumor shows extensive calcification with a few viable tumor cells (Fig. 9.41).

Patterns of Growth in Retinoblastoma The tumors may show 4 patterns of growth. In endophytic growth pattern the tumor grows towards the vitreous. In exophytic growth pattern the tumor cells grow towards the choroid. In mixed patterns of tumor growth, there is both endophytic and exophytic growth pattern. The fourth pattern is diffuse infiltrating retinoblastoma where the tumor cells infiltrate the retina and there could be intraocular inflammation like presentation [219, 220].

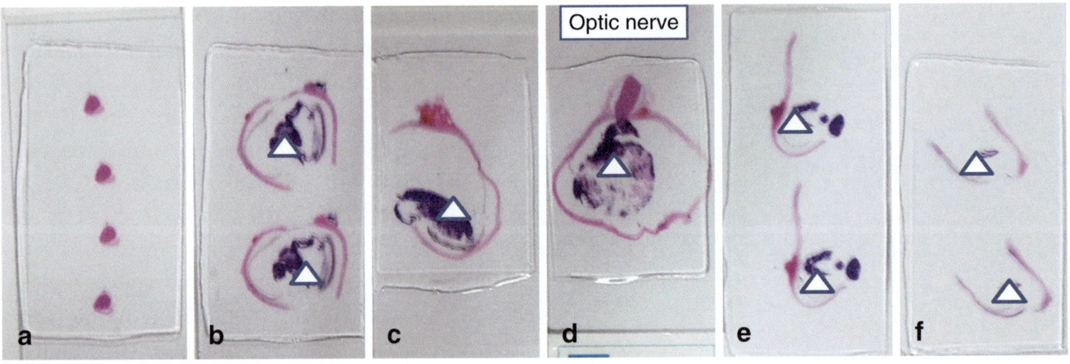

Fig. 9.37 Photomicrograph of the glass slide of the enucleated eye ball showing the sections taken according to International Retinoblastoma Staging Working Group (IRSWG) guidelines. (**a**) Surgical end of optic nerve. (**b**, **c**, **e**) Lateral portion of the globe. (**d**) Pupil optic nerve axis sections of the eye ball and (**f**) bread loaf sections from the lateral calotte showing sclera and choroid. The tumor is shown by the triangle cartoon

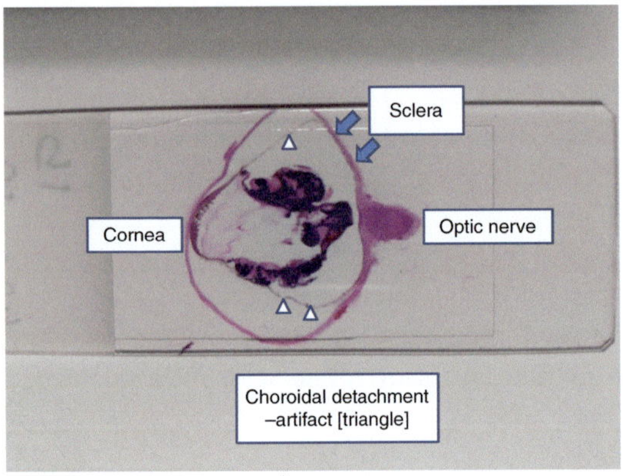

Fig. 9.38 Photomicrograph of the glass slide of the enucleated eye ball showing a retinoblastoma infiltrating the retina in a diffuse pattern

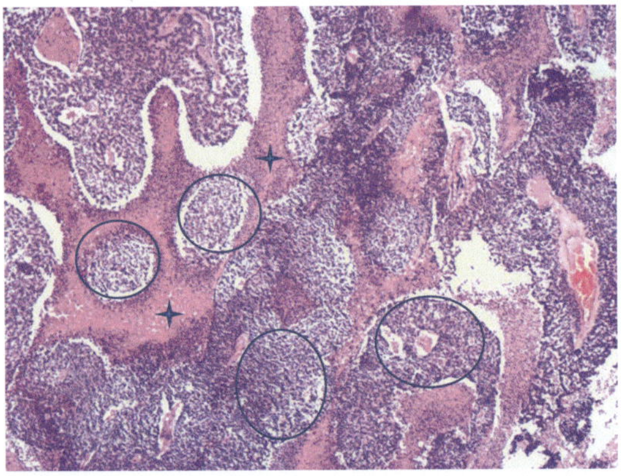

Fig. 9.39 Posterior segment of the enucleated eye ball showing a retinoblastoma with tumor cells arranged in lobules and showing areas of necrosis (arrow) and viable tumor cells (circle)

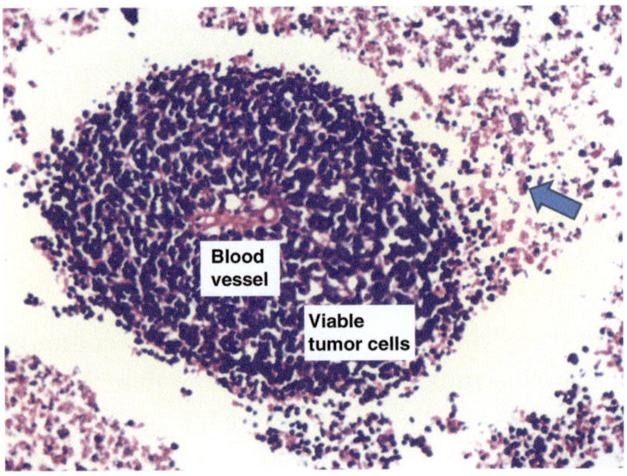

Fig. 9.40 Retinoblastoma tumor cells arranged around central blood vessel. Viable cells are seen close to the blood vessel and necrotic cells are seen in the peripheral portion (arrow). This pattern of arrangement of tumor cells around central blood vessel is known as pseudorosettes

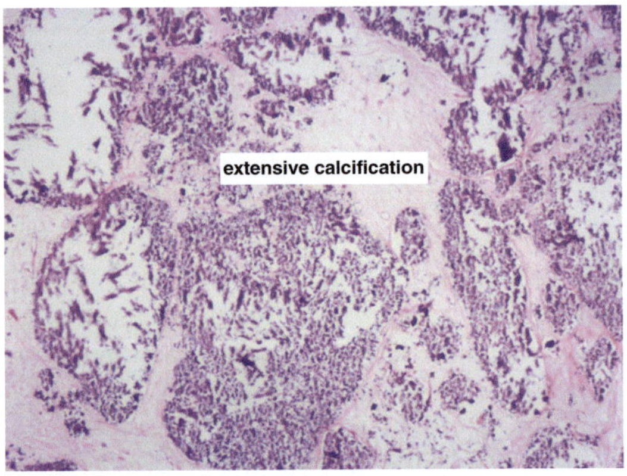

Fig. 9.41 Retinoblastoma with extensive calcification of the tumor lobules in the posterior segment

9.6.6 Invasiveness of Tumor Cells

Choroid The bread loaf sections from the lateral portion of the eye ball are looked at to comment on the choroidal invasion and sclera invasion. The sections from the pupil optic nerve axis and slightly lateral to the pupil optic nerve axis are looked at to comment on the choroidal invasion of the tumor. The tumor cells show various levels of retinal pigment epithelial invasion (Fig. 9.42) and choroidal invasion. When the tumor cells invading the choroid are 3 mm and less and not touching the sclera fibers it is known as focal choroidal invasion (Fig. 9.43).

When the tumor cells have invaded the choroid more than 3 mm and touching the sclera fibers it is massive choroidal invasion of choroid (Fig. 9.44).

Optic Nerve The optic nerve is looked for tumor cell invasion in the laminar portion and post laminar portion of the optic nerve and the transected end of the optic nerve is screened for tumor cells both in the optic nerve and in the meningeal sheath of the optic nerve (Fig. 9.45).

Anterior Segment There could be anterior segment invasion in the form of iris surface lining of

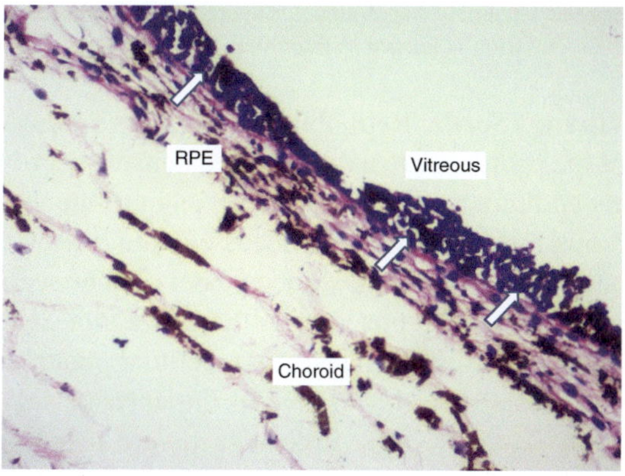

Fig. 9.42 Retinoblastoma tumor cells invading the retinal pigment epithelium. The arrows show the retinal pigment epithelium (RPE)

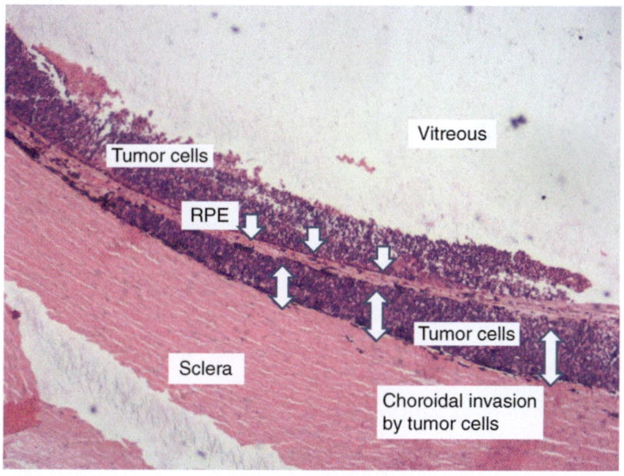

Fig. 9.44 Retinoblastoma with invasion of choroid by tumor cells >3 mm. The double arrowhead shows the choroidal space invaded by the tumor. The line of single arrow shows the retinal pigment epithelium (RPE)

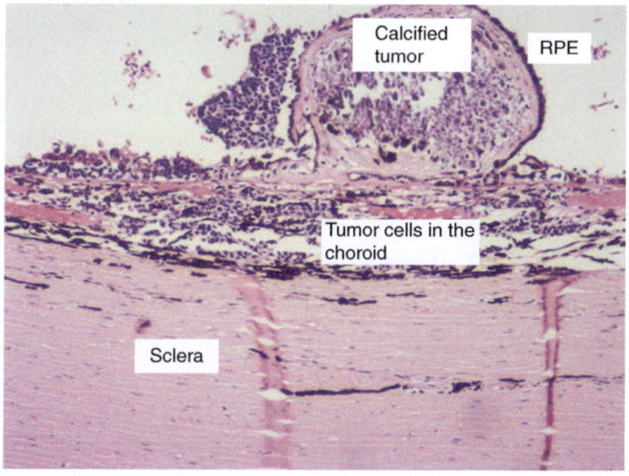

Fig. 9.43 Retinoblastoma with focal invasion of choroid by tumor cells. There is calcified tumor nodule below the retinal pigment epithelial cells

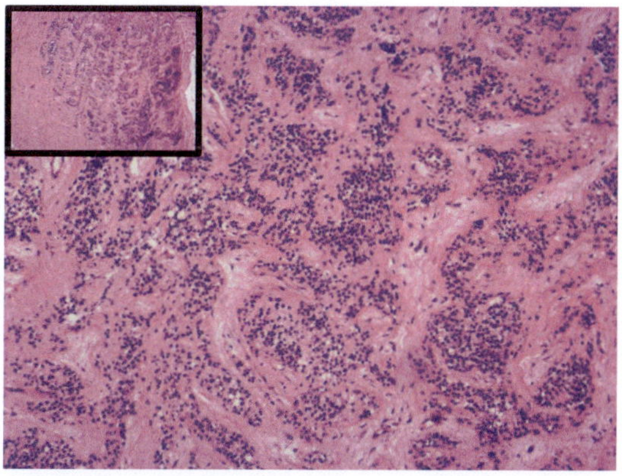

Fig. 9.45 Retinoblastoma with invasion of laminar and post laminar portion of the optic nerve. Inset showing the optic nerve showing the post laminar portion

tumors, iris stroma showing tumors, anterior chamber angle invaded by tumor cells. Prognosis based on anterior segment invasion is evolving. High risk retinoblastoma suggests that there is choroid invasion >3 mm and invasion of the post laminar portion/surgical end of optic nerve.

Differentiation The tumor cells also show some pattern formation. These are called as rosettes. The tumor cells may be arranged around a central neural material or around a lumen. The former is called as homer-wright rosettes (Fig. 9.46) and the latter one is called as Flexner–wintersteiner rosettes (Fig. 9.47). Tumor cells can also show extensive photoreceptor differentiation and have arrangement like bouquet. This is known as fleurettes (Fig. 9.48).

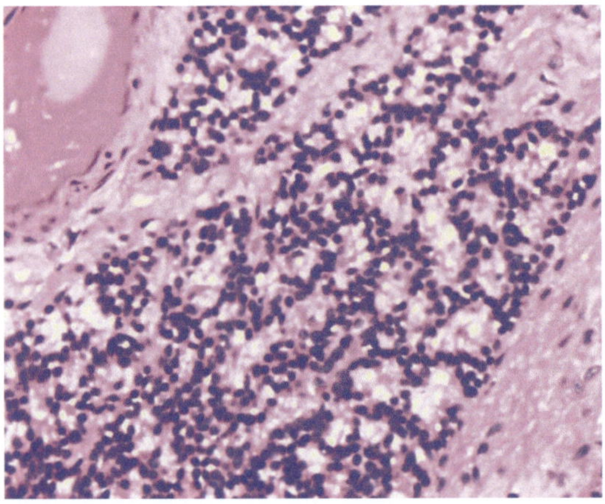

Fig. 9.48 The lobule of retinoblastoma shows tumor cells with extensive photoreceptor differentiation with and have arrangement like bouquet. This pattern of tumor cell differentiation is known as fleurettes

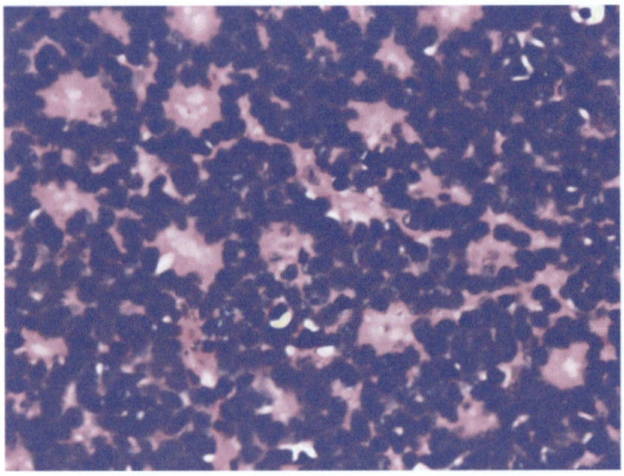

Fig. 9.46 Retinoblastoma tumor cells showing Flexner-Wintersteiner rosettes with central lumen

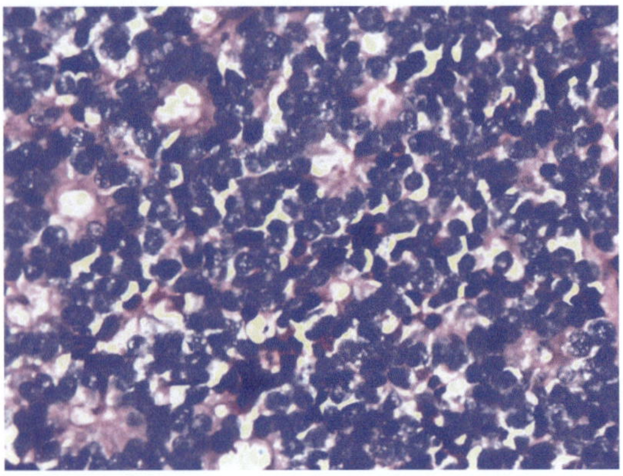

Fig. 9.47 Retinoblastoma tumor cells showing Homer Wright rosettes with central neuropil

Vitreous Seeds Retinoblastoma tumors because of the proliferative nature show extensive necrosis and tumor cellular debris seeps in to the vitreous fluid. The vitreous seeds contain necrotic and viable cells, Some blood vessels can be seen within the vitreous seeds, there are not real blood vessels are just extracellular matrix. Vitreous seeds may escape to the anterior segment. Tumors with vitreous seeds are respond to poorly to systemic chemotherapy [221]. Histopathologically vitreous seeds are of three types. Vitreous seeds can be single viable tumor cells, clumps of cells which may contain viable and necrotic cells and finally the necrotic cells and inflammatory cells post chemotherapy such as melphalan (Fig. 9.49).

MYCN Retinoblastoma RB1 mutation is negative in this category of tumor and these are unilateral RB. These tumors are seen in young children and are invasive. Morphologically these tumors are different. These tumor cells are large with multiple nucleoli and necrosis and there is no differentiation and no calcification. It is important to identify these tumors because they may need aggressive therapy and may not respond to platinum based therapy [217].

Molecular Profiling Gene expression profiling showed that retinoblastoma tumors could be clas-

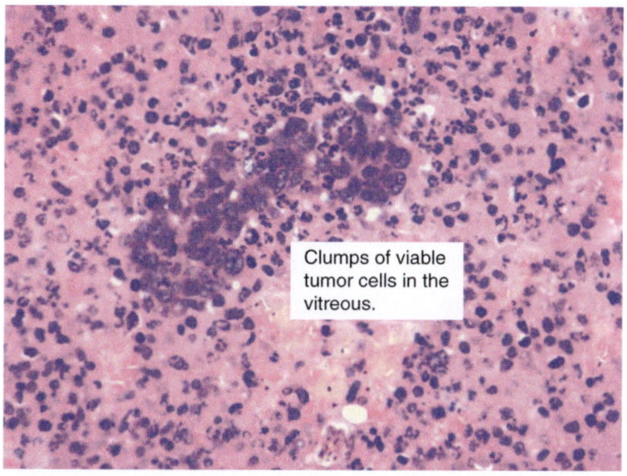

Fig. 9.49 Clumps of viable tumor cells in the vitreous. The vitreous contains numerous cellular debris some viable and majority appear necrotic

sified in to 2 groups [4]. Group 1 retinoblastoma showed an invasive pattern of growth while Group 2 retinoblastoma were found to have proliferating tumor cells retaining cone photoreceptor cells [4].

Anaplasia Anaplasia is considered a bad prognosis and in general indicates the poorly differentiated tumor cells. Grading of anaplasia is important in retinoblastoma as patients with retinoblastoma who do not have invasion of choroid or optic nerve and if the tumor shows severe anaplasia there is increased risk for metastasis. The anaplastia is based on tumor size, shape, nuclear atypia and molding. Three grades of anaplasia have been identified such as mild, moderate, or severe anaplasia [222, 223] (Figs. 9.50 and 9.51).

Retinoblastoma tumors with high risk histopathology features metastasize rapidly to the brain if there is extensive optic nerve invasion and tumor cells spread through the cerebrospinal fluid. If the tumors show extensive choroidal invasion, they metastasize to the bone marrow and the regional nodes. Metastases after 3 years are rare and secondary tumors such as osteogenic sarcoma, peripheral neuroectodermal tumor/Ewing's sarcoma should be ruled out.

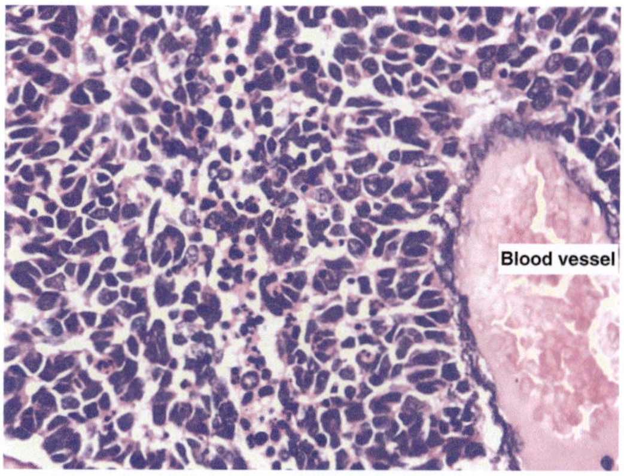

Fig. 9.50 Retinoblastoma tumor cells elongated and molding-moderate atypia. There is no rosettes formation by the tumor cells

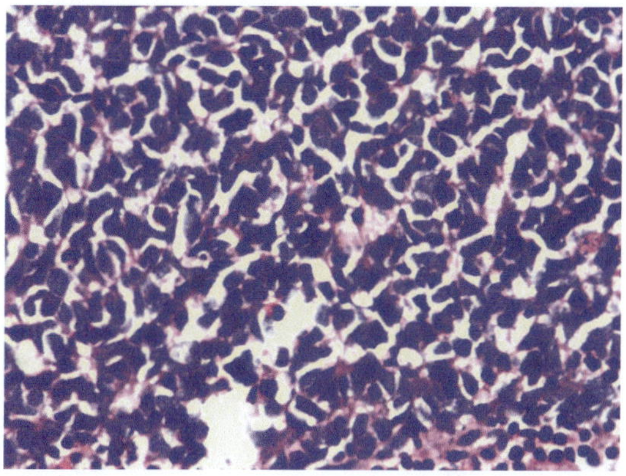

Fig. 9.51 Retinoblastoma tumor cells severe anaplasia with tumor cells elongated and molding-severe atypia. There is no rosettes formation by the tumor cells

Immunohistochemistry Synaptophysin is helpful in staining retinoblastoma tumor cells, it can help to document the choroidal invasion and help to identify the suspicious foci of tumor cells in the post laminar portion of the optic nerve (Figs. 9.52 and 9.53).

Update Recently, tumor-derived cell-free DNA from anterior chamber aspirate in retinoblastoma patients has shown 6p gain in the aqueous humor is a potential prognostic biomarker for poor clinical response to therapy and this has a lot of potential to prognosticate Retinoblastoma tumors [224].

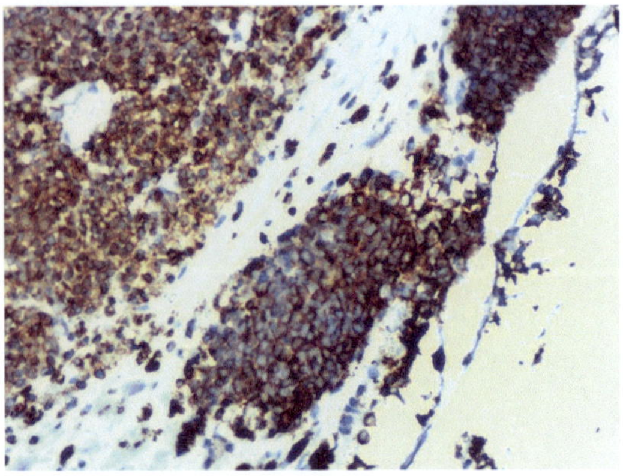

Fig. 9.52 Retinoblastoma with focal invasion of choroid by tumor cells showing synaptophysin positivity in the tumor cells showing a membrane positivity

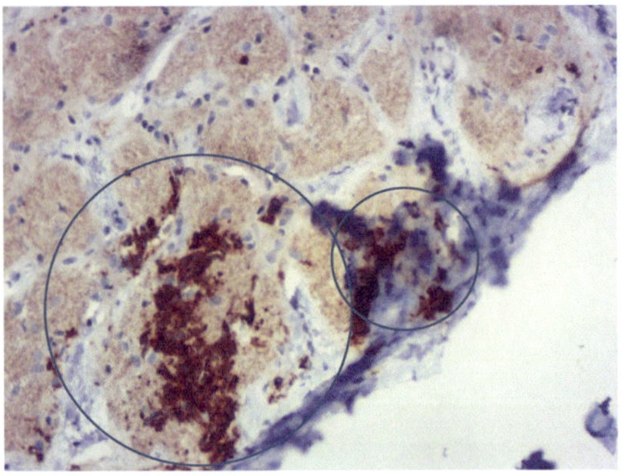

Fig. 9.53 Surgical end of optic nerve showing foci of retinoblastoma tumor cells showing synaptophysin positivity. The tumor cells are enclosed in the circle

9.6.7 Vitreo Retinal Lymphoma

It is a high grade lymphoproliferative disorder where atypical lymphocytes infiltrate the retina and vitreous. The topic is discussed detail under lymphomas.

9.6.8 Secondary Tumors of Retina

Local intraocular tumors such as medulloepithelioma can secondarily invade the retina [84, 147, 225] (Fig. 9.54). Retina is also involved in tumors that originate from other organs. They are uncommon and simulate inflammation of the retina.

9.6.9 Rare Primary Intraocular Tumors

9.6.9.1 Primitive Neuroectodermal Tumor/Ewing's Sarcoma of the Retina

Clinical Notes Primitive neuroectodermal tumors/Ewing's sarcoma is a malignant round cell tumor that usually arises in the bone and soft tissues. First, these tumors could arise in the extremities or pelvis of children with unilateral and bilateral retinoblastoma post chemotherapy [226–228]. Here, important differential diagnosis in osteogenic sarcoma, bone metastasis from retinoblastoma. In the second category, Ewing's sarcoma can present as an intraocular mass from the peripheral retina [229]. In the third category Ewing's sarcoma metastatic to choroid has been reported [230, 231].

Histopathology Tumor is cellular and is composed of round cells, with areas of necrosis and rosettes. Both Homer-Wright rosette and Flexner-Wintersteiner rosettes can be seen, however the former is more predominant. Cells could show nuclear atypia and there is no calcification.

Histopathology Differential Diagnosis This tumor closely mimics retinoblastoma as it has round cells, necrosis and rosettes and anaplastic retinoblastoma.

Immunohistochemistry and Molecular Testing Membranous staining of CD99 and molecular testing for EWS/FLI-1 fusion transcript in the tumor confirms the diagnosis.

9.6.9.2 Primary Intraocular Synovial Sarcoma

Clinical Notes Synovial sarcoma is a malignant tumor of soft tissues and rare in the intraocular portion of the eye. There are a few cases where synovial sarcoma has been reported in the conjunctiva [232]; and orbit [233, 234] and one case has been reported with origin from intraocular location post retinal surgery [235].

Histopathology The tumor is cellular and shows spindle cells arranged in a fascicular pattern. The spindle cells show nuclear atypia and mitotic activity.

Immunohistochemistry and Molecular Testing IHC and molecular studies are a must for diagnosis. Tumor cells are positive for TLE1, EMA and the t(X; 18) translocation and the *SYT-SSX* fusion gene are specific markers for synovial sarcoma.

9.6.9.3 Malignant Extra Renal Rhabdoid Tumor

Clinical Notes Malignant extrarenal rhabdoid tumor is a rare and highly aggressive tumor of childhood. Intraocular involvement by malignant extrarenal rhabdoid tumor is rare. It had been reported in the Lid [236], orbit [237–240]. There have been 2 cases of primary intraocular tumor [58, 60] and one with intraocular mass simulating retinoblastoma as a result of metastasis [59].

Histopathology The tumor is cellular and composed of large tumor cells with nucleus pushed to one side with eosinophilic cytoplasm and having prominent nucleoli. The tumor shows mitosis and areas of necrosis.

Histopathology Differential Diagnosis Retinoblastoma, Peripheral neuroectodermal tumor/ Ewing's sarcoma are to be considered.

Immunohistochemistry Tumor cells are focal positive for CD99, neuron specific enolase and neurofilament. There negative staining for desmin and myoD1 and there is loss of nuclear staining for SMARCB1/INI1 protein in the tumor cells.

9.6.10 Retinal Pigment Epithelium

The retinal pigment epithelium (RPE) is a special layer between the retina and choroid. The RPE rests on a membrane called Bruch's membrane [241].

RPE cells show reactive proliferation in phthisical eye and in chronic inflammations. However, the RPE is also frequently involved in tumors.

Primary tumors arising from the RPE

9.6.11 Tumors of the Retinal Pigment Epithelium

Benign tumor
Classification of RPE tumors based on clinical behaviour
Primary tumors of RPE

- Reactive hyperplasia of the RPE
- Simple and combined hamartoma of the RPE
- Congenital hypertrophy of RPE
- Adenoma of RPE

Primary malignant tumor

- Adenocarcinoma arising from the Retinal Pigment Epithelium

9.6.11.1 Benign Tumor

Reactive Hyperplasia of the Retinal Pigment Epithelium

Clinical Notes It presents as [pigmented patches. Nodular RPE hyperplasia can simulate a choroidal melanoma. There is some amount of vision loss because of secondary retinal detachment [242, 243].

Histopathology Reactive hyperplasia of the retinal pigment epithelium is a non-neoplastic proliferation. RPE proliferation could be small foci or present in considerable amount. There could be associated osseous metaplasia of the RPE too.

Histopathology Differential Diagnosis Nodular Hyperplasia of the RPE cells can have a pseudo glandular pattern and mimic adenocarcinoma. There is no atypia and mitotic activity. The epithelial cells are surrounded by PAS positive basement membrane.

Simple and Combined Hamartoma of the Retinal Pigment Epithelium

Clinical Notes Hamartomas of the retinal pigment epithelium are rare.

Histopathology The cells are heavily pigmented due to the presence of large melanosomes.

Congenital Hypertrophy of the Retinal Pigment Epithelium

Clinical Note Congenital hypertrophy of the retinal pigment epithelium as the name mentions is a focal hypertrophic benign retinal pigment epithelial cell. The cells are heavily pigmented due to the presence of large melanosomes.

Adenoma of the Retinal Pigment Epithelium

Clinical Note It is seen as a pigmented nodule in the choroid and may mimic melanoma.

Histopathology Adenoma of the RPE arises from the RPE. These tumors can invade the adjacent structures such as the choroid and retina. The tumor shows cords and tubular arrangements of cells which are closely arranged and the tumor cells are surrounded by PAS positive basement membrane like material and the tumor cells can also show vacuolar pattern or a combined pattern.

Histopathology Differential Diagnosis If there is atypia or mitotic activity the tumor should be considered as RPE adenocarcinoma.

Immunohistochemistry The neoplastic RPE cells are positive for Melan A, MITF, SOX-10 cytokeratin and vimentin.

9.6.11.2 Primary Malignant Tumors

Adenocarcinoma Arising from the Retinal Pigment Epithelium

Clinical Notes Adenocarcinoma is a rare tumor from the RPE. There are some predisposing factors such as a chorioretinal scar, congenital hypertrophy of the RPE and a pthisical eye [244, 245]. The tumor if pigmented could mimic a melanoma and if amelanotic a metastatic tumor [246].

Histopathology The tumor arises from the retinal pigment epithelium. The tumor because of its location can invade the retina causing secondary retinal detachment. It can invade the choroid and the adjacent structures such as optic nerve. The tumor cells are heavily pigmented. Bleaching is needed to study the tumor. The tumor shows varied patterns like tubular, papillary, multiple vacuolations in the cells or combined patterns (Figs. 9.54 and 9.55). The tumor cells are surrounded by PAS positive material. The tumor cells show nuclear atypia and mitotic activity [247]. Extra scleral extension could be seen rarely [248].

Histopathology Differential Diagnosis The tubular and papillary patterns can be seen in reactive hyperplasia and adenoma. However there is usually no atypia and mitotic activity. Epithelioid cell melanoma can mimic RPE adenocarcinoma.

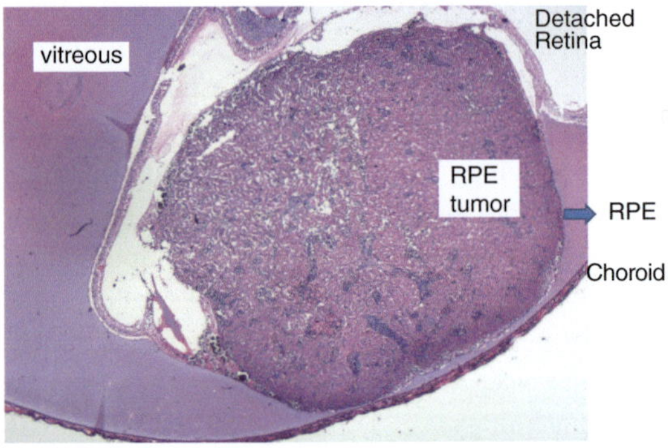

Fig. 9.54 RPE adenocarcinoma arising from the retinal pigment epithelium

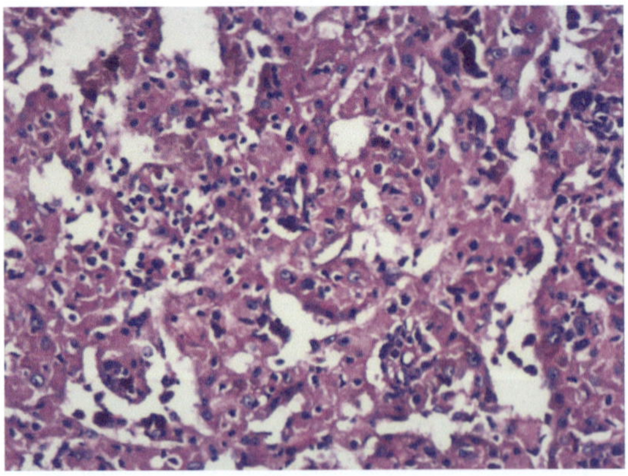

Fig. 9.55 RPE adenocarcinoma showing tubular and glandular arrangement of tumor cells

Immunohistochemistry The tumor cells express both melanocyte markers and epithelial markers. Ki-67 can be low to high [249].

9.6.12 Optic Disc and Optic Nerve Tumors

We mainly discuss those tumors that can have an intraocular tumor like presentation

Primary tumors

- Melanocytoma of the optic disc and Optic nerve
- Medulloepithelioma of the optic disc and optic nerve
- Astrocytoma of the optic nerve
- Meningioma of the optic disc and optic nerve
- Atypical teratoid/rhabdoid tumors

Secondary tumors of the optic nerve

- Metastatic tumors

9.6.12.1 Primary Tumors

Optic Disc Melanocytoma

Clinical Notes It is a benign melanocytic tumor arising from the optic disc and optic nerve. The tumor is usually asymptomatic. However visual testing may show abnormal visual fields.

Histopathology It is a densely pigmented tumor and bleaching shows the tumor is composed of oval cells. The tumor cells have a low nucleo-cytoplasmic ratio and have tiny nucleoli. There is extensive necrosis with inflammation. Melanophages are seen scattered within the tumor.

Histopathology Differential Diagnosis Melanoma to be ruled out with serial sections.

Optic Nerve Medulloepithelioma

Clinical Notes Optic nerve medulloepitheliomas have been reported [250]. They can mimic intraocular tumors.

Histopathology The histopathology and grading is similar to ciliary body medulloepithelioma discussed earlier.

Atypical Teratoid/Rhabdoid Tumors

Clinical Notes These are very rare tumors and seen in young children. They can present as proptosis. There are 3 cases reported earlier with involvement of the optic nerve [251].

Histopathology The tumor cells are large epithelioid with cytoplasm showing eosinophilic globular inclusions. The nucleus is slightly eccentric and there are prominent nucleoli in the tumor cells. Mitotic activity and areas of necrosis are seen. Serial sections are recommended and clinical correlation and immunohistochemistry and genetic testing is suggested.

Histopathological Differential Diagnosis Anaplastic Retinoblastoma; Teratoid medulloepithelioma with Rhabdomyoblastic component.

Immunohistochemistry The tumor is usually positive for EMA, vimentin, S-100 protein and negative for desmin, myogenin, INI1, chromogranin, synaptophysin, CD34 and CD99 [250].

9.7 Conclusion

Thus, in this chapter on intraocular tumors I have tried to classify the tumors based on anatomical site of origin and also list the primary and secondary tumors that have occured based on the published literature. I have also tried to classify these tumors based on their clinical behaviour as benign, intermediate and malignant. The classification given above is slightly from the recently published WHO classification of intraocular tumors [252]. The chapters would enable the ophthalmologist and Pathologist with little knowledge of Ophthalmic pathology to diagnose the complex intraocular tumors.

References

1. Grossniklaus HE. Ophthalmic pathology: history, accomplishments, challenges, and goals. Ophthalmology. 2015;122(8):1539–42. https://doi.org/10.1016/j.ophtha.2015.04.001.
2. Bonzheim I, Giese S, Deuter C, Süsskind D, Zierhut M, Waizel M, et al. High frequency of MYD88 mutations in vitreoretinal B-cell lymphoma: a valuable tool to improve diagnostic yield of vitreous aspirates. Blood. 2015;126(1):76–9. https://doi.org/10.1182/blood-2015-01-620518.
3. Onken MD, Worley LA, Tuscan MD, Harbour JW. An accurate, clinically feasible multi-gene expression assay for predicting metastasis in uveal melanoma. J Mol Diagn. 2010;12(4):461–8. https://doi.org/10.2353/jmoldx.2010.090220.
4. Kapatai G, Brundler M-A, Jenkinson H, Kearns P, Parulekar M, Peet AC, McConville CM. Gene expression profiling identifies different sub-types of retinoblastoma. Br J Cancer. 2013;109(2):512–25. https://doi.org/10.1038/bjc.2013.283.
5. Dogrusöz M, Bagger M, van Duinen SG, Kroes WG, Ruivenkamp CAL, Böhringer S, et al. The prognostic value of AJCC staging in uveal melanoma is enhanced by adding chromosome 3 and 8q status. Invest Ophthalmol Vis Sci. 2017;58(2):833–42. https://doi.org/10.1167/iovs.16-20212.
6. Morrison PJ. The iris - a window into the genetics of common and rare eye diseases. Ulster Med J. 2010;79(1):3–5.
7. Borrás T. The cellular and molecular biology of the iris, an overlooked tissue: the iris and pseudoexfoliation glaucoma. J Glaucoma. 2014;23(8 Suppl 1):S39–42. https://doi.org/10.1097/IJG.0000000000000104.
8. Otsuka F, Kawashima T, Imakado S, Usuki Y, Hon-Mura S. Lisch nodules and skin manifestation in neurofibromatosis type 1. Arch Dermatol. 2001;137(2):232–3.
9. Meyer P, Graeff E, Kohler C, Munier F, Bruder E. Juvenile xanthogranuloma involving concurrent iris and skin: clinical, pathological and molecular pathological evaluations. Am J Ophthalmol Case Rep. 2018;9:10–3. https://doi.org/10.1016/j.ajoc.2017.09.004.
10. Murthy KR, Dammalli M, Pinto SM, Murthy KB, Nirujogi RS, Madugundu AK, et al. A comprehensive proteomics analysis of the human iris tissue: ready to embrace postgenomics precision medicine in ophthalmology OMICS. 2016;20(9):510–9. https://doi.org/10.1089/omi.2016.0100.
11. Wagner AH, Anand VN, Wang W-H, Chatterton JE, Sun D, Shepard AR, et al. Exon-level expression profiling of ocular tissues. Exp Eye Res. 2013;111:105–11. https://doi.org/10.1016/j.exer.2013.03.004.
12. Zhang P, Kirby D, Dufresne C, Chen Y, Turner R, Ferri S, et al. Defining the proteome of human iris, ciliary body, retinal pigment epithelium, and choroid. Proteomics. 2016;16(7):1146–53. https://doi.org/10.1002/pmic.201500188.
13. Shah S, Koban Y, Le BHA, Bechtold M, Zolfaghari E, Kim JW, Berry JL. Iris hypoplasia as the presenting sign of retinoblastoma in a child with a 13q deletion. J Pediatr Ophthalmol Strabismus. 2018;55:e10–3. https://doi.org/10.3928/01913913-20180215-02.
14. Shields JA, Shields CL. Tumors and related lesions of the pigmented epithelium. Asia-Pacific J Ophthalmol. 2017;6(2):215–23. https://doi.org/10.22608/APO.201705.
15. Novakovic P, Kellie SJ, Taylor D. Childhood leukaemia: relapse in the anterior segment of the eye. Br J Ophthalmol. 1989;73(5):354–9.
16. Googe PB, Harris DJ, Powers T, Rosenberg AE, Eagle RC, Gapp J. Iris melanocytic nevus with rosettes. J Cutan Pathol. 2014;41(7):620–2. https://doi.org/10.1111/cup.12331.
17. Morcos MW, Odashiro A, Bazin R, Pereira PR, O'Meara A, Burnier MN. Balloon cell nevus of the iris. Pathol Res Pract. 2014;210(12):1160–3. https://doi.org/10.1016/j.prp.2014.04.026.
18. Shields CL, Kaliki S, Hutchinson A, Nickerson S, Patel J, Kancherla S, et al. Iris nevus growth into melanoma: analysis of 1611 consecutive eyes: the ABCDEF guide. Ophthalmology. 2013;120(4):766–72. https://doi.org/10.1016/j.ophtha.2012.09.042.
19. Margo CE, Groden L. Balloon cell nevus of the iris. Am J Ophthalmol. 1986;102(2):282–3.
20. Naumann G, Ruprecht KW. Xanthoma of the iris. A clinicopathological report. Ophthalmologica. 1972;164(4):293–305. https://doi.org/10.1159/000306764.
21. Shome D, Honavar SG, Gupta P, Vemuganti GK, Reddy PVA. Metastasis to the eye and orbit from renal cell carcinoma--a report of three cases and review of literature. Surv Ophthalmol. 2007;52(2):213–23. https://doi.org/10.1016/j.survophthal.2006.12.004.
22. Sharma V, Finger PT, Sidoti PA, Semenova E, Iacob CE. Rapidly growing iris melanocytoma with secondary glaucoma in a 6-year-old child. Eur J Ophthalmol. 2016;26(4):e71–3. https://doi.org/10.5301/ejo.5000726.
23. de Alves LF, Fernandes BF, Menezes MS, Ribeiro AS, Leal MM, Burnier JV, Burnier MN. Management of glaucoma in an eye with diffuse iris melanocytoma. Br J Ophthalmol. 2011;95(10):1471–9. https://doi.org/10.1136/bjo.2009.175638.
24. Fineman MS, Eagle RC, Shields JA, Shields CL, De Potter P. Melanocytomalytic glaucoma in eyes with necrotic iris melanocytoma. Ophthalmology. 1998;105(3):492–6. https://doi.org/10.1016/S0161-6420(98)93033-0.
25. Bodson A, Zografos L, Schalenbourg A. Spontaneous regression of iris melanocytoma: a case report. Klin Monatsblatter Augenheilkd. 2018;235(4):473–5. https://doi.org/10.1055/s-0043-123642.
26. Harbour JW, Augsburger JJ, Eagle RC. Initial management and follow-up of melanocytic iris tumors. Ophthalmology. 1995;102(12):1987–93.
27. Cialdini AP, Sahel JA, Jalkh AE, Weiter JJ, Zakka K, Albert DM. Malignant transformation of an iris melanocytoma. A case report. Graefes Arch Clin Exp Ophthalmol. 1989;227(4):348–54.

28. Inoue R, Saishin Y, Shima C, Yoshikawa H, Ohguro N, Tano Y. A case of iris melanocytoma transformed to malignant melanoma. Jpn J Ophthalmol. 2009;53(3):271–3. https://doi.org/10.1007/s10384-008-0649-0.
29. Sagoo MS, Mruthyunjaya P, Cree I, Luthert PJ, Hungerford JL. Malignant transformation of iris melanocytoma to iris ring melanoma. Br J Ophthalmol. 2007;91(11):1571–2. https://doi.org/10.1136/bjo.2006.105858.
30. Shields JA, Shields CL, Mercado G, Gündüz K, Eagle RC. Adenoma of the iris pigment epithelium: a report of 20 cases: the 1998 Pan-American Lecture. Arch Ophthalmol. 1999;117(6):736–41.
31. Singh AD, Rundle PA, Longstaff S, Jacques R, Rennie IG. Iris pigment epithelial adenoma: resection and repair. Eye. 2006;20(3):385–6. https://doi.org/10.1038/sj.eye.6701851.
32. Offret H, Saraux H. Adenoma of the iris pigment epithelium. Arch Ophthalmol. 1980;98(5):875–83.
33. Mayro EL, Surakiatchanukul T, Shields JA, Shields CL. Distinguishing midzonal iris pigment epithelial cyst from adenoma and ciliary body melanoma. Oman J Ophthalmol. 2018;11(2):161–3. https://doi.org/10.4103/ojo.OJO_226_2017.
34. Yeaney GA, Platt S, Singh AD. Primary iris leiomyoma. Surv Ophthalmol. 2017;62(3):366–70. https://doi.org/10.1016/j.survophthal.2016.11.007.
35. Chalam KV, Cutler Peck CM, Grover S, Radhakrishnan R. Lenticular meridional astigmatism secondary to iris mesectodermal leiomyoma. J Cataract Refract Surg. 2012;38(1):170–3. https://doi.org/10.1016/j.jcrs.2011.10.016.
36. Tuncer S, Peksayar G, Demiryont M, Gozum N. Longterm follow-up of a patient with iris leiomyoma treated with partial lamellar iridocyclectomy. Acta Ophthalmol Scand. 2004;82(1):112–4.
37. Eide N, Farstad IN, Røger M. A leiomyoma of the iris documented by immunohistochemistry and electron microscopy. Acta Ophthalmol Scand. 1997;75(4):470–3.
38. Li ZY, Tso MO, Sugar J. Leiomyoepithelioma of iris pigment epithelium. Arch Ophthalmol. 1987;105(6):819–24.
39. Richetta A, Giustini S, Recupero SM, Pezza M, Carlomagno V, Amoruso G, Calvieri S. Lisch nodules of the iris in neurofibromatosis type 1. J Eur Acad Dermatol Venereol. 2004;18(3):342–4. https://doi.org/10.1111/j.1468-3083.2004.00915.x.
40. van Poppelen NM, Vaarwater J, Mudhar HS, Sisley K, Rennie IG, Rundle P, et al. Genetic background of iris melanomas and iris melanocytic tumors of uncertain malignant potential. Ophthalmology. 2018;125(6):904–12. https://doi.org/10.1016/j.ophtha.2017.12.022.
41. Yu L, Aldave AJ, Glasgow BJ. Epstein-Barr virus-associated smooth muscle tumor of the iris in a patient with transplant: a case report and review of the literature. Arch Pathol Lab Med. 2009;133(8):1238–41. https://doi.org/10.1043/1543-2165-133.8.1238.
42. Suankratay C, Shuangshoti S, Mutirangura A, Prasanthai V, Lerdlum S, Shuangshoti S, et al. Epstein-Barr virus infection-associated smooth-muscle tumors in patients with AIDS. Clin Infect Dis. 2005;40(10):1521–8. https://doi.org/10.1086/429830.
43. Bergeron E, Lihimdi N, Bergeron D, Landreville S. Orbital recurrence of iris melanoma 21 years after enucleation. BMJ Case Rep. 2017;2017:221137. https://doi.org/10.1136/bcr-2017-221137.
44. Fabian ID, Thaung C, AlHarby L, Sisley K, Mudhar HS, Doherty RE, et al. Late solitary extraocular recurrence from previously resected iris melanoma. Am J Ophthalmol. 2017;181:97–105. https://doi.org/10.1016/j.ajo.2017.06.025.
45. Shields CL, Ramasubramanian A, Ganguly A, Mohan D, Shields JA. Cytogenetic testing of iris melanoma using fine needle aspiration biopsy in 17 patients. Retina. 2011;31(3):574–80. https://doi.org/10.1097/IAE.0b013e3181f57e62.
46. Harbour JW, Wilson D, Finger PT, Worley LA, Onken MD. Gene expressing profiling of iris melanomas. Ophthalmology. 2013;120(1):213, 213.e1–3. https://doi.org/10.1016/j.ophtha.2012.08.016.
47. Spraul CW, d'Heurle D, Grossniklaus HE. Adenocarcinoma of the iris pigment epithelium. Arch Ophthalmol. 1996;114(12):1512–7.
48. Dryja TP, Zakov ZN, Albert DM. Adenocarcinoma arising from the epithelium of the iris and ciliary body. Int Ophthalmol Clin. 1980;20(2):177–90.
49. Martin V, Cuenca X, Lopez S, Albertini A-F, Lang P, Simon J-M, et al. Iris metastasis from prostate carcinoma: a case report and review of the literature. Cancer Radiother. 2015;19(5):331–3. https://doi.org/10.1016/j.canrad.2014.12.008.
50. de Mello PC, Brasil OFM, Vidoris A, Morales MC, Belfort RN. Iris metastases from systemic cancer: a report of three cases. Arq Bras Oftalmol. 2016;79(6):407–10. https://doi.org/10.5935/0004-2749.20160115.
51. Hernández-Da Mota SE, Ulaje-Nuñez JM, Salinas-Gallegos JL, Rodríguez-Reyes A. Iris metastasis as a first manifestation of lung adenocarcinoma. Arch Soc Esp Oftalmol. 2018;93(7):357–9. https://doi.org/10.1016/j.oftal.2018.02.007.
52. Celebi ARC, Kilavuzoglu AE, Altiparmak UE, Cosar CB, Ozkiris A. Iris metastasis of gastric adenocarcinoma. World J Surg Oncol. 2016;14:71. https://doi.org/10.1186/s12957-016-0840-6.
53. Yoshikawa T, Miyata K, Nakai T, Ohbayashi C, Kaneko M, Ogata N. Iris metastasis preceding diagnosis of gastric signet ring cell adenocarcinoma: a case report. BMC Ophthalmol. 2018;18(1):125. https://doi.org/10.1186/s12886-018-0795-1.
54. Woyke S, Chwirot R. Rhabdomyosarcoma of the iris. Report of the first recorded case. Br J Ophthalmol. 1972;56(1):60–4.
55. Elsas FJ, Mroczek EC, Kelly DR, Specht CS. Primary rhabdomyosarcoma of the iris. Arch Ophthalmol. 1991;109(7):982–4.
56. Font RL, Zimmerman LE. Electron microscopic verification of primary rhabdomyosarcoma of the iris. Am J Ophthalmol. 1972;74(1):110–7.

57. Fabian ID, Hildebrand GD, Wilson S, Foord T, Sagoo MS. Alveolar rhabdomyosarcoma of the foot metastasizing to the iris: report of a rare case. BMC Cancer. 2016;16:447. https://doi.org/10.1186/s12885-016-2496-6.
58. Ayala Barroso E, Tapia Bahamondes A, Sánchez España JC, Alós L, Medel Jiménez R. Primary intraocular malignant rhabdoid tumor without extrascleral compromise. J Pediatr Ophthalmol Strabismus. 2018;55:e7–9. https://doi.org/10.3928/01913913-20180215-01.
59. Akhtar M, Ali MA, Sackey K, Bakry M, Johnson T. Malignant rhabdoid tumor of the kidney presenting as intraocular metastasis. Pediatr Hematol Oncol. 1991;8(1):33–43.
60. Shah SJ, Ali MJ, Mulay K, Honavar SG, Reddy VA. Primary intraocular malignant extrarenal rhabdoid tumor: a clinicopathological correlation. J Pediatr Ophthalmol Strabismus. 2013;50:e18–20. https://doi.org/10.3928/01913913-20130423-03.
61. Roukens AH, Kroep JR, Marinkovic M, Nout RA, Bovée JVMG, Vasylenko Y, et al. Primary Ewing sarcoma of the iris. Lancet. 2014;383(9913):256. https://doi.org/10.1016/S0140-6736(13)60183-X.
62. Gündüz K, Shields JA, Shields CL, De Potter P, Wayner MJ. Ewing sarcoma metastatic to the iris. Am J Ophthalmol. 1997;124(4):550–2.
63. de Alava E. Ewing sarcoma, an update on molecular pathology with therapeutic implications. Surg Pathol Clin. 2017;10(3):575–85. https://doi.org/10.1016/j.path.2017.04.001.
64. Krohn J, Tvenning A-O, Kjersem B, Høvding G. Iris cavernous haemangioma associated with recurrent hyphaema treated by laser photocoagulation. Acta Ophthalmol. 2017;95(1):e80–1. https://doi.org/10.1111/aos.12967.
65. Chien JL, Sioufi K, Ferenczy S, Say EAT, Shields CL. Optical coherence tomography angiography features of iris racemose hemangioma in 4 cases. JAMA Ophthalmol. 2017;135(10):1106–10. https://doi.org/10.1001/jamaophthalmol.2017.3390.
66. Shields CL, Atalay HT, Wuthisiri W, Levin AV, Lally SE, Shields JA. Sector iris hemangioma in association with diffuse choroidal hemangioma. J AAPOS. 2015;19(1):83–6. https://doi.org/10.1016/j.jaapos.2014.09.012.
67. Reid JP, Puglis CL, Slagle WS. Intraocular mantle cell lymphoma of the iris. Optom Vis Sci. 2014;91(4 Suppl 1):S25–9. https://doi.org/10.1097/OPX.0000000000000218.
68. Demirci H, Grant JS, Elner VM. Intralesional rituximab for primary iris lymphoma. JAMA Ophthalmol. 2015;133(1):104–5. https://doi.org/10.1001/jamaophthalmol.2014.3303.
69. Economou MA, Kopp ED, All-Ericsson C, Seregard S. Mantle cell lymphoma of the iris. Acta Ophthalmol Scand. 2007;85(3):341–3. https://doi.org/10.1111/j.1600-0420.2006.00845.x.
70. Agarwal A, Sadiq MA, Rhoades WR, Jack LS, Hanout M, Bierman PJ, et al. Combined systemic and ocular chemotherapy for anterior segment metastasis of systemic mantle cell lymphoma. J Ophthalmic Inflammation Infect. 2015;5(1):30. https://doi.org/10.1186/s12348-015-0060-1.
71. Park CY, Hwang SW, Kim DY, Huh HJ, Oh J-H. Anaplastic large cell lymphoma involving anterior segment of the eye. Korean J Ophthalmol. 2014;28(1):108–12. https://doi.org/10.3341/kjo.2014.28.1.108.
72. Stacey AW, Lavric A, Thaung C, Siddiq S, Sagoo MS. Solitary iris plasmacytoma with anterior chamber crystalline deposits. Cornea. 2017;36(7):875–7. https://doi.org/10.1097/ICO.0000000000001222.
73. Shields CL, Shields JA, Gross NE, Schwartz GP, Lally SE. Survey of 520 eyes with uveal metastases. Ophthalmology. 1997;104(8):1265–76.
74. Jurecka T, Skorkovská S, Coupková H, Postránecká V. Iris metastasis as the first sign of small-cell lung carcinoma with metastatic involvement of the mediastinum. Klin Onkol. 2009;22(4):179–82.
75. Liu S-L, Nie Y-H, He T, Yan X-X, Xing Y-Q. Iris metastasis as the first sign of small cell lung cancer: a case report. Oncol Lett. 2017;13(3):1547–52. https://doi.org/10.3892/ol.2017.5648.
76. Koshy J, John MJ, Thomas S, Kaur G, Batra N, Xavier WJ. Ophthalmic manifestations of acute and chronic leukemias presenting to a tertiary care center in India. Indian J Ophthalmol. 2015;63(8):659–64. https://doi.org/10.4103/0301-4738.169789.
77. Al-Salam S, Algawi K, Alashari M. Malignant non-teratoid medulloepithelioma of ciliary body with retinoblastic differentiation: a case report and review of literature. Neuropathology. 2008;28(5):551–6. https://doi.org/10.1111/j.1440-1789.2008.00886.x.
78. Sreelakshmi KV, Chandra A, Krishnakumar S, Natarajan V, Khetan V. Anterior chamber invasion in retinoblastoma: not an indication for adjuvant chemotherapy. Invest Ophthalmol Vis Sci. 2017;58(11):4654–61. https://doi.org/10.1167/iovs.17-22111.
79. Zamir E, Smith RE, See RF, Yiu SC, Burnstine M, Rao NA. Squamous cell carcinoma of the limbus extending into the anterior segment. Arch Ophthalmol. 2002;120(8):1106–7.
80. Cable MM, Lyon DB, Rupani M, Matta CS, Hidayat AA. Case reports and small case series: primary basal cell carcinoma of the conjunctiva with intraocular invasion. Arch Ophthalmol. 2000;118(9):1296–8.
81. Wenkel H, Rummelt V, Naumann GO. Malignant melanoma of the conjunctiva with intraocular extension. Arch Ophthalmol. 2000;118(4):557–60.
82. Sandinha T, Russell H, Kemp E, Roberts F. Malignant melanoma of the conjunctiva with intraocular extension: a clinicopathological study of three cases. Graefes Arch Clin Exp Ophthalmol. 2007;245(3):431–6. https://doi.org/10.1007/s00417-006-0401-8.
83. Goel R, Murthy KR, Srikanth SM, Pinto SM, Bhattacharjee M, Kelkar DS, et al. Characterizing the normal proteome of human ciliary body. Clin Proteomics. 2013;10(1):9. https://doi.org/10.1186/1559-0275-10-9.

84. Ahmad MT, Zhang P, Dufresne C, Ferrucci L, Semba RD. The human eye proteome project: updates on an emerging proteome. Proteomics. 2018;18(5–6):e1700394. Review. https://doi.org/10.1002/pmic.201700394.
85. Taban M, Sears JE, Singh AD. Ciliary body naevus. Eye. 2007;21(12):1528–30. https://doi.org/10.1038/sj.eye.6702622.
86. Koch KR, Ortmann M, Heindl LM. Extraocular extension of a benign ciliary body nevus. JAMA Ophthalmol. 2015;133(12):e153137. https://doi.org/10.1001/jamaophthalmol.2015.3137.
87. Hale PN, Allen RA, Straatsma BR. Benign melanomas (nevi) of the choroid and ciliary body. Arch Ophthalmol. 1965;74(4):532–8.
88. LoRusso FJ, Boniuk M, Font RL. Melanocytoma (magnocellular nevus) of the ciliary body: report of 10 cases and review of the literature. Ophthalmology. 2000;107(4):795–800.
89. Odashiro M, Odashiro A, Leite L, Melo M, Odashiro P, Miiji L, et al. Melanocytoma of ciliary body and choroids simulating melanoma. Pathol Res Pract. 2010;206(2):130–3. https://doi.org/10.1016/j.prp.2009.03.006.
90. Al-Hinai A, Edelstein C, Burnier MN. Unusual case of melanocytoma. Can J Ophthalmol. 2004;39(4):461–3.
91. McLean IW, Burnier MN, Zimmerman LE, Jakobiec FA. Tumors of the eye and ocular adnexa. In: McLean IW, Burnier MN, Zimmerman LE, Jakobiec FA, editors. Atlas of tumor pathology. Washington, DC: Armed Forces Institute of Pathology; 1994. p. 161–5.
92. Mohamed MD, Gupta M, Parsons A, Rennie IG. Ultrasound biomicroscopy in the management of melanocytoma of the ciliary body with extrascleral extension. Br J Ophthalmol. 2005;89(1):14–6. https://doi.org/10.1136/bjo.2004.048967.
93. Li HK, Shields CL, Shields JA, Eagle RC, Mason JO. Iridociliochoroidal melanoma arising from melanocytoma in a black teenager. J AAPOS. 2010;14(2):178–80. https://doi.org/10.1016/j.jaapos.2010.01.007.
94. Font RL, Croxatto JO, Rao NA. Tumors of the eye and ocular adnexa. Washington, DC: American Registry of Pathology; 2006. p. 124–6.
95. Loeffler KU, Seifert P, Spitznas M. Adenoma of the pigmented ciliary epithelium: ultrastructural and immunohistochemical findings. Hum Pathol. 2000;31(7):882–7.
96. Shields JA, Shields CL, Eagle RC, Friedman ES, Wheatley HM. Age-related hyperplasia of the nonpigmented ciliary body epithelium (Fuchs adenoma) simulating a ciliary body malignant neoplasm. Arch Ophthalmol. 2009;127(9):1224–5. https://doi.org/10.1001/archophthalmol.2009.217.
97. Pecorella I, Ciocci L, Modesti M, Appolloni R. Adenoma of the non-pigmented ciliary epithelium: a rare intraocular tumor with unusual immunohistochemical findings. Pathol Res Pract. 2009;205(12):870–5. https://doi.org/10.1016/j.prp.2009.02.009.
98. Yan J, Liu X, Zhang P, Li Y. Acquired adenoma of the nonpigmented ciliary epithelium: analysis of five cases. Graefes Arch Clin Exp Ophthalmol. 2015;253(4):637–44. https://doi.org/10.1007/s00417-014-2928-4.
99. Elizalde J, Ubia S, Barraquer RI. Adenoma of the nonpigmented ciliary epithelium. Eur J Ophthalmol. 2006;16(4):630–3.
100. Shields JA, Augsburger JJ, Wallar PH, Shah HG. Adenoma of the nonpigmented epithelium of the ciliary body. Ophthalmology. 1983;90(12):1528–30.
101. Murphy MF, Johnston PB, Lyness RW. Adenoma of the non-pigmented epithelium of the ciliary body. Eye. 1997;11(Pt 3):419–20. https://doi.org/10.1038/eye.1997.89.
102. Shields JA, Eagle RC, Shields CL. Adenoma of nonpigmented ciliary epithelium with smooth muscle differentiation. Arch Ophthalmol. 1999;117(1):117–9.
103. Mansoor S, Qureshi A. Ciliary body adenoma of nonpigmented epithelium. J Clin Pathol. 2004;57(9):997–8. https://doi.org/10.1136/jcp.2004.017871.
104. Shields JA, Shields CL, Eagle RC, De Potter P. Observations on seven cases of intraocular leiomyoma. The 1993 Byron Demorest lecture. Arch Ophthalmol. 1994;112(4):521–8.
105. Peyman GA, Martinez CE, Hew A, Peralta E, Kraut RJ. Endoresection of a ciliary body leiomyoma. Can J Ophthalmol. 1998;33(1):32–4.
106. Biswas J, Kumar SK, Gopal L, Bhende MP. Leiomyoma of the ciliary body extending to the anterior chamber: clinicopathologic and ultrasound biomicroscopic correlation. Surv Ophthalmol. 2000;44(4):336–42.
107. Chotiner EA, Shields CL, Shields JA, Gündüz K, Eagle RC. Ciliary body leiomyoma with anterior chamber invasion. Arch Ophthalmol. 2001;119(8):1218–9.
108. Remmer MH, Kaliki S, Eagle RC, Shields CL, Shields JA. Giant leiomyoma of the ciliary body. Oman J Ophthalmol. 2014;7(2):81–3. https://doi.org/10.4103/0974-620X.137165.
109. Richter MN, Bechrakis NE, Stoltenburg-Didinger G, Foerster MH. Transscleral resection of a ciliary body leiomyoma in a child: case report and review of the literature. Graefes Arch Clin Exp Ophthalmol. 2003;241(11):953–7. https://doi.org/10.1007/s00417-003-0766-x.
110. Kiratli H, Bilgiç S, Söylemezoglu F. Ciliary body leiomyomas. Three case reports. J Fr D'ophtalmol. 2005;28(10):1105–9.
111. Shields JA, Shields CL, Eagle RC. Mesectodermal leiomyoma of the ciliary body managed by partial lamellar iridocyclochoroidectomy. Ophthalmology. 1989;96(9):1369–76.
112. Kiratli H, Ağın A, Önder S. Ciliary body mesectodermal leiomyoma diagnosed by fine needle aspiration biopsy. Ocul Oncol Pathol. 2017;3(3):199–203. https://doi.org/10.1159/000454863.
113. Koletsa T, Karayannopoulou G, Dereklis D, Vasileiadis I, Papadimitriou CS, Hytiroglou

P. Mesectodermal leiomyoma of the ciliary body: report of a case and review of the literature. Pathol Res Pract. 2009;205(2):125–30. https://doi.org/10.1016/j.prp.2008.06.004.
114. Schlötzer-Schrehardt U, Jünemann A, Naumann GOH. Mitochondria-rich epithelioid leiomyoma of the ciliary body. Arch Ophthalmol. 2002;120(1):77–82.
115. Saavedra E, Singh AD, Sears JE, Ratliff NB. Plexiform pigmented schwannoma of the uvea. Surv Ophthalmol. 2006;51(2):162–8. https://doi.org/10.1016/j.survophthal.2005.12.004.
116. Kim IT, Chang SD. Ciliary body schwannoma. Acta Ophthalmol Scand. 1999;77(4):462–6.
117. Thaller VT, Perinti A, Perinti A. Benign schwannoma simulating a ciliary body melanoma. Eye. 1998;12(Pt 1):158–9. https://doi.org/10.1038/eye.1998.33.
118. Pineda R, Urban RC, Bellows AR, Jakobiec FA. Ciliary body neurilemoma. Unusual clinical findings intimating the diagnosis. Ophthalmology. 1995;102(6):918–23.
119. Freedman SF, Elner VM, Donev I, Gunta R, Albert DM. Intraocular neurilemmoma arising from the posterior ciliary nerve in neurofibromatosis. Pathologic findings. Ophthalmology. 1988;95(11):1559–64.
120. Spencer WH, Jesberg DO. Glioneuroma (choristomatous malformation of the optic cup margin). A report of two cases. Arch Ophthalmol. 1973;89(5):387–91.
121. Addison DJ, Font RL. Glioneuroma of iris and ciliary body. Arch Ophthalmol. 1984;102(3):419–21.
122. Kumar KS, Shetty KB. Glioma of ciliary body presenting as episcleral nodule. Indian J Ophthalmol. 1995;43(2):76–8.
123. Kuhlenbeck H, Haymaker W. Neuroectodermal tumors containing neoplastic neuronal elements; ganglioneuroma, spongioneuroblastoma and glioneuroma; with a clinicopathologic report of 11 cases and a discussion of their origin and classification. Mil Surg. 1946;99:273–304.
124. Naeser P, Möller P. Astrocytoma of the ciliary body. A clinicopathological case report. Acta Ophthalmol. 1985;63(1):28–30.
125. Mei H, Xing Y, Yang A, Wang J, Xu Y, Wang Z, Heiligenhaus A. Astrocytoma of the ciliary body. Ophthalmologica. 2009;223(1):72–4. https://doi.org/10.1159/000175924.
126. Goto H, Usui Y, Nagao T. Perivascular epithelioid cell tumor arising from ciliary body treated by local resection. Ocul Oncol Pathol. 2015;1(2):88–92. https://doi.org/10.1159/000369330.
127. Furusato E, Cameron JD, Newsom RW, Fujishiro T, Kojima T, Specht CS, et al. Ocular perivascular epithelioid cell tumor: report of 2 cases with distinct clinical presentations. Hum Pathol. 2010;41(5):768–72. https://doi.org/10.1016/j.humpath.2009.12.006.
128. Mai KT, Belanger EC. Perivascular epithelioid cell tumor (PEComa) of the soft tissue. Pathology. 2006;38(5):415–20. https://doi.org/10.1080/00313020600922504.
129. Costache M, Patrascu OM, Adrian D, Costache D, Sajin M, Ungureanu E, Simionescu O. Ciliary body melanoma - a particularly rare type of ocular tumor. Case report and general considerations. Maedica. 2013;8(4):360–4.
130. Demirci H, Shields CL, Shields JA, Honavar SG, Eagle RC. Ring melanoma of the ciliary body: report on twenty-three patients. Retina. 2002;22(6):698–706.
131. Plasseraud KM, Wilkinson JK, Oelschlager KM, Poteet TM, Cook RW, Stone JF, Monzon FA. Gene expression profiling in uveal melanoma: technical reliability and correlation of molecular class with pathologic characteristics. Diagn Pathol. 2017;12(1):59. https://doi.org/10.1186/s13000-017-0650-3.
132. Kumar JB, Proia AD, Mruthyunjaya P, Sharma S. Primary adenocarcinoma of pigmented ciliary epithelium in a phthisical eye. Surv Ophthalmol. 2016;61(4):502–5. https://doi.org/10.1016/j.survophthal.2015.11.001.
133. Sukeda A, Mori T, Suzuki S, Ochiai A. Adenocarcinoma of the pigmented ciliary epithelium. BMJ Case Rep. 2014;2014:bcr2014204534. https://doi.org/10.1136/bcr-2014-204534.
134. Nicolò M, Nicolò G, Zingirian M. Pleomorphic adenocarcinoma of the ciliary epithelium: a clinicopathological, immunohistochemical, ultrastructural, DNA-ploidy and comparative genomic hybridization analysis of an unusual case. Eur J Ophthalmol. 2002;12(4):319–23.
135. Papale JJ, Akiwama K, Hirose T, Tsubota K, Hanaoka K, Albert DM. Adenocarcinoma of the ciliary body pigment epithelium in a child. Arch Ophthalmol. 1984;102(1):100–3.
136. Rodrigues M, Hidayat A, Karesh J. Pleomorphic adenocarcinoma of ciliary epithelium simulating an epibulbar tumor. Am J Ophthalmol. 1988;106(5):595–600.
137. Bhandari AP, Swami SY, Gadkari RU. Papillary adenocarcinoma of ciliary body. Oman J Ophthalmol. 2013;6(2):132–4. https://doi.org/10.4103/0974-620X.116663.
138. Günalp I, Sertçelik A, Uğurbaş SH, Astarci M. Papillary adenocarcinoma of the ciliary body simulating retinoblastoma. Am J Ophthalmol. 1997;123(2):268–9.
139. Grossniklaus HE, Zimmerman LE, Kachmer ML. Pleomorphic adenocarcinoma of the ciliary body. Immunohistochemical and electron microscopic features. Ophthalmology. 1990;97(6):763–8.
140. Meyer P, Arnold-Wörner N. Metastasis of the ciliary body and iris from an oropharyngeal carcinoma. Ophthalmologe. 2014;111(6):565–7. https://doi.org/10.1007/s00347-013-2898-7.
141. Lieb WE, Shields JA, Shields CL, Spaeth GL. Mucinous adenocarcinoma metastatic to the iris, ciliary body, and choroid. Br J Ophthalmol. 1990;74(6):373–6.
142. Cajaiba MM, Chojniak MM, Cunha IW. Unusual primary ocular neoplasm in a child: leiomyosarcoma of the ciliary body. Pediatr Dev Pathol. 2008;11(6):479–81. https://doi.org/10.2350/07-02-0231.1.

143. Park S-W, Kim H-J, Chin H-S, Tae K-S, Han J-Y. Mesectodermal leiomyosarcoma of the ciliary body. AJNR. 2003;24(9):1765–8.
144. Gopal L, Babu EK, Gupta S, Krishnakumar S, Biswas J, Rao NA. Pigmented malignant medulloepithelioma of the ciliary body. J Pediatr Ophthalmol Strabismus. 2004;41(6):364–6.
145. Manjandavida FP, Honavar SG, Mulay K, Reddy VAP, Vemuganti GK. Malignant teratoid ciliary body medulloepithelioma in a neonate. J Pediatr Ophthalmol Strabismus. 2013;50:e37–40. https://doi.org/10.3928/01913913-20130730-01.
146. Shah PK, Meeralakshmi P, Shanthi R, Saravanan VR, Kalpana N, Narendran V. Pigmented ciliary body medulloepithelioma in a newborn infant. Oman J Ophthalmol. 2017;10(3):257–8. https://doi.org/10.4103/ojo.OJO_1_2017.
147. Font RL, Rishi K. Diffuse retinal involvement in malignant nonteratoid medulloepithelioma of ciliary body in an adult. Arch Ophthalmol. 2005;123(8):1136–8. https://doi.org/10.1001/archopht.123.8.1136.
148. Burris CKH, Papastefanou VP, Thaung C, Hay G, Grantham M, Cohen VML. Nonteratoid medulloepithelioma presenting in a 78-year-old male. Ocul Oncol Pathol. 2016;2(4):218–21. https://doi.org/10.1159/000445209.
149. Zimmerman LE. The remarkable polymorphism of tumors of the ciliary epithelium. Trans Aust Coll Ophthalmol. 1970;2:114–25.
150. Ho YF, Tsai Y-J, Wu S-Y. Malignant ciliary body medulloepithelioma with brain and parotid metastasis. J Pediatr Ophthalmol Strabismus. 2017;54:e18–22.https://doi.org/10.3928/01913913-20170201-05.
151. Jakobiec FA, Borkar DS, Stagner AM, Lee NG. Intraocular teratoid medulloepithelioma presenting with a completely rhabdomyosarcomatous distant metastasis. JAMA Ophthalmol. 2016;134(8):919–23. https://doi.org/10.1001/jamaophthalmol.2016.1515.
152. Kaliki S, Shields CL, Eagle RC, Vemuganti GK, Almeida A, Manjandavida FP, et al. Ciliary body medulloepithelioma: analysis of 41 cases. Ophthalmology. 2013;120(12):2552–9. https://doi.org/10.1016/j.ophtha.2013.05.015.
153. Verdijk RM. On the classification and grading of medulloepithelioma of the eye. Ocul Oncol Pathol. 2016;2(3):190–3. https://doi.org/10.1159/000443963.
154. Konstantinidis L, Angi M, Coupland SE, Damato B. Primary B-cell lymphoma of the ciliary body with 360° ('ring'-like) growth pattern. Eye. 2014;28(3):355–6. https://doi.org/10.1038/eye.2013.282.
155. Mashayekhi A, Shields CL, Shields JA. Iris involvement by lymphoma: a review of 13 cases. Clin Exp Ophthalmol. 2013;41(1):19–26. https://doi.org/10.1111/j.1442-9071.2012.02811.x.
156. Pei M, Zhao C, Gao F, Zhang M. Bilateral mantle cell lymphoma of the ciliary body that responded to a combined local radiotherapy and chemotherapy regimen: a case report. BMC Cancer. 2019;19(1):355. https://doi.org/10.1186/s12885-019-5530-7.
157. Krishnamurthy A, Singh SS, Majhi U, Ramshankar V, Krishnamurthy A. A rare case of a recurrent giant solitary fibrous tumor of the ciliary body of the orbit. J Maxillofac Oral Surg. 2016;15(Suppl 2):378–81. https://doi.org/10.1007/s12663-016-0926-2.
158. Das D, Deka P, Verma G, Kuri GC, Bhattacharjee H, Bharali G, et al. IgG4-related intraocular inflammation masquerading as ciliary body melanoma in a young girl. Indian J Ophthalmol. 2016;64(8):601–3. https://doi.org/10.4103/0301-4738.191510.
159. Guo Q, Hao J, Sun SB, Xu SP, Yang Q, Guo QL, Cui GD. Oligodendroglioma of the ciliary body: a unique case report and the review of literature. BMC Cancer. 2010;10:579. https://doi.org/10.1186/1471-2407-10-579.
160. Ahmad SS, Lad L, Ghani SA. A case of choroidal melanocytoma mimicking a choroidal melanoma. Saudi J Ophthalmol. 2015;29(3):242–5. https://doi.org/10.1016/j.sjopt.2015.02.002.
161. Robertson DM, Campbell RJ, Salomão DR. Mushroom-shaped choroidal melanocytoma mimicking malignant melanoma. Arch Ophthalmol. 2002;120(1):82–5.
162. Shields JA, Shields CL, Eagle RC. Melanocytoma (hyperpigmented magnocellular nevus) of the uveal tract: the 34th G. Victor Simpson lecture. Retina. 2007;27(6):730–9. https://doi.org/10.1097/IAE.0b013e318030e81e.
163. Kurli M, Finger PT, Manor T, McCormick SA, Grossniklaus HE. Finding malignant change in a necrotic choroidal melanocytoma: a clinical challenge. Br J Ophthalmol. 2005;89(7):921–2. https://doi.org/10.1136/bjo.2004.060038.
164. Brownstein S, Dorey MW, Mathew B, Little JM, Lindley JI. Melanocytoma of the choroid: atypical presentation and review of the literature. Can J Ophthalmol. 2002;37(4):247–52.
165. Mittal R, Cherepanoff S, Thornton S, Kalirai H, Damato B, Coupland SE. Bilateral diffuse uveal melanocytic proliferation: molecular genetic analysis of a case and review of the literature. Ocul Oncol Pathol. 2015;2(2):94–9. https://doi.org/10.1159/000440766.
166. Pefkianaki M, Agrawal R, Desai P, Pavesio C, Sagoo MS. Bilateral diffuse uveal melanocytic proliferation (BDUMP) associated with B-cell lymphoma: report of a rare case. BMC Cancer. 2015;15:23. https://doi.org/10.1186/s12885-015-1020-8.
167. Höh AE, Holz FG, Dithmar S. Bilateral diffuse uveal melanocytic proliferation in a patient with metastatic breast cancer. Ophthalmologe. 2014;111(10):961–4. https://doi.org/10.1007/s00347-014-3019-y.
168. Chiang W-Y, Lin J-W, Yang I-H, Kuo H-K. Posterior choroidal leiomyoma: a rare case report and literature review. APMIS. 2015;123(6):540–5. https://doi.org/10.1111/apm.12384.
169. Shields JA, Shields CL, Eagle RC Jr, De Potter P. Observations on seven cases of intraocular leio-

myoma. The 1993 Byron Demorest Lecture. Arch Ophthalmol. 1994;112(4):521–8. Review.
170. Perri P, Paduano B, Incorvaia C, Costagliola C, Parmeggiani F, Rossi S, et al. Mesectodermal leiomyoma exclusively involving the posterior choroid. Am J Ophthalmol. 2002;134(3):451–4.
171. Ceballos EM, Aaberg TM, Halpern RL, Grossniklaus HE. Choroidal leiomyoma: report of a case. Retina. 1999;19(4):349–51.
172. Shanmugam PM, Ramanjulu R. Vascular tumors of the choroid and retina. Indian J Ophthalmol. 2015;63(2):133–40. https://doi.org/10.4103/0301-4738.154387.
173. Rinaldo L, Xu SCY, Eggers SD, Salomão DR, Chen JJ, Raghunathan A. Rare occurrence of an intraocular choroidal solitary fibrous tumor/hemangiopericytoma. Ocul Oncol Pathol. 2018;4(4):213–9. https://doi.org/10.1159/000481947.
174. Jaffee IM, Char DH. Myomelanocytic choroidal tumor: cytopathologic diagnosis. Retina. 2017;37(2):413–6. https://doi.org/10.1097/IAE.0000000000001387.
175. Dhupper M, Biswas J, Gopal L, Kumar SK, Khetan V. Clinicopathological correlation of choroidal melanoma in Indian population: a study of 113 cases. Oman J Ophthalmol. 2012;5(1):42–5. https://doi.org/10.4103/0974-620X.94766.
176. Kaliki S, Shields CL, Shields JA. Uveal melanoma: estimating prognosis. Indian J Ophthalmol. 2015;63(2):93–102. https://doi.org/10.4103/0301-4738.154367.
177. Folberg R, Hendrix MJ, Maniotis AJ. Vasculogenic mimicry and tumor angiogenesis. Am J Pathol. 2000;156(2):361–81. https://doi.org/10.1016/S0002-9440(10)64739-6.
178. Onken MD, Lin AY, Worley LA, Folberg R, Harbour JW. Association between microarray gene expression signature and extravascular matrix patterns in primary uveal melanomas. Am J Ophthalmol. 2005;140(4):748–9. https://doi.org/10.1016/j.ajo.2005.04.024.
179. Dimaras H, Parulekar MV, Kwok G, Simpson ER, Ali A, Halliday W, et al. Molecular testing prognostic of low risk in epithelioid uveal melanoma in a child. Br J Ophthalmol. 2013;97(3):323–6. https://doi.org/10.1136/bjophthalmol-2012-302561.
180. Onken MD, Worley LA, Ehlers JP, Harbour JW. Gene expression profiling in uveal melanoma reveals two molecular classes and predicts metastatic death. Cancer Res. 2004;64(20):7205–9. https://doi.org/10.1158/0008-5472.CAN-04-1750.
181. Harbour JW, Chen R. The DecisionDx-UM gene expression profile test provides risk stratification and individualized patient care in uveal melanoma. PLoS Currents. 2013;5:618. https://doi.org/10.1371/currents.eogt.af8ba80fc776c8f1ce8f5dc485d4a618.
182. Harbour JW. A prognostic test to predict the risk of metastasis in uveal melanoma based on a 15-gene expression profile. Methods Mol Biol. 2014;1102:427–40. https://doi.org/10.1007/978-1-62703-727-3_22.
183. Plasseraud KM, Cook RW, Tsai T, Shildkrot Y, MiddlebrookB,MaetzoldD,etal.Clinicalperformance and management outcomes with the DecisionDx-UM gene expression profile test in a prospective multicenter study. J Oncol. 2016;2016:5325762. https://doi.org/10.1155/2016/5325762.
184. Klufas MA, Itty S, McCannel CA, Glasgow BJ, Moreno C, McCannel TA. Variable results for uveal melanoma-specific gene expression profile prognostic test in choroidal metastasis. JAMA Ophthalmol. 2015;133(9):1073–6. https://doi.org/10.1001/jamaophthalmol.2015.1790.
185. Miller AK, Benage MJ, Wilson DJ, Skalet AH. Uveal melanoma with histopathologic intratumoral heterogeneity associated with gene expression profile discordance. Ocul Oncol Pathol. 2017;3(2):156–60. https://doi.org/10.1159/000453616.
186. Coupland SE, Kalirai H, Ho V, Thornton S, Damato BE, Heimann H. Concordant chromosome 3 results in paired choroidal melanoma biopsies and subsequent tumor resection specimens. Br J Ophthalmol. 2015;99(10):1444–50. https://doi.org/10.1136/bjophthalmol-2015-307057.
187. Damato B, Coupland SE. Translating uveal melanoma cytogenetics into clinical care. Arch Ophthalmol. 2009;127(4):423–9. https://doi.org/10.1001/archophthalmol.2009.40.
188. Shields CL, Ganguly A, Bianciotto CG, Turaka K, Tavallali A, Shields JA. Prognosis of uveal melanoma in 500 cases using genetic testing of fine-needle aspiration biopsy specimens. Ophthalmology. 2011;118(2):396–401. https://doi.org/10.1016/j.ophtha.2010.05.023.
189. Shields CL, Say EAT, Hasanreisoglu M, Saktanasate J, Lawson BM, Landy JE, et al. Cytogenetic abnormalities in uveal melanoma based on tumor features and size in 1059 patients: the 2016 W. Richard green lecture. Ophthalmology. 2017;124(5):609–18. https://doi.org/10.1016/j.ophtha.2016.12.026.
190. Shields CL, Say EAT, Hasanreisoglu M, Saktanasate J, Lawson BM, Landy JE, et al. Personalized prognosis of uveal melanoma based on cytogenetic profile in 1059 patients over an 8-year period: The 2017 Harry S. Gradle lecture. Ophthalmology. 2017;124(10):1523–31. https://doi.org/10.1016/j.ophtha.2017.04.003.
191. Mensink HW, Vaarwater J, Kiliç E, Naus NC, Mooy N, Luyten G, et al. Chromosome 3 intratumor heterogeneity in uveal melanoma. Invest Ophthalmol Vis Sci. 2009;50(2):500–4. https://doi.org/10.1167/iovs.08-2279.
192. Alameddine RM, Mansour AM, Kahtani E. Review of choroidal osteomas. Middle East Afr J Ophthalmol. 2014;21(3):244–50. https://doi.org/10.4103/0974-9233.134686.
193. Shields CL, Sun H, Demirci H, Shields JA. Factors predictive of tumor growth, tumor decalcification, choroidal neovascularization, and visual outcome in 74 eyes with choroidal osteoma. Arch Ophthalmol. 2005;123:1658–66. https://doi.org/10.1001/archopht.123.12.1658.
194. Aylward GW, Chang TS, Pautler SE, Gass JD. A long-term follow-up of choroidal osteoma. Arch Ophthalmol. 1998;116(10):1337–41.

195. Mizota A, Tanabe R, Adachi-Usami E. Rapid enlargement of choroidal osteoma in a 3-year-old girl. Arch Ophthalmol. 1998;116(8):1128–9.
196. Shields CL, et al. Uveal metastasis: clinical features and survival outcome of 2214 tumors in 1111 patients based on primary tumor origin. Middle East Afr J Ophthalmol. 2018;25(2):81–90.
197. Shields JA, Shields CL. Intraocular tumors: an atlas and textbook. 3rd ed. Philadelphia: Lippincott Williams & Wilkins; 2008.
198. Shields JA, Shields CL. An atlas and textbook. 3rd ed. Philadelphia: Lippincott, Wolters Kluwer; 2016. p. 213–45.
199. Krishna M. Diagnosis of metastatic neoplasms: an immunohistochemical approach. Arch Pathol Lab Med. 2010;134(2):207–15. https://doi.org/10.1043/1543-2165-134.2.207.
200. Dabbs DJ. Diagnostic immunohistochemistry: theranostic and genomic applications. 5th ed. Philadelphia: Elsevier; 2018.
201. Wing GL, Weiter JJ, Kelly PJ, Albert DM, Gonder JR. von Hippel-Lindau disease: angiomatosis of the retina and central nervous system. Ophthalmology. 1981;88(12):1311–4.
202. Park S, Chan C-C. Von Hippel-Lindau disease (VHL): a need for a murine model with retinal hemangioblastoma. Histol Histopathol. 2012;27(8):975–84. https://doi.org/10.14670/HH-27.975.
203. Chan CC, Collins AB, Chew EY. Molecular pathology of eyes with von Hippel-Lindau (VHL) disease: a review. Retina. 2007;27(1):1–7.
204. Gass JD. Cavernous hemangioma of the retina. A neuro-oculo-cutaneous syndrome. Am J Ophthalmol. 1971;71(4):799–814.
205. Yamaguchi K, Yamaguchi K, Tamai M. Cavernous hemangioma of the retina in a pediatric patient. Ophthalmologica. 1988;197(3):127–9. https://doi.org/10.1159/000309932.
206. Shields JA, Shields CL. A textbook and atlas. These vascular tumors may be associated with vitreous hemorrhage. Philadelphia: WB Saunders Co; 1992.
207. Irvine F, O'Donnell N, Kemp E, Lee WR. Retinal vasoproliferative tumors: surgical management and histological findings. Arch Ophthalmol. 2000;118(4):563–9.
208. Eagle RC Jr, Shields JA, Donoso L, Milner RS. Malignant transformation of spontaneously regressed retinoblastoma, retinoma/retinocytoma variant. Ophthalmology. 1989;96(9):1389–95.
209. Gallie BL, Ellsworth RM, Abramson DH, Phillips RA. Retinoma: spontaneous regression of retinoblastoma or benign manifestation of the mutation? Br J Cancer. 1982;45(4):513–21.
210. Lueder GT, Héon E, Gallie BL. Retinoma associated with vitreous seeding. Am J Ophthalmol. 1995;119(4):522–3.
211. Abouzeid H, Balmer A, Moulin AP, Mataftsi A, Zografos L, Munier FL. Phenotypic variability of retinocytomas: preregression and postregression growth patterns. Br J Ophthalmol. 2012;96(6):884–9. https://doi.org/10.1136/bjophthalmol-2011-300896.
212. Dimaras H, Khetan V, Halliday W, Orlic M, Prigoda NL, Piovesan B, et al. Loss of RB1 induces non-proliferative retinoma: increasing genomic instability correlates with progression to retinoblastoma. Hum Mol Genet. 2008;17(10):1363–72. https://doi.org/10.1093/hmg/ddn024.
213. Eagle RC. High-risk features and tumor differentiation in retinoblastoma: a retrospective histopathologic study. Arch Pathol Lab Med. 2009;133(8):1203–9. https://doi.org/10.1043/1543-2165-133.8.1203.
214. Margo C, Hidayat A, Kopelman J, Zimmerman LE. Retinocytoma. A benign variant of retinoblastoma. Arch Ophthalmol. 1983;101(10):1519–31.
215. Federico S, Brennan R, Dyer MA. Childhood cancer and developmental biology a crucial partnership. Curr Top Dev Biol. 2011;94:1–13. https://doi.org/10.1016/B978-0-12-380916-2.00001-2.
216. Thériault BL, Dimaras H, Gallie BL, Corson TW. The genomic landscape of retinoblastoma: a review. Clin Exp Ophthalmol. 2014;42(1):33–52. https://doi.org/10.1111/ceo.12132.
217. Rushlow DE, Mol BM, Kennett JY, Yee S, Pajovic S, Thériault BL, et al. Characterisation of retinoblastomas without RB1 mutations: genomic, gene expression, and clinical studies. Lancet. 2013;14(4):327–34. https://doi.org/10.1016/S1470-2045(13)70045-7.
218. Sastre X, Chantada GL, Doz F, Wilson MW, de Davila MTG, Rodríguez-Galindo C, et al. Proceedings of the consensus meetings from the International Retinoblastoma Staging Working Group on the pathology guidelines for the examination of enucleated eyes and evaluation of prognostic risk factors in retinoblastoma. Arch Pathol Lab Med. 2009;133(8):1199–202. https://doi.org/10.1043/1543-2165-133.8.1199.
219. Rao R, Honavar SG, Mulay K, Reddy VAP. Eye salvage in diffuse anterior retinoblastoma using systemic chemotherapy with periocular and intravitreal topotecan. J AAPOS. 2018;22(3):235–237.e2. https://doi.org/10.1016/j.jaapos.2017.11.013.
220. Fernandez MP, Al-Holou SN, Fischer O, Murray T, Harbour JW, Dubovy SR, Berrocal AM. Fluorescein angiography findings in diffuse retinoblastoma: two case reports with clinicopathologic correlation. J AAPOS. 2017;21(4):337–339.e2. https://doi.org/10.1016/j.jaapos.2017.03.013.
221. Amram AL, Rico G, Kim JW, Chintagumpala M, Herzog CE, Gombos DS, Chévez-Barrios P. Vitreous seeds in retinoblastoma: clinicopathologic classification and correlation. Ophthalmology. 2017;124(10):1540–7.
222. Hudson LE, Mendoza P, Hudson WH, Ziesel A, Hubbard GB, Wells J, et al. Distinct gene expression profiles define anaplastic grade in retinoblastoma. Am J Pathol. 2018;188(10):2328–38. https://doi.org/10.1016/j.ajpath.2018.06.013.
223. Mendoza PR, Specht CS, Hubbard GB, Wells JR, Lynn MJ, Zhang Q, et al. Histopathologic grading of anaplasia

in retinoblastoma. Am J Ophthalmol. 2015;159(4):764–76. https://doi.org/10.1016/j.ajo.2014.12.014.
224. Berry JL, Xu L, Kooi I, Murphree AL, Prabakar RK, Reid M, et al. Genomic cfDNA analysis of aqueous humor in retinoblastoma predicts eye salvage: the surrogate tumor biopsy for retinoblastoma. Mol Cancer Res. 2018;16:1701–12. https://doi.org/10.1158/1541-7786.MCR-18-0369.
225. Gorham JP, Szalai E, Wells JR, Grossniklaus HE. Retinoinvasive uveal melanoma: report of 2 cases and review of the literature. Ocul Oncol Pathol. 2017;3(4):292–5. https://doi.org/10.1159/000468940.
226. Mittal R, Al Awadi S, Sahar O, Behbehani AM. Ewing's sarcoma as second malignant neoplasm after retinoblastoma: a case report. Med Princ Pract. 2008;17(1):84–5. https://doi.org/10.1159/000109597.
227. Helton KJ, Fletcher BD, Kun LE, Jenkins JJ, Pratt CB. Bone tumors other than osteosarcoma after retinoblastoma. Cancer. 1993;71(9):2847–53.
228. Tahasildar N, Goni V, Bhagwat K, Tripathy SK, Panda BB. Ewing's sarcoma as second malignancy following a short latency in unilateral retinoblastoma. J Orthop Traumatol. 2011;12(3):167–71. https://doi.org/10.1007/s10195-011-0152-0.
229. Grossniklaus HE, Shehata B, Sorensen P, Bergstrom C, Hubbard GB. Primitive neuroectodermal tumor/Ewing sarcoma of the retina. Arch Pathol Lab Med. 2012;136(7):829–31. https://doi.org/10.5858/arpa.2011-0403-CR.
230. Jampol LM, Cottle E, Fischer DS, Albert DM. Metastasis of Ewing's sarcoma to the choroid. Arch Ophthalmol. 1973;89(3):207–9.
231. Chan CC, Pack S, Pak E, Tsogos M, Zhuang Z. Translocation of chromosomes 11 and 22 in choroidal metastatic Ewing sarcoma detected by fluorescent in situ hybridization. Am J Ophthalmol. 1999;127(2):226–8.
232. Votruba M, Hungerford J, Cornes PGS, Mabey D, Luthert P. Primary monophasic synovial sarcoma of the conjunctiva. Br J Ophthalmol. 2002;86(12):1453–4.
233. Hartstein ME, Silver F-L, Ludwig OJ, O'Connor DM. Primary synovial sarcoma. Ophthalmology. 2006;113(11):2093–6. https://doi.org/10.1016/j.ophtha.2006.04.037.
234. O'Sullivan MJ, Kyriakos M, Zhu X, Wick MR, Swanson PE, Dehner LP, et al. Malignant peripheral nerve sheath tumors with t(X;18). A pathologic and molecular genetic study. Mod Pathol. 2000;13(12):1336–46. https://doi.org/10.1038/modpathol.3880247.
235. Ito J, Suzuki S, Yoshida A, Mori T. Primary intraocular synovial sarcoma in the post retinal detachment operative state. BMJ Case Rep. 2015;2015:bcr2015209919. https://doi.org/10.1136/bcr-2015-209919.
236. Prívarová E, Griščíková L, Lokaj M, Vokurková J, Mazánek P, Autrata R. Eye manifestation of extrarenal malignant rhabdoid tumor. Cesk Slov Oftalmol. 2014;70(2):62–5.
237. Rootman J, Damji KF, Dimmick JE. Malignant rhabdoid tumor of the orbit. Ophthalmology. 1989;96(11):1650–4.
238. Gündüz K, Shields JA, Eagle RC, Shields CL, De Potter P, Klombers L. Malignant rhabdoid tumor of the orbit. Arch Ophthalmol. 1998;116(2):243–6.
239. Walford N, Deferrai R, Slater RM, Delemarre JF, Dingemans KP, Van den Bergh Weerman MA, Voute PA. Intraorbital rhabdoid tumor following bilateral retinoblastoma. Histopathology. 1992;20(2):170–3.
240. Watanabe H, Watanabe T, Kaneko M, Suzuya H, Onishi T, Okamoto Y, et al. Treatment of unresectable malignant rhabdoid tumor of the orbit with tandem high-dose chemotherapy and gamma-knife radiosurgery. Pediatr Blood Cancer. 2006;47(6):846–50. https://doi.org/10.1002/pbc.20699.
241. Bok D. The retinal pigment epithelium: a versatile partner in vision. J Cell Sci. 1993;17:189–95.
242. Wei W, Mo J, Jie Y, Li B. Adenoma of the retinal pigment epithelium: a report of 3 cases. Can J Ophthalmol. 2010;45(2):166–70. https://doi.org/10.3129/i09-249.
243. Shields JA, Shields CL, Gündüz K, Eagle RC. Neoplasms of the retinal pigment epithelium: the 1998 Albert Ruedemann, Sr, memorial lecture, part 2. Arch Ophthalmol. 1999;117(5):601–8.
244. Shields JA, Eagle RC, Barr CC, Shields CL, Jones DE. Adenocarcinoma of retinal pigment epithelium arising from a juxtapapillary histoplasmosis scar. Arch Ophthalmol. 1994;112(5):650–3.
245. Trichopoulos N, Augsburger JJ, Schneider S. Adenocarcinoma arising from congenital hypertrophy of the retinal pigment epithelium. Graefes Arch Clin Exp Ophthalmol. 2006;244(1):125–8. https://doi.org/10.1007/s00417-005-0011-x.
246. Klein KA, Lally DR, Taney LS, Laver NV, Duker JS. Retinal pigment epithelial adenocarcinoma presenting as an amelanotic mass. Ophthalmic Surg Lasers Imaging Retina. 2015;46(3):369–72.
247. Sommacal A, Campbell RJ, Helbig H. Adenocarcinoma of the retinal pigment epithelium. Arch Ophthalmol. 2003;121(10):1481–3. https://doi.org/10.1001/archopht.121.10.1481.
248. Loeffler KU, Kivelä T, Borgmann H, Witschel H. Malignant tumor of the retinal pigment epithelium with extraocular extension in a phthisical eye. Graefes Arch Clin Exp Ophthalmol. 1996;234(Suppl 1):S70–5.
249. Grossniklaus HE, Eberhart CG, Kivelä TT. WHO classification of tumors, vol. 12. 4th ed. Lyon: IARC; 2018.
250. Mahdi Y, Kharmoum J, Alouan A, Elouarradi H, Elkhiyat I, Maher M, Benchrif MZ, Kili A, Daoudi R, Cherradi N. Primary atypical teratoid/rhabdoid tumor of the optic nerve: a rare entity in an exceptional location. Diagn Pathol. 2015;10:47.
251. Allen JC, Judkins AR, Rosenblum MK, Biegel JA. Atypical teratoid/rhabdoid tumor evolving from an optic pathway ganglioglioma: case study. Neuro-Oncology. 2006;8(1):79–82.
252. Grossniklaus HE, Eberhart CG, Kivelä TT. WHO classification of tumours of the eye, IARC WHO classification of tumours, vol. 12. 4th ed. Lyon: IARC; 2018.

Ocular Von Hippel-Lindau Disease 10

Abhilasha Maheshwari, Hadas Newman,
and Paul T. Finger

Von Hippel-Lindau (VHL) disease is an autosomal dominant, multisystem disorder with a predilection for the central nervous system (CNS) and the retina. The incidence of VHL disease is approximately 1 in 40,000 to 1 in 54,000 live births [1]. Retinal capillary hemangioblastoma is the most common and often the earliest manifestation of VHL disease [2]. Therefore, ophthalmologists play a crucial role in the early diagnosis and management of these patients.

10.1 History

Eugen von Hippel, a German ophthalmologist, coined the term angiomatosis retinae in 1904 which later came to be known as retinal hemangioblastoma (retinal hemangioma) [3]. Lindau, a Swedish pathologist, established the relationship between cerebellar and retinal hemangioblastomas. In 1964, Melmon and Rosen reported cases of "von Hippel's disease" and "Lindau's disease" with overlapping ophthalmic, CNS, and visceral manifestations, establishing the clinical spectrum of "von Hippel–Lindau" disease [4].

Supported by The Eye Cancer Foundation, Inc. http://eyecancercure.com

A. Maheshwari · H. Newman · P. T. Finger (✉)
The New York Eye Cancer Center,
New York, NY, USA
e-mail: pfinger@eyecancer.com

10.2 Ophthalmic Manifestations

Retinal capillary hemangioma, a slow growing benign hamartoma, is the most common and earliest presentation in VHL. The mean age at diagnosis of retinal capillary hemangioma in VHL disease is 25 years and most patients present between their 10th and 40th years [5, 6]. The frequency of occurrence of retinal capillary hemangioma in VHL disease has been reported to vary from 49% to 85% [7–9]. It usually manifests as a solitary tumor but one-third of patients have multiple hemangiomas [10]. Half of the patients have bilateral involvement [11].

Retinal capillary hemangiomas are usually orange-red circumscribed, round vascular tumors supplied by a pair of dilated and tortuous feeder vessels (Fig. 10.1).

They can be asymptomatic. In cases with exudation, they can present with diminution of vision or metamorphopsia. They can be classified (Table 10.1) based on the location, morphology, effects on the retina and relationship to VHL disease [12, 13].

Most of the retinal capillary hemangiomas are in the temporal periphery and accompanied by at least one pair of dilated retinal vessels [2, 14, 15]. Juxtapapillary retinal capillary hemangiomas are less common (11–15% of cases) and their appearance can vary depending on whether the lesion is endophytic, exophytic or sessile. The endophytic variant appears as an orange red protrusion from the anterior surface of the optic disk and adjacent

V. Khetan (ed.), *Intraocular Tumors*, https://doi.org/10.1007/978-981-15-0395-5_10

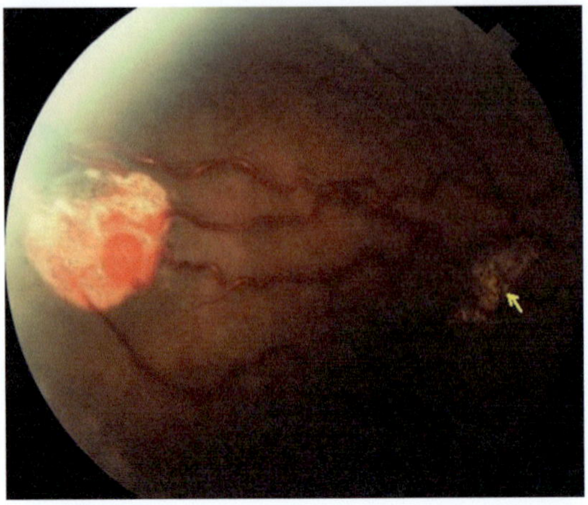

Fig. 10.1 Fundus photograph showing a round orange retinal lesion with prominent dilated retinal vessels typical of retinal capillary hemangioma. Note the presence of exudation (arrow)

Table 10.1 Classification system for retinal hemangioma [3]

Basis	Classification
Retinal distribution	1. Peripheral 2. Juxtapapillary 3. Bilateral
Effects of retina exudative	a. Vascular dilation/ exudation b. Retinal detachment c. Vitreoretinal traction
Systemic involvement	L-. Without VHL L+. With VHL

retina [2]. The exophytic tumor is adjacent to or surrounding the optic disk and can simulate chronic papilledema [2]. The sessile variant of juxtapapillary retinal capillary hemangioma is subtle in appearance and can be difficult to diagnose [2].

Secondary effects are predominantly exudative (25%) or tractional (9%) [2]. Intraretinal and subretinal exudation are limited to the vicinity of the hemangioma, but can also produce a macular star exudate leading to visual deterioration. Secondary glial proliferation on the retina and in the vitreous can lead to tractional retinal detachment [2]. The anterior segment is rarely involved secondarily with complications such as neovascular glaucoma and cataract.

10.3 Natural History of Disease

The retinal capillary hemangioma probability increases progressively with age. Classification systems aiding in staging the clinical progression have been developed by Vail [16].

The natural course of retinal capillary hemangiomas can be either of progression, stability or spontaneous regression [5]. Small lesions may remain stable for years, may show gliosis without leakage, or enlarge. In late stage, they may cause massive exudation and retinal detachment, uveitis, neovascular glaucoma and phthisis bulbi.

10.4 Differential Diagnosis (Table 10.2)

The fundus findings of retinal capillary hemangioma are typically diagnostic and can be observed during ophthalmoscopic examination. However, the following conditions should be ruled out:

Coat's Disease: Intraretinal exudation and collection of subretinal fluid is present, both, in Coat's disease and retinal capillary hemangioma. The vascular abnormality, however, is diffuse in Coats's and localized in retinal capillary hemangioma. Prominent feeder vessels, circumscribed round retinal angioma, family history and systemic features of VHL disease are also absent [2].

Wyburn–Mason Syndrome (Racemose Angioma): The dilated vessels of racemose angioma do not have an intervening orange red circumscribed retinal capillary hemangioma. They do not leak blood, serum or exudate.

Retinal Cavernous Hemangioma: This is a cluster of small, saccular vascular dilations around a central vein, but there are no prominent feeder vessels or exudation.

Retinal Macroaneurysm: Presents with subretinal, intraretinal or vitreous hemorrhage. It is centered on a retinal arteriole and feeder vessels are absent. There is often a history of systemic hypertension.

Vasoproliferative Tumor: Presents with retinal capillary hemangioma, orange color and presence of exudation. The differentiating feature is the absence of prominent feeder vessels and extreme peripheral retinal location of VPRT.

Astrocytic Hamartoma: Prominent vascularity makes the differentiation from retinal capillary hemangioma difficult. However, astrocytic hamartoma

Table 10.2 Diagnostic features of retinal vascular tumors

Type	Location	Appearance	Feeder vessels	Exudation
Retinal capillary hemangioma	Juxtapapillary/ peripheral	Round reddish mass	Prominent	Present
Coat's disease	Peripheral	Irregular dilatations with telangiectasia	Absent	Present
Cavernous hemangioma	Non-specific	Saccular grape like clusters	Absent	Absent
Racemose angioma	Diffuse	Dilated tortuous retinal vessels	Absent	Absent
Vasoproliferative tumor	Periphery	Orange globular mass	Absent	Present
Retinal macroaneurysm	Posterior	Round red lesion	Absent	Present
Astrocytic hamartoma	Posterior pole	Translucent or white mass	Absent	Usually absent

is usually translucent, does not have feeder vessels and is calcified.

Others: RPA adenoma or uveal melanoma with prominent feeder vessels can sometimes resemble capillary hemangioma. Juxtapapillary retinal capillary hemangioma can also simulate unilateral disc edema, juxtapapillary choroiditis, choroidal neovascularization, choroidal hemangioma and amelanotic choroidal melanoma.

10.5 Diagnostic Methods

Fluorescein angiography is the most informative diagnostic tool to detect retinal capillary hemangioma. Due the vascular nature of the tumor and endophytic growth pattern it exhibits a dramatic and relatively unique pattern of hyperfluorescence [17]. Obtaining early-phase images is critically important. Fluorescein is evident in the early arterial phase in the dilated feeder arteriole, the tumor has fine capillary homogeneous filling, and the draining vein becomes prominent in the venous phase. The tumor demonstrates progressively intense hyper-fluorescence with late leakage of dye into the overlying vitreous humor (Fig. 10.2). Fluorescein angiography is helpful in establishing the diagnosis of juxtapapillary hemangioma and can be an adjunct to treatment planning by differentiating the feeder arteriole from the draining vein. Fluorescein angiography is particularly helpful for assessment of the tumor's response the treatment.

Other diagnostic modalities may be employed but have a minimal role. ICG can help differentiate choroidal lesions, such as choroidal hemangioma or choroidal neovascular membrane from retinal capillary hemangioma [2, 18].

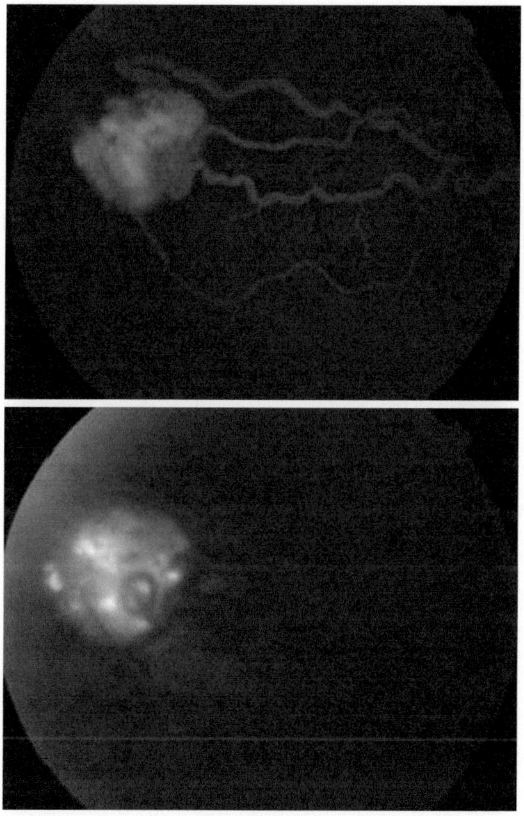

Fig. 10.2 Fluorescein angiogram demonstrating (top) progressive and complete filling of the hemangioma, retinal artery and the vein and (bottom) late leakage of the retinal capillary hemangioma

Ultrasonography can help measure the tumor thickness. A-scan shows an initial spike followed by high internal reflectivity and B-scan shows a well-demarcated retinal lesion without choroidal invasion [19]. If present, B-scan can also document secondary exudative retinal detachment.

MRI can detect associated CNS hemangiomas. Color Doppler imaging and laser scanning tomography can be used to document tumor blood flow and angiographic changes in feeder vessels after treatment [2, 20].

10.6 Treatment

Treatment depends upon the location, size and related complications, presence of bilateral multiple tumors and the likelihood of new tumor formation. Despite treatment, 25% of patients show permanent visual loss (vision of 20/40 in one or both eyes) and 20% have visual acuity less than 20/100 in at least one eye [2].

Treatment modalities include observation, cryotherapy, plaque radiotherapy and vitreoretinal surgery. Understanding of VHL protein function and tumorigenesis have led to new treatment that target the biology of the disease, as opposed to ablative or surgical approaches. Molecules upregulated in the VHL mutation, such as VEGF and PDGF, have been targeted in investigational anti-angiogenic therapies, both in systemic and ocular manifestation of the disease [10].

10.6.1 Observation

It can be considered if the retinal capillary hemangioma is very small (up to 500 microns), not associated with exudation, does not threaten the vision or has undergone spontaneous regression with gliosis, sheathing and lack of feeder vessels [2]. Juxtapapillary hemangiomas are more commonly treated with primary observation in that they can remain stable for years. Treatment should only be taken when tumor progresses or causes a threat to visual acuity, due to the adverse effect of treatment on the optic nerve and major vessels [13, 21].

10.6.2 Laser Photocoagulation

To treat small to medium-sized retinal capillary hemangiomas in eyes with clear media. At The New York Eye Cancer Center, we typically first close the arterial feeder vessel(s). If such indirect tumor devascularization is not achieved, we encircle the posterior 180° of the tumor to avascular scar. If complete vascular regression has still not been achieved, then we apply laser directly to the hemangioma (Fig. 10.3). A response rate of 91–100% has been shown with laser treatment [22, 23]. In general, response to laser treatment is evaluated in 4–6-week intervals (Fig. 10.4).

10.6.3 Cryotherapy

Anterior location of the hemangioma, subretinal fluid which can reduce the laser energy uptake and diameter greater than 3 mm are indications of cryotherapy. Double freeze-thaw technique is employed under indirect ophthalmoscopy [5]. The cryotherapy is applied until the ice ball completely encloses the hemangioma before thawing is initiated [2]. A 15-year review found that all hemangiomas under 3.75 mm in diameter successfully responded to cryotherapy. However, there is a risk of cryotherapy-related exudative detachment.

10.6.4 Plaque Brachytherapy

A recent study proved that plaque treatment was efficacious for retinal capillary hemangiomas that were 5 mm or less in diameter [2]. Radiation complications can be related to tumor location and radiation dose to the fovea and optic nerve [24, 25].

10.6.5 Anti-Angiogenic Medications

Drugs like bevacizumab and ranibizumab, have been used, but do not provide long-term cessation of tumor growth or reduction in subretinal fluid

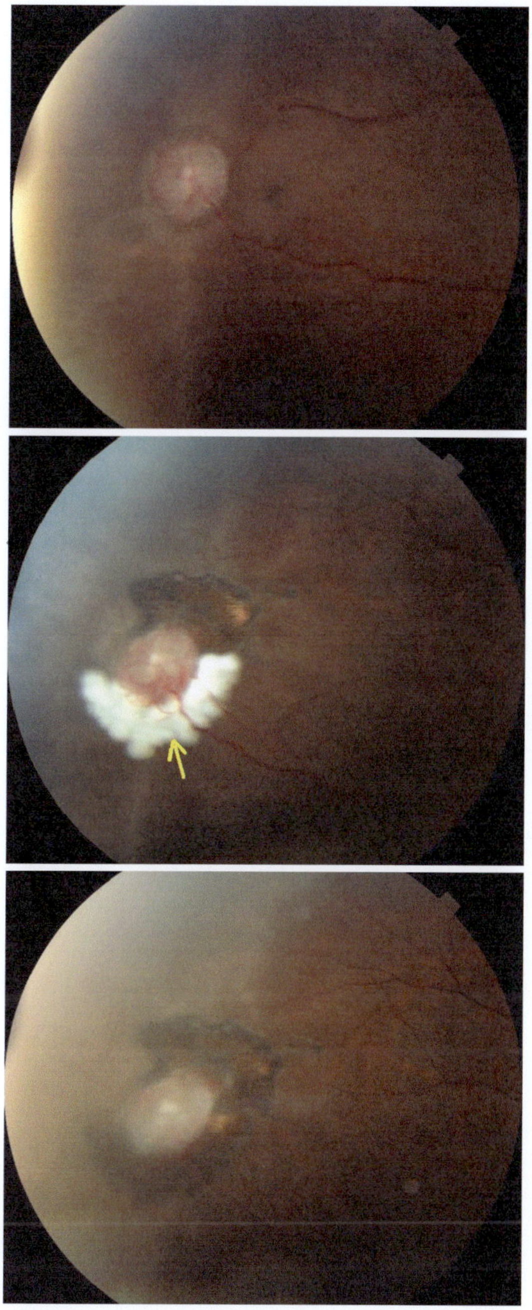

Fig. 10.3 Fundus photograph showing (top) retinal capillary hemangioma measuring 2.0 × 2.0 mm in size before and (middle) immediately after placement of photocoagulation on the feeding artery delimiting the lesion. Argon green laser was used with spot size of 250–500 microns, duration of 0.20 s, and power of 250–500 mW. Total of 200 spots (arrow) were applied. (Bottom) Delineated stable lesion after 6 weeks of treatment

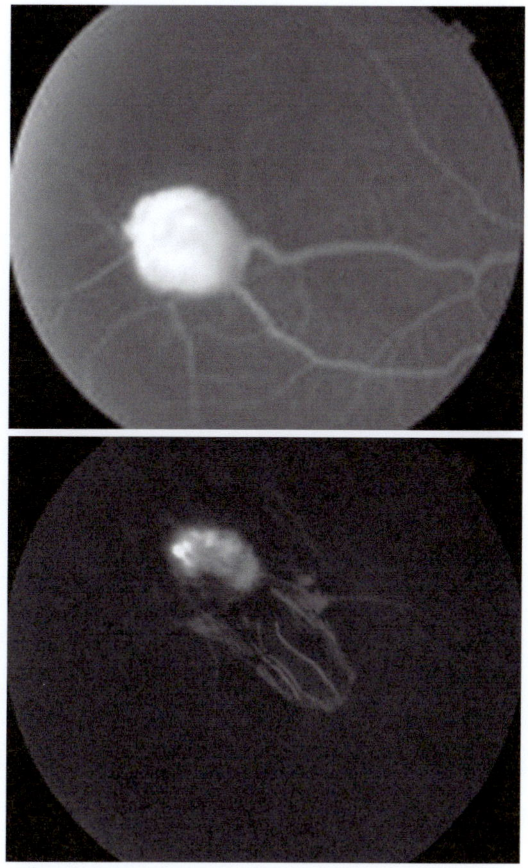

Fig. 10.4 Fluorescein angiogram (top) prior to treatment with laser photocoagulation and (bottom) 6 weeks after treatment. Note the presence of sclerosed vessels

[26–28]. A prospective study of intravitreal pegaptanib, an aptamer that inhibits VEGF isoform 165, found that pegaptanib did not influence lesion regression, but can minimally decrease exudation in some cases [29]. A small case series of oral propranolol was studied in 7 patients, the hemangiomas showed stability of the lesions during treatment [28].

10.6.6 Others

Transpupillary thermotherapy (TTT), photodynamic therapy, proton beam radiation have also been described with inconsistent results. Pars plana vitrectomy may become necessary for advanced and complicated cases [5]. Enucleation is performed for blind-painful eyes unresponsive to conservative therapy.

10.7 Systemic Manifestations

The systemic manifestations of VHL include CNS hemangiomas of the brain and spinal cord, renal cell carcinomas, renal cysts, pheochromocytomas, pancreatic cysts, islet cell tumors, epididymal cystadenomas, endolymphatic sac tumors of the inner ear and adnexal papillary cystadenomas of the broad ligament [30]. About 50% of VHL patients manifest only one feature of VHL disease, and very few develop all the manifestations [2, 8]. After retinal capillary hemangioma, the most frequently affected organ systems are the CNS, kidneys and adrenal glands, many of them occurring years after the initial presentation with retinal capillary hemangiomas [30].

The diagnosis of VHL disease is based on retinal capillary hemangioma or CNS hemangioma, visceral lesions and a family history of similar lesions (Table 10.3). After the diagnosis is made, both ophthalmic and systemic screening protocols should be followed. At The New York Eye Cancer Center, we perform brain and abdominal imaging at diagnosis and every 2 years thereafter. Initial and yearly medical physical, neurologic examinations are obtained.

According to National Cancer institute, VHL disease can be classified, on clinical grounds, into two main types: Type I (pheochromocytoma absent) and Type II (pheochromocytoma present) [2].

Table 10.3 Diagnostic criteria for von Hippel-Lindau disease [2]

Family history	Features
Positive	Any one of the following: 1. Retinal capillary hemangioma 2. CNS hemangioma 3. Visceral lesions[a]
Negative	Any one of the following: 1. Two or more retinal capillary hemangiomas 2. Two or more CNS hemangiomas 3. Single retinal or CNS hemangioma with a visceral lesion[a]

[a]Visceral lesions include renal cysts, renal carcinoma, pheochromocytoma, pancreatic cysts, islet cell tumors, epididymal cystadenoma, endolymphatic sac tumor, and adnexal papillary cystadenoma

10.8 Genetics

VHL disease is an autosomal dominant disease, due to heterozygous mutation of VHL tumor suppressor gene located on chromosome 3p25-26. The protein product of the VHL gene forms a complex with other proteins that targets hypoxia inducible factors (HIFs) for degradation. Mutations in the VHL gene result in stabilization of the HIFs, which bind to specific enhancer in elements in the VEGF gene and stimulate angiogenesis.

Patients with a suspicion or diagnosis of VHL should undergo both genetic testing and counseling. With a near complete penetrance of the disease, genetic testing has been proven to be helpful in early diagnosis and clinical screening for disease manifestations.

References

1. Maher ER, Iselius L, Yates JR, et al. Von Hippel-Lindau disease: a genetic study. J Med Genet. 1991;28(7):443–7.
2. Singh AD, Shields CL, Shields JA. von Hippel-Lindau disease. Surv Ophthalmol. 2001;46(2):117–42.
3. Singh AD, Rundle PA, Rennie I. Retinal vascular tumors. Ophthalmol Clin N Am. 2005;18(1):167–76. x
4. Melmon KL, Rosen SW. Lindau's disease. Review of the literature and study of a large kindred. Am J Med. 1964;36:595–617.
5. Magee MA, Kroll AJ, Lou PL, Ryan EA. Retinal capillary hemangiomas and von Hippel-Lindau disease. Semin Ophthalmol. 2006;21(3):143–50.
6. Lonser RR, Glenn GM, Walther M, et al. von Hippel-Lindau disease. The Lancet. 2003;361(9374):2059–67.
7. Lamiell JM, Salazar FG, Hsia YE. von Hippel-Lindau disease affecting 43 members of a single kindred. Medicine (Baltimore). 1989;68(1):1–29.
8. Maher ER, Yates JR, Harries R, et al. Clinical features and natural history of von Hippel-Lindau disease. Q J Med. 1990;77(283):1151–63.

9. Neumann HP, Wiestler OD. Clustering of features of von Hippel-Lindau syndrome: evidence for a complex genetic locus. The Lancet. 1991;337:1052.
10. Salazar FG, Lamiell JM. Early identification of retinal angiomas in a large kindred von Hippel-Lindau disease. Am J Ophthalmol. 1980;89(4):540–5.
11. Carr RE, Noble KG. Retinal angiomatosis. Ophthalmology. 1980;87(9):956–9.. 961
12. Augsburger JJ, Shields JA, Goldberg RE. Classification and management of hereditary retinal angiomas. Int Ophthalmol. 1981;4(1–2):93–106.
13. Gass JD, Braunstein R. Sessile and exophytic capillary angiomas of the juxtapapillary retina and optic nerve head. Arch Ophthalmol. 1980; 98(10):1790–7.
14. Schmidt D, Natt E, Neumann HP. Long-term results of laser treatment for retinal angiomatosis in von Hippel-Lindau disease. Eur J Med Res. 2000;5(2):47–58.
15. Webster AR, Maher ER, Moore AT. Clinical characteristics of ocular angiomatosis in von Hippel-Lindau disease and correlation with germline mutation. Arch Ophthalmol. 1999;117(3):371–8.
16. Vail D. Angiomatosis retinae, eleven years after diathermy coagulation. Am J Ophthalmol. 1958;46(4):525–34.
17. Haining WM, Zweifach PH. Fluorescein angiography in von Hippel-Lindau disease. Arch Ophthalmol. 1967;78(4):475–9.
18. Shields CL, Shields JA, De Potter P. Patterns of indocyanine green videoangiography of choroidal tumours. Br J Ophthalmol. 1995;79(3):237–45.
19. Goes F, Benozzi J. Ultrasonography of haemangioma of the optic disc. Bull Soc Belge Ophtalmol. 1980;190:87–97.
20. Lieb WE, Shields JA, Cohen SM, et al. Color Doppler imaging in the management of intraocular tumors. Ophthalmology. 1990;97(12):1660–4.
21. Kremer I, Gilad E, Ben-Sira I. Juxtapapillary exophytic retinal capillary hemangioma treated by yellow krypton (568 nm) laser photocoagulation. Ophthalmic Surg. 1988;19(10):743–7.
22. Lane CM, Turner G, Gregor ZJ, Bird AC. Laser treatment of retinal angiomatosis. Eye. 1989;3:33–8.
23. Bonnet M, Garmier G. Treatment of retinal capillary angiomas of von Hippel's disease. J Fr Ophtalmol. 1984;7(8–9):545–55.
24. Finger PT, Chin KJ, Yu G-P, Palladium-103 for Choroidal Melanoma Study Group. Risk factors for radiation maculopathy after ophthalmic plaque radiation for choroidal melanoma. Am J Ophthalmol. 2010;149(4):608–15.
25. Kreusel KM, Bornfeld N, Lommatzsch A, Wessing A, Foerster MH. Ruthenium-106 brachytherapy for peripheral retinal capillary hemangioma. Ophthalmology. 1998;105(8):1386–92.
26. von Buelow M, Pape S, Hoerauf H. Systemic bevacizumab treatment of a juxtapapillary retinal haemangioma. Acta Ophthalmol Scand. 2007;85(1):114–6.
27. Slim E, Antoun J, Kourie HR, Schakkal A, Cherfan G. Intravitreal bevacizumab for retinal capillary hemangioblastoma: a case series and literature review. Can J Ophthalmol. 2014;49(5):450–7.
28. Albiñana V, Escribano RMJ, Soler I, et al. Repurposing propranolol as a drug for the treatment of retinal haemangioblastomas in von Hippel-Lindau disease. Orphanet J Rare Dis. 2017;12(1):122.
29. Dahr SS, Cusick M, Rodriguez-Coleman H, et al. Intravitreal anti-vascular endothelial growth factor therapy with pegaptanib for advanced von Hippel-Lindau disease of the retina. Retina. 2007;27(2):150–8.
30. Choyke PL, Glenn GM, Walther MM, Patronas NJ, Linehan WM, Zbar B. von Hippel-Lindau disease: genetic, clinical, and imaging features. Radiology. 1995;194(3):629–42.

11 Intraocular Lymphomas

Kaustubh Mulay, Santosh G. Honavar, Santosh U. Kafle, and Sarah E. Coupland

11.1 Background

Lymphoma is a malignant neoplasm derived from monoclonal proliferations of B- or T-lymphocytes and rarely, natural killer (NK) cells. Ophthalmic involvement is relatively rare and may involve the ocular adnexa, orbit or intraocular structures. The intraocular lymphomas represent about 0.01% of ophthalmic diseases [1, 2]. They may arise as primary tumours within the eye, either within the vitreoretinal or uveal tract, or occur as secondary manifestations of a systemic Non-Hodgkin lymphoma (NHL). Vitreoretinal lymphomas (VRL) often occur in association with central nervous system (CNS) disease and are aggressive tumours. In contrast, primary uveal lymphomas tend to be low-grade B-NHL, and have a good prognosis. Secondary lymphomas represent an intraocular manifestation of a systemic NHL, and commonly occur in the choroid. Given their rarity and ability to masquerade clinically as inflammatory processes, the clinical diagnosis of intraocular lymphoma (both VRL and uveal lymphoma) is generally challenging, and typically requires a vitrectomy/chorioretinal biopsy for histopathological confirmation. Treatment of VRL is controversial and varies between centres, particularly in the absence of a concurrent CNS disease [2]. Although the earlier recognition of VRL has improved in recent times, the prognosis remains poor. Here, we summarize the available literature on both VRL and uveal lymphomas.

11.2 Primary Vitreoretinal Lymphoma (PVRL)

11.2.1 Definition

Vitreoretinal lymphoma is defined as a malignant lymphocytic neoplasm affecting the retina with or without involvement of the vitreous or the optic nerve. It is considered a subset of PCNSL, and can occur concurrently, subsequent to- or antedate the cerebral disease. In the case of the latter, the primary site is considered to be the eye. VRL is a high-grade B-cell NHL, often running a rapid clinical course.

K. Mulay
National Reporting Centre for Ophthalmic Pathology (NRCOP), Centre For Sight, Hyderabad, India

S. G. Honavar
Department of Ophthalmic and Facial Plastic Surgery and Ocular Oncology, Centre For Sight, Hyderabad, India

S. U. Kafle
Department of Ophthalmic Pathology and Laboratory Medicine, Eastern Regional Eye Care Program, Biratnagar Eye Hospital, Biratnagar, Nepal

Department of Molecular and Clinical Cancer Medicine, Institute of Translational Medicine, University of Liverpool, Liverpool, UK

S. E. Coupland (✉)
Department of Molecular and Clinical Cancer Medicine, Institute of Translational Medicine, University of Liverpool, Liverpool, UK
e-mail: s.e.coupland@liverpool.ac.uk

V. Khetan (ed.), *Intraocular Tumors*, https://doi.org/10.1007/978-981-15-0395-5_11

11.2.2 Historical Perspective, Nomenclature and, Classification of the Intraocular Lymphomas

Triebenstein, in 1920, first reported an intraocular lymphoma, which on further examination was most likely to have been a primary choroidal lymphoma [3]. Three decades later, first Cooper and Riker, and then Givner described Triebenstein's disease as 'malignant lymphoma of the uveal tract' [4, 5]. In 1975, Klingele and Hogan called it 'ocular reticulum sarcoma' [6]. The term 'reticulum cell sarcoma' was first used by Vogel in 1968 to also describe the retinal form of this disease [7]. This terminology was soon shown to be a misnomer and, with the advent of World Health Organization (WHO) lymphoma classification in 2001, this disease entity was renamed as "intraocular lymphoma" with a specific subtyping as a diffuse large B-cell lymphoma [8, 9]. Whilst the terminology 'primary intraocular lymphoma' or 'PIOL' was proposed [10, 11], it became clear that choroidal and vitreoretinal lymphomas differed significantly from each other (each histologically, genetically and clinically) and should not be subsumed under the same term of 'PIOL'. Hence, the term 'primary vitreoretinal lymphoma (PVRL)' was proposed to differentiate this entity from 'primary uveal (choroidal) lymphoma', and it is currently the accepted terminology to describe this subset of intraocular lymphomas [12–15]. It has been recommended that the intraocular lymphomas be subtyped according to their location and whether they are primary or secondary to CNS or systemic involvement [13]. Any further classification of the lymphomas are based on the subsequent revision of the WHO Lymphoma classification [16].

11.2.3 Epidemiology of VRL

VRL is rare, but its exact incidence is unknown with most data relating to PCNSL [17]. PCNSL with ocular involvement and PVRL represent 1% of non-Hodgkin lymphoma (NHL), 1% of all intracranial tumors and less than 1% of intraocular malignancies [18]. In recent times, a true increase in the incidence of VRL and PCNSL has been noted in both immunodeficient and immunosuppressed patients [1, 19, 20]. Although rare cases have been reported in infants and adolescents, VRL is usually a disease of adults [1, 13, 17, 21–23]. Patients are usually older than 40 years with the mean age of presentation being the fifth and sixth decade [1, 14, 17]. Many reports in the literature suggest females to be affected more frequently than males [24–26].

11.2.4 Pathogenesis of VRL

The exact etiology of VRL remains very unclear with several hypotheses being proposed but most of these being far from proven. For example, these include the role of infectious agents, the chemokine hypothesis, selective homing of malignant lymphocytes to the eye and clonal transformation of local polyclonal inflammatory cells.

In anecdotal cases, infectious agents such as Epstein-Barr virus (EBV), Human herpes virus-8 (HHV8) and *Toxoplasma gondii* have been proposed to be involved in the pathogenesis of VRL [27, 28]. EBV transforms human B-lymphocytes eventually leading to continuous proliferation while HHV8 viral genome expresses genes responsible for inhibition of apoptosis, cell cycle entry and angiogenesis with proliferation of B-lymphocytes [20, 29]. The role of *Toxoplasma gondii* in lymphomagenesis is unknown. However, It is possible that a chronic immunological response to ocular *T. gondii* infection could lead in some cases to VRL development [28].

Chemokines and chemokine receptors selective for B-lymphocytes were identified in retinal pigment epithelium (RPE) and malignant B-cells, respectively [30]. It has been suggested that B-cell chemokines may be involved in the pathogenesis of VRL by selectively attracting lymphoma cells to the RPE from the choroidal circulation [30]. Another hypothesis on the infiltration of malignant lymphocytes from the systemic circulation into the eye and brain suggests that permissive retinal endothelial cell receptors and lack of robust immune surveillance may allow preferential entry of malignant lymphocytes to the retina than the choroid with subsequent clonal proliferation in the eye [2, 12, 31].

One group suggested that VRL develop subsequent to an infectious uveitis [28]. This opens up another hypothesis that initial polyclonal proliferation of inflammatory lymphocytes may undergo mutagenesis leading to a monoclonal proliferation characteristic of VRL. Endoantigens from a non-infectious uveitis may produce the same phenomenon [2].

11.2.5 Clinical Features of VRL

Diagnosis of PVRL is difficult and based on clinical features, investigations and microscopic evaluation. While clinical signs aid the diagnosis of VRL to some extent and investigative tools help differentiating it from mimics, it is the microscopic evaluation that remains the diagnostic cornerstone in such patients [2, 32–61]. Between 64% and 83% cases of PVRL are bilateral with a frequent tendency to mimic posterior chronic uveitis [13, 14, 17]. Most are insidious in onset and in many, timely diagnosis is marred by diagnostic difficulties. Blurring of vision and/or floaters are presenting symptoms. Yet, visual acuity can be relatively well preserved [17]. Vitreous floaters may be noticed long before VRL is suspected, and are often attributed to normal degenerative changes or uveitis [13]. Steroids may temporarily benefit the patient, but thereby delay the diagnosis of VRL. Anterior segment inflammation is usually absent [13, 32]. Keratic precipitates and cells may be seen in the anterior chamber but infiltrating cells are usually confined to the vitreous cavity [13, 33]. Pseudohypopyon is a rare presentation. Sheets and clusters of lymphomatous cells may be seen in the vitreous. These cells are larger than inflammatory cells and may not cluster with the reactive cells, resulting in an 'aurora borealis' appearance from cells lining along the vitreous fibrils [13]. A mild to moderate haze may be seen which, at times is accentuated at the periphery or superiorly (Fig. 11.1a, b) [13, 17]. Lymphoma cells may grow along the Bruch's membrane under the RPE. These may be seen as creamy lesions with orange-yellow infiltrates deep to the retina (Fig. 11.1a, b) [17]. Islands of dislodged RPE lie over these deposits, which with early or diffuse involvement gives rise to a characteristic 'leopard-skin' pigmentation (Fig. 11.2) [13]. RPE atrophy and subretinal fibrosis may result from spontaneous resolution [35]. Optic nerve and orbital involvement are rare but may occur [36, 37].

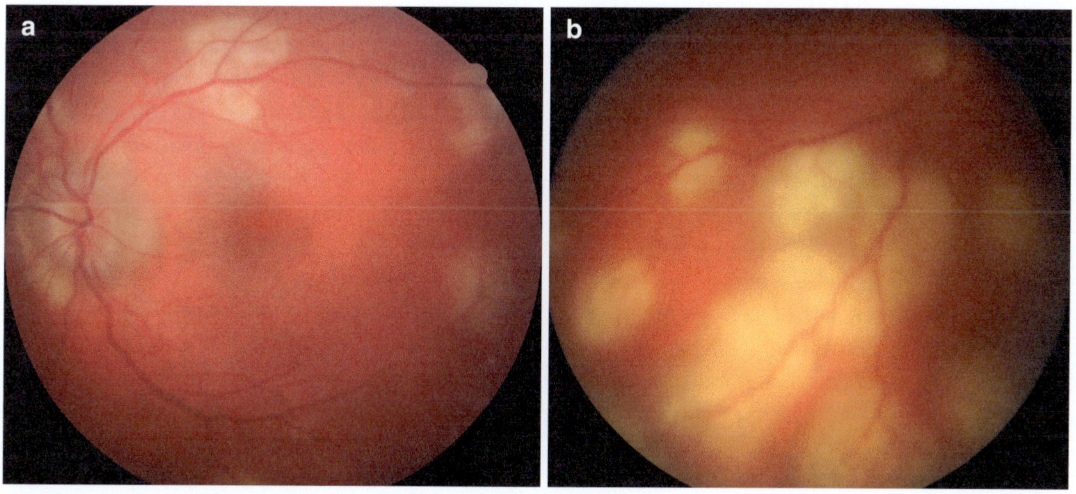

Fig. 11.1 Pathognomic subretinal and vitreal infiltrates involving the (**a**) left and (**b**) right of an elderly female with VRL and simultaneous CNS disease. There is additional optic nerve involvement of the left eye. Images care of Stefan Seregard, Sweden

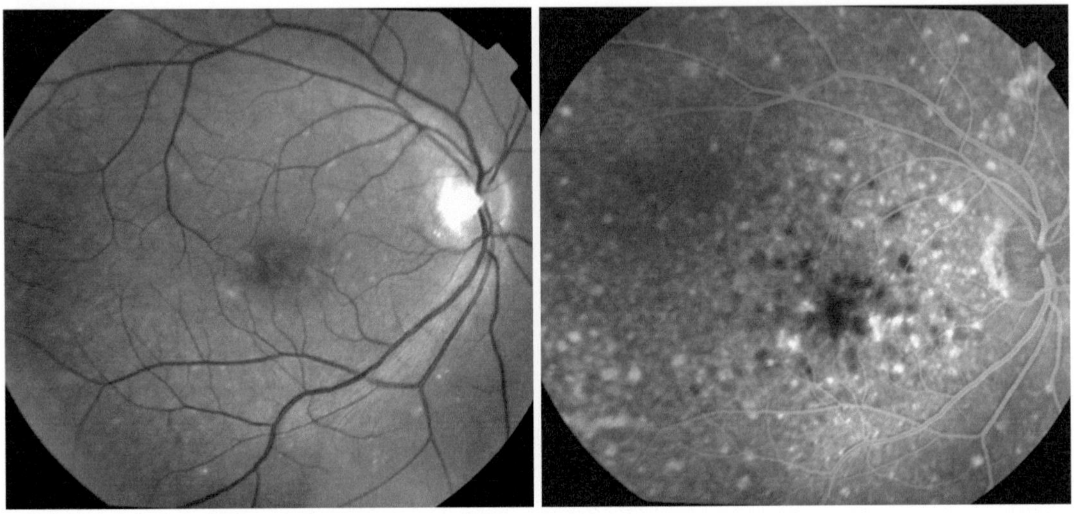

Fig. 11.2 Typical leopard skin alterations seen on the later phase of the fluorescein angiography, in a patient with subsequently diagnosed VRL. Images care of Nathalie Cassoux, France

Concomitant CNS involvement is present in 16–34% of patients with VRL [17]. Subsequent PCNSL occurs in 42–92% patients of VRL within a mean interval of 8–29 months [17]. Hemiparesis, ataxia and new-onset seizures common presentation of CNS involvement [36, 38].

11.2.6 Diagnosis of VRL

As mentioned previously, although clinical examination and ocular imaging are help in the diagnosis of VRL, the gold standard for its diagnosis is demonstration of neoplastic lymphocytes in the eye.

11.2.6.1 Optical Coherence Tomography (OCT)

Direct infiltration of retinal by lymphomatous cells with focal growth creates a semi-opaque gray spot that appears homogenous on OCT. Lymphomatous infiltration can be seen as nodular, hyper-reflective signals in the form of dots, bands and nodules at or above the level of RPE in the eyes of patients with VRL using spectral-domain OCT (SD-OCT) [39, 40]. However, these hyper-reflective spots need to be differentiated from those seen in age related macular degeneration or diabetic macular edema [41, 42].

11.2.6.2 Fluorescein Angiography (FA)

FA shows early and late hypofluorescent lesions in cases with outer retinal involvement [2]. Punctuate hyperfluorescent window defects, round hypofluorescent lesions and vasculitis were observed by Cassoux et al. in their study on 44 patients with VRL [32]. Leakage of fluorescein along retinal veins and periarteriolar staining has been demonstrated in PVRL [41].

11.2.6.3 Indocyanine Green Angiography(IGA)

In the early phase of VRL, small hypofluorescent lesions are seen while such lesions become less apparent in the later phases [17]. FA and IGA when used together, have a positive- and negative- predictive value of 89% and 85%, respectively, for VRL [44].

11.2.6.4 Fundus Autofluorescence (FAF)

FAF is a non-invasive technique that can acquire a topographic map of the lipofuscin distribution in the RPE cells. One of the characteristic FAF findings in eyes with VRL is a granular pattern consisting of hyperautofluorescent spots surrounded by a hypoautofluorescent ring [45]. Lymphomatous infiltration in the sub-RPE space alters RPE metabolism leading to hyperautofluorescence [40]. On the other hand, lymphomatous infiltration above the RPE may block autofluorescence from RPE cells resulting in a granular pattern of hypoautofluorescent spots surrounded by hyperautofluorescent rings [40]. Hypofluorescent spots ('leopard spots') seen on FA correspond to hyperautofluorescent spots on FAF [40, 45]. Whitish areas of retinal infiltration appear hypoautofluorescent on FAF and hyperfluorescent on FA [45].

11.2.6.5 Ultrasound B Scan (UBS)

Although UBS findings are not specific for VRL, it can be used in cases where posterior segment is difficult to visualize [17]. Findings on UBS include vitreous debris, retinal detachment, elevated chorioretinal lesions, and widening of optic nerve [17].

11.2.6.6 Vitreous Sampling

Although lymphoma cells are typically located between the RPE and the Bruch's membrane, they may invade the vitreous. Vitreous biopsy (VB) and pars plana vitrectomy (PPV) are the 2 methods practised to sample the vitreous. VB targets the core vitreous resulting in the collection of 1–2 mL of sample while PPV targets the core and cortical vitreous resulting in collection of 50–100 mL of fluid [46]. In order to ensure adequate and maximum cellular viability, samples need to be transported to the laboratory without delay, and preferably with prior notification of the laboratory. A number of soft fixative solutions can be used to send the sample when suspecting VRL [47]. We use 'Shandon' cytofix (also called Cytolyt) or HEPES-glutamic acid buffer mediated Organic solvent Protection Effect (HOPE) solution [17, 46].

In addition to maximizing sample size, PPV also improves vision by clearance of vitreous debris. The greater cellularity of a PPV as compared to a core vitreous biopsy also permits performance of additional tests such as the immunophenotyping of the cells using immunohistochemistry (IHC) or flow cytometry, DNA extraction for IgH monoclonality and polymerase chain reaction (PCR) studies (see below) [46]. Retinal tears and tumour seeding through the sclerectomy port to the epibulbar space may occur very rarely [46, 48].

11.2.6.7 Neuroimaging, CSF Examination and Brain Biopsy

Since VRL is a subset of PCNSL, it is crucial that CNS lesions be excluded with the help of contrast enhanced magnetic resonance imaging (MRI). CNS lesions may be uni- or multifocal that appear hypodense on T1-weighted and hyperdense on T2-weighted images [17, 49]. Identification of lymphoma cells in CSF in a patient with concurrent oculocerebral lymphoma can spare the patient from an additional invasive procedure, such as vitrectomy. However, it must be noted that the yield of lymphoma cells in the Cerebral Spinal Fluid (CSF) is low, with a false negative rate of 25% in patients with CNS lesions [8, 50]. Stereotactic brain biopsies need to be performed in patients with suspicious MRI lesions but a negative CSF cytology.

11.2.6.8 Light Microscopy of VRL

Although malignant lymphoid cells can be visualised using a Papanicolou or Hematoxylin-eosin stain, a Giemsa or Diff-Quick stain of a cytospin is preferred since they outline the characteristics of lymphoma cells better. VRL cells are typically fragile and can be tightly packed in the sub-RPE, and appear as large lymphoid cells with scanty basophilic cytoplasm and large nuclei, which may be round, oval, bean-shaped or hypersegmented with prominent nucleoli and mitoses (Fig. 11.3a) [52–54]. Inflammatory background with admixed macrophages and small T-cells or necrotic lymphoma cells may be seen [51, 55].

11.2.6.9 Immunohistochemistry and Flow Cytometry

Demonstration of a dominant B-cell infiltrate within the vitreous and of monoclonality of the B-cells, either as kappa or lambda chain restriction, supports the diagnosis of a lymphoma. As above, most VRL are of B-cell origin and thus express CD19, CD20, CD22 and CD79a (Fig. 11.3b) [56]. Aberrant concomitant expression of MUM1 and BCL-6 has also

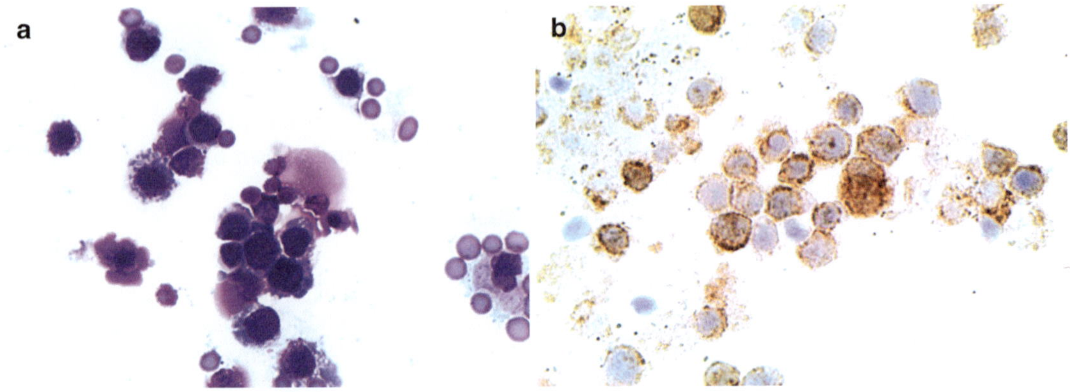

Fig. 11.3 (**a**) May Grunewald Giemsa staining of a vitrecitmy specimen, demonstrating large atypical lymphocyte blasts with a small rim of cytoplasm, and some smaller scattered erythrocytes (MMG, ×60 objective). (**b**) CD79 immunostaining of the same vitrectomy sample showing the clear positivity of the neoplastic lymphocytes for this marker (DAB, ×60 objective)

been reported [55]. Exceptionally rare cases of anaplastic large cell and T-cell types of VRL have been described [57, 58]. T-cell lymphomas express CD3 and thus make differentiation from a reactive infiltrate difficult. In such cases, PCR studies for T-cell receptor gene rearrangements can help in establishing the diagnosis of T-cell type VRL.

11.2.6.10 Other Laboratory Tests

Analysis of interleukin (IL) ratios is used in some centres to provide additional information in the diagnosis of lymphoma. Malignant B-cells express high levels of IL10 while inflammatory cells express high levels of IL6 [59–61]. A raised IL10:IL6 ratio is therefore suggestive of an intraocular manifestation of a B-cell NHL.

More commonly, diagnostic laboratories assess the B-cell infiltrate for monoclonality using polymerase chain reaction, directed against the immunoglobulin heavy chain gene (IgH-PCR). This test requires good quality DNA to be extracted from the cells within the vitreous infiltrate [62].

Blood tests for human immunodeficiency virus, complete blood count and test to exclude unusual causes of uveitis may also be useful.

11.2.6.11 Genetics of VRL

Molecular studies have demonstrated that VRL arise from a post-germinal centre B-cell with the immunoglobulin gene demonstrating a highly mutated pattern, similar to that observed in PCNSL [63]. The Myeloid differentiation primary response 88 (*MYD88*) gene is mutation in about 70% of cases of VRL, and hence this can be used to confirm the diagnosis of VRL [64]. The chromosomal translocation t(14;18) involving the *bcl2* gene has been reported in some PVRL, although this is not used in the diagnostic arena [20, 65].

11.2.6.12 Differential Diagnosis

The differential diagnosis of VRL, a challenging masquerade syndrome, includes a variety of infectious and non-infectious lesions. These include viral retinitis, extensive retinochoroidal toxoplasmosis, syphilitic retinitis, Whipple's disease, sarcoidosis, tuberculosis, Behcet's disease, idiopathic uveitis and metastatic carcinomas [66].

11.2.6.13 Treatment of VRL

There are no consensus international guidelines to date for VRL treatment. The ultimate goal of eradicating the VRL cells within the eye to reduce the risk of relapse in the form of CNS infiltration has to be balanced with preserving sight and the treatment toxicities. Hence, it is clear that treatment of PCNSL/PVRL requires a multidisciplinary approach, and that each patient's case must be discussed in detail and in a timely manner, prior to treatment commencement [67–69].

Ocular radiotherapy, intravitreal methotrexate and/or rituximab, administration of high-dose systemic methotrexate (HD-MTX), myeloablative chemotherapy, and immunotherapy have been reported to achieve remission of PVRL, although many patients relapse with the recurrent disease occurring either in the form of ocular disease (even in the contralateral eye) or CNS lymphoma [70].

When whole brain radiotherapy (WBRT), either as CNS prophylaxis or for consolidation for existent disease, should be administered remains unclear. When HD-MTX is given with WBRT for consolidation, delayed neurotoxicity, most particularly dementia, has been reported as an important complication. Studies suggest that WBRT could be deferred until relapse without compromising survival in elderly patients. Alternatives to HD-MTX include dose-reduced WBRT and consolidative high-dose cytarabine (HD-Ara-C), high-dose chemotherapy and autologous stem cell transplantation for selected patients, pomalidomide or ibrutinib, in conjunction with local therapy. The reader is referred to recent reviews on PVRL treatment, which understandably does overlap with CNSL management [70–72].

11.2.6.14 Prognosis of VRL

With an overall 5-year survival rate of less than 25%, the prognosis of VRL remains poor despite advancements in new treatments [73, 74]. However, promising new therapies are on the horizon with new generation anti-CD20 antibodies [75], kinase inhibitors [76], chimeric antigen receptor therapy using T-cells [77], and with targeted new therapies directed against mutant cells, including MYD88 mutant B-lymphocytes [78]. Hence, we have to remain hopeful rather than fatalistic.

11.3 Uveal Lymphomas

Uveal lymphomas can be subdivided into 'primary' neoplasms of the choroid, iris and ciliary body as well as 'secondary' uveal lymphomas in patients with disseminated disease. These lymphomas mainly involve the choroid.

11.3.1 Primary Uveal Lymphomas

Epidemiology The cause of primary uveal lymphomas is unknown. The exact incidence of primary uveal lymphomas is also unclear, although it appears that there are at least 100 cases in the literature since first described by Triebenstein in 1920 (see above). Various terms have been given to uveal lymphoma in the literature, including uveal pseudotumour, reactive lymphoid hyperplasia, and then uveal lymphoproliferative neoplasia. It was only in 2002 that it was convincingly established that most uveal lymphomas represented 'extranodal marginal zone B-cell lymphomas' (EMZL), according to the WHO Lymphoma Classification [79].

Clinical Features Primary uveal lymphoma usually occurs unilaterally, and is more common in men than women. Presentation is in the sixth and seventh decades of life. Typical presenting symptoms include recurrent, painless episodes of blurred vision and metamorphopsia, caused by secondary serous retinal detachment involving the fovea. The key early signs of primary uveal lymphoma involving predominantly the choroid include multifocal, yellow-pink choroidal swellings on fundus examination (Fig. 11.4). The vitreous usually remains clear. In some patients, subconjunctival or episcleral extensions may become apparent as 'salmon patches [17, 80].

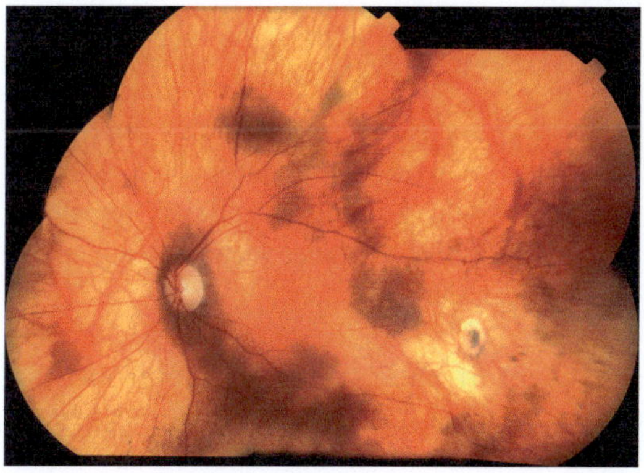

Fig. 11.4 Montage of a fundoscopy demonstrating an extensive primary choroidal lymphoma. Image care of Bertil Damato, San Francisco

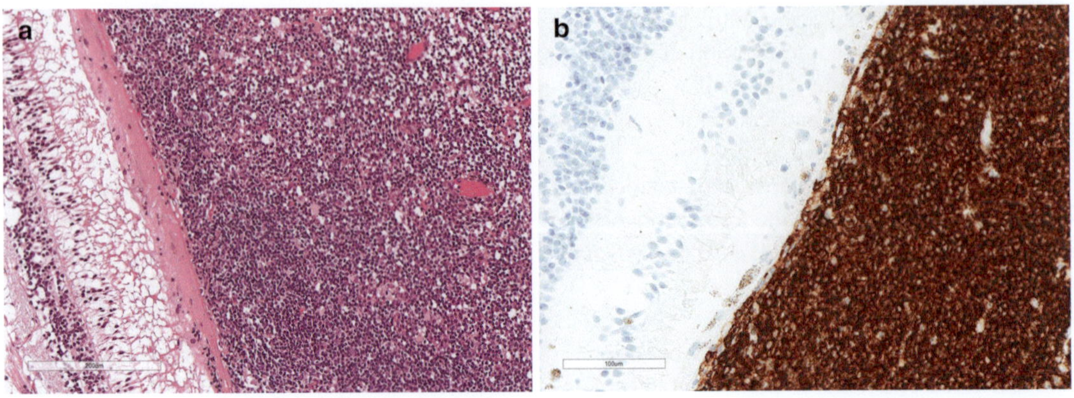

Fig. 11.5 (**a**) Enucleated eye of another case of primary choroidal lymphoma, demonstrating the location of the tumour cells within the choroid and their relationship to Bruch's membrane, the retinal pigment epithelium, and the overlying atrophic retina (H&E stain; scale bar on image). (**b**) Immunostaining for the same case demonstrating the positivity for CD20 (scale bar on image)

Pathology On microscopy, the uvea is filled with a dense infiltrate of monocytoid and plasmacytoid lymphoma cells (Fig. 11.5a). These are typically small, and are located in the so-called 'marginal zone', surrounding reactive germinal centres. The number of mitoses is small. The infiltrate can be extensive, involving the whole uvea, and also extending into the extraocular space by using the scleral exit routes. On immunohistochemistry, the B-cells express CD20, CD79a and PAX5 (Fig. 11.5b). The plasmacellular differentiation can be highlighted in the immunoglobulin light and heavy chains immunostains. Monoclonality can also be demonstrated using IgH-PCR [79]. The overlying Bruch's membrane is not infiltrated by the primary uveal lymphoma cells, but the retina may demonstrate atrophy of the photoreceptors.

Genetics Very few genetic studies have been undertaken of uveal lymphomas. It is assumed that they would demonstrate similar translocations to the EMZL of other locations, e.g. those of the ocular adnexa.

Treatment If untreated, uveal lymphoma can cause glaucoma through extensive involvement of the iris and ciliary body, and retinal detachment, ultimately making the eye blind and painful. Treatment with low-dose radiotherapy induces complete tumour regression with few if any residual effects and good improvement in vision. The survival prognosis is usually good (*cf.* VRL).

11.4 Secondary Uveal Lymphoma

Secondary uveal lymphomas are neoplasms that arise outside the central nervous system and then spread to the eye [12]. The incidence of this is not clear, as most Stage IV systemic NHL patients are not examined systematically for ophthalmological changes. Many patients with secondary uveal lymphoma are elderly, in their sixth decades although cases in young individuals have been described [81–83]. The choroid is the most frequent intraocular structure to be involved; exceptionally rarely, additional infiltration of the anterior chamber, optic nerve and even the retina is seen [81–88]. Presenting features and findings of ocular examination depend on the structures involved. Histologically, the majority of the secondary uveal lymphomas described in literature are of diffuse large B-cell lymphomas (Fig. 11.6a, b) [89]; rare cases of anaplastic large cell lymphoma and peripheral T-cell lymphoma have also been described [81–88, 90, 91]. In cases where the ocular manifestation is concurrent to the systemic lymphoma, management revolves around treatment of the systemic lymphoma, and usually includes a combination of surgical exci-

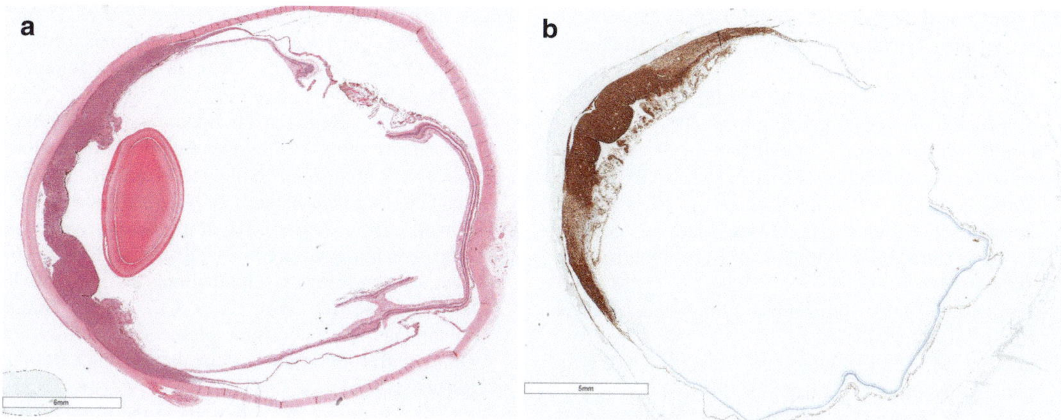

Fig. 11.6 (**a**) Low power of an enucleated eye demonstrating extensive anterior uveal involvement by a secondary lymphoma (scale bar on image). (**b**) CD20 immunostaining of the same case (scale bar on image)

sion, chemotherapy and radiotherapy. In ocular lesions which are subsequent to the primary, chemotherapy and/or radiotherapy is advocated.

11.5 Summary

Intraocular lymphomas are a heterogeneous group of neoplasms, which essentially can be divided into where they occur in the eye, and their pathological subtype. The VRL are the most common of these tumours and are the most aggressive, with poor survival often being associated with CNS involvement. The uveal lymphomas can be divided into those that are primary and secondary. The former are low-grade B-cell NHL with a very good response rate to low-dose radiotherapy, and a minimal risk of CNS involvement. Secondary uveal lymphomas represent manifestations of systemic NHL in the eye, usually in patients with very advanced disease. The outcomes of these patients is dependent on the particular subtype and the response to systemic therapy.

References

1. Mochizuki M, Singh AD. Epidemiology and clinical features of intraocular lymphoma. Ocul Immunol Inflamm. 2009;17:69–72.
2. Davis J. Intraocular lymphoma: a clinical perspective. Eye. 2013;27:153–62.
3. Triebenstein O. Ein Beitrag zur Frage der aleukämischen Augenveränderungen. Klin Monatsbl Augenheilkd. 1920;64:825–36.
4. Cooper EL, Riker JL. Malignant lymphoma of the uveal tract. Am J Ophthalmol. 1951;34:1153–8.
5. Givner I. Malignant lymphoma with ocular involvement: a clinico-pathologic report. Am J Ophthalmol. 1955;39:29–32.
6. Klingele TG, Hogan MJ. Ocular reticulum cell sarcoma. Am J Ophthalmol. 1975;79:39–47.
7. Vogel MH, Font RL, Zimmerman LE, Levine RA. Reticulum cell sarcoma of the retina and uvea. Report of six cases and review of the literature. Am J Ophthalmol. 1968;66:205–15.
8. Chan CC, Sen HN. Current concepts in diagnosis and managing primary vitreoretinal (intraocular) lymphoma. Discov Med. 2013;15:93–100.
9. Char DH, Ljung BM, Miller T, Phillips T. Primary intraocular lymphoma (ocular reticulum cell sarcoma) diagnosis and management. Ophthalmology. 1988;95:625–30.
10. Char DH, Ljung BM, Deschenes J, Miller TR. Intraocular lymphoma: immunological and cytological analysis. Br J Ophthalmol. 1988;72:905–11.
11. Qualman SL, Mendelsohn G, Mann RB, Green WR. Intraocular lymphomas. Natural history based on a clinicopathologic study of eight cases and review of the literature. Cancer. 1983;52:878–86.
12. Coupland SE, Damato B. Understanding intraocular lymphomas. Clin Exp Ophthalmol. 2008;36:564–78.
13. Chan CC, Rubenstein JL, Coupland SE, et al. Primary vitreoretinal lymphoma: a report from an international primary central nervous system lymphoma collaborative group symposium. Oncologist. 2011;16:1589–99.
14. Mulay K, Narula R, Honavar SG. Primary vitreoretinal lymphoma. Indian J Ophthalmol. 2015;63:180–6.

15. Coupland SE, Chan CC, Smith J. Pathophysiology of retinal lymphoma. Ocul Immunol Inflamm. 2009;17:227–37.
16. Jaffe ES, Harris NL, Stein H, Vardman JS. Tumours of hematologic and lymphoid tissues 2007. In: World Health Organization. classification of tumours. pathology and genetics. 4th ed. Lyon: IARC Press; 2008.
17. Sagoo MS, Mehta H, Swampillai AJ, et al. Primary intraocular lymphoma. Surv Ophthalmol. 2014;59:503–16.
18. Bardenstein DS. Intraocular lymphoma. Cancer Control. 1998;5:317–25.
19. Schabet M. Epidemiology of primary CNS lymphoma. J Neuro-Oncol. 1999;43:199–201.
20. Chan CC. Molecular pathology of primary intraocular lymphoma. Trans Am Ophthalmol Soc. 2003;101:275–92.
21. Chan SM, Hutnik CM, Heathcote JG, et al. Iris lymphoma in a pediatric cardiac transplant recipient: clinicopathologic findings. Ophthalmology. 2000;107:1979–82.
22. Wender A, Adar A, Maor E, et al. Primary B-cell lymphoma of the eyes and brain in a 3-year-old boy. Arch Ophthalmol. 1994;112:450–1.
23. Sobrin L, Dubovy SR, Davis JL, et al. Isolated, bilateral intraocular lymphoma in a 15-year-old girl. Retina. 2005;25:370–3.
24. Berenbom A, Davila RM, Lin HS, et al. Treatment outcomes for primary intraocular lymphoma: implications for external beam radiotherapy. Eye. 2007;21:1198–201.
25. Buettner H, Bolling JP. Intravitreal large cell lymphoma. Mayo Clin Proc. 1993;68:1101–5.
26. Peterson K, Gordon KB, Heinmann MH, et al. The clinical spectrum of ocular lymphoma. Cancer. 1993;72:843–9.
27. Chan CC, Shen DF, Whitcup SM, et al. Detection of human herpesvirus-8 and Epstein-Barr virus DNA in primary intraocular lymphoma. Blood. 1999;93:2749–51.
28. Sauer TC, Meyers SM, Shen D, Vegh S, Vygantas C, Chan CC. Primary intraocular (retinal) lymphoma following ocular toxoplasmosis. Retin Cases Brief Rep. 2010;4:160–3.
29. Kaplan LD. Human herpesvirus-8: Kaposi sarcoma, multicentric Castleman disease, and primary effusion lymphoma. Hematology Am Soc Hematol Educ Program. 2013;2013:103–8.
30. Chan CC, Shen D, Hackett JJ, Buggage RR, Tuaillon N. Expression of chemokine receptors, CXCR4 and CXCR5, and chemokines, BLC and SDF-1, in the eyes of patients with primary intraocular lymphoma. Ophthalmology. 2003;110:421–6.
31. McCann KJ, Ashton-Key M, Smith K, Stevenson FK, Ottensmeier CH. Primary central nervous system lymphoma: tumor-related clones exist in the blood and bone marrow with evidence for separate development. Blood. 2009;113:4677–88.
32. Cassoux N, Merle-Beral H, Leblond V, et al. Ocular and central nervous system lymphoma: clinical features and diagnosis. Ocul Immunol Inflamm. 2000;8:243–50.
33. Coupland SE, Heimann H, Bechrakis NE. Primary intraocular lymphoma: review of clinical, histopathological and molecular biological features. Graefes Arch Clin Exp Ophthalmol. 2004;242:901–13.
34. Lobo A, Larkin G, Clark BJ, et al. Pseudo-hypopyon as the presenting feature in B-cell and T-cell intraocular lymphoma. Clin Exp Ophthalmol. 2003;31:155–8.
35. Dean JM, Novak MA, Chan CC, et al. Tumor detachments of the retinal pigment epithelium in ocular/central nervous system lymphoma. Retina. 1996;16:47–56.
36. Gill MK, Jampol LM. Variations in the presentation of primary intraocular lymphoma: case reports and a review. Surv Ophthalmol. 2001;45:463–71.
37. Matzkin DC, Slamovits TL, Rosenbaum PS. Simultaneous intraocular and orbital non-Hodgkin lymphoma in the acquired immune deficiency syndrome. Ophthalmology. 1994;101:850–5.
38. Hochberg FH, Miller DC. Primary central nervous system lymphoma. J Neurosurg. 1988;68:835–53.
39. Jang HS, Sepah YJ, Sophie R, et al. Longitudinal spectral domain optical coherence tomography changes in eyes with intraocular lymphoma. J Ophthalmic Inflamm Infect. 2013;3:59.
40. Egawa M, Mitamura Y, Hayashi Y, Naito T. Spectral-domain optical coherence tomographic and fundus autofluorescence findings in eyes with primary intraocular lymphoma. Clin Ophthalmol. 2014;8:335–41.
41. Folgar FA, Chow JH, Farsiu S, et al. Spatial correlation between hyperpigmentary changes on color fundus photography and hyperreflective foci on SDOCT in intermediate AMD. Invest Ophthalmol Vis Sci. 2012;53:4626–33.
42. Ota M, Nishijima K, Sakamoto A, et al. Optical coherence tomographic evaluation of foveal hard exudates in patients with diabetic maculopathy accompanying macular detachment. Ophthalmology. 2010;117:1996–2002.
43. Fardeau C, Lee CP, Merle-Beral H, et al. Retinal fluorescein, indocyanine green angiography, and optic coherence tomography in non-Hodgkin primary intraocular lymphoma. Am J Ophthalmol. 2009;147:886–94.
44. Fardeau C, Lee CP, Merle-Beral H, et al. Retinal fluorescein, indocyanine green angiography, and optical coherence tomography in non-Hodgkin primary intraocular lymphoma. Am J Ophthalmol. 2009;147:886–94.
45. Casady M, Faia L, Nazemzadeh M, Nussenblatt R, Chan CC, Sen HN. Fundus autofluorescence patterns in primary intraocular lymphoma. Retina. 2014;34:366–72.
46. Mudhar HS, Sheard R. Diagnostic cellular yield is superior with full pars plana vitrectomy compared with core vitreous biopsy. Eye (Lond). 2013;27:50–5.

47. Whitcup SM, Chan CC, Buggage RR, et al. Improving the diagnostic yield of vitrectomy for intraocular lymphoma. Arch Ophthalmol. 2000;118:446.
48. Cursiefen C, Holbach LM, Lafaut B, et al. Oculocerebral non-Hodgkin's lymphoma with uveal involvement: development of an epibulbar tumor after vitrectomy. Arch Ophthalmol. 2000;118:1437–40.
49. Jack CR Jr, O'Neil BP, Banks PM, et al. Central nervous system lymphoma: histologic types and CT appearance. Radiology. 1988;167:211–5.
50. DeAngelis LM. Primary central nervous system lymphomas. Curr Treat Options in Oncol. 2001;2:309–18.
51. Gonzales JA, Chan CC. Biopsy techniques and yields in diagnosing primary intraocular lymphoma. Int Ophthalmol. 2007;27:241–50.
52. Whitcup SM, de Smet MD, Rubin BI, et al. Intraocular lymphoma. Clinical and histopathologic diagnosis. Ophthalmology. 1993;100:1399–406.
53. Michels RG, Knox DL, Erozan YS, et al. Intraocular reticulum cell sarcoma. Diagnosis by pars plana vitrectomy. Arch Ophthalmol. 1975;93:1331–5.
54. Chan CC, Buggage RR, Nussenblatt RB. Intraocular lymphoma. Curr Opin Ophthalmol. 2002;13:411–8.
55. Chan CC, Wallace DJ. Intraocular lymphoma: update on diagnosis and management. Cancer Control. 2004;11:285–95.
56. Chan CC, Gonzalez JA. Primary intraocular lymphoma. Hackensack, NJ: World Scientific; 2007.
57. Mihaljević B, Sretenović A, Jaković L, et al. A case of primary peripheral T-cell type non-Hodgkin lymphoma originating in the iris—clinicopathological findings. Vojnosanit Pregl. 2010;67:1025–8.
58. Park CY, Hwang SW, Kim do Y, Huh HJ, Oh JH. Anaplastic large cell lymphoma involving anterior segment of the eye. Korean J Ophthalmol. 2014;28:108–12.
59. Blay JY, Favrot M, Rossi JF, Wijdenes J. Role of interleukin-6 in paraneoplastic thrombocytosis. Blood. 1993;82:2261–2.
60. Chan CC, Whitcup SM, Solomon D, Nussenblatt RB. Interleukin-10 in the vitreous of patients with primary intraocular lymphoma. Am J Ophthalmol. 1995;120:671–3.
61. Cassoux N, Merle-Beral H, Lehoang P, et al. Interleukin-10 and intraocular-central nervous system lymphoma. Ophthalmology. 2001;108:426–7.
62. Coupland SE, Bechrakis NE, Anastassiou G, et al. Evaluation of vitrectomy specimens and chorioretinal biopsies in the diagnosis of primary intraocular lymphoma in patients with Masquerade syndrome. Graefes Arch Clin Exp Ophthalmol. 2003;241(10):860–70.
63. Coupland SE, Hummel M, Müller HH, et al. Molecular analysis of immunoglobulin genes in primary intraocular lymphoma. Invest Ophthalmol Vis Sci. 2005;46(10):3507–14.
64. Bonzheim I, Giese S, Deuter C, et al. High frequency of MYD88 mutations in vitreoretinal B-cell lymphoma: a valuable tool to improve diagnostic yield of vitreous aspirates. Blood. 2015;126(1):76–9. https://doi.org/10.1182/blood-2015-01-620518.
65. Wallace DJ, Shen D, Reed GF, et al. Detection of the bcl-2 t(14;18) translocation and proto-oncogene expression in primary intraocular lymphoma. Invest Ophthalmol Vis Sci. 2006;47:2750–6.
66. Jaehne D, Coupland SE. Primary vitreoretinal lymphoma. Ophthalmologe. 2018;115:343–56. https://doi.org/10.1007/s00347-018-0681-5.
67. Hoang-Xuan K, Bessell E, Bromberg J, et al. Diagnosis and treatment of primary CNS lymphoma in immunocompetent patients: guidelines from the European Association for Neuro-Oncology. Lancet Oncol. 2015;16(7):e322–32. https://doi.org/10.1016/S1470-2045(15)00076-5.
68. Nguyen DT, Houillier C, Choquet S, et al. Primary oculocerebral lymphoma: MTX polychemotherapy alone on intraocular disease control. Ophthalmology. 2016;123(9):2047–50. https://doi.org/10.1016/j.ophtha.2016.03.043.
69. Soussain C, Suzan F, Hoang-Xuan K, et al. Results of intensive chemotherapy followed by hematopoietic stem-cell rescue in 22 patients with refractory or recurrent primary CNS lymphoma or intraocular lymphoma. J Clin Oncol. 2001;19(3):742–9.
70. Fend F, Ferreri AJ, Coupland SE. How we diagnose and treat vitreoretinal lymphoma. Br J Haematol. 2016;173(5):680–92.
71. Deckert M, Engert A, Brück W, et al. Modern concepts in the biology, diagnosis, differential diagnosis and treatment of primary central nervous system lymphoma. Leukemia. 2011;25(12):1797–807.
72. Ferreri AJ, Zucca E, Armitage J, et al. Ten years of international primary CNS lymphoma collaborative group studies. J Clin Oncol. 2013;31(27):3444–5.
73. Itty S, Olson JH, O'Connell DJ, et al. Treatment of primary intraocular lymphoma (PIOL) has involved systemic, intravitreal or intrathecal chemotherapy and/or radiotherapy. Retina. 2009;29(3):415–6.
74. Grimm SA, McCannel CA, Omuro AM, et al. Primary CNS lymphoma with intraocular involvement: international PCNSL Collaborative Group Report. Neurology. 2008;71(17):1355–60.
75. Marshall MJE, Stopforth RJ, Cragg MS. Therapeutic antibodies: what have we learnt from targeting CD20 and where are we going? Front Immunol. 2017;8:1245.
76. Lionakis MS, Dunleavy K, Roschewski M, et al. Inhibition of B cell receptor signaling by ibrutinib in primary CNS lymphoma. Cancer Cell. 2017;31(6):833–43.
77. Onea AS, Jazirehi AR. CD19 chimeric antigen receptor (CD19 CAR)-redirected adoptive T-cell immunotherapy for the treatment of relapsed or refractory B-cell non-Hodgkin's lymphomas. Am J Cancer Res. 2016;6(2):403–24.
78. Shiratori E, Itoh M, Tohda S. MYD88 inhibitor ST2825 suppresses the growth of lymphoma and Leukaemia cells. Anticancer Res. 2017;37(11):6203–9.
79. Coupland SE, Foss HD, Hidayat AA. Extranodal marginal zone B cell lymphomas of the uvea: an analysis of 13 cases. J Pathol. 2002;197(3):333–40.

80. Neudorfer M, Kessler A, Anteby I, et al. Co-existence of intraocular and orbital lymphoma. Acta Ophthalmol Scand. 2004;108:426–7.
81. Karakawa A, Taoka K, Kaburaki T, et al. Clinical features and outcomes of secondary intraocular lymphoma. Br J Haematol. 2017;183:668–71. https://doi.org/10.1111/bjh.15005.
82. Kim JL, Mendoza P, Rashid A, Hayek B, Grossniklaus HE. Optic nerve lymphoma. Report of two cases and review of the literature. Surv Ophthalmol. 2015;60:153–65.
83. Savino G, Petroni S, Balia L, et al. Secondary orbital and intraocular lymphoma treated with immunochemotherapy. Retin Cases Brief Rep. 2013;7:267–70.
84. Park CY, Hwang SW, Kim DY, Huh HJ, Oh JH. Anaplastic large cell lymphoma involving anterior segment of the eye. Korean J Ophthalmol. 2014;28:108–12.
85. Say EA, Knupp CL, Gertsch KR, Chavala SH. Metastatic B-cell lymphoma masquerading as infectious retinitis and vasculitis. Oncol Lett. 2012;3:1245–8.
86. Chi M, Bucher N, Gabrielian A, MacCumber MW, Zdunek T. Subcutaneous diffuse large B-cell lymphoma with intraocular involvement. Future Oncol. 2012;8:757–60.
87. Corrêa ZM, Augsburger JJ, Dalal MD, Spaulding A. Secondary intraocular uveal involvement by primary paranasal sinus lymphoma. Int Ophthalmol. 2012;32:397–400.
88. Cao X, Shen D, Callanan DG, Mochizuki M, Chan C-C. Diagnosis of systemic metastatic retinal lymphoma. Acta Ophthalmol. 2011;89:149–54.
89. Salomão DR, Pulido JS, Johnston PB, et al. Vitreoretinal presentation of secondary large B-cell lymphoma in patients with systemic lymphoma. JAMA Ophthalmol. 2013;131(9):1151–8.
90. Iwase T, Sugiyama K, Takahira M, Uchiyama A. Intraocular lymphoma metastasis from larynx. Eur J Ophthalmol. 2007;17:133–5.
91. Wallace DJ, Altemare CR, Shen DF, et al. Primary testicular and intraocular lymphomas: two case reports and a review of the literature. Surv Ophthalmol. 2006;51:41–50.

Choroidal Hemangioma and Its Management

12

Shweta Gupta and Swathi Kaliki

12.1 Introduction

Choroidal hemangioma is the most common vascular tumor of the uveal tract. It is a benign tumor, which is either circumscribed (Fig. 12.1) or diffuse (Fig. 12.2) based on the extent of choroidal involvement. The circumscribed type is usually sporadic and is not associated with systemic abnormalities, whereas diffuse type is associated with facial naevus flammeus or encephalofacial angiomatosis, e.g. Sturge-Weber (SW) syndrome [1].

12.2 Circumscribed Choroidal Hemangioma

Circumscribed choroidal hemangiomas (CCHs) are relatively rare hamartomatous vascular tumors [1]. They often manifest as unifocal lesions and commonly present uniocularly with extemely rare bilateral involvement [2–4].

12.2.1 Clinical Features

Symptoms

Majority of the tumors remain asymptomatic till 2nd to 5th decades. Patients with parafoveal tumors present with either gradual or sudden onset diminution in visual acuity, defect in the visual field, floaters, photopsis and metamorphopsia secondary to exudation of fluid [1, 5]. Subfoveal tumors cause central vision loss due to serous macular detachment or cystoid macular edema [6]. They may also produce hyperopic shift secondary to the anterior displacement of the retina [1].

Signs

Majority of circumscribed choroidal hemangioma are easily diagnosed with Indirect ophthalmoscopy. They appear as a discrete, indistinct, smooth, round or oval, orange-red lesion with homogenous surface usually located behind the equator usually at the macula or surrounding the optic disc [7–9]. Associated clinical features include overlying retinal edema, pigmentary changes within the retinal pigment epithelium, orange pigment deposition, subretinal fluid, exudative retinal detachment, subretinal fibrosis and macular edema [1]. Sometimes a total RD can occur which may lead to neovascular glaucoma.

S. Gupta · S. Kaliki (✉)
The Operation Eyesight Universal Institute for Eye Cancer (SG, SK), L V Prasad Eye Institute, Hyderabad, India

V. Khetan (ed.), *Intraocular Tumors*, https://doi.org/10.1007/978-981-15-0395-5_12

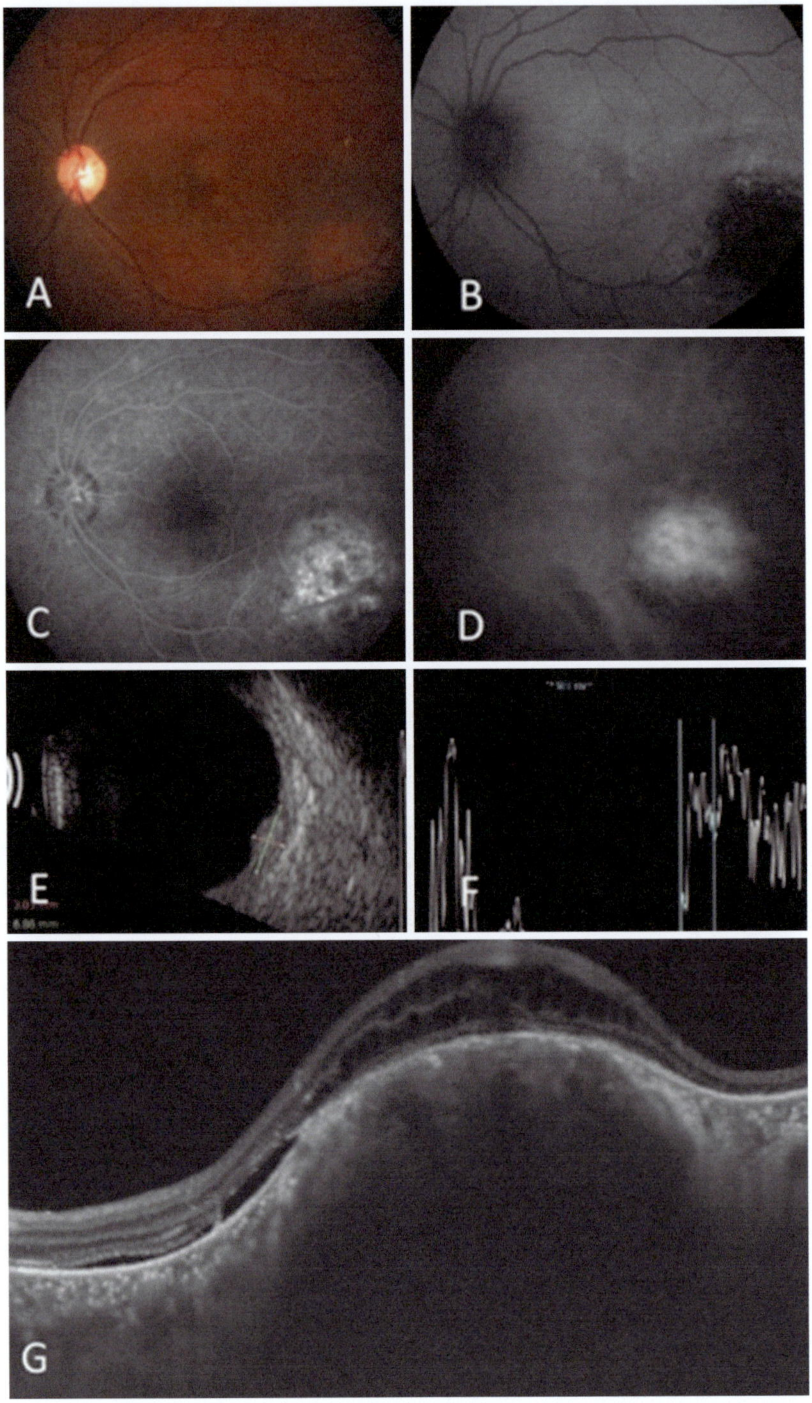

Fig. 12.1 Circumscribed choroidal hemangioma. (**a**) Fundus photograph showing reddish orange lesion in the inferotemporal quadrant. (**b**) Autofluorescence showing hypoautofluorescence of the lesion with mild hyperautofluorescence of the cuff of subretinal fluid. (**c**) Fluorescein angiography showing early mottled hyperfluorescence. (**d**) Indocyanine green angiography showing early hyperfluorescence. (**e**) B-scan ultrasonography showing a acoustically solid choroidal lesion with (**f**) high internal reflectivity on A-scan. (**g**) Enhanced depth imaging Optical coherence tomography showing retinal edema, subretinal fluid, choroidal lesion with widening of choroidal vessels

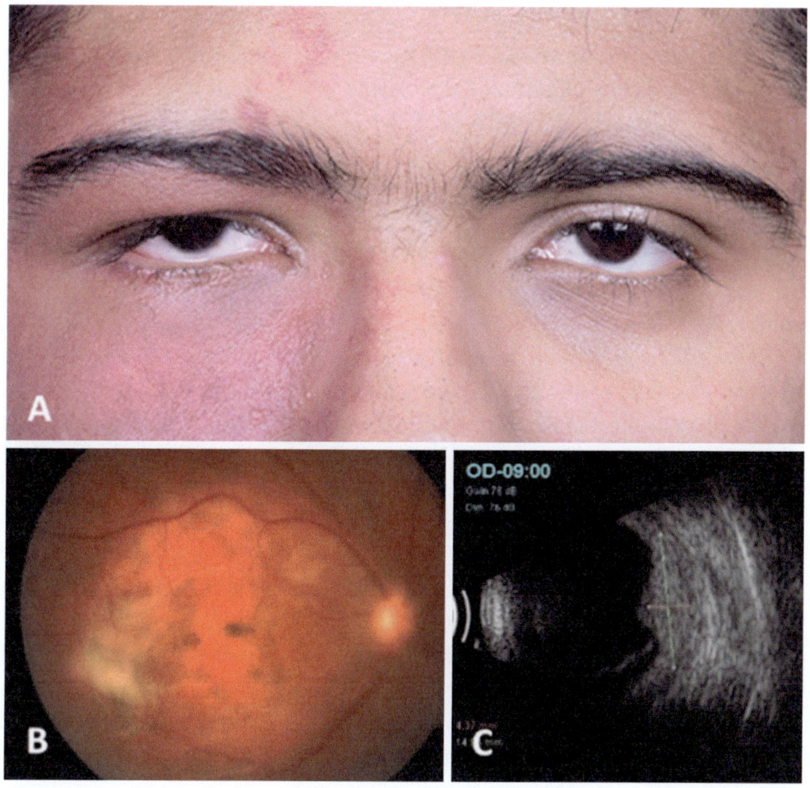

Fig. 12.2 Diffuse choroidal hemangioma in Sturge-Weber syndrome. (**a**) External photograph showing port-wine stain involving the right periocular region. (**b**) Tomato catsup fundus with nodular component of the lesion in the macular area. (**c**) B-scan showing diffuse choroidal thickening with central nodular component

12.2.2 Ancillary Investigations

12.2.2.1 Ultrasonography

Circumscribed choroidal hemangioma shows high anterior spike as well as typical homogenous high internal reflectivity similar to the surrounding choroid on A scan and acoustic solidity without significant shadowing on B scan [1, 7, 8]. Ultrasonography also helps in measuring the tumor dimensions [10].

12.2.2.2 Fluorescein Angiography

Fundus fluorescein angiography (FFA) adds little information to the diagnosis of choroidal hemangioma, as it shows some typical but non-pathognomic features [1, 2, 5, 7, 8]. Prearterial/early arterial phases display irregular linear hyperfluorescence due to filling of choroidal vasculature and large tumor vessels before the retinal vessels [8]. Profuse accelerating leakage originating from a tiny hyperfluorescent foci is noticed due to intrinsic vasculature in the arterial and venous phase [1]. Intraretinal hyperfluorescence can be seen in late phases secondary to widespread leakage of the dye in the intraretinal cystic spaces [5].

12.2.2.3 Indocyanine Green Angiography (ICGA)

Indocyanine Green (ICG) angiography is more important than FFA in the diagnosis of choroidal hemangioma. Typical angiographic feature is the appearance of lacy, diffuse and strong hyperfluorescence in arterial phase at an average of 1.2 min after injection due to 'early filling' of intratumoral vessels within 30 s of dye injection. This is followed by a characteristic late 'wash out' which appears as hypofluorescence relative to surrounding tumor at 30–60 min [9]. The tumor shows characteristic 'Mulberry appearance" with a surrounding rim of hyperfluorescence in the late frames [1, 11].

12.2.2.4 Spectral Domain and Enhanced Depth Imaging Optical Coherence Tomography (SD-OCT and EDI-OCT)

SD-OCT helps in identification and evaluation of secondary retinal changes in choroidal tumors and has replaced traditional FFA and ICGA to monitor activity of these tumors following treatment [12].

EDI-OCT is useful in assessment of lesion with 0.1 mm thickness which are very thin to get measured with the help of conventional ultrasonography [13]. Circumscribed choroidal hemangioma on EDI scans shows a homogenous hyporeflective appearance resulting from enlarged vascular interfaces across the layers of the choroid and typical multilobular pattern corresponding to the intrinsic spaces of intratumoral vessels [14, 15]. A sloping anterior surface without choriocapillaries compression and a hyper-reflective halo surrounding the tumor is also seen [13, 16].

The evaluation of integrity of RPE and the inner segment/outer segment photoreceptor junction is useful while considering various treatment options. They are also important prognostic factors for potential visual outcome following treatment. At baseline, it helps to distinguish acute leakage (subretinal fluid with normal retinal thickness and preserved architecture of photoreceptors and) from chronic leakage (subretinal fluid with intraretinal edema, retinoschisis, retinal atrophy and photoreceptors loss [17, 18].

It is worthwhile for monitoring treatment response based on decrease in central foveal thickness, regression of macular edema or exudative retinal detachment and restoration of foveal anatomy [12, 19]. OCT can detect early as well as recurrent sub-retinal and intraretinal fluid following treatment, before it becomes clinically apparent and causes deterioration in vision [19, 20].

12.2.2.5 Autofluorescence

It further evaluates the status of overlying RPE and allows detection of subtle subretinal fluid (SRF). Choroidal hemangiomas appear hypo or isofluorescent in comparison to the perilesional choroid. Overlying lipofuscin and fresh SRF shows hyper-autofluorescence and RPE hyperplasia, chronic SRF, localized fibrosis and atrophy shows hypo-autofluorescence [21].

12.2.2.6 Magnetic Resonance Imaging (MRI)

Choroidal hemangiomas appear hyperintense to the vitreous in T1-weighted images and isointense in T2-weighted images, unlike most of the intraocular tumors, which are hypointense on T2. On gadolinium administration, the tumor shows a marked enhancement [8, 22].

12.2.2.7 Histopathology

Choroidal hemangiomas are histopathologically classified into three types as capillary, cavernous and mixed type based on predominant type of vessel [23]. Majority of the circumscribed hemangiomas are cavernous and mixed type. Large, thin-walled blood-filled endothelium lined vascular channels and separated by thin intervascular septa constitute the cavernous type. The capillary type consists of small blood vessels with indistinct endothelial cells and intervening loose connective tissue [1].

Extensive cystic changes, in the outer retinal layers overlying the tumor may coalesce to form retinoschisis. The pigmented rim seen clinically is caused by irregularly compressed choroidal melanocytes at the periphery of the hemangioma [1].

12.2.3 Differential Diagnosis

Amelanotic Choroidal Melanoma

Choroidal hemangioma is a typical orange-red lesion unlike a choroidal melanoma. It demonstrates high internal reflectivity on A scan as opposed to low-medium reflectivity in melanoma. The characteristic findings of acoustic hollowness and choroidal excavation seen in melanoma on ultrasonography are almost never seen with a hemangioma [6].

Choroidal Metastasis

Choroidal metastasis usually appears dull or creamy yellow and is frequently multifocal and bilateral as compared to unifocal, unilateral and orange-red color of a hemangioma [24].

Posterior Scleritis

Posterior scleritis can be confused sometimes with choroidal hemangioma but is usually accompanied by inflammatory signs and choroidal folds [25].

12.2.4 Management

Treatment of circumscribed choroidal hemangioma differs for each case and depends on the severity of symptoms, presence or absence of subretinal fluid and potential for visual recovery [8, 26].

Treatment is not necessary for asymptomatic cases with extramacular lesions, without any evidence of subretinal fluid as there is low risk of progression in size or visual deterioration. These lesions can be safely observed with periodic review [1, 5].

Various treatment options have been described for tumors in which intervention is indicated. The treatment for circumscribed choroidal hemangioma has advanced considerably in recent years from cryotherapy [27], conventional photocoagulation, external beam radiation therapy to new options including photodynamic therapy, proton beam radiotherapy, episcleral plaque radiotherapy, transpupillary thermotherapy (TTT) and anti-VEGF pharmacotherapy.

Current treatment strategy is to treat the primary tumor and the subsequent secondary effects concurrently from the onset. Detailed peripheral fundus examination by indirect ophthalmoscopy and panoramic imaging modalities is imperative [10].

12.2.4.1 Laser Photocoagulation

Argon green laser (514 mm) is used to create whitish appearance at the surface of the tumor. This creates a chorioretinal adhesion and subsequently helps to resolve the SRF [8]. Scatter photocoagulation to the tumor surface on one or more occasions for vision threatening exudative RD results in resolution of SRF with retinal reattachment and temporary visual improvement, but tumor regression may not be seen [21]. Post treatment SRF recurrence and need for additional treatment was observed in 40% of the patients [8]. Final visual acuity is often poor with laser photocoagulation [28]. Numerous complications have been described in association with laser photocoagulation such as cataract, bleeding, secondary choroidal neovascularization and retinal ablation resulting in visual field defects [1, 29, 30].

12.2.4.2 Transpupillary Thermotherapy (TTT)

TTT is an appropriate treatment option for extrafoveal tumors (Fig. 12.3). A diode laser (810-nm) with 300–1200 mW power, 2–14 min exposure time and 2–3 mm spot size is used to create confluent greyish spots over the entire tumor surface [31]. This raises temperature inside the tumor above 45 °C but below 60 °C. It leads to the formation of less evident chorioretinal scar in comparison to photocoagulation. ICG has also been described to enhance the effect of TTT [32]. It helps in subretinal fluid resolution and induces tumor regression leading to preservation or improvement in vision [31, 33]. TTT can cause certain complications such as cystoid macular edema (CME), preretinal fibrosis and retinal vascular occlusion making it unsuitable for subfoveal and peripapillary tumors [31].

12.2.4.3 Photodynamic Therapy (PDT)

PDT is safe and effective therapy for circumscribed choroidal hemangioma. Currently, it has been recommended as the first line treatment for subfoveal and juxtafoveal tumors [1, 21, 34–37]. It offers the advantage of tissue-specific vascular occlusion and tumor destruction while sparing adjacent neurosensory retina [27]. Verteporfin is sequestered in abnormal large caliber vessels and selective occlusion of choroidal neovascularization can be achieved. Thus, the overlying neurosensory retinal layers and Bruch membrane are almost unaffected, leaving retinal function intact [29].

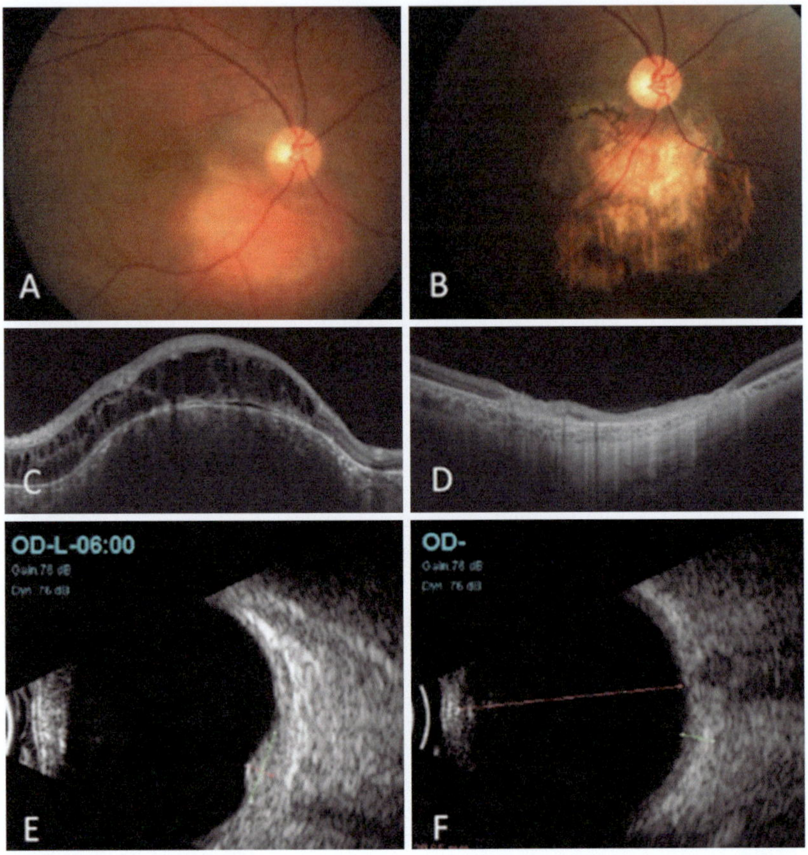

Fig. 12.3 Treatment with transpupillary thermotherapy. (**a**) Pre-treatment fundus photograph showing choroidal hemangioma inferior to the optic disc. (**b**) Post-treatment fundus photograph showing chorioretinal atrophy with sparing of retinal vessels. (**c**) Pre-treatment enhanced depth imaging optical coherence tomography (EDI-OCT) showing retinal edema, subretinal fluid, and choroidal lesion. (**d**) Post-treatment EDI-OCT showing resolution of retinal edema, subretinal fluid, and choroidal lesion with chorioretinal scar. (**e**) Pre-treatment B-scan showing dome shaped choroidal elevation. (**f**) Post-treatment B-scan showing resolution of the choroidal lesion

There are numerous treatment protocols including verteporfin injection parameters (Injection over 10 min versus bolus injection), total number of treatment sessions (1–5 sessions), laser power (50–100 J/cm^2), duration of exposure (83–186 s), and number of laser spots (single or overlapping multiple spots). Similar results have been observed with different protocols but more RPE and retinal changes were noticed with bolus injections. It is preferable to wait for 4–6 months after PDT for resolution of SRF, before additional treatment sessions as repeat or over treatment may result in RPE atrophy and adverse visual outcomes [38–47].

Excellent anatomical outcome in terms of resolution of subretinal fluid and induction of tumor regression as well as functional outcomes in terms of visual improvement or stabilization have been reported in 73–100% of patients with a single treatment in majority of cases [12, 46–48]. Few unusual and transient complications have been described including vascular occlusion, choroidal effusion, choroidal atrophy and perifoveal hemorrhage [39, 45, 49, 50].

12.2.4.4 External Beam Radiation Therapy

Efficacy of external beam radiotherapy (EBRT) in cases of circumscribed hemangioma is varying between different case series. Ritland et al. demonstrated complete resolution of RD and tumor regression along with visual acuity improvement in 90% of eyes (dose 20–24 Gy) [51]. Schilling and Kong et al. have reported good anatomical and functional outcomes [23, 52, 53]. Madreperla et al. described EBRT as less effective in treatment of circumscribed hemangioma in comparison to diffuse ones [28].

12.2.4.5 Proton Beam Radiotherapy

Proton beam radiotherapy is a useful therapeutic alternative for larger choroidal hemangiomas with extensive exudative retinal detachment. Before introduction of PDT, proton beam radiotherapy was mostly preferred to treat macular and juxtapapillary CCH as charged particles have a highly localized and uniform dose distribution. There are conflicting reports regarding the usage of proton beam therapy in such situations. Zografos et al. [54] and Hannouche et al. [55] described it as ideal for treatment in this critical region (dose 16–18 Gy) while Lee and Hungerford [56] found only slight advantage over EBRT in terms of optic neuropathy or maculopathy.

12.2.4.6 Plaque Radiotherapy

Episcleral plaque radiotherapy with I-125 [5, 28], Co-60 [57], Ru-106 [28, 51] (Fig. 12.4) is an effective treatment for large circumscribed hemangiomas with extensive SRF where PDT would not be possible and juxta-papillary tumors unresponsive to PDT or TTT [28]. Low-dose radiation delivery (20–40 Gy) to the tumor apex is sufficient. Tumor regression, resorption of SRF and regression of iris neovascularization have been reported with I-125 and palladium-103 plaque radiotherapy [58, 59]. Vision deterioration

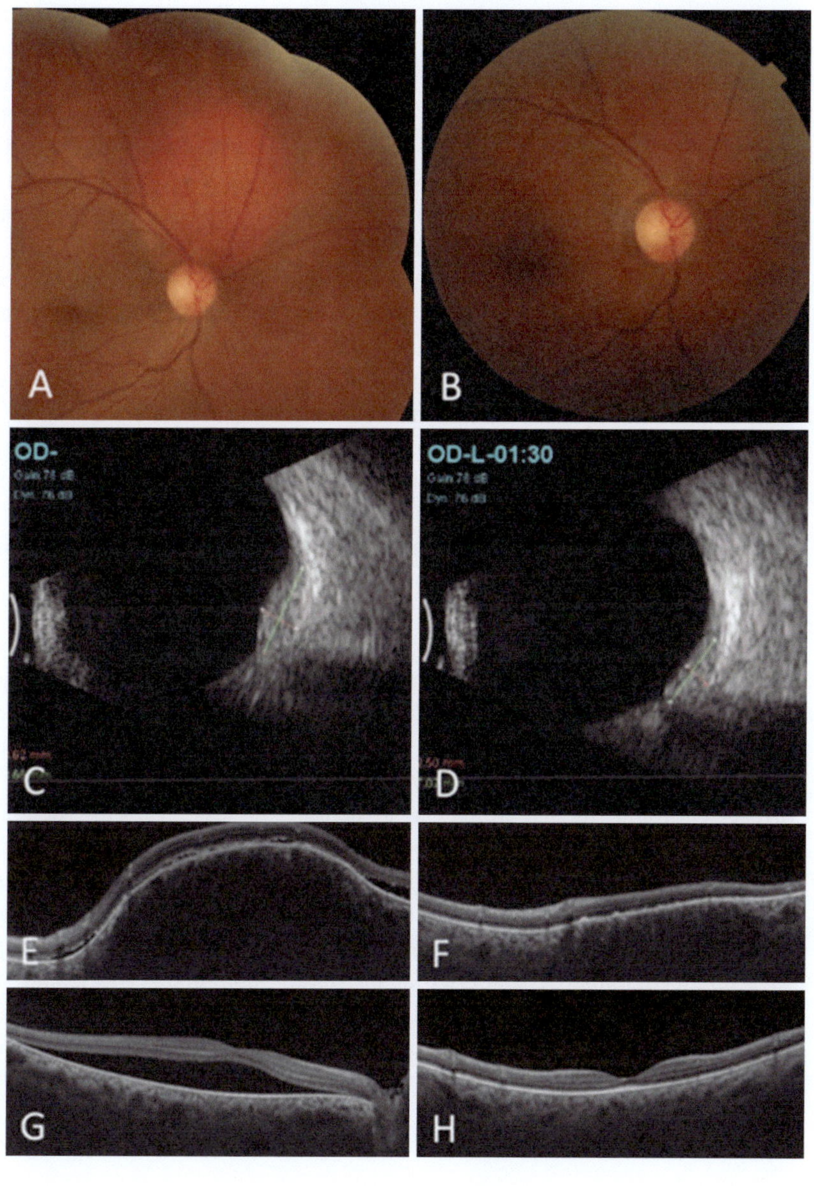

Fig. 12.4 Treatment with plaque radiotherapy. (**a**) Pre-treatment fundus photograph showing choroidal hemangioma superior to the optic disc. (**b**) Post-treatment fundus photograph showing resolution of the choroidal lesion. (**c**) Pre-treatment B-scan showing dome shaped choroidal elevation. (**d**) Post-treatment B-scan showing resolution of the choroidal lesion. (**e**) Pre-treatment enhanced depth imaging optical coherence tomography (EDI-OCT) showing subretinal fluid and choroidal lesion. (**f**) Post-treatment EDI-OCT showing resolution subretinal fluid and flattening of the choroidal lesion. (**g**) Pre-treatment EDI-OCT showing subretinal fluid involving fovea. (**h**) Post-treatment EDI-OCT showing healthy fovea with no subretinal fluid

secondary to radiation retinopathy and optic neuropathy may occur in up to 30% of patients [58].

12.2.4.7 Anti-VEGF Treatment

Single or multiple intravitreal injections of anti vascular endothelial growth factor (VEGF) e.g. Bevacizumab with or without PDT or TTT has been tried to resolve SRF [60, 61].

12.2.4.8 Oral Beta Blockers

Oral propranolol has been recently found to be efficacious for partial or complete resolution of SRF associated with CCH [62, 63].

12.2.5 Visual and Anatomical Prognosis

Shields et al. have noticed complete resolution of SRF in patients with shorter duration of symptoms and tumor location in inferior quadrant. Poor initial visual acuity, delay in referral and failed prior laser photocoagulation are predictors of poor final visual acuity [5]. According to Schilling et al., a successful functional outcome is dependent on the time interval between the onset and commencement of therapy and formation of subretinal fibrosis. Subretinal fibrosis has been described as consistent finding after the treatment, which was seen irrespective of the treatment choice or duration of treatment and was responsible for poor visual prognosis [53].

12.3 Diffuse Choroidal Hemangioma

Diffuse choroidal hemangioma is a benign vascular tumor with ill-defined borders and widespread extension in the posterior choroid involving almost entire choroid [1]. It is associated with Sturge-Weber syndrome, an encephalotrigeminal angiomatosis that is a triad of facial, ocular and cerebral vascular malformations. Diffuse choroidal hemangioma can be present in 30–50% of patients with Sturge-Weber Syndrome [3, 64].

12.3.1 Clinical Features

Symptoms

Diagnosis of diffuse choroidal hemangioma is usually forthright in the presence of Sturge-Weber syndrome. The typical cutaneous features in the syndrome encourage an early ocular examination in these patients. Thus it is frequently diagnosed at a young age in the eye ipsilateral to the nevus flammeus [64]. The choroidal involvement is mostly unilateral, however bilateral diffuse choroidal hemangioma have been described in association with bilateral facial nevus flammeus [3].

Patient with diffuse lesions may also present with visual deterioration caused by amblyopia. Significant amblyopia can either occur due to hyperopic refractive error, foveal distortion or from a secondary exudative retinal detachment [1]. The pupil shows a bright red reflex in the involved eye in contrast to the normal reflex in the opposite pupil [65].

However, if asymptomatic or in presence of subtle clinical features at presentation, diagnosis may be delayed.

Signs

Diffuse choroidal hemangioma shows an extensive orange-red thickening of the posterior choroid, classically described as ‘tomato-catsup fundus’, which is predominantly seen in the macular area. These are very large lesions and often extend anterior to the equator. There may be concomitant exudative retinal detachment with macular involvement, cystoid degeneration in the sensory retina over the tumor surface with RPE disruption and photoreceptor loss [23].

An exhaustive ocular examination is crucial to assess various ocular signs in a neuro-oculocutaneous hemangiomatosis. These include ipsilateral congenital or developmental glaucoma (70%), asymmetry of the optic cup with enlargement of optic disc, conjunctival/episcleral hemangioma (70%) and choroidal hemangiomas (50%) [64, 66]. Other ocular manifestations such as retinal vascular tortuosity, iris heterochromia, retinal detachment, and strabismus are also described [64, 67].

12.3.2 Ancillary Investigations

Diagnosis is predominantly clinical but sometimes, posterior polar lesions may not be instantaneously discernable on fundus examination due to diffuse boundaries of the tumor [68]. The anterior extension of the lesion can be easily recognized on indirect ophthalmoscopy, wide-angle photography and angiography.

Ultrasonography reveals a diffuse thickening of choroid with medium to high internal reflectivity. FFA demonstrates extensive involvement with persistent hyperfluorescence over the late phases of the angiogram. No 'washout' phenomenon is noticed on ICG angiography as in circumscribed choroidal hemangiomas. Diffuse lesions share similar features as CCH on SD-OCT, autofluoresence and MRI [10].

12.3.3 Histopathology

Proliferation of small along with the large blood vessels is seen in diffuse choroidal hemangioma and is usually classified as a mixed hemangioma [1].

12.3.4 Management

Treatment of diffuse choroidal hemangioma is challenging. Decision for treatment is taken after assessment of visual symptoms and potential for visual recovery.

Asymptomatic cases that lack subretinal fluid and lesions with subtle clinical features at presentation are usually considered for observation. These untreated lesions may present later in life with advanced disease or complications and poor visual prognosis [68].

Currently, radiotherapy and photodynamic therapy are the preferred modalities of treatment.

12.3.4.1 Radiotherapy (External Beam Radiotherapy and Proton Beam Radiotherapy)

These tumors are classically treated with lens sparing EBRT (1250–2000 cGy). However, EBRT takes months for absorption of subretinal fluid and there is probability of recurrence or persistence of fluid requiring additional radiotherapy [23, 36, 37, 53, 69, 70]. EBRT and proton beam radiotherapy [54, 71] have been demonstrated as an effective treatment of these lesions with regression of tumor and resolution of subretinal fluid. The potential side effects secondary to radiation exposure and damage to overlying retina with subsequent decrease in vision need to be considered.

12.3.4.2 Plaque Radiotherapy

More targeted radiation can also be utilized to treat these lesions with the plaque (Cobalt-60 and Ruthenium-106) placement over the thickest part of the tumor [57, 72]. These treatment modalities help in tumor regression and complete resolution of the exudation in majority along with glaucoma control in some cases [73]. Prompt clinical response and lesser complication rate make this a safe and effective alternative for diffuse lesions [72].

12.3.4.3 Photodynamic Therapy

Photodynamic therapy is a relatively non-invasive and efficient treatment for diffuse choroidal hemangioma in lesions with shallow SRF. Similar results, in terms of regression of the tumor and resolution of exudative RD, are noted after a single spot over the thickest part of the tumor or multiple non-overlapping spots in single or multiple sessions. Variable improvement in visual acuity is expected depending upon the degree of amblyopia [68, 74–77]. However, following PDT the exudative response of the tumor may increase [78]. There are certain advantages of PDT over various forms of radiotherapy such as no radiation exposure, minimal side effects and ease of delivery. Thus, it can be considered in selected cases of diffuse hemangiomas.

12.3.4.4 Miscellaneous

Novel treatment options has been recently initiated in treatment of diffuse choroidal hemangioma such as anti-VEGF pharmacotherapy and beta blockers.

Shoeibi et al. demonstrated that an early single injection of intravitreal bevacizumab is effective in choroidal hemangiomas associated with

Sturge-Weber syndrome [79]. The effect of single injection of pegaptanib has also been described in post-EBRT persistent Exudative RD in a patient with SWS [80].

Propranolol (2 mg/kg/day) has also been shown to hasten the absorption of exudative RD. It is hypothesized that the Propranolol alters the endothelial cells, vascular tone, angiogenesis, and apoptosis [81]. Extensive secondary RD may require drainage of SRF and/ or scleral buckling with pars plana vitrectomy and injection of gas and endolaser [1].

12.3.4.5 Supportive Treatment

Amblyopia can be tackled with refractive correction and amblyopia therapy [1]. Glaucoma management is challenging in patients with diffuse choroidal hemangioma. Medical treatment is effective in few patients and majority of patients require surgical intervention [82]. Prostaglandin analogs should be avoided while treating associated glaucoma in patients with Sturge-Weber syndrome, as they can precipitate or worsen the exudative complications. Risk of postoperative serous or hemorrhagic choroidal detachment following glaucoma filtering surgery is also present [83].

12.3.5 Prognosis

According to Schilling et al., associated secondary glaucoma in cases of diffuse choroidal hemangioma is a predictor of post treatment poor visual outcome [53].

12.4 Conclusion

Choroidal hemangioma, though rare, is the most common vascular tumor of the uveal tract. It can be accurately diagnosed by a good clinical examination and ancillary investigations. It is associated with good visual outcomes when detected early and treated appropriately.

References

1. Shields JA, Shields CL. Intraocular tumors: a text and atlas. Philadelphia: W.B. Saunders Company; 1992.
2. Schepens CL, Schwartz A. Intraocular tumors: I. Bilateral hemangioma of the choroid. Arch Ophthalmol. 1958;60(1):72–83.
3. Lindsey PS, Shields JA, Goldberg RE, Augsburger JJ, Frank PE. Bilateral choroidal hemangiomas and facial nevus flammeus. Retina. 1981;1(2):88–95.
4. Fukuda T, Shimada N, Ishida T, Furuse Y, Tobita H, Ohno-Matsui K. Bilateral circumscribed choroidal hemangioma with retinal and choroidal venous abnormalities. Jpn J Ophthalmol. 2011;55(6):688–90.
5. Shields CL, Honavar SG, Shields JA, Cater J, Demirci H. Circumscribed choroidal hemangioma: clinical manifestations and factors predictive of visual outcome in 200 consecutive cases. Ophthalmology. 2001;108(12):2237–48.
6. Turell ME, Singh AD. Vascular tumors of the retina and choroid: diagnosis and treatment. Middle East Afr J Ophthalmol. 2010;17(3):191–200.
7. Bonnet M, Francoz-Taillanter N. Cavernous hemangioma of the choroid (clinical review of 10 cases). Bull Soc Ophtalmol Fr. 1980;81(4-5):455–8.
8. Anand R, Augsburger JJ, Shields JA. Circumscribed choroidal hemangiomas. Arch Ophthalmol. 1989;107(9):1338–42.
9. Shields CL, Shields JA, De Potter P. Patterns of indocyanine green videoangiography of choroidal tumours. Br J Ophthalmol. 1995;79(3):237–45.
10. Heimann H, Jmor F, Damato B. Imaging of retinal and choroidal vascular tumours. Eye. 2013 ;27(2):208–16.
11. Schalenbourg A, Piguet B, Zografos L. Indocyanine green angiographic findings in choroidal hemangiomas: a study of 75 cases. Ophthalmologica. 2000;214(4):246–52.
12. Blasi MA, Tiberti AC, Scupola A, Balestrazzi A, Colangelo E, Valente P, et al. Photodynamic therapy with verteporfin for symptomatic circumscribed choroidal hemangioma: five-year outcomes. Ophthalmology. 2010 Aug;117(8):1630–7.
13. Shields CL, Pellegrini M, Ferenczy SR, Shields JA. Enhanced depth imaging optical coherence tomography of intraocular tumors: from placid to seasick to rock and rolling topography—the 2013 Francesco Orzalesi lecture. Retina. 2014;34(8):1495–512.
14. Torres VLL, Brugnoni N, Kaiser PK, Singh AD. Optical coherence tomography enhanced depth imaging of choroidal tumors. Am J Ophthalmol. 2011;151(4):586–593.e2.
15. Filloy A, Caminal JM, Arias L, Jordán S, Català J. Swept source optical coherence tomography imaging of a series of choroidal tumours. Can J Ophthalmol. 2015;50(3):242–8.
16. Flores-Moreno I, Caminal JM, Arias-Barquet L, Rubio-Caso MJ, Catala-Mora J, Vidal-Martí M, et al. En face mode of swept-source optical coherence tomography in circumscribed choroidal haemangioma. Br J Ophthalmol. 2016;100(3):360–4.
17. Sayanagi K, Pelayes DE, Kaiser PK, Singh AD. 3D spectral domain optical coherence tomography findings in choroidal tumors. Eur J Ophthalmol. 2011;21(3):271–5.

18. Shields CL, Materin MA, Shields JA. Review of optical coherence tomography for intraocular tumors. Curr Opin Ophthalmol. 2005;16(3):141–54.
19. Kwon HJ, Kim M, Lee CS, Lee SC. Treatment of serous macular detachment associated with circumscribed choroidal hemangioma. Am J Ophthalmol. 2012;154(1):137–45.
20. Zhang Y, Liu W, Fang Y, Qian J, Xu G, Wang W, et al. Photodynamic therapy for symptomatic circumscribed macular choroidal hemangioma in Chinese patients. Am J Ophthalmol. 2010;150(5):710–715.e1.
21. Ramasubramanian A, Shields CL, Harmon SA, Shields JA. Autofluorescence of choroidal hemangioma in 34 consecutive eyes. Retina. 2010;30(1):16–22.
22. De Potter P, Shields JA, Shields CL. Tumors of the uvea. In: MRI of the eye and orbit. Philadelphia, PA: JB Lippincott Company; 1995. p. 304.
23. Witschel H, Font RL. Hemangioma of the choroid. A clinicopathologic study of 71 cases and a review of the literature. Surv Ophthalmol. 1976;20(6):415–31.
24. Stephens RF, Shields JA. Diagnosis and management of cancer metastatic to the uvea: a study of 70 cases. Ophthalmology. 1979;86(7):1336–49.
25. Benson WE, Shields JA, Tasman W, Crandall AS. Posterior scleritis a cause of diagnostic confusion. Arch Ophthalmol. 1979;97(8):1482–6.
26. Newman DK. Photodynamic therapy: current role in the treatment of chorioretinal conditions. Eye. 2016;30(2):202–10.
27. Humphrey WT. Choroidal hemangioma: response to cryotherapy. Ann Ophthalmol. 1979;11(1):100–4.
28. Madreperla SA, Hungerford JL, Plowman PN, Laganowski HC, Gregory PT. Choroidal hemangiomas: visual and anatomic results of treatment by photocoagulation or radiation therapy. Ophthalmology. 1997;104(11):1773–8; discussion 1779
29. Sanborn GE, Augsburger JJ, Shields JA. Treatment of circumscribed choroidal hemangiomas. Ophthalmology. 1982;89(12):1374–80.
30. Shields JA. The expanding role of laser photocoagulation for intraocular tumors: the 1993 H. Christian Zweng memorial lecture. Retina. 1994;14(4):310–22.
31. Gündüz K. Transpupillary thermotherapy in the management of circumscribed choroidal hemangioma. Surv Ophthalmol. 2004;49(3):316–27.
32. Kamal A, Watts AR, Rennie IG. Indocyanine green enhanced transpupillary thermotherapy of circumscribed choroidal haemangioma. Eye. 2000;14(5):701–5.
33. García-Arumí J, Sararols Ramsay L, Corcostegui Guraya B. Transpupillary thermotherapy for circumscribed choroidal hemangiomas. Ophthalmology. 2000;107(2):351–6.
34. Elizalde J, Vasquez L, Iyo F, Abengoechea S. Photodynamic therapy in the management of circumscribed choroidal hemangioma. Can J Ophthalmol. 2012;47(1):16–20.
35. Pilotto E, Urban F, Parrozzani R, Midena E. Standard versus bolus photodynamic therapy in circumscribed choroidal hemangioma: functional outcomes. Eur J Ophthalmol. 2011;21(4):452–8.
36. Scott TA, Augsburger JJ, Brady LW, Hernandez C, Woodleigh R. Low dose ocular irradiation for diffuse choroidal hemangiomas associated with bullous nonrhegmatogenous retinal detachment. Retina. 1991;11(4):389–93.
37. Alberti WE. Clinical features and management of choroidal hemangiomas, including those occurring in association with Sturge-Weber syndrome. In: Albert WE, Sagerman RH, editors. Radiotherapy of intraocular and orbital tumors. Berlin: Springer; 1993. p. 87–92.
38. Madreperla SA. Choroidal hemangioma treated with photodynamic therapy using verteporfin. Arch Ophthalmol. 2001;119(11):1606–10.
39. Landau IME, Steen B, Seregard S. Photodynamic therapy for circumscribed choroidal haemangioma. Acta Ophthalmol Scand. 2002;80(5):531–6.
40. Porrini G, Giovannini A, Amato G, Ioni A, Pantanetti M. Photodynamic therapy of circumscribed choroidal hemangioma. Ophthalmology. 2003;110(4):674–80.
41. Barbazetto I, Schmidt-Erfurth U. Photodynamic therapy of choroidal hemangioma: two case reports. Graefes Arch Clin Exp Ophthalmol. 2000;238(3):214–21.
42. Jurklies B, Anastassiou G, Ortmans S, Schüler A, Schilling H, Schmidt-Erfurth U, et al. Photodynamic therapy using verteporfin in circumscribed choroidal haemangioma. Br J Ophthalmol. 2003;87(1):84–9.
43. Schmidt-Erfurth UM, Michels S, Kusserow C, Jurklies B, Augustin AJ. Photodynamic therapy for symptomatic choroidal hemangioma: visual and anatomic results. Ophthalmology. 2002;109(12):2284–94.
44. Verbraak FD, Schlingemann RO, Keunen JEE, de Smet MD. Longstanding symptomatic choroidal hemangioma managed with limited PDT as initial or salvage therapy. Graefes Arch Clin Exp Ophthalmol. 2003;241(11):891–8.
45. Singh AD, Kaiser PK, Sears JE, Gupta M, Rundle PA, Rennie IG. Photodynamic therapy of circumscribed choroidal haemangioma. Br J Ophthalmol. 2004;88(11):1414–8.
46. Boixadera A, Arumí JG, Martínez-Castillo V, Encinas JL, Elizalde J, Blanco-Mateos G, et al. Prospective clinical trial evaluating the efficacy of photodynamic therapy for symptomatic circumscribed choroidal hemangioma. Ophthalmology. 2009;116(1):100–105.e1.
47. Singh AD. Ocular phototherapy. Eye. 2013;27(2):190–8.
48. Jurklies B, Bornfeld N. The role of photodynamic therapy in the treatment of symptomatic choroidal hemangioma. Graefes Arch Clin Exp Ophthalmol. 2005;243(5):393–6.
49. Schmidt-Erfurth UM, Kusserow C, Barbazetto IA, Laqua H. Benefits and complications of photodynamic therapy of papillary capillary hemangiomas. Ophthalmology. 2002;109(7):1256–66.
50. Xiao Y, Guo X, Ouyang P. Branch retinal artery occlusion associated with photodynamic therapy in a circumscribed choroidal haemangioma. Photodiagn Photodyn Ther. 2013;10(4):644–6.

51. Ritland JS, Eide N, Tausjø J. External beam irradiation therapy for choroidal haemangiomas. Visual and anatomical results after a dose of 20 to 25 Gy. Acta Ophthalmol Scand. 2001;79(2):184–6.
52. Karimi S, Nourinia R, Mashayekhi A. Circumscribed choroidal hemangioma. J Ophthalmic Vis Res. 2015;10(3):320–8.
53. Schilling H, Sauerwein W, Lommatzsch A, Friedrichs W, Brylak S, Bornfeld N, et al. Long term results after low dose ocular irradiation for choroidal haemangiomas. Br J Ophthalmol. 1997;81(4):267–73.
54. Zografos L, Egger E, Bercher L, Chamot L, Munkel G. Proton beam irradiation of choroidal hemangiomas. Am J Ophthalmol. 1998;126(2):261–8.
55. Hannouche D, Frau E, Desjardins L, Cassoux N, Habrand JL, Offret H. Efficacy of proton therapy in circumscribed choroidal hemangiomas associated with serious retinal detachment. Ophthalmology. 1997;104(11):1780–4.
56. Lee V, Hungerford JL. Proton beam therapy for posterior pole circumscribed choroidal haemangioma. Eye. 1998;12(6):925–8.
57. Zografos L, Bercher L, Chamot L, Gailloud C, Raimondi S, Egger E. Cobalt-60 treatment of choroidal hemangiomas. Am J Ophthalmol. 1996;121(2):190–9.
58. Lopez-Caballero C, Saornil MA, De Frutos J, Bianciotto C, Muiños Y, Almaraz A, et al. High-dose iodine-125 episcleral brachytherapy for circumscribed choroidal haemangioma. Br J Ophthalmol. 2010;94(4):470–3.
59. Aizman A, Finger PT, Shabto U, Szechter A, Berson A. Palladium 103 (103Pd) plaque radiation therapy for CircumscribedChoroidal hemangioma with retinal detachment. Arch Ophthalmol. 2004;122(11):1652–6.
60. Mandal S, Naithani P, Venkatesh P, Garg S. Intravitreal bevacizumab (avastin) for circumscribed choroidal hemangioma. Indian J Ophthalmol. 2011;59(3):248–51.
61. Sagong M, Lee J, Chang W. Application of intravitreal bevacizumab for circumscribed choroidal hemangioma. Korean J Ophthalmol. 2009;23(2):127–31.
62. Sanz-Marco E, Gallego R, Diaz-Llopis M. Oral propranolol for circumscribed choroidal hemangioma. Case Rep Ophthalmol. 2011;2(1):84–90.
63. Tanabe H, Sahashi K, Kitano T, Tomita Y, Saito AM, Hirose H. Effects of oral propranolol on circumscribed choroidal hemangioma: a pilot study. JAMA Ophthalmol. 2013;131(12):1617–22.
64. Sullivan TJ, Clarke MP, Morin JD. The ocular manifestations of the Sturge-Weber syndrome. J Pediatr Ophthalmol Strabismus. 1992;29(6):349–56.
65. Susac JO, Smith JL, Scelfo RJ. The tomato-catsup fundus in Sturge-Weber syndrome. Arch Ophthalmol. 1974;92(1):69–70.
66. Shanmugam PM, Ramanjulu R. Vascular tumors of the choroid and retina. Indian J Ophthalmol. 2015;63(2):133–40.
67. Abdolrahimzadeh S, Scavella V, Felli L, Cruciani F, Contestabile MT, Recupero SM. Ophthalmic alterations in the Sturge-Weber syndrome, Klippel-Trenaunay syndrome, and the Phakomatosis Pigmentovascularis: an independent group of conditions? Biomed Res Int. 2015;2015:1–11.
68. Hussain RN, Jmor F, Damato B, Heimann H. Verteporfin photodynamic therapy for the treatment of choroidal haemangioma associated with Sturge-Weber syndrome. Photodiagn Photodyn Ther. 2016;15(Supplement C):143–6.
69. Grant LW, Anderson C, Macklis RM, Singh AD. Low dose irradiation for diffuse choroidal hemangioma. Ophthalmic Genet. 2008;29(4):186–8.
70. Gottlieb JL, Murray TG, Gass JDM. Low-dose external beam irradiation for bilateral diffuse choroidal hemangioma. Arch Ophthalmol. 1998;116(6):815–7.
71. Yonekawa Y, MacDonald SM, Shildkrot Y, Mukai S. Standard fractionation low-dose proton radiotherapy for diffuse choroidal hemangiomas in pediatric Sturge-Weber syndrome. J Am Assoc Pediatr Ophthalmol Strabismus. 2013;17(3):318–22.
72. Murthy R, Hanovar S, Naik M, Gopi S, Reddy VA. Ruthenium-106 plaque brachytherapy for the treatment of diffuse choroidal haemangioma in Sturge-Weber syndrome. Indian J Ophthalmol. 2005;73:274–5.
73. Arepalli S, Shields CL, Kaliki S, Emrich J, Komarnicky L, Shields JA. Diffuse choroidal hemangioma management with plaque radiotherapy in 5 cases. Ophthalmology. 2013;120(11):2358–9.
74. Tsipursky MS, Golchet PR, Jampol LM. Photodynamic therapy of choroidal hemangioma in Sturge-Weber syndrome, with a review of treatments for diffuse and circumscribed choroidal hemangiomas. Surv Ophthalmol. 2011;56(1):68–85.
75. Monteiro S, Casal I, Santos M, Meireles A. Photodynamic therapy for diffuse choroidal hemangioma in Sturge-Weber syndrome [internet]. Case Rep Med. 2014;2014:452372. https://www.hindawi.com/journals/crim/2014/452372/abs/
76. Anand R. Photodynamic therapy for diffuse choroidal hemangioma associated with Sturge weber syndrome. Am J Ophthalmol. 2003;136(4):758–60.
77. Cacciamani A, Scarinci F, Parravano M, Giorno P, Varano M. Choroidal thickness changes with photodynamic therapy for a diffuse choroidal hemangioma in Sturge-Weber syndrome. Int Ophthalmol. 2014;34(5):1131–5.
78. Singh AD, Rundle PA, Vardy SJ, Rennie IG. Photodynamic therapy of choroidal haemangioma associated with Sturge-Weber syndrome. Eye (Lond). 2005;19(3):365–7.
79. Shoeibi N, Ahmadieh H, Abrishami M, Poorzand H. Rapid and sustained resolution of serous retinal detachment in Sturge-Weber syndrome after single injection of intravitreal bevacizumab. Ocul Immunol Inflamm. 2011;19(5):358–60.
80. Paulus Y, Jain A, M Moshfeghi D. Resolution of persistent exudative retinal detachment in a case of Sturge-Weber syndrome with anti-VEGF administration. Ocul Immunol Inflamm. 2009;17:292–4.
81. Arevalo JF, Arias JD, Serrano MA. Oral propranolol for exudative retinal detachment in

diffuse choroidal hemangioma. Arch Ophthalmol. 2011;129(10):1373–5.
82. Mandal AK. Primary combined trabeculotomy-trabeculectomy for early-onset glaucoma in Sturge-Weber syndrome. Ophthalmology. 1999;106(8):1621–7.
83. Addison PKF, Papadopoulos M, Nischal KK, Hykin PG. Serous retinal detachment induced by topical bimatoprost in a patient with Sturge–Weber syndrome. Eye. 2011;25(1):124–5.

Metastatic Tumors of the Uvea

13

Yusra F. Shao, Jose J. Echegaray,
and Arun D. Singh

13.1 Introduction

Tumor metastasis to the eye is a rare phenomenon. Some malignant tumors such as breast and lung cancer are most frequent primary tumors to metastasize to the eye [1–4]. More rarely, cutaneous melanomas, gastrointestinal, thyroid, renal and prostate cancers metastasize to the eye. Ocular metastasis may present in the setting of a known primary malignancy or in absence of a known primary tumor [1–3]. Uveal metastasis may be the presenting feature at the time of diagnosis of lung cancer in up to 44% of cases [5]. In rare cases, the history of prior cancer may be so remote that the patients may not readily recall details of prior cancer treatment [6]. In all suspected cases of metastases, a thorough work up is necessary to diagnose the primary malignancy. Intraocular metastasis is predominantly uveal in location, most frequently to the choroid (88%) but also to the iris (7.8–9%) and ciliary body (2%) [3], with rare exception of retinal metastasis [7]. In the chapter, we will explore the common presenting symptoms, findings, and diagnostic work up for uveal metastasis.

Y. F. Shao · J. J. Echegaray · A. D. Singh (✉)
Department of Ophthalmic Oncology, Cole Eye Institute, Cleveland Clinic, Cleveland, OH, USA
e-mail: SHAOY3@ccf.org; JJEchegaray@med.miami.edu; singha@ccf.org

13.2 Presenting Symptoms

The presenting symptoms may vary according to the site of tumor metastasis within the uvea. Choroidal metastasis may present with blurred vision, floaters and/or photopsia. Metastasis to the anterior uveal segment (ciliary body and iris) may present as iritis, hyphema or as secondary glaucoma [8]. In exceptional cases, patients may be asymptomatic, and a tumor is visualized during ocular exam for other diagnostic purposes [9].

13.3 Examination

Visual acuity may be significantly decreased if the tumor involves the macula. There may be an accompanying visual field defect. Intraocular pressure may also be elevated in the setting of large tumor. Slit lamp exam may reveal edema and inflammation of the anterior chamber and iritis. Hyphema or pseudohypopyon may also be present where tumor cells layer in the anterior chamber [8].

Iris metastases present as yellow-to-white nodule with visible intrinsic vessels and frequent seeding in the angle. Ciliary body metastases present as yellow sessile or dome shaped lesions with visible episcleral sentinel vessel. Choroidal metastatic tumors often appear pale-yellow, placoid or dome (Fig. 13.1) shaped lesion with indistinct margins and overlying

V. Khetan (ed.), *Intraocular Tumors*, https://doi.org/10.1007/978-981-15-0395-5_13

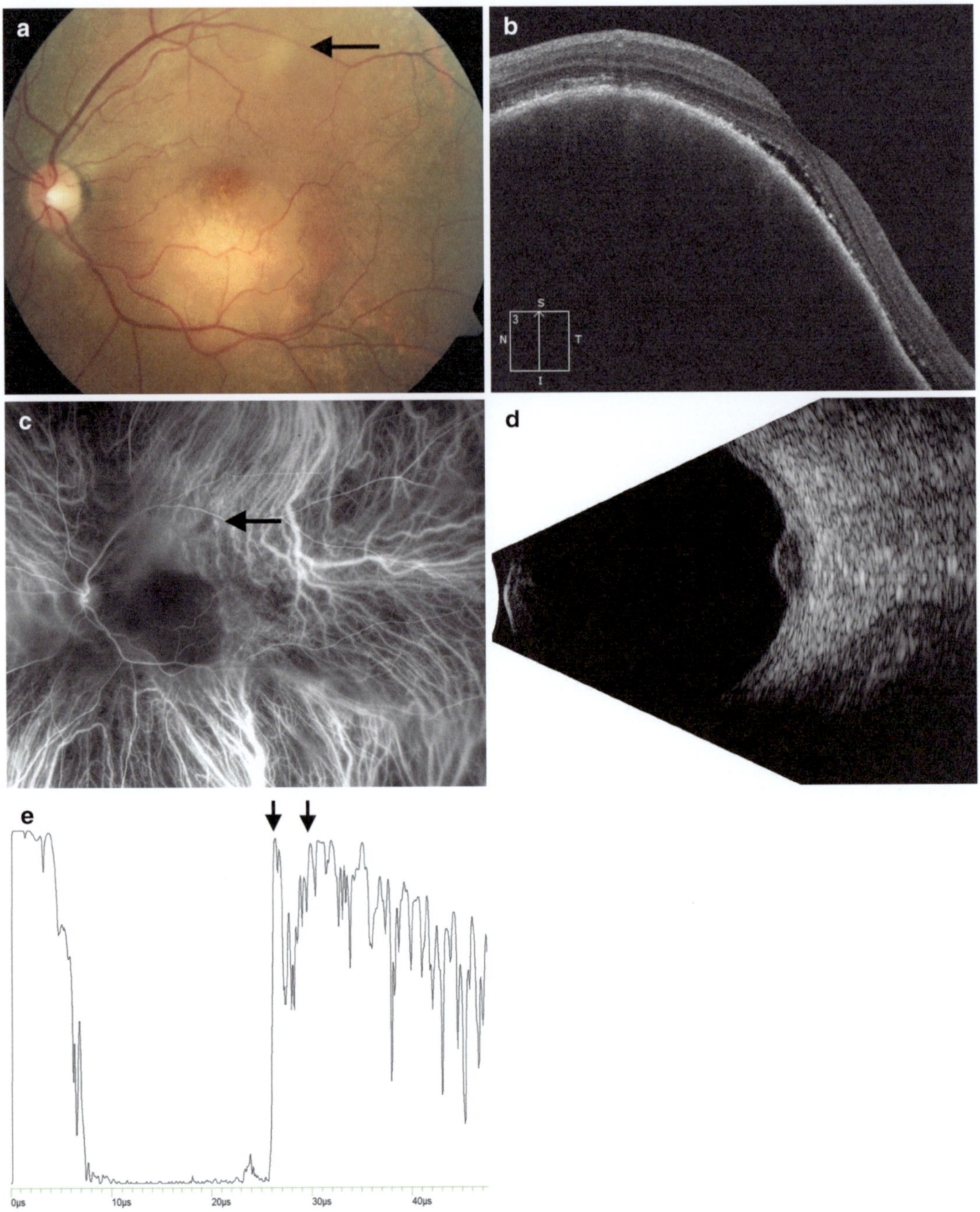

Fig. 13.1 A 67 year old female with stage 4 adenocarcinoma of the lung, positive for EGFR mutation, presented with blurred vision in the left eye (20/50). Right eye fundus examination was normal. In the left eye, a yellow choroidal mass (**a**) involving the macula (6.0 × 6.9 × 1.5 mm). Note a smaller lesion (1.0 × 1.0 × flat) in the superior macula (arrow). Associated shallow sub retinal fluid was confirmed by OCT (**b**). ICG revealed hypofluorescence (lack of intrinsic vascularity) in all phases of the angiogram (**c**). USG B-scan shows a placoid shape (**d**) with medium high internal reflectivity on A-scan (**e**, between arrows). MRI of the brain excluded intracranial lesions. In consultation with her oncologist, she he will be treated with osimertinib

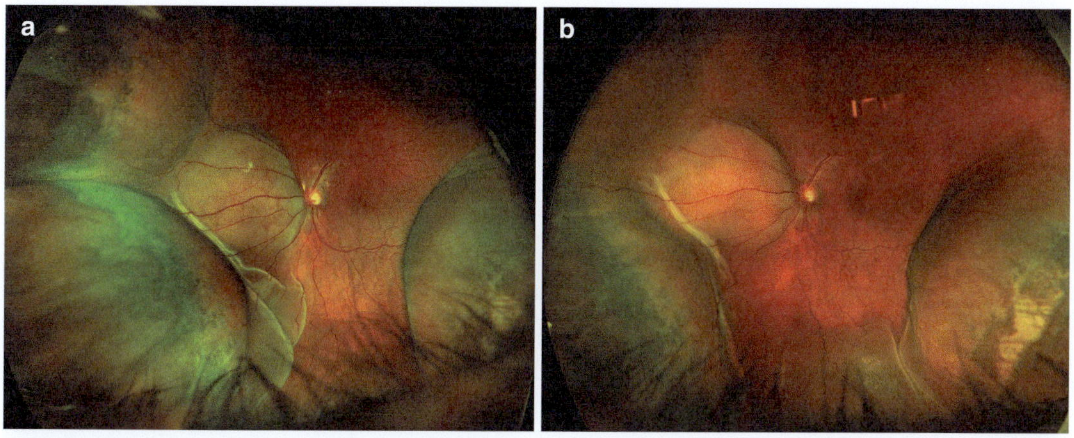

Fig. 13.2 A 60 year old male with stage 3b poorly differentiated lung adenocarcinoma, diagnosed 5 months ago, status post chemotherapy, radiation and targeted therapy presented with pain, blurred vision, redness and tearing of the left eye. Most recent CT scan showed progression of disease. On exam, visual acuity was 20/20 bilaterally. Slit lamp exam was significant for chemosis of the left eye and narrow angle. Dilated fundus exam revealed a dome shaped lesion nasal to the disc (10.5 × 9.5 × 4.9 mm) with associated ciliochoroidal and exudative retinal detachment (**a**). Ultrasound showed the lesion to be slightly irregular and highly reflective. The left eye was treated with radiation (30 Gy,10 fx), prednisone taper for secondary scleral inflammation. Fifteen days after completion of radiation therapy, ciliochoroidal and retinal detachment were partially resolved (**b**). However, systemic disease progressed and the patient was transitioned to hospice and expired

retinal pigment layer may have a leopard-spot-like appearance. Exudative retinal detachment (Fig. 13.2) and subretinal fluid (Fig. 13.3) is often present with choroidal metastasis. Carcinoid, renal cancer and thyroid cancer metastasis, being orange colored, may simulate a choroidal hemangioma. Melanocytic dome shaped tumor is typical for metastatic cutaneous melanoma [10].

13.4 Differential Diagnosis

Appearance of the tumor can help delineate metastatic lesions from primary ocular tumors. The differential diagnosis of uveal metastasis includes primary ocular tumors such as amelanotic uveal melanoma, choroidal hemangioma, scleritis, and inflammatory granuloma. Primary ocular tumors such as uveal melanoma is typically well vascularized while metastatic lesions are typically avascular. Primary tumors are often unifocal while metastatic tumors tend to be multifocal or bilateral (Fig. 13.1). Careful examination of the unaffected eye to detect subclinical metastasis is therefore of importance to establish the diagnosis of uveal metastases.

13.5 Diagnostic Testing

Optical coherence tomography (OCT) can detect shallow sub retinal fluid (Figs. 13.1 and 13.3), demonstrates an irregular (lumpy-bumpy) anterior surface, and, in smaller lesions reveal internal composition of the chordal mass [11, 12]. Angiography, particularly ICG can help differentiate between primary uveal tumor from a metastatic lesion. Primary tumors often have intrinsic vasculature whereas metastatic tumors are usually avascular (Fig. 13.1). Ultrasonography B reveals a placoid or dome shaped uveal mass (Fig. 13.1) with exudative retinal detachment. Internal reflectivity (A scan) can range from medium to high reflectivity (Fig. 13.1).

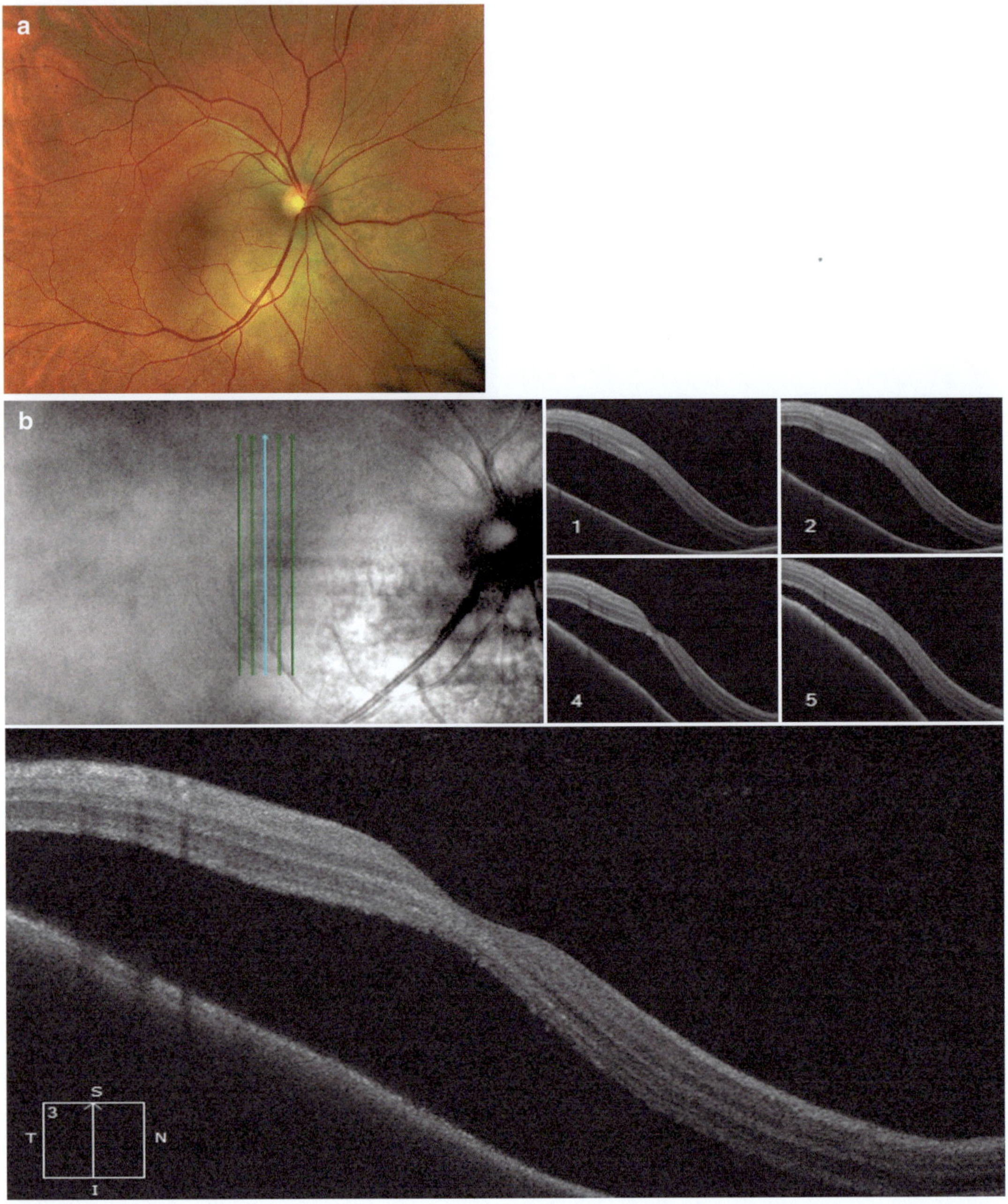

Fig. 13.3 A 61 year old female with stage 4 adenocarcinoma of the lung, positive for EML4-ALK gene translocation diagnosed 2 years ago and complicated by malignant pleural effusion status post chemotherapy and targeted therapy, currently on Crizotinib, presented with blurry vision in the right eye of 3 weeks. Most recent staging CT showed slight increase in pleural metastasis. Ophthalmic exam showed decreased vision in the right (20/400) compared to left (20/20) with normal anterior segment findings. Right eye fundus examination revealed a circumpapillary, amelanotic choroidal mass (**a**) involving the fovea (13.0 × 8.5 × 2.6 mm) with associated shallow sub retinal fluid (**b**). MRI of the brain excluded intracranial lesions. Per oncologist, Crizotinib was switched to Alectinib. Repeat eye exam in 1 month showed improved vision in the right (20/60), interval decrease in tumor height to 1 mm (**c**) and resolution of subretinal fluid involving the fovea (**d**). Similarly, interval decrease in size of pleural nodules was observed. Patient continues to be followed with serial exams

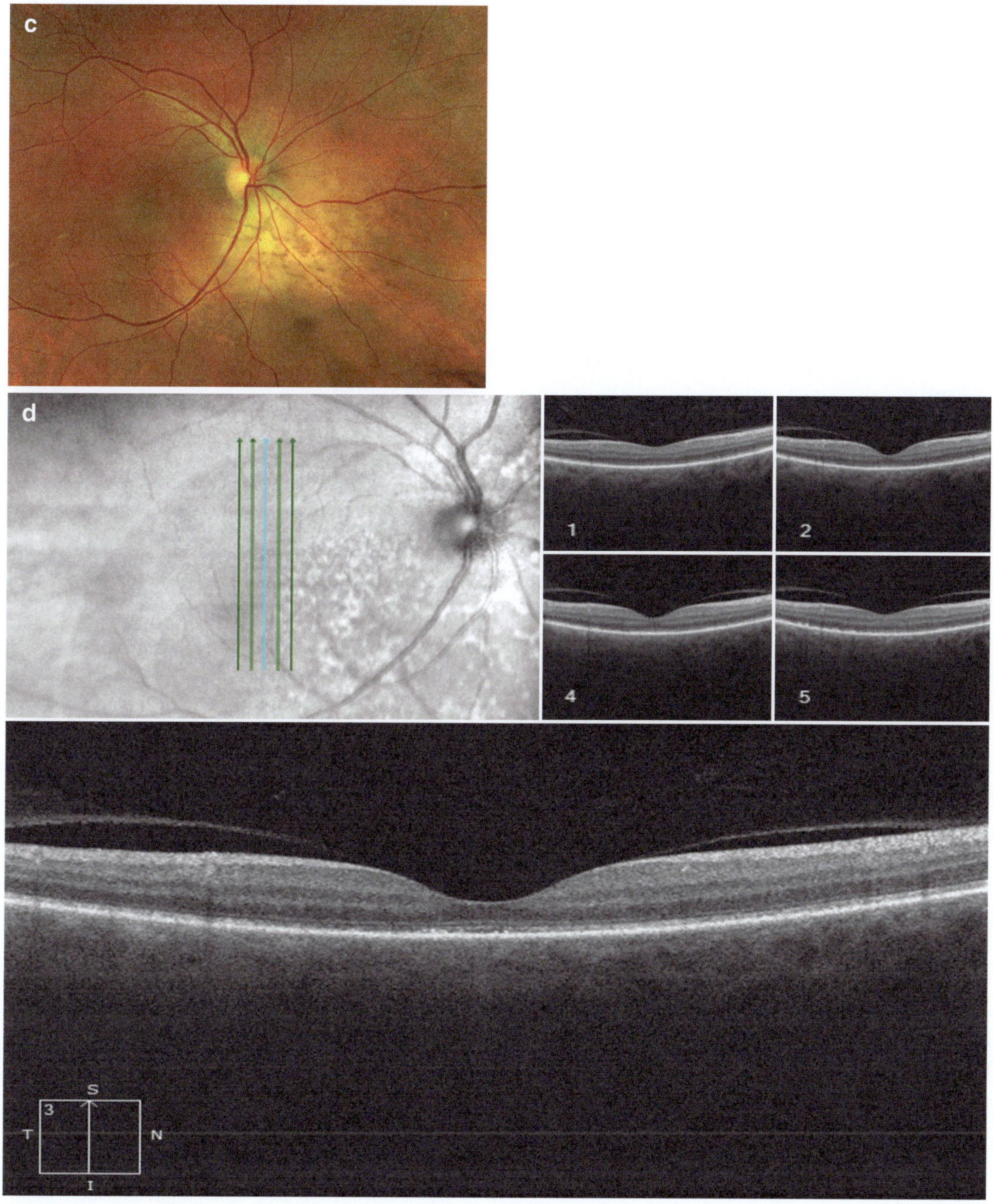

Fig. 13.3 (continued)

13.5.1 Systemic Evaluation

If the primary tumor is known, CT brain, chest, abdomen, and pelvis may be indicated to evaluate for systemic progression of the primary tumor. In most cases, metastatic disease is revealed on further imaging [4]. If the primary tumor is unknown, a search is undertaken using full body PET/CT to identify the primary malignancy, keeping in mind that breast and lung are the most frequent site of primary tumor in case with uveal metastases [1, 3]. Discussion with the primary oncologist may help further guide diagnostic imaging. Biopsy of the uveal metastasis is considered, if the initial imaging studies are inconclusive [13, 14].

13.6 Treatment

Multiple treatment options exist. In general, the treatment is guided by the type of primary tumor and extent of metastasis within the eye and elsewhere. Treatment decisions are also made in consultation with the primary oncologist. Systemic therapy is a preferred option particularly in presence of systemic disease or when the primary tumor is known to be chemotherapy or immunotherapy sensitive, such a lung cancer (Figs. 13.1 and 13.3) [5, 15]. Hormonal therapy can be used for metastatic breast cancer [6].

Radiation therapy is often successful for both focal and diffuse lesions. External beam radiation and proton beam irradiation can be used especially for multiple diffuse lesions (Fig. 13.2) [16–18]. Episcleral plaque brachytherapy is indicated for focal solitary lesions [18–20]. Transpupillary thermotherapy and photodynamic therapy are effective for small, solitary, choroidal lesions with thickness of less than 3.5 mm and minimal subretinal fluid, if systemic therapy has failed or intolerable due to toxicity [21].

Successful systemic and radiation therapy decreases tumor size and associated subretinal fluid and retinal detachment (Figs. 13.2 and 13.3). Enucleation is considered a last resort for local tumors and is an option in patients with a blind painful eye [5]. Advanced cases of systemic metastasis, with low chance of recovery, are considered for supportive hospice care.

13.7 Prognosis

With local therapy, which is palliative in intent, complete or partial vision can often be restored, intraocular pressure decreased, and exudative retinal detachment partially or completely resolved in majority of the cases. Overall survival prognosis depends on the nature of primary malignancy, extent of spread, and available treatment options as determined in consultation with the primary oncologist.

References

1. Bornfeld N. Uveal metastatic tumors. In: Damato BE, Singh AD, editors. Clinical ophthalmic oncology: Uveal tumors. Heidelberg: Springer; 2014, chap. 28. p. 355–63.
2. Eliassi-Rad B, Albert DM, Green WR. Frequency of ocular metastases in patients dying of cancer in eye bank populations. Br J Ophthalmol. 1996;80(2):125–8.
3. Shields CL, Shields JA, Gross NE, et al. Survey of 520 eyes with uveal metastases. Ophthalmology. 1997;104(8):1265–76.
4. Kreusel KM, Bechrakis NE, Krause L, et al. Incidence and clinical characteristics of symptomatic choroidal metastasis from breast cancer. Acta Ophthalmol Scand. 2007;85(3):298–302.
5. Shah SU, Mashayekhi A, Shields CL, et al. Uveal metastasis from lung cancer: clinical features, treatment, and outcome in 194 patients. Ophthalmology. 2014;121(1):352–7.
6. Levison AL, Erenler F, Zhao Y, et al. Late-onset choroidal metastasis from breast cancer. Retin Cases Brief Rep. 2018;12:342.
7. Vajzovic L, Mruthyunjaya P. Retinal metastatic tumors. In: Singh AD, Damato BE, editors. Clinical ophthalmic oncology: retinal tumors. Heidelberg: Springer; 2014, chap. 5. p. 91–102.
8. Shields JA, Shields CL, Kiratli H, de Potter P. Metastatic tumors to the iris in 40 patients. Am J Ophthalmol. 1995;119(4):422–30.
9. Wiegel T, Kreusel KM, Bornfeld N, et al. Frequency of asymptomatic choroidal metastasis in patients with disseminated breast cancer: results of a prospective screening programme. Br J Ophthalmol. 1998;82(10):1159–61.
10. Grajewski RS, Schuler-Thurner B, Mauch C, et al. Ocular diseases in metastatic cutaneous melanoma: review of 108 consecutive patients in two German tertiary centers. Graefes Arch Clin Exp Ophthalmol. 2014;252(4):679–85.
11. Torres VL, Brugnoni N, Kaiser PK, Singh AD. Optical coherence tomography enhanced depth imaging of choroidal tumors. Am J Ophthalmol. 2011;151(4):586–93.e2.
12. Al-Dahmash SA, Shields CL, Kaliki S, et al. Enhanced depth imaging optical coherence tomography of choroidal metastasis in 14 eyes. Retina. 2014;34(8):1588–93.
13. Aziz HA, Martel JN, Biscotti CV, et al. This, that, or something different? Surv Ophthalmol. 2015;60(5):495–9.
14. Biscotti CV, Singh AD. Uveal metastases. Monogr Clin Cytol. 2012;21:17–30.

15. Feng Y, Singh AD, Lanigan C, et al. Choroidal metastases responsive to crizotinib therapy in a lung adenocarcinoma patient with ALK 2p23 fusion identified by ALK immunohistochemistry. J Thorac Oncol. 2013;8(12):e109–11.
16. Wiegel T, Bottke D, Kreusel KM, et al. External beam radiotherapy of choroidal metastases—final results of a prospective study of the German Cancer Society (ARO 95-08). Radiother Oncol. 2002;64(1):13–8.
17. Tsina EK, Lane AM, Zacks DN, et al. Treatment of metastatic tumors of the choroid with proton beam irradiation. Ophthalmology. 2005;112(2):337–43.
18. Seregard S, Pelayes DE, Singh AD. Radiation therapy: uveal tumors. Dev Ophthalmol. 2013; 52:36–57.
19. Shields CL, Shields JA, De Potter P, et al. Plaque radiotherapy for the management of uveal metastasis. Arch Ophthalmol. 1997;115(2):203–9.
20. Lim JI, Petrovich Z. Radioactive plaque therapy for metastatic choroidal carcinoma. Ophthalmology. 2000;107(10):1927–31.
21. Ghodasra DH, Demirci H. Photodynamic therapy for choroidal metastasis. Am J Ophthalmol. 2016;161:104–9.e1-2.

14 Miscellaneous Intra-Ocular Tumours

Bikramjit P. Pal and Abhinav Dhami

Uveal melanomas are the most common primary intraocular tumors in adults and account for total of 79–81% of all the ocular melanomas. They can be divided as anterior tumors (iris) and posterior tumors (ciliary body and choroid). The most common neoplasm is observed in the choroid accounting for 80% of all uveal melanomas followed by ciliary body (10%) and iris (10%). Uveal melanomas account for 75% malignanacy of the intraocular tumors. The incidence in 6 per 100,000, about 0.003% of all cancers. The mean reported age of diagnosed uveal melanoma is 43.7 years in Chinese, 51.6 years in American blacks, 55.2 years in Japanese, and 52.4 years in the Hispanic population [1–7].

Ciliary body tumors remain asymptomatic for a long period of time as most often they go undetected. Primary tumors of the ciliary epithelium are classified as congential and acquired. The *congenital* tumors include: Glioneuroma and medulloepithelioma; *Acquired* tumors include Fuchs adenoma(psuedoepitheliomatous hyperplasia and ciliary body non pigmented, pigmented or mixed epithelial tumours: adenoma and adenocarcinoma [8].

B. P. Pal (✉)
Vitreoretina and Ocular Oncology Services, Pals Retina Care, Ranchi, Jharkhand, India

H M Diwan Eye Foundation, Kolkata, India

A. Dhami
Vitreoretinal Services, Dhami Eye Care, Ludhiana, Punjab, India

Medulloepithelioma: is an embryonal neoplasm arising from the primitive medullary epithelium or inner layer of optic cup and apperares in the first deacde of life. Zimmerman classified it into teratoid and nonteratoid types. The non teratoid medulloepithelioma (Diktyoma) is a proliferation of cells of the medullary epithelium. The teratoid medulloepithelioma has hetroplastic appendages like cartilage, skeletal muscle and brain tisse. Both the types can be either as benign or malignant [9]. There is no population based information on the incidence or prevalance of these tumors and majorly consists of single case reports in literature [8, 9]. These tumors are slow growing tumors and are mostly overlooked due to the secondary complications and usually go undetected.

On slit lamp evalution they appear as irregular shaped, with smooth surface and grey to fleshy pink colour. Visual loss is attributed to cataract formation (lens notch) and secondary glaucoma (neovascular glaucoma). It has a characteristic cyclitic membrane giving the apperance of PHPV. It can distinguished as it appears a sheet of neoplastic membrane that migrated from the main retina to the anterior vitreous. The major differential diagnosis that need to be ruled out are retinoblastoma and Persistant hyperplastic primary vitreous.

Histopathology: Medulloepitheliomas are characterized by cords of primitive neuroepithelial cells that resemble the embryonic retina or neural tube surrounded by a loose mesenchy-

V. Khetan (ed.), *Intraocular Tumors*, https://doi.org/10.1007/978-981-15-0395-5_14

mal tissue rich in hyaluronic acid. The teratoid medulloepithelioma is characterized by the presence of heteroplastic tissue, neuroblastic tissue [10].

They may present with cysts inside the tumor, chalky white opacities with calcification on USG. The diagnosis of medulloepithelioma can be made best by clinical recognition in the first decade of life. Fine needle aspiration biopsy plays an important role in the diagnosis of medulloepithelioma [11].

MRI and ultrasound have limited role in diagnosis [9, 10].

Treatment:

(a) Local Resection of tumour is considered if tumour is small, well circumscribed(<3-clock hour), as initial management but has high recurrence rate.
(b) Iridocyclectomy
(c) Enucleation is indicated if the tumour has a friable apperance or there is adjacent free floating cyst [9].

14.1 Acquired Neoplasm

These are tumours of the pigmented and non pigmented ciliary epithelium. They are divided into benign (adenoma) and malignant (adenocarcinoma). The clinical onset occurs in adulthood with a mean age of 45 years, with no sex predeliction.

The patients remain either asymptomatic or present with painless loss of vision, with a white to tan coloured, irregular, multilobular mass. The patient can present with anterior chamber flare and cells, focal cataract and a subluxed lens. A sentinel vessel can occur in episceral tissue overlying the tumor.

Hisopathologically acquied neoplams are of 5 types:

Psuedoadenomatous, hyperplasia, adenoma, adenocarcinoma. The latter two are further classifed as solid, pappilary and pleomorphic. The tumour of non pigmented epithelium of ciliary body occur internal to the pigment epithelium whereas a melanoma is located external to pigment epithelium and are pigmented with a smooth surface and has a mushroom shaped appearence.

The main consideration in the differential diagnosis are ciliary body melanoma, medulloepithelioma, adenoma or adenocarcinoma of the ciliary pigment epithelium, leiomyoma, neurilemoma, metastatic carcinoma, and granuloma. Medulloepithelioma is a congenital tumor in onset and tends to be more cystic with an associated lens notch, iris neovacularization and persistent primary vitreous Leiomyoma occurs in younger patients and have a smooth surface and is less likely to cause cells in the vitreous. Metastatic carcinoma will have a positive history of tumour elsewhere. The granuloma of ciliary body is associated with severe uveal inflammation.

The diagnosis can be ascertained by transillumination as the tumour transmits light well, whereas melanoma will block the transmission. In B-scan ultrasonography the tumour shows abrupt elevation,acoustic solidity and high internal reflectivity. Magnetic resonance imaging offers limited knowledge at diffrentiating adenoma from melanoma due to similar imaging features.

The treatment options includes local resection and enucleation [12].

14.2 Retinal Astrocytoma

A variety of benign and malignant tumors are known to involve the retina, the more common tumors include retinoblastoma, primary intraocular lymphoma and angiomatosis retinae, however, astrocytic tumors of the retina are quite rare. These tumors sometimes are found to be solitary without the stigmata of phakomatosis or may present with multiple tumors in association with tuberous sclerosis complex (TSC) or neurofibromatosis. It has been rarely associated with retinitis pigmentosa [13]. The finding of more than one retinal hamartoma has been determined to be significant and specific to retain as a major feature for diagnosis of TSC, as the lesions have similar histologic features to the tubers located in the brains of TSC patients [14].

They are classified as massive retinal gliosis (MRG), astrocytic hamartoma, or acquired astrocytoma.

MRG is a non-neoplastic tissue that occurs in response to eye disorders such as inflammation, trauma or infection. They tend to occur in the peripheral retina. The presence of MRG pathology indicates previous retinal inflammation, retinal pigment epithelial proliferation and calcification [13, 15].

Astrocytic hamartoma are benign and stable tumor and can be either solitary or multiple in numbers, most often associated with tuberous sclerosis or neurofibromatosis. The hamartoma contain giant astrocytes that are often nonreactive or weakly positive for glial fibrillary acidic protein, and there is a high frequency of calcification [15].

Acquired retinal astrocytoma is a benign tumor that occurs sporadically and is not associated with TSC. They generally arise from the optic disc or retinal juxtapapillary area. They are of two types, one being progressive and cause intraocular damage that includes exudative retinal detachment, neovascular glaucoma, central retinal vein occlusion and tumor necrosis with secondary intraocular inflammation, which ultimately can result in a painful blind eye [16] while the other is a stationery type of tumor.

Retinal traction, retinal pigment epithelial alterations, and extensive yellow retinal exudation are typically found with astrocytic tumors. Differential diagnoses that need to be ruled out are retinoblastoma, choroidal melanoma or other malignant tumors [15, 16].

Serafino et al. described EDI-OCT features in 86 eyes of 47 patients with retinal astrocytic hamartoma and classified the tumors into type I (42%), type II (26%), type III (20%), and type IV (12%). They described:

- Type I as flat and generally in the nerve fiber layer
- Type II with slight elevation of the nerve fiber layer and retinal traction
- Type III with "moth-eaten" lucent areas suggestive of calcification involving inner and outer retina
- Type IV with optically empty intralesional cavities [17].

The treatment options include enucleation, endoresection, brachytherapy and photodynamic therapy and unfortunately all of these therapies are associated with some risk for potential visual acuity damage [13–15].

14.3 Conclusion

While it may be difficult to differentiate astrocytic tumors or medulloepitheliomas on clinical evaluation itself due to rare occurrence and late detection of such tumors and thus may masquerade other tumor phenotypes. A thorough comprehensive examination in entitled that take into account the clinical findings, along with the medical histories and the type of complications associated with each tumor that can assist in making the correct diagnosis.

References

1. Shields CL, et al. Review of cystic and solid tumours of irs. Oman J Ophthalmol. 2013;6:159–64.
2. Sheilds CL, et al. Clinical survey of 3680 iris tumor based on the patient age of presentation. Ophthalmology. 2012;119:407–14.
3. Shields JA. Primary cysts of the iris. Trans Am Ophthalmol Soc. 1981;79:771–809.
4. Grutzmacher R, et al. Congential cyst. Br J Ophthalmol. 1987;71:227–34.
5. Lois N, et al. Primary cysts of the iris pigment epithelium. Clinical features and natural course in 234 patients. Ophthalmology. 1998;105(10):1879–85.
6. Margio FA, et al. Anterior segment tumors current concept and innovations. Surv Ophthalmol. 2003;48:569–93.
7. Kaliki S, et al. Uveal melanoma: estimating prognosis. Indian J Ophthalmol. 2015;63:93–102.
8. Romanowska-Dixon B, et al. Adenoma of iris and ciliary body. Case report. Pol J Pathol. 2003; 54(3):187–90.

9. Shields AJ, et al. Congenital neoplasms of non-pigmented ciliary epithelium (medulloepithelioma). Ophthalmology. 1996;103(12):1998–2006.
10. Saunders T, et al. Intraocular medulloepithelioma. Arch Pathol Lab Med. 2012;136:212–6.
11. Rishi P, Dhami A, Biswas J. Biopsy techniques for intraocular tumors. Indian J Ophthalmol. 2016 Jun;64(6):415–21.
12. Shields JA, et al. Acquired neoplasms of the non pigmented ciliary epithelium. Ophthalmology. 1996;103:2007–16.
13. Fuchino T, Hayashi T, Suzuma K, Taneoka A, Abe K, Kinoshita N, Yasui H, Kitaoka T, Fukuoka J. Solitary retinal astrocytoma: a case series. Open J Pathol. 2013;03(2):60–4.
14. Northrup H, Krueger DA, International Tuberous Sclerosis Complex Consensus Group. Tuberous sclerosis complex diagnostic criteria update: recommendations of the 2012 International Tuberous Sclerosis Complex Consensus Conference. Pediatr Neurol. 2013;49(4):243–54.
15. Deshmukh SD, Ashturkar AV, Babanagare SV, Gokhale SK, Deshpande AA. Massive retinal gliosis: an unusual case with immunohistochemical study. Indian J Ophthalmol. 2011;59:246–8.
16. Tomida M, Mitamura Y, Katome T, Eguchi H, Naito T, Harada T. Aggressive retinal astrocytoma associated with tuberous sclerosis. Clin Ophthalmol. 2012;6:715.
17. Serafino M, Pichi F, Giuliari GP, Shields CL, Ciardella AP, Nucci P. Retinal astrocytic hamartoma: spectral-domain optical coherence tomography classification and correlation with tuberous sclerosis complex. J Am Assoc Pediatr Ophthalmol Strabismus. 2013;17(1):e27.

15 Various Syndromes with Benign Intraocular Tumors

Mahesh Shanmugam Palanivelu and Pradeep Sagar

15.1 Introduction

A selected group of benign intraocular tumors are part of neuro-oculo-cutaneous syndromes (syn: phakomatoses) with the common features of familial inheritance, variable expressivity, multi-system involvement with potential for malignant transformation. They are often associated with a genetic defect, commonly a loss of function of a tumor suppressor gene.

Neuro-oculo-cutaneous syndromes are often associated with benign vascular tumors of the retina and choroid, benign glial cell tumors and hamartomas involving the retina and retinal pigment epithelial cells.

The following conditions will be discussed in this chapter:

(a) von-Hippel Lindau Syndrome
(b) Wyburn Mason Syndrome
(c) Cavernous hemangioma of the retina
(d) Sturge-Weber Syndrome
(e) Tuberous sclerosis
(f) Neurofibromatosis type 1
(g) Syndromes associated with combined hamartoma of the retina and retinal pigment epithelium (CHRRPE)
(h) Syndromes associated with congenital hypertrophy of retinal pigment epithelium (CHRPE)

15.2 von-Hippel Lindau Syndrome

von-Hippel Lindau (VHL) syndrome is characterized by retinal and central nervous system (CNS) hemangioblastomas, pheochromocytomas, multiple pancreatic, renal and epididymal cysts. Renal cysts have the potential of malignant transformation to renal cell carcinoma. VHL syndrome is distinct from other phakomatoses in that it does not have major cutaneous features, with the occasional occurrence of dermal nevi or café au lait spots [1].

15.2.1 Epidemiology [2]

Incidence—1:32000 live births.

No sexual predilection.

Age at diagnosis: infancy to 70 years (Average age-26 years).

15.2.2 Genetics and Pathophysiology

Inheritance—Autosomal dominant. It has almost 100% penetrance by 65 years of age [3]. An individual inherits a germline mutation wherein one

The original version of this chapter was revised. The correction to this chapter can be found at https://doi.org/10.1007/978-981-15-0395-5_22

M. S. Palanivelu (✉) · P. Sagar
Department of Vitreo-Retina and Ocular Oncology, Sankara Eye Hospital, Bangalore, India

V. Khetan (ed.), *Intraocular Tumors*, https://doi.org/10.1007/978-981-15-0395-5_15

copy of the VHL allele is inactive in all the cells of the body. A somatic mutation of the other allele increases the probability of tumor development (Knudson's two-hit hypothesis) [4].

The VHL gene is located on the short arm of chromosome 3 (3p25.3). The VHL gene is a tumor suppressor gene and encodes a 213 amino acid protein (pVHL).

The major function of pVHL is its role in oxygen sensing pathway. Hypoxia inducible factor-α (HIF-α) undergoes hydroxylation under normoxic conditions. Once modified by the –OH group, HIF-α is captured by pVHL and delivers HIF-α to an E3-ubiquitin ligase complex, and subsequent proteasomal degradation. Mutation in VHL results in inappropriate stabilization of HIF-α, and leads to over expression of hypoxic signaling even in the presence of oxygen [5].

Various genes involved in oxygen transport, angiogenesis, and anaerobic energy metabolism are up regulated in the absence of pVHL. pVHL is also involved in regulation of senescence, cytokine signaling, collagen IV assembly into the extracellular matrix, regulation of a normal extracellular fibronectin matrix and tumor suppression [5].

Increase in vascular endothelial growth factor (VEGF) in VHL syndrome is believed to heighten formation and growth of retinal capillary hemangioblastoma [6], and renal cell carcinoma [7].

15.2.3 Systemic Features

Systemic manifestations of VHL include CNS hemangioblastoma (Fig. 15.1), pheochromocytoma, clear cell renal cell carcinoma, renal cysts (Fig. 15.2), pancreatic cysts, endolymphatic sac tumor and several other tumors and cysts. Renal cell carcinoma is the leading cause of mortality in patients with VHL, occurring in 5% of patients by age 30 and 40% by 60 years of age.

Systemic features of VHL syndrome is summarized in Table 15.1 [8–13].

The management options for the systemic features of VHL syndrome are summarized in Table 15.2 [8–13].

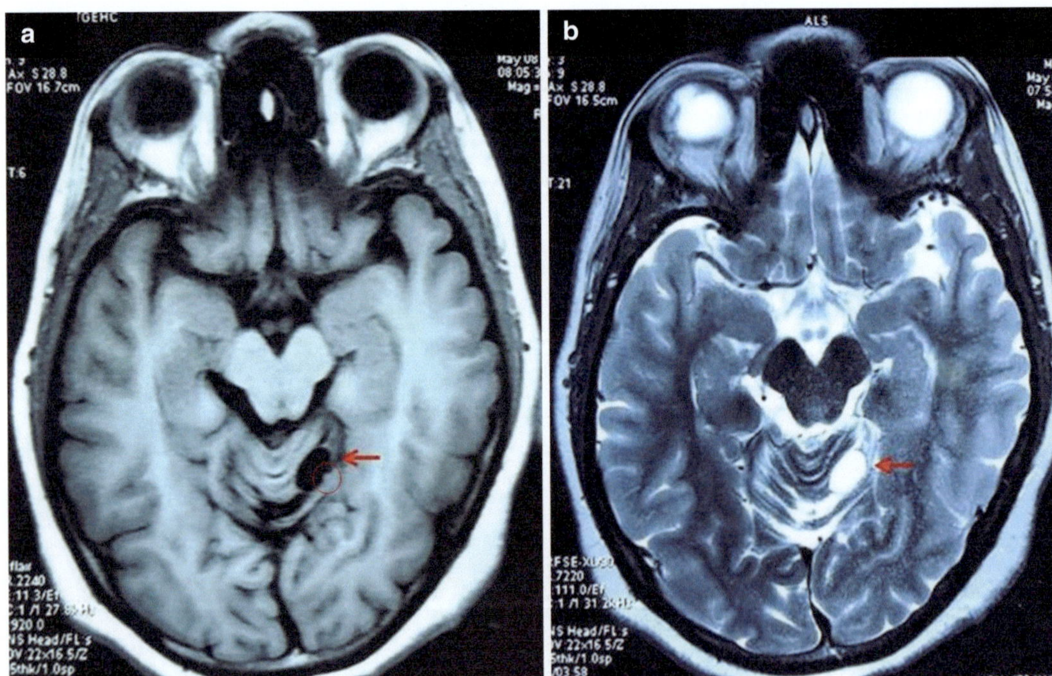

Fig. 15.1 MRI brain of a patient with VHL. Oval shaped lesion (arrow) hypo intense on T1 (**a**) and hyper intense on T2 weighted image (**b**) suggestive of a cyst. Tiny hyper intense nodule (red circle) is seen at the wall of cyst suggestive of hemangioblastoma

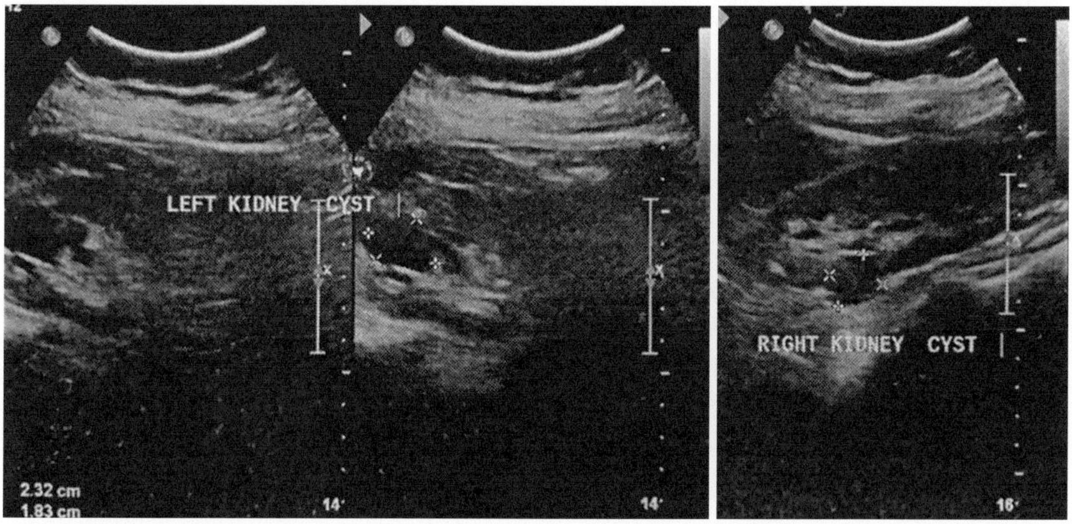

Fig. 15.2 Abdominal ultrasound image of a patient with VHL showing bilateral renal cysts

15.2.4 Ocular Features

Retinal capillary hemangioblastoma (RCH) is the hallmark of VHL syndrome in the eye. RCH may occur as an isolated lesion or as a part of VHL [14]. The mean age at diagnosis is 18 years in patients with VHL and 36 years for sporadic cases [15].

In a patient with solitary RCH, the risk of developing VHL is 45% if the patient is <10 years of age and decreases to 1% if the age at diagnosis is >60 years [9].

RCH can also be associated with other systemic conditions such as Marshall-Stickler syndrome [16].

15.2.4.1 Clinical features

Symptoms

Patients can present with decreased vision due to macular exudation, tractional or combined tractional-rhegmatogenous retinal detachment involving the posterior pole. Rarely vitreous hemorrhage may cause floaters.

Signs

The smaller RCHs appear as yellow spot between a feeding arteriole and a draining venule (Fig. 15.3). The larger ones appear as orange-red circumscribed lesions with a dilated tortuous feeding arteriole and a draining venule (Fig. 15.4). Presence of dilated pair of vessels in the posterior pole with macular exudation should prompt one to examine the periphery for presence of RCH (Fig. 15.5). The most common retinal location of these tumors is in the superotemporal quadrant (42%) and in the midperiphery (58%) [17].

Some authors believe that two forms of disease exist—the exudative form and the vitreoretinal form (Fig. 15.6) [18]. Exudation at the macular region is due to subretinal migration of lipid from the peripheral tumor. The proliferation of the epimacular membranes in the vitreoretinal form causes tractional detachment of macula and decreased vision (Fig. 15.7). Traction on the RCH can lead to "free floating" angioma in the vitreous, vitreous hemorrhage and a combined traction-rhegmatogenous retinal detachment.

Juxtapapillary RCHs are ill defined and involves an eccentric part of the optic disc. It differs from the peripheral RCH in that no definite feeder arteriole or a draining venule is seen. It can be endophytic, sessile or exophytic [18].

Endophytic tumor appears as an orange-red lesion (Fig. 15.8). But the sessile and the exophytic tumors does not show the characteristic fundus appearance (Fig. 15.8) and can be misdiagnosed as papillitis, unilateral papilledema, choroiditis,

Table 15.1 Systemic features of VHL syndrome

	CNS hemangioblastoma	Renal cell carcinoma	Pheochromocytoma	Endolymphatic sac tumor	Pancreatic neuroendocrine tumors (PNET) or cyst	Epididymal cystadenoma	Cystadenoma of broad ligament
Prevalence	60–80%	70% (In type 1 and 2B)	10–20%	6–15%	35–70%	26–60%	Unknown
Mean age at presentation	33 years	40 years	30 years	31 years	36 years	Unknown	Unknown
Location	Cerebellum (16–69%), brainstem (5–22%), spinal cord (13–53%), Cauda equina (11%), supratentorial (1–7%), pituitary (2–4%)	Multifocal and bilateral	Multifocal and bilateral			Unilateral or bilateral	Unilateral or bilateral
Clinical features	Based on the anatomical location, associated edema, cyst and tumor size • Cerebellum: cerebellar impairment and increased intracranial pressure, gait ataxia, dysmetria, headaches diplopia, vertigo, and emesis • Spinal cord: radiculopathy and myelopathy-hypesthesia, weakness, gait ataxia, hyper-reflexia, pain, and incontinence • Brain stem: cranial nerve impairment-dysphagia • Rare cases: intra-parenchymal or subarachnoid hemorrhage	Usually detected pre-symptomatically during annual imaging	Excessive norepinephrine production leading to hypertension, tachycardia, palpitations, headaches, sweating, pallor, and nausea	Ear fullness, disequilibrium, and hearing loss Larger lesions (>3 cm) can result in facial paresis	Pancreatic exocrine and endocrine deficiency Compression of intestine and bile duct can lead to symptoms	Asymptomatic and detected incidentally	Mostly asymptomatic Rarely present as abdominopelvic mass with symptoms of abdominal discomfort
Clinical course	50% of tumors will increase in size over 5 years	Small renal tumors enlarge slowly (mean < 2 cm/year) Advanced RCC (>3 cm) develop metastatic disease. Leading cause of mortality in VHL	Rarely undergo malignant transformation	Benign but locally aggressive Can erode temporal bone	Neuroendocrine tumors can undergo malignant transformation (8%)	Benign	Benign

Table 15.2 The management options for the systemic features of VHL syndrome

	CNS hemangioblastoma	Renal cell carcinoma	Pheochromocytoma	Endolymphatic sac tumor	Pancreatic neuroendocrine tumors (PNET) or cyst	Epididymal cystadenoma	Cystadenoma of broad ligament
Diagnosis	Contrast enhanced magnetic resonance imaging (MRI) is the modality of choice Can identify tumors as small as 2 mm	Abdominal ultrasonography and MRI	Plasma free metanephrines is the most sensitive method (97%) Contrast-enhanced MRI of the abdomen is the preferred modality of identifying tumor	Pre and post contrast MRI Audiogram to assess hearing loss	MRI Additional tests: Endoscopic ultrasound and somatostatin receptor scintigraphy	Ultrasonography is the modality of choice	MRI of the abdomen or pelvic ultrasound
Treatment	Surgical resection of symptomatic tumors. Stereotactic radio surgery in inoperable cases	Individual renal lesions are kept under regular surveillance until it reaches 3 cm diameter when partial nephrectomy is required Renal transplantation would be required as repeated renal surgery will compromise renal function	Surgical resection with partial adrenalectomy Perioperative management with a combination of alpha-adrenergic and beta-adrenergic blockade is necessary	Surgical resection of detectable tumors Complete resection is indicated if intralabyrinthine hemorrhage is noted even in absence of visible tumors on imaging (hemorrhage indicate presence of microscopic tumors)	Observation of asymptomatic tumors Surgical decompression in patients with obstructive symptoms Whipple procedure for PNETs with a potential for metastatic disease	Observation	Observation Surgical resection if symptomatic

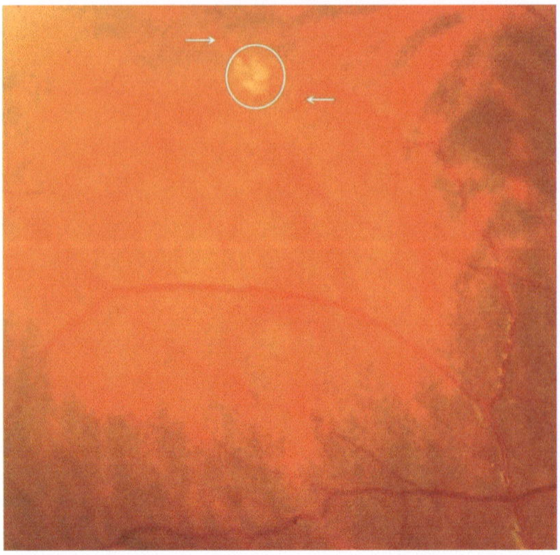

Fig. 15.3 Fundus photograph of a small RCH seen as a yellow spot (within circle) between a feeding arteriole and a draining venule (arrows)

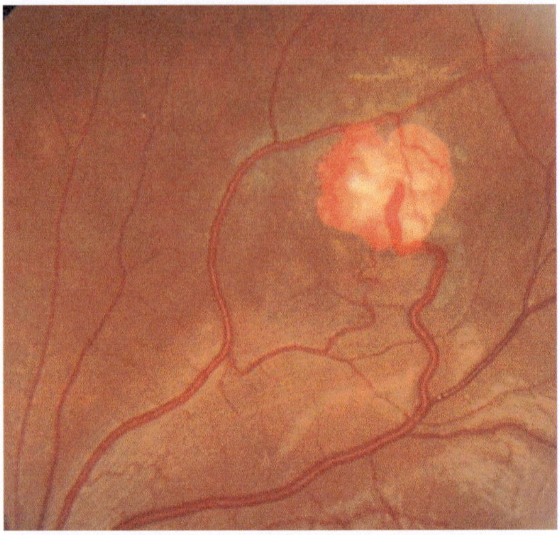

Fig. 15.4 Fundus photograph of a large RCH. Tumor is orange red in colour with dilated and tortuos feeding arteriole and a draining venule

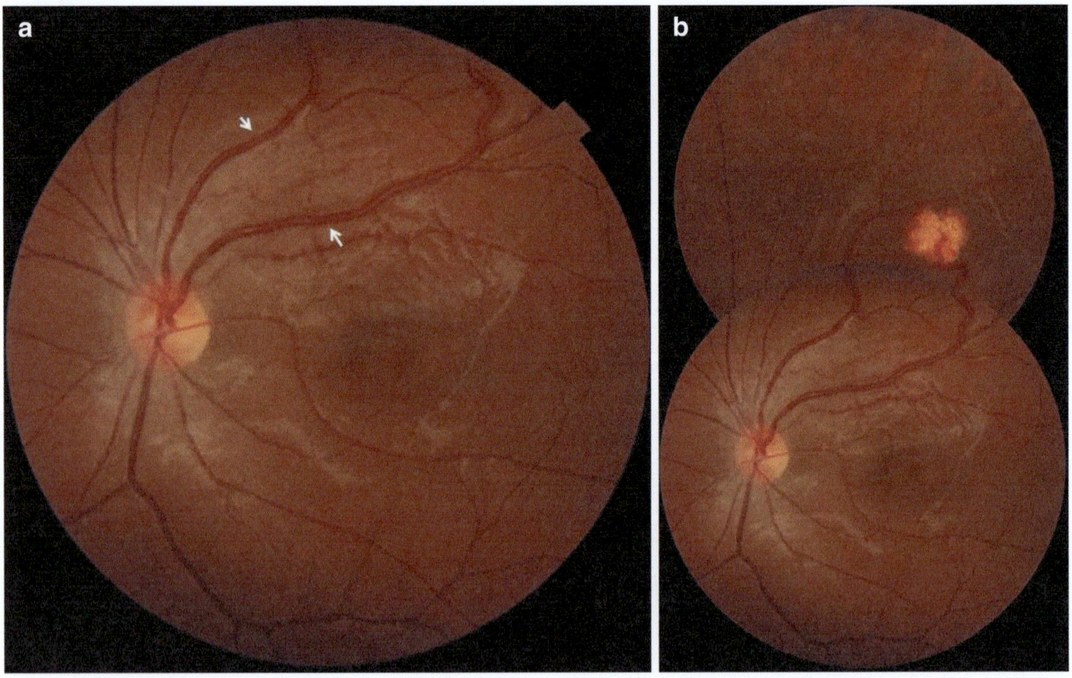

Fig. 15.5 Fundus photograph of posterior pole (**a**) showing dilated pair of vessels (arrow). Montage (**b**) shows a RCH communicating with this pair of vessels

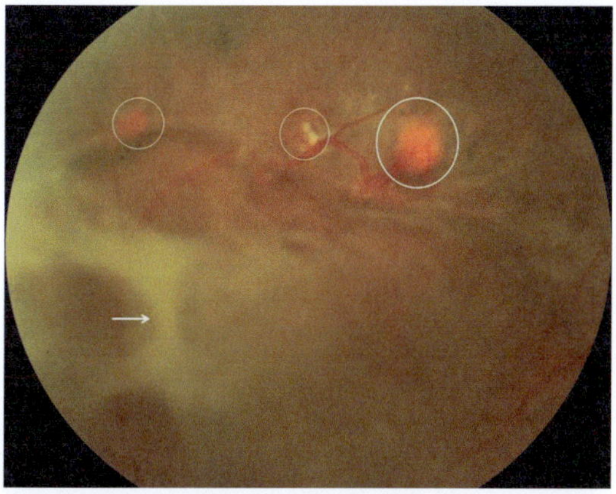

Fig. 15.6 Fundus photograph of vitreo-retinal form showing extensive fibrous proliferation (arrow) with multiple RCH (circles) in adjacent area

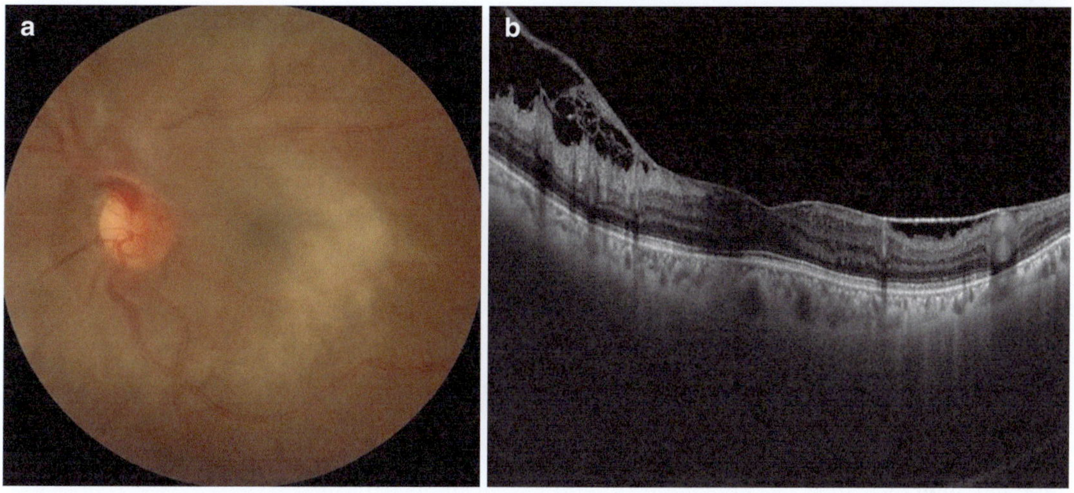

Fig. 15.7 Fundus photograph (**a**) and OCT (**b**) of the posterior pole of the same eye in Fig. 15.6. Extensive proliferation of the posterior hyaloid with partial detachment is seen on OCT

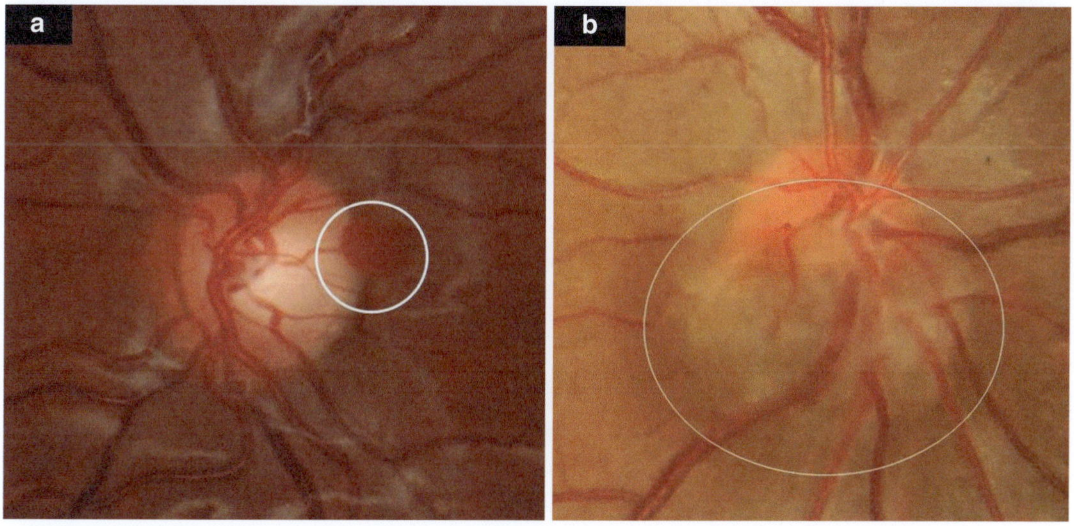

Fig. 15.8 Fundus photograph of juxtapapillary RCHs. Endophytic form (**a**) and exophytic form (**b**)

choroidal hemangioma or choroidal neovascularization [19]. It can be asymptomatic or can lead to peripapillary exudation.

Without treatment, most eyes with RCH progress to total retinal detachment, neovascular glaucoma and painful blind eye. Anterior hyaloid proliferation resulting in ciliary body traction and subsequent hypotony can result in phthisis bulbi.

15.2.5 Diagnosis

The diagnosis can be made most often on slit lamp biomicroscopy and indirect ophthalmoscopy with the classic picture of an orange red tumor with a feeding arteriole, draining venule associated with macular exudates. A fundus fluorescein angiogram may be necessary to identify early lesions that are not visible on clinical examination. On fundus fluorescein angiography (FFA) these lesions show intense early phase hyperfluorescence and in late phases tumors either leak profusely (Fig. 15.9) or stain without significant leak. The paired vessels are well delineated as well.

Optical coherence tomography (OCT) aids detection of small RCHs that appear as retinal thickening with mild shadowing of the underlying structures [20]. Tumor exudation results in intra and subretinal fluid, accumulation of hard exudate and photoreceptor layer rips close to the lesion, that can be demonstrated by the OCT (Fig. 15.10) [21].

OCT aids in assessment of response to the treatment such as resolution of edema (Fig. 15.11).

Optical coherence tomography angiography (OCTA) allows visualization of the depth of the lesion in the retina in addition to its vascularity. Our preliminary experience of imaging RCH showed that these tumors appear to arise from the superficial retinal capillary plexus and appear bright on OCTA due to their rich vascularity (unpublished data) (Fig. 15.12). Tumors that were indistinct to clinical examination were picked up by OCTA, similar to fluorescein angiography (FFA). Current technological limitations of OCTA such as small field and difficulty in imaging the retinal periphery limit its role as a screening tool in lieu of FFA but it may aid in follow-up of treated lesions [22].

15.2.6 Differential Diagnosis

The peripheral RCH may be mistaken for

- Coat's disease: paired dilated vessels are not seen in coat's disease

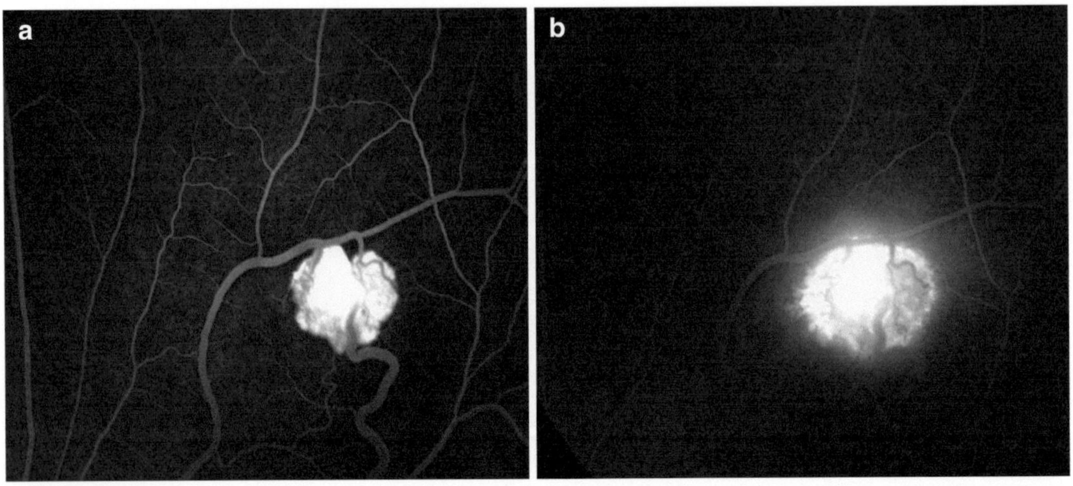

Fig. 15.9 Fundus fluorescein angiography (FFA) of RCH. Early phase (**a**) shows hyperfluorescence and late phase (**b**) shows leak

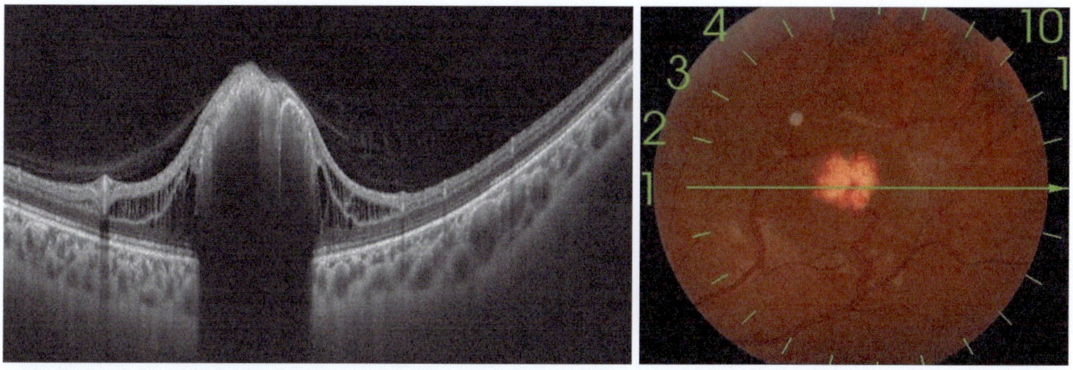

Fig. 15.10 OCT of RCH. Tumor is seen as a hyperreflective lesion with shadowing. Adjacent retina shows schisis of inner retina due to exudation

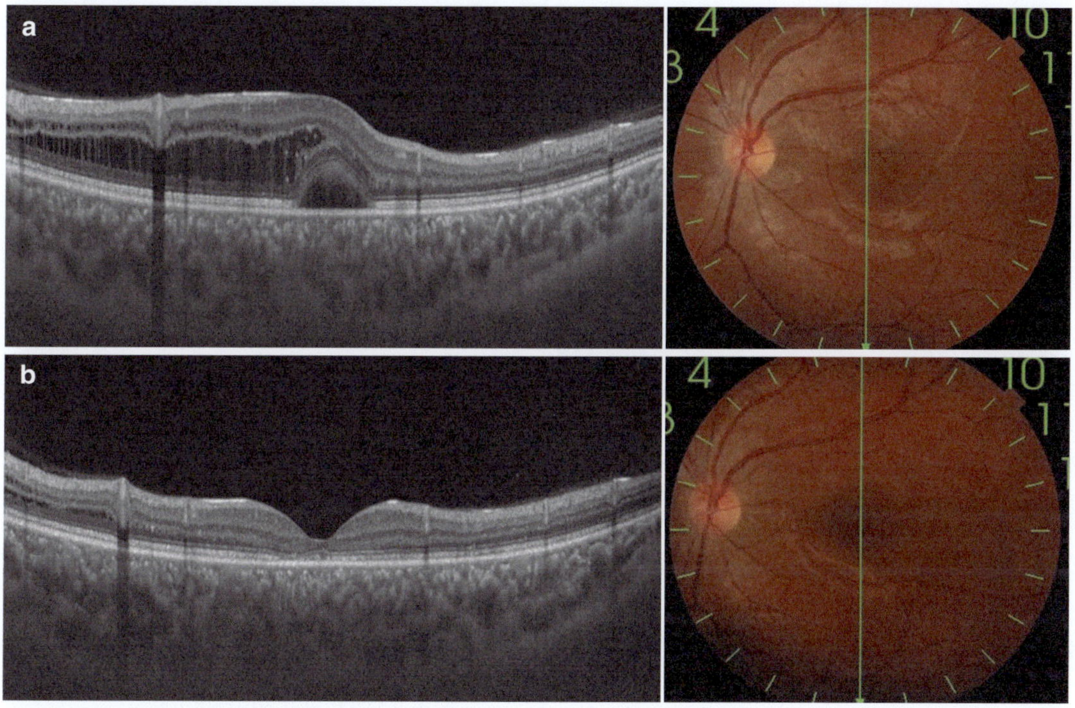

Fig. 15.11 Macular OCT of the same eye in Fig. 15.10. Pre-treatment image (**a**) shows macular edema with subfoveal fluid. Resolution of subretinal fluid (**b**) after laser photocoagulation of the tumor

- Racemose angioma: no tumor is seen between the arteriole and venule in racemose angioma (Fig. 15.13).
- Vasoproliferative tumor: usually seen in inferior retina; minimally dilated feeder vessels; usually solitary.
- Retinal macroaneurysm: occurs along a arteriole without a draining venule
- Retinal cavernous hemangioma: no feeder vessels; multiple sac like aneurysmal dilatations (grape like clusters).
- Familial exudative vitreoretinopathy
- Nematode endophthalmitis.

Peripapillary RCH: Simulate papilledema, optic neuritis, peripapillary choroidal neovascular membrane and optic disc granuloma.

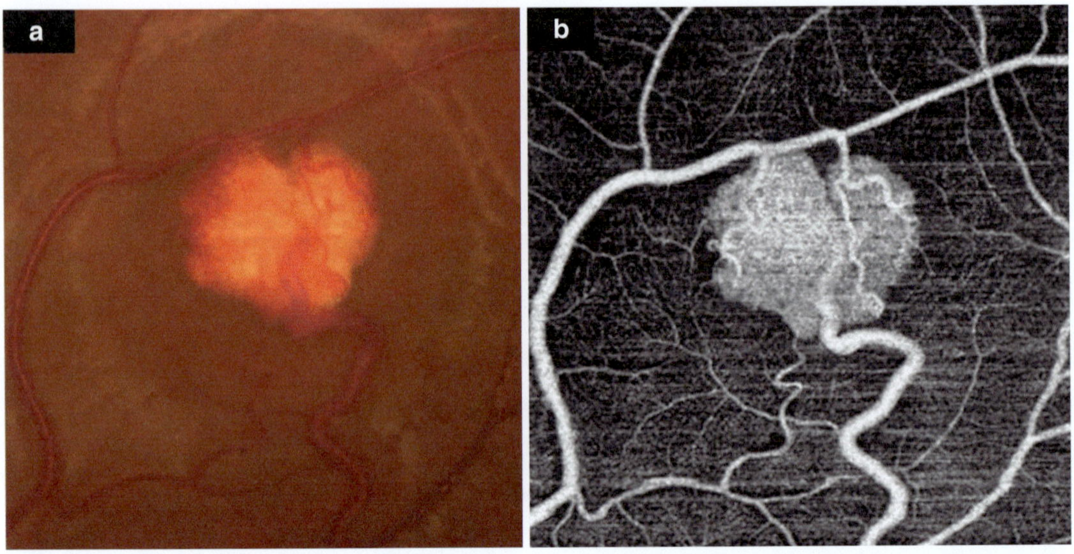

Fig. 15.12 OCTA of RCH. Tumor shows compact vascularity. Feeding and draining vessels can be identified

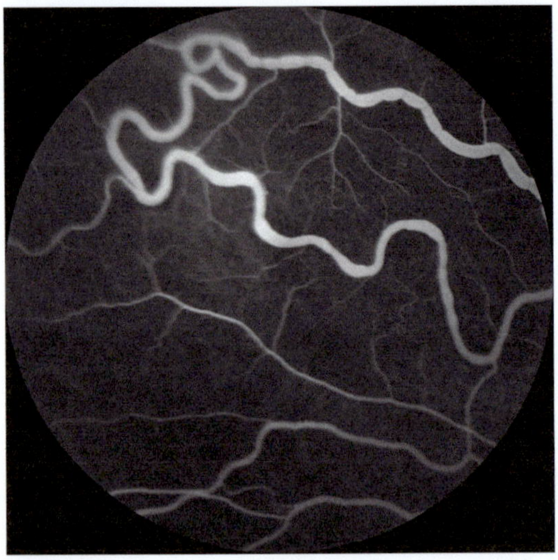

Fig. 15.13 FFA of a patient with racemose angioma. No tumor is seen between the arteriole and venule

15.2.7 Histopathology

The lesions are composed of benign proliferation of spindle and endothelial cells, pericytes, small blood vessels and clear stromal cells. The foamy stromal cells between the capillaries stain positive for glial fibrillary acid protein and neuron-specific enolase [23].

15.2.8 Diagnostic Criteria

15.2.8.1 VHL: (Old Criteria)

1. Positive family history
   - One or more of the following typical lesions
     - Hemangioblastoma of the CNS or eye
     - Multiple renal, pancreatic or hepatic cysts
     - Pheochromocytoma
     - Renal cell carcinoma
2. No family history
   - Two or more hemangioblastomas of the retina, spine or brain.

     or
   - a single hemangioblastoma in association with a visceral manifestation.

15.2.8.2 VHL: (New Criteria)

Definitive diagnosis: Positive for VHL gene.

15.2.8.3 Classification [24]

Type 1: VHL without pheochromocytoma.

Type 2: VHL with pheochromocytoma.

2A: Without renal cell carcinoma.

2B: With renal cell carcinoma and pancreatic involvement.

2C: With risk for pheochromocytoma only

Table 15.3 Surveillance of individuals with VHL syndrome

Sl. No	Condition	1st screening	Investigations	Frequency
1	Retinal hemangioblastoma	Infancy or early childhood (1 year)	Ophthalmoscopic examination	Annually
2	CNS hemangioblastoma	16 years of age	MRI brain and spine	2 yearly
3	Renal cell carcinoma	16 years of age	Ultrasound abdomen	Annually
			MRI abdomen	2 yearly
4	Pancreatic tumor	16 years of age	Ultrasound abdomen	Annually
			MRI abdomen	2 yearly
5	Pheochromocytoma	8 years of age	Blood pressure	Annually
			Urinary fractionated metanephrines	Annually
			Plasma normetanephrine levels[a], Adrenal imaging[a]	Annually

[a]In families at high-risk for pheochromocytoma

15.2.9 Surveillance

Surveillance should be considered in:

1. Individuals with VHL syndrome.
2. Those with a VHL pathogenic variant.
3. At-risk relatives of unknown genetic status.

Guidelines for surveillance is summarized in Table 15.3 [25].

15.2.10 Treatment

The choice of treatment is determined by the size, location, and associated findings such as subretinal fluid, retinal traction, and the visual potential of the eye.

It is proven that early treatment of RCH leads to better visual results [26].

Careful observation in a compliant patient can be recommended if the RCH is very small (up to 500 microns) and not associated with exudation or subretinal fluid and not visually threatening. Juxtapapillary tumors can be observed as they tend to remain stable [27].

Peripheral RCH without retinal detachment are treated with laser photocoagulation. It is preferable to use green, yellow or blue green wavelength to treat these lesions, as red or infrared lasers may not be absorbed well by the tumor.

Tumors <2 mm in diameter are treated with direct laser photocoagulation (Fig. 15.14).

For tumors 3–5 mm in diameter, it is preferable to try occlusion of the communicating vessels—the arteriole first, followed by the tumor and the venule. The RCH can be treated in multiple sessions. Complications such as hemorrhage from the tumor and secondary retinal detachment may occur after laser photocoagulation.

For tumors larger than 5 mm, it is preferable to use triple freeze thaw cryotherapy. Complications such as exudative retinal detachment and hemorrhage can occur after cryotherapy. Treatment of peripheral large tumors can result in vitreoretinal proliferation, resulting in traction or traction-rhegmatogenous retinal detachment, vitreous hemorrhage and in some cases circumferential fibrovascular proliferation of the vitreous base. The development of fibrovascular proliferation is multifactorial and is due to VEGF secretion by the tumor, altered vitreoretinal interface and increase in inflammation.

Transpupillary thermotherapy [28] and plaque brachytherapy have been employed in the management of retinal and disc angiomas [29].

Plaque brachytherapy of peripheral large tumors is a viable option and offers the ability to treat tumors elevated from the retinal surface due to vitreous traction. A radiation dose of 1250–2500 cGY delivered to the apex of the tumor (500–800 Gy scleral dose) results in regression of the tumor [30, 31].

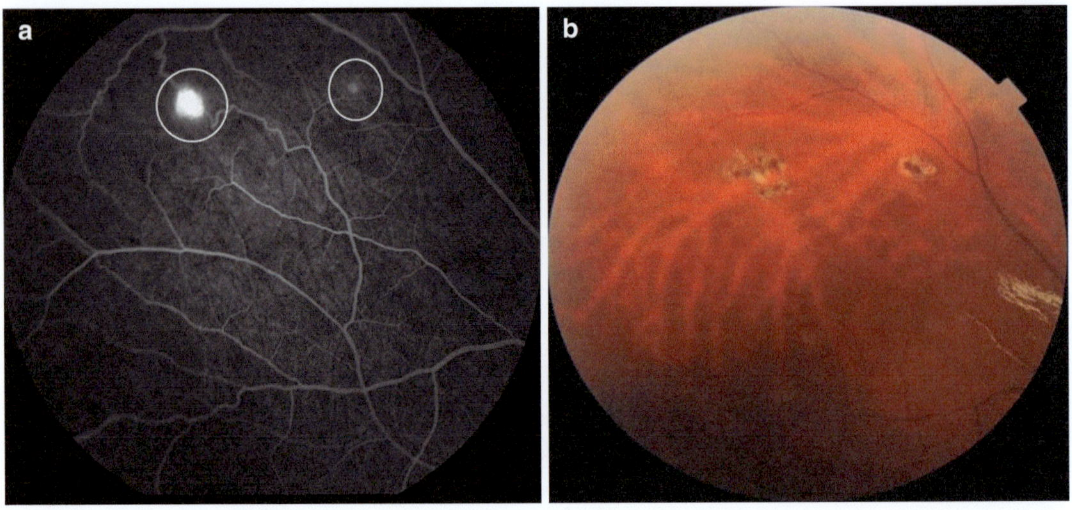

Fig. 15.14 Pre-treatment FFA of small RCHs (**a**). Tumors replaced by scarring after laser photocoagulation (**b**)

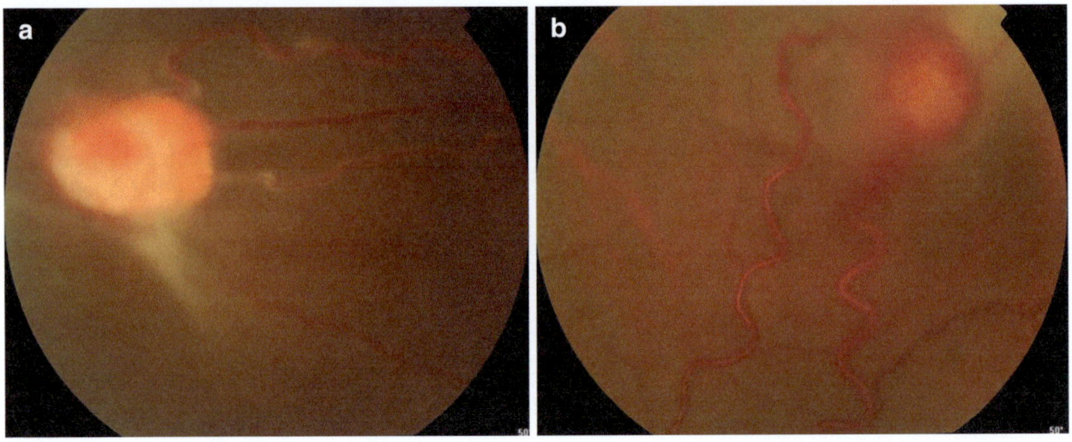

Fig. 15.15 Fundus photograph of a patient with multiple large RCH. Both the tumors; one in nasal quadrant (**a**) and one in superior quadrant (**b**) were treated with plaque brachytherapy in a single session. Initially the nasal tumor was treated with desired radiation dose. Then the plaque was shifted to the superior quadrant to treat the other tumor

Multiple large tumors in an eye can be treated in a single session by rotating the plaque to treat an untreated tumor once the desired dose of radiation has been delivered to one tumor (Fig. 15.15). A low penetrance plaque such as ruthenium 106 is preferable in such situations to limit the overall radiation dose delivered to the eye (Fig. 15.16).

Proton beam irradiation and external beam radiotherapy are used as salvage therapy when other treatments fail [32].

Photodynamic therapy (PDT) is preferred modality to treat peripapillary RCH. Standard fluence PDT leads to regression of the tumor and resolution of macular detachment. However it may be associated with risk of retinal vascular occlusion and optic disc ischemia [33].

Trans-retinal feeder vessel ligation combined with vitrectomy and photocoagulation has been reported in literature [34] and is performed infrequently by the authors.

While a successful ligation of the feeder vessel could be achieved and the tumor appeared to regress on short-term follow-up, the tumor generated new feeder vessels over time. Vitrectomy

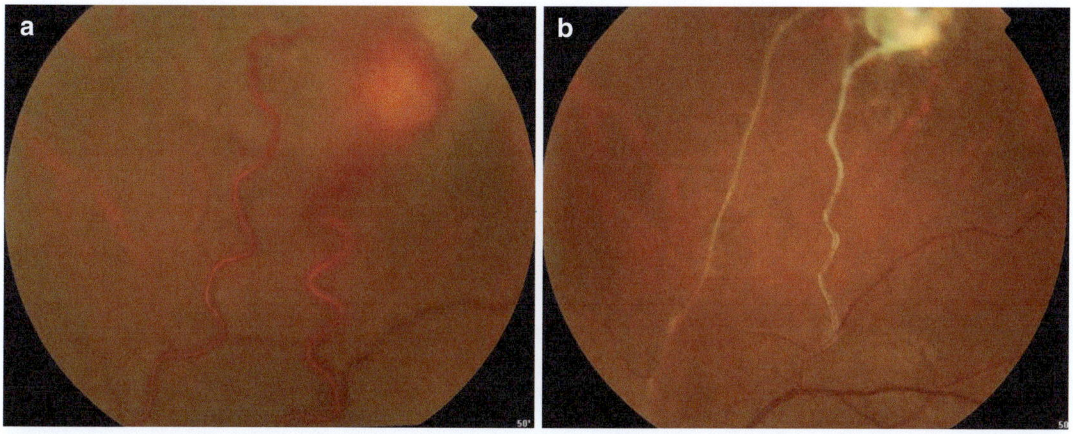

Fig. 15.16 Fundus photograph of same eye in Fig. 15.16. Pre brachytherapy (**a**) and post brachytherapy (**b**) images. Complete regression of tumor with sclerosis of feeding and draining vessels is evident

with excision of the tumor and extensive intraocular diathermy are other techniques that have been attempted to treat recalcitrant tumors. However, these extensive surgeries will not yield long-lasting results due to the severe vitreous base proliferation that occurs over time resulting in chronic hypotony.

If the tumors are associated with bullous retinal detachment, drainage of sub retinal fluid, cryotherapy and scleral buckling may be necessary. Advanced vitreoretinal form of the disease may need vitrectomy to treat tractional or rhegmatogenous retinal detachment [35] (Fig. 15.17).

Overtime we have moved away from aggressive vitreoretinal surgical techniques to multimodal therapy to treat advanced disease with multiple large hemangioblastomas with vitreoretinal complications. We employ brachytherapy to treat elevated or large tumors that could not be treated with cryotherapy or laser photocoagulation. Judicious vitrectomy to remove relevant vitreoretinal traction, such as that exerting traction on the posterior pole is employed. Scleral buckling is employed to support elevated RCH and peripheral vitreoretinal traction (rather than resort to resection of tumors or retinectomy). We are successful in stabilizing a subset of advanced vitreoretinal pathology associated with VHL with this technique.

Bevacizumab and ranibizumab have shown some beneficial effect on subretinal exudation and cystoid macular edema associated with juxtapapillary RCH and some peripheral retinal hemangioblastoma. Multiple injections are required and treatment is often combined with PDT and intravitreal or sub-tenon triamcinolone. The efficacy appears to be limited to the exudative component and does not bear any significance in decreasing the size of the lesions or the occurrence of newer ones. Anti- VEGF agents are useful to treat small lesions and as adjuncts in treating exudation associated with larger lesions [36, 37].

15.2.11 Prognosis

The high incidence of clear cell renal cell carcinoma associated with VHL syndrome results in an average life expectancy of 49 years in affected individuals. Other causes of morbidity and mortality are CNS hemangioblastomas, pheochromocytomas and pancreatic tumors. Protocol based surveillance followed by prompt treatment can however increase life expectancy.

Ocular prognosis depends on the number of tumors and activity. Many VHL patients progress rapidly with the development of numerous RCH leading to exudation and vitreoretinal complications resulting in bilateral blindness. Early and prompt treatment of small retinal tumors and regular monitoring can alleviate the associated morbidity to some extent.

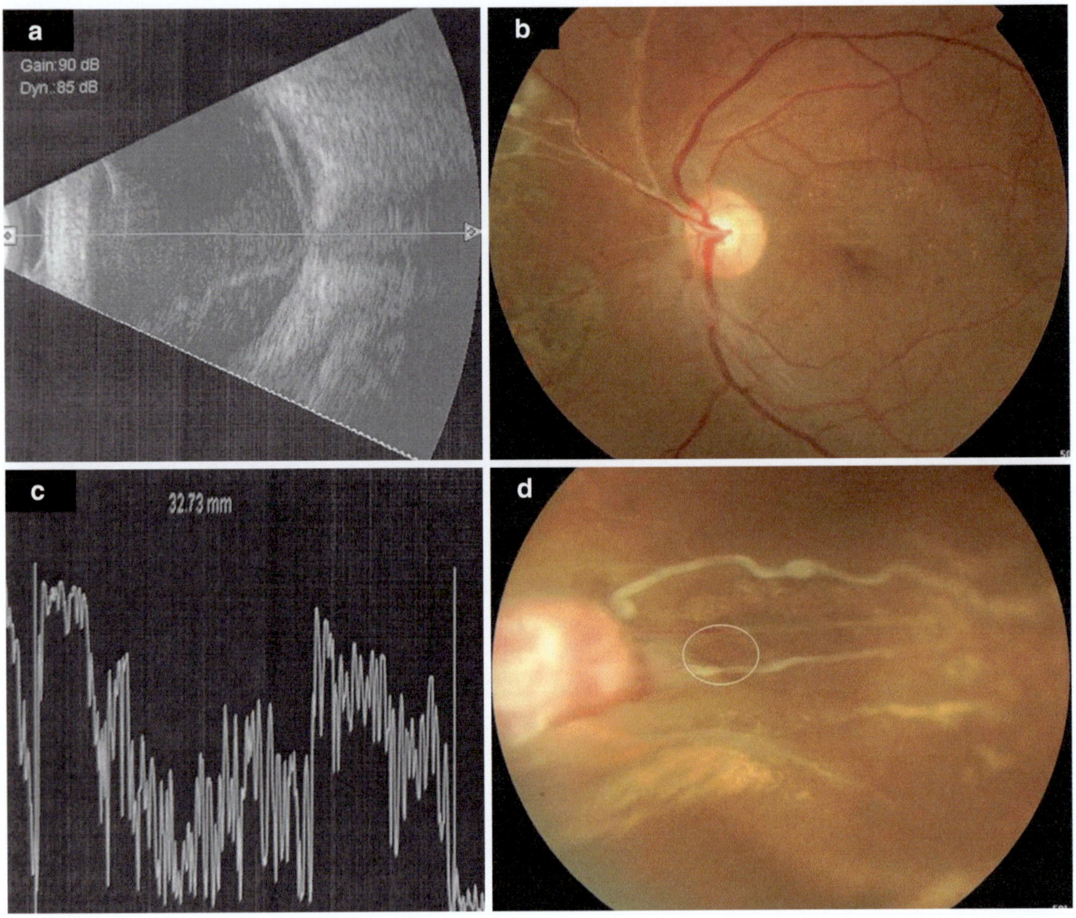

Fig. 15.17 Ultrasound image of the same eye in Fig. 15.15 after the development of retinal detachment with vitreous hemorrhage (**a**, **b**). Patient underwent vitreo-retinal intervention with encirclage. Post-operative images (**c**, **d**) showing attached retina. Rhegma (within circle) can be seen posterior to the tumor

15.3 Wyburn-Mason Syndrome

Wyburn-Mason syndrome (also known as Bonnet–Dechaumme–Blanc syndrome or retino-encepalofacial angiomatosis) was first described in 1943 when an association between racemose hemangiomatosis of the retina and arteriovenous malformations (AVMs) of the brain was noted [38, 39].

It is characterized by AVMs affecting the retina, visual pathways, midbrain and facial structures.

15.3.1 Epidemiology

It is extremely rare with no sexual or racial predilection.

Age at presentation: The AVMs are congenital; however asymptomatic small lesions may be diagnosed only later in life. Larger AVMs causing visual or neurologic impairment are diagnosed early in life.

Wyburn Mason syndrome is unilateral in most of the cases, but intracranial AVM can be located in the midline extending into both the sides.

15.3.2 Genetics and Pathophysiology

Inheritance: No definite hereditary pattern is seen.

The etiology and risk factors are unknown, but genetic factors may play a role. Vascular dysgenesis of the embryological anterior plexus occurring in the early gestational period may result in AVMs of Wyburn Mason syndrome. Depending on the timing of the insult during embryogenesis, the severity of the AVM varies [40].

15.3.3 Systemic Features

Wyburn Mason syndrome in its complete form is characterized by the presence of AVMs in the cranial cavity, orbit, along the visual pathway, facial skin, oropharynx and nasopharynx. Rarely AVMs involving the lung, spinal cord may co-exist [41].

AVM involving the bones of the skull, maxilla, and mandible may lead to massive bleeding during dental extraction. Intraocular AVM communicating with intramuscular facial AVM has been reported [42].

The clinical features and management of systemic features is summarized in Table 15.4 [43–45].

15.3.4 Ocular Features

15.3.4.1 Clinical Features

Symptoms

The macular location of the AVM can result in vision loss and the congenital nature of the disease leads to strabismus. In the absence of macular involvement, vision may be normal or minimally affected.

Signs

Arteriovenous communications in Wyburn Mason syndrome have been classified in to three types [46].

Table 15.4 Clinical features and management of systemic manifestations of Wyburn Mason syndrome

	Intracranial AVM	Orbital AVM	AVM of visual pathway	Facial skin	Oronasopharynx
Incidence	30–81%	Unknown	Unknown	Less common	Rarely reported
Location	Hypothalamus, thalamus, basal ganglion, midbrain		Optic chiasma, occipital lobe, optic nerve, Optic tract	Eyelids, cheeks, forehead	
Clinical features	Neuropsychiatric changes, headaches, seizures, stroke, hemiparesis, subarachnoid hemorrhage, intracerebral hemorrhages, increased intracranial pressure, papilledema, cranial neuropathies, hydrocephalus	Pulsating proptosis	visual-field abnormalities (homonymous hemianopia)	Present as a faint cutaneous discoloration to high-flow maxillofacial or mandibular AVMs Can cause life-threatening hemorrhage. Severe cosmetic and psychological problems	Potentially life-threatening oral hemorrhages or epistaxis
Management	Symptomatic management is preferred as lesions are diffuse and not amenable to surgical resection Endovascular embolization in an attempt to reduce the risk of bleeding or re-bleeding is reported	Observation			Intractable oronasal bleeding can be controlled by endovascular embolization of the vascular malformation

- Type 1: An abnormal capillary plexus is interposed between the arteriole and the venule. These lesions do not cause symptoms and are not usually associated with cerebral involvement.
- Type 2: No capillary bed is found and direct arteriovenous communication exists; patients experience few visual symptoms. Associated cerebral vascular malformation may be found.

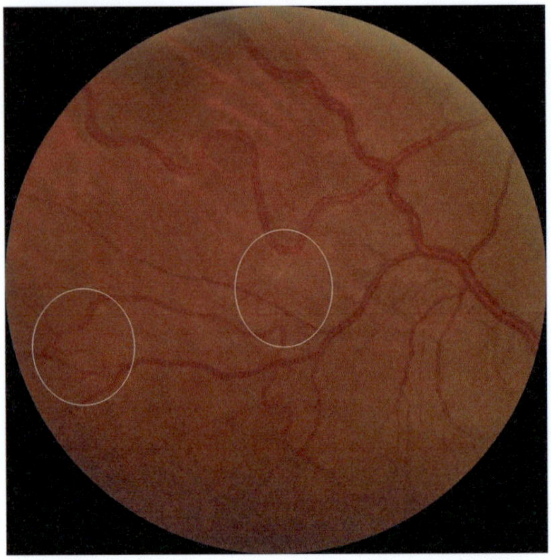

Fig. 15.18 Fundus photograph of a patient with racemose angioma showing direct arteriovenous communications (within circles) without intervening capillary bed

- Type 3: Patients have more complex and extensive arteriovenous malformation with visual loss and increased risk of cerebral disease. One or more dilated arterioles emanate from the disc, travel for a variable distance in the retina, form arteriovenous communication and return to the disc (Figs. 15.18 and 15.19). Exudation or retinal detachment usually does not occur. Visual loss may occur due to vaso-occlusion, nerve fiber loss caused by pressure on the optic nerve or the anterior visual pathway by the AVM, intra-retinal and vitreous hemorrhage and rarely macular exudation [47–49].

15.3.5 Diagnosis

The clinical appearance is characteristic and a fluorescein angiogram may show rapid filling of the arteriovenous communication without leakage (Fig. 15.20).

Racemose angioma may appear as large intraretinal cystic mass and rarely retinal changes such as atrophy, edema may be seen on the OCT.

15.3.6 Differential Diagnosis

RCH—Presence of a tumor between the feeding retinal arteriole and venule is suggestive of RCH.

Fig. 15.19 Fundus photograph of a patient with racemose angioma showing multiple dilated tortuous vessels arising from the disc. Occlusion with subsequent sclerosis of an arteriovenous malformation is seen (arrow)

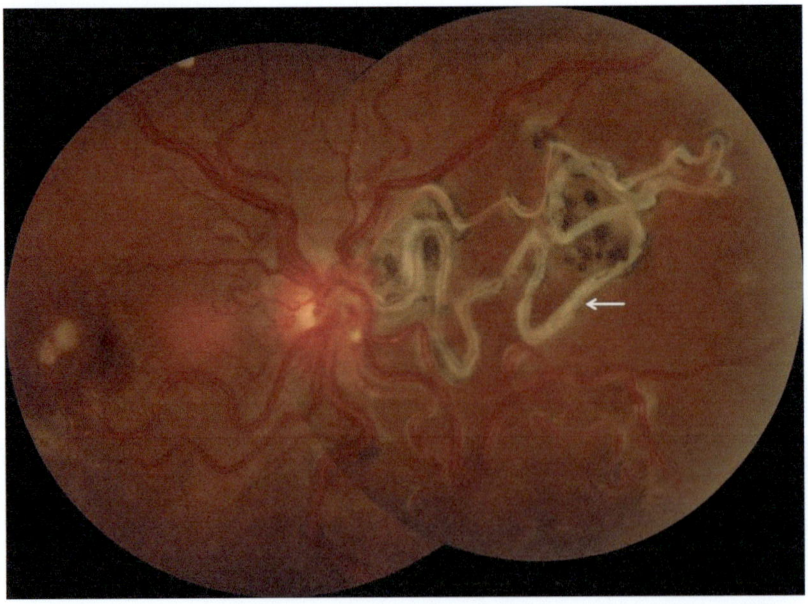

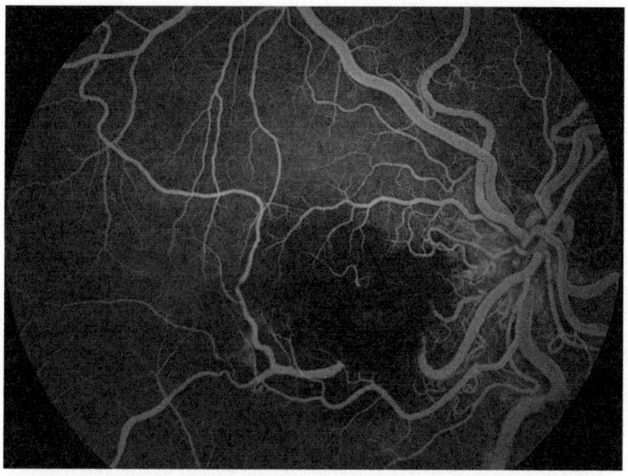

Fig. 15.20 FFA of the same eye in Fig. 15.19 showing macroaneurysm with adjacent blocked fluorescence due to hemorrhage

15.3.7 Treatment

Most lesions are stable and do not need treatment. However, the visual prognosis is poor. Rarely vitreous hemorrhage, subretinal hemorrhage and macular exudation have been described in racemose angioma. Vitrectomy has been employed for clearing non resolving vitreous hemorrhage [50]. Anti-VEGF agents have been employed to treat macular exudation [51].

15.4 Cavernous Hemangioma of the Retina

Cavernous hemangioma of the retina is also recognized as a phakomatoses with involvement of the retina, skin and the central nervous system.

15.4.1 Epidemiology

It is a rare tumor and is more prevalent in females [52].

The average age at presentation is 23 years. It is mostly unilateral with few reports of bilateral occurrences.

15.4.2 Genetics and Pathophysiology

Inheritance: Autosomal dominant. Penetrance and expressivity are variable.

The causative gene is localized to the region 7q11-q22 [53–55]. Its pathogenesis is largely unknown.

15.4.3 Systemic Features

Cavernous hemangioma of retina is so rare that our knowledge about its systemic features is restricted to a few case reports.

15.4.3.1 Cutaneous Cavernous Hemangioma

Multiple reddish purple lesions in skin described variably as capillary malformation, vascular lesion, angioma, vascular hamartoma, cavernous hemangioma are reported to occur in scalp, trunk, neck and arm [56].

Cutaneous vascular hamartoma without ocular lesions was described in an identical twin of patient with cavernous hemangioma of retina suggesting a common genetic defect underlying both cutaneous and retinal lesions [52].

Skin lesions are minimally elevated and do not blanch on pressure and are typical of mature cavernous hemangioma. Histopathological examination of the cutaneous lesion is consistent with cavernous hemangioma.

Vascular lesion is also reported under the tongue [57].

15.4.3.2 Intracranial Cavernous Hemangioma

Multiple intracranial cavernous hemangiomas are reported to occur in cerebrum, midbrain, pons and cerebellum. Affected individuals can develop seizures (most common manifestation), cranial nerve palsies and intracranial hemorrhage resulting in death [52, 58].

Hepatic cavernous angiomas may also occur [59].

15.4.3.3 Treatment

Surgical excision of intracranial cavernous hemangioma is employed with good results [60].

15.4.4 Ocular Features

Cavernous hemangioma may affect the macular or peripheral retina. Although retinal cavernous hemangioma is usually considered to be the only ocular manifestation of this autosomal dominant condition, other rarely reported ocular features include choroidal hemangioma [57] and ocular melanocytosis [61]. Cone dystrophy was noted in a patient with superonasal cavernous hemangioma [62].

15.4.4.1 Symptoms

Peripheral tumors are asymptomatic. Macular location of the tumor or complications such as intra-retinal hemorrhage at the macula, macular distortion due to epiretinal membrane proliferation, vitreous hemorrhage and amblyopia in children may lead to decrease in vision [63, 64].

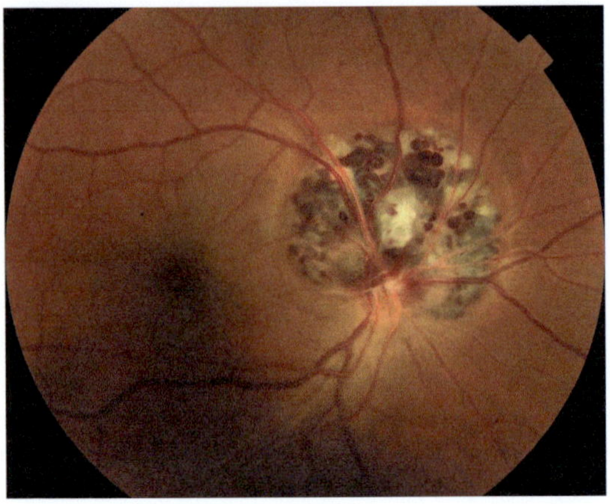

Fig. 15.21 Fundus photograph of cavernous hemangioma of optic disc. (Image courtesy: Dr. Madhukumar and Dr. Surabhi Ruia)

15.4.4.2 Signs

Cavernous hemangioma appears as a cluster of dark red saccules with associated fibroglial proliferation within the inner retinal layers or on the surface of the optic disc (Fig. 15.21). The lesions are variable in size and location, and frequently follow the course of a major retinal vein. No feeder arteriole or draining venule is usually seen though some authors have noted twin vessels to be associated with this tumor [65].

They are usually non-progressive. A few may enlarge and cause vitreous hemorrhage.

Exudation is not a feature of cavernous hemangioma of the retina. Epiretinal membranes and fibroglial proliferation may result in foveal ectopia and visual loss [64].

Massive growth of the tumor up to the iris root with concomitant vitreous hemorrhage and hyphema has been reported rarely [17].

15.4.5 Diagnosis

The diagnosis is evident on fundus examination and FFA is quite characteristic. Cavernous hemangioma has a sluggish circulation, which leads to the separation of the blood cells from the plasma, which settles down inferiorly within the saccule. Fluorescein enters the saccule slowly and fills the supernatant plasma, giving an appearance of 'fluorescein cap' (Fig. 15.22).

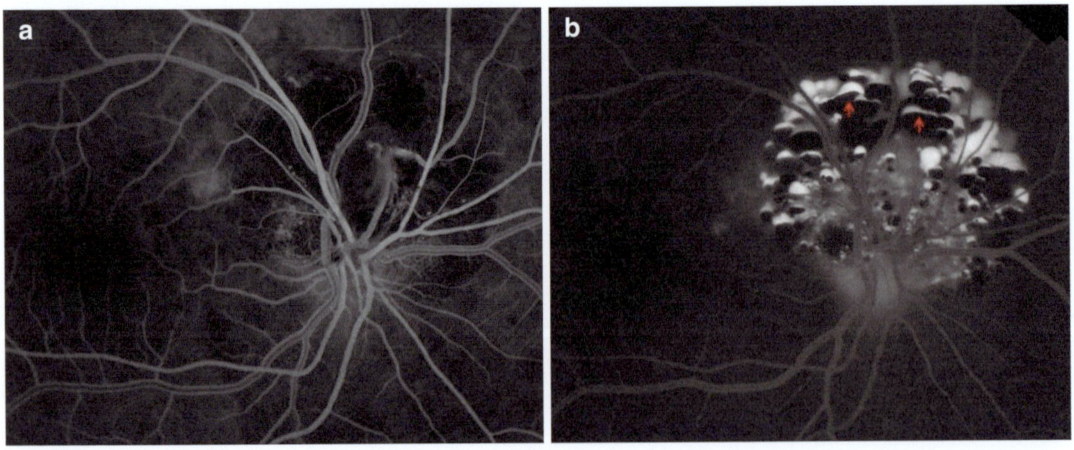

Fig. 15.22 Early (**a**) and late (**b**) phase FFA images of cavernous hemangioma of optic disc. Late phase image shows typical 'fluorescein caps' (arrows). (Image courtesy: Dr. Madhukumar and Dr. Surabhi Ruia)

Magnetic resonance image (MRI) of brain may be considered to rule out presence of intracranial lesions.

15.4.6 Differential Diagnosis

Coat's disease.

Leber multiple miliary aneurysm.

15.4.7 Treatment

Cavernous hemangioma of the retina is usually stable and does not require treatment. Some cases can develop vitreous hemorrhage. In such cases cryotherapy, laser photocoagulation, low energy plaque and vitrectomy to clear the vitreous hemorrhage may be employed. Vitrectomy may be considered for removing epimacular membranes. Associated retinal changes such as cystoid macular edema may however limit vision recovery [66].

We treated a patient with recurrent subretinal and vitreous hemorrhage secondary to a cavernous hemangioma of the optic disc with standard photodynamic therapy (PDT) after the resolution of hemorrhage. The cavernous hemangioma regressed after PDT [67] (Fig. 15.23).

15.5 Sturge-Weber Syndrome

Sturge-Weber syndrome (SWS) is a neurocutaneous syndrome affecting the leptomeninges, facial skin in the ophthalmic and maxillary distributions

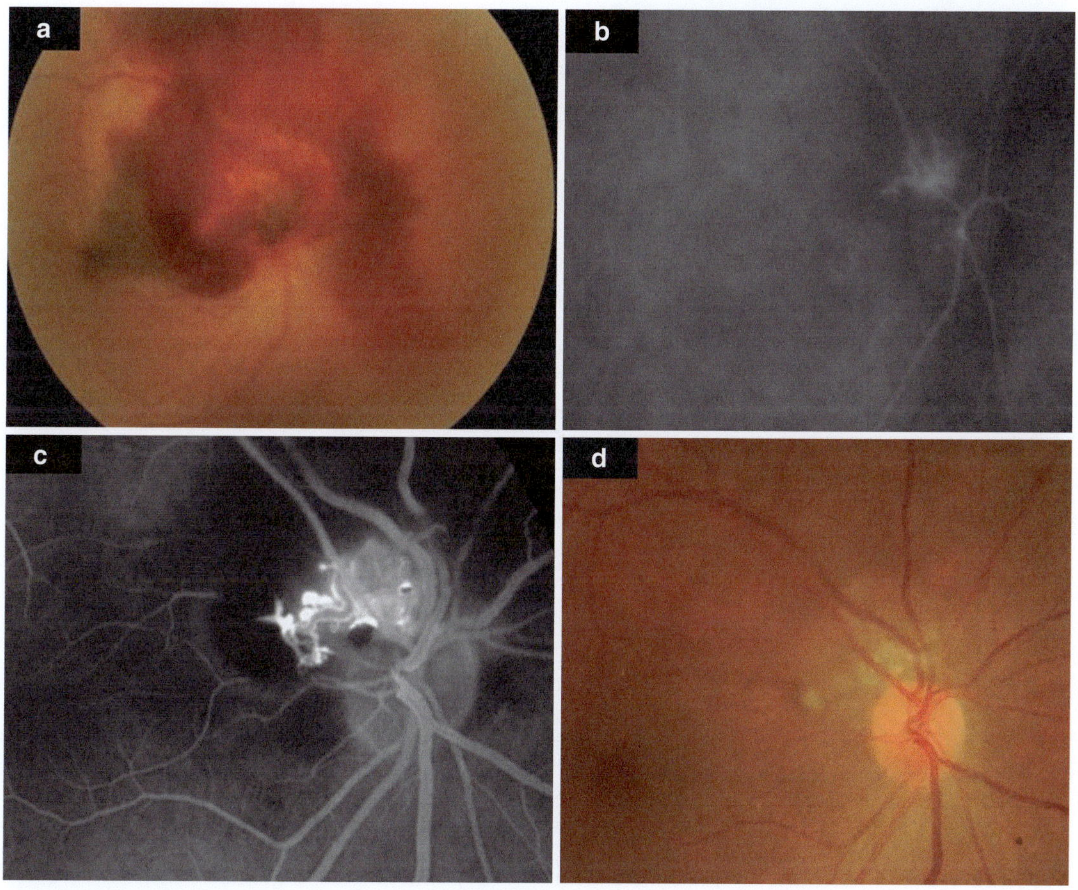

Fig. 15.23 Color photograph (**a**), FFA (**b**), indocyanine green angiography (**c**) of cavernous hemangioma of disc showing subretinal and vitreous hemorrhage. Complete resolution of the tumor with gliosis after photodynamic therapy (**d**)

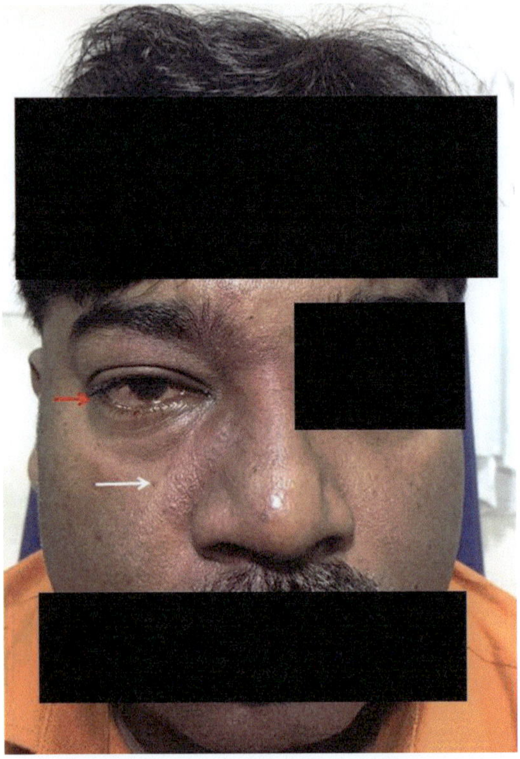

Fig. 15.24 Face photograph of a patient with SWS. Port wine stain is seen involving the skin of upper lid, lower lid, nose and upper lip (white arrow). Conjunctival congestion (red arrow) is seen due to episcleral and conjunctival vessels. Fundus examination of the patient showed a solitary choroidal hemangioma

of the trigeminal nerve (encephalotrigeminal angiomatosis) (Fig. 15.24). It is associated with leptomeningeal angioma, facial port-wine stain (PWS) and glaucoma in its complete form.

15.5.1 Epidemiology [68]

Incidence: 1 in 50,000.

No sexual or racial predilection.

15.5.2 Genetics and Pathogenesis

Inheritance is sporadic.

Sturge-Weber syndrome is associated with somatic mosaicism. A gain of function mutation (p.Arg183Gln) in GNAQ gene on chromosome 9q21 is seen in skin and brain samples. GNAQ encodes guanine nucleotide binding protein which is involved in activation of mitogen-activated protein kinase (MAPK) pathway. The MAPK pathway is a chain of proteins in the cell that communicates a signal from a cell surface receptor to the DNA. The somatic substitutions in GNAQ encoding p.Gln209Leu and p. Arg183Gln are found in patients with uveal melanoma. p.Gln209Leu is more commonly seen in uveal melanoma. But he MAPK signal transduction induced by p.Arg183Gln (seen in SWS) is weaker and less promiscuous than the effect of the substitution p.Gln209Leu (seen in uveal melanoma) [69].

Before the discovery of GNAQ mutation, SWS was assumed to be due to failure of normal regression of the vascular plexus around the cephalic portion of the neural tube that is destined to become facial skin. This residual vascular tissue would form the angiomas of the leptomeninges, face and ipsilateral eye [70].

15.5.3 Classification (Roach) [71]

Type 1: Facial PWS and leptomeningeal angiomatosis, with or without associated glaucoma.

Type 2: Facial PWS and no leptomeningeal involvement, with or without glaucoma (most common form).

Type 3: Only leptomeningeal angiomatosis (least common).

15.5.4 Systemic Features

Systemic manifestations of SWS are restricted to facial skin and cranial cavity.

Facial port-wine stain is present at birth in a typical patient. A child with a port-wine stain on the face has 6% chance of having the SWS [72]. If the port-wine stain is located in the distribution of the ophthalmic branch of the trigeminal nerve the risk increases to 26% [73].

Leptomeningeal angioma commonly involves the parietal and occipital cortex resulting in progressive, characteristic calcifications in the external layers of the cerebral cortex and cortical atrophy underlying the angioma.

Clinical features and management of systemic manifestations of SWS is summarized in Table 15.5 [74–76].

15.5.5 Ocular Features

The bulbar conjunctiva may show diffuse or localized area of pinkish discoloration related to increased conjunctival vascularization. Episcleral vessel dilatation can be observed in approximately 50% of SWS patients [77].

Secondary glaucoma is the most common ocular manifestation. It occurs most commonly in early life (60% presenting at birth or early infancy; 30% in childhood). Glaucoma is often ipsilateral to the facial port-wine stain but may develop in contralateral eye rarely.

Theories explaining glaucoma in SWS are [77, 78]:

- Increased episcleral venous pressure due to AV shunts in episcleral hemangioma
- Congenital malformation of anterior chamber angle

Table 15.5 Clinical features and management of systemic manifestations of SWS

	Location	Age at presentation	Clinical features	Clinical course	Diagnosis	Treatment
Port-wine stain	Along V1 distribution: Upper lid, frontal region[a] Less often in V2 distribution Usually unilateral, but can also be bilateral	Birth	Color varies from pink to purple	Soft tissue hypertrophy, bony hypertrophy, formation of proliferative nodules or progressive ectasia, excessive growth of jaw and maxilla, facial deformation	Clinical	Pulsed dye laser is the treatment of choice Hemoporfin photodynamic therapy is also reported to be effective
Leptomeningeal angiomatosis[b]	Ipsilateral to PWS Occipital and occipito-parietal lobe Usually unilateral but can also be bilateral	First year of life	Seizures, slowly progressive hemiparesis, migraine-like vascular headaches, delayed neuropsychological development, episodes similar to cerebrovascular events with acute transient hemiplegia, visual field defects, behavioral problems	Progressive neurological deterioration. Recurrent seizures can lead to cognitive decline	Contrast enhanced MRI is the modality of choice	Anticonvulsant therapy to prevent and treat seizures Aspirin in anti-platelet dose to prevent episodes of ischemia resulting from venous stasis and thrombotic events Excision of the lesion Corpus callosotomy and hemispherectomy in intractable cases

V1 = Ophthalmic branch of trigeminal nerve; V2 = Maxillary branch of trigeminal nerve

[a]V1 involvement is associated with high risk of leptomeningeal angioma

[b]Symptoms are due to secondary changes in underlying brain due to hypoxia. It may be atrophic and show neuronal loss, astrocytosis, cortical dysgenesis, and calcifications distributed perivascularly or in the cerebral cortex

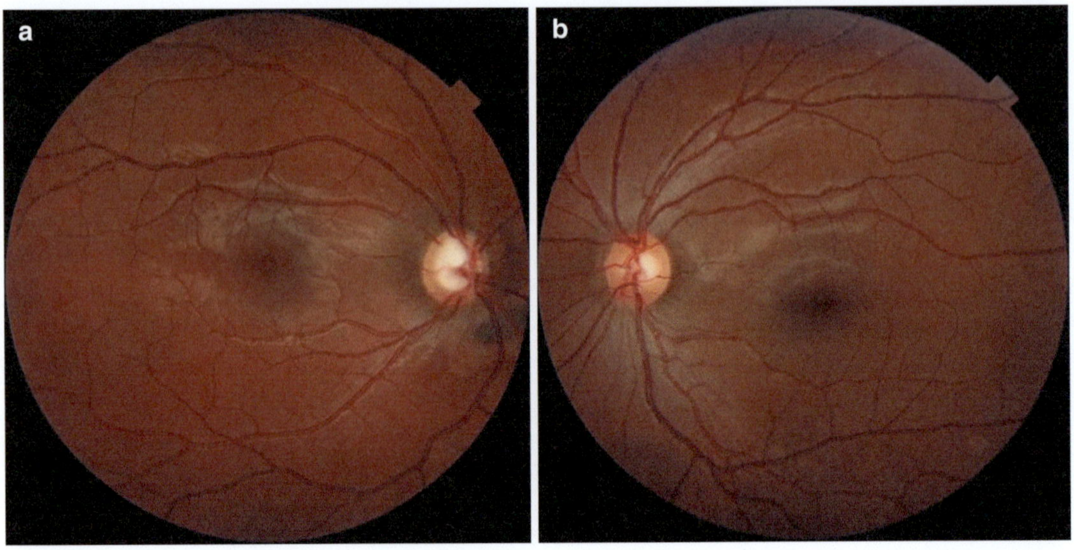

Fig. 15.25 Fundus photograph of right (**a**) and left eye (**b**) of a patient with port wine stain involving right side of face. Asymmetry of optic disc is evident

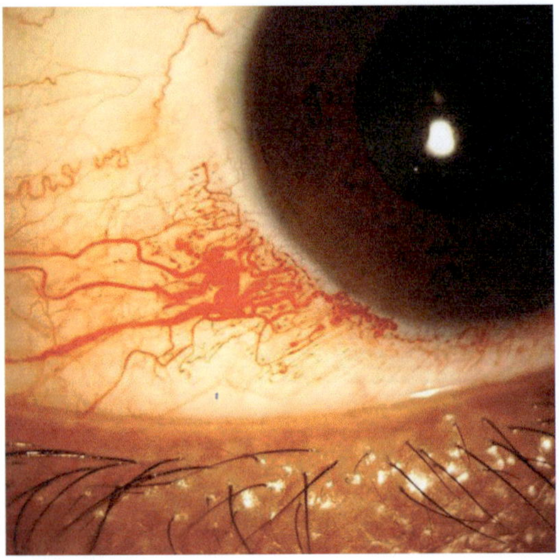

Fig. 15.26 Slit lamp photograph of patient in Fig. 15.24 showing dilated, tortuous episcleral and conjunctival vessels

- Increased fluid production from the ciliary body
- Premature aging of the trabecular meshwork–Schlemm's canal complex.

Ipsilateral congenital glaucoma can develop, particularly when port wine stain involves the upper lid. Asymmetry of optic disc with enlargement of the optic cup can be seen [79] (Fig. 15.25).

Other ocular manifestations include diffuse choroidal hemangioma, conjuntival or episcleral hemangiomas [80] (Fig. 15.26).

15.5.5.1 Diffuse Choroidal Hemangioma

Clinical Features

Symptoms

Diffuse choroidal hemangiomas are usually recognized in early childhood as they can cause visual impairment due to hyperopic amblyopia, exudative retinal detachment or glaucomatous optic nerve damage. However, the presence of facial PWS may prompt a fundus examination in an otherwise asymptomatic patient.

Signs

The pupil shows a brilliant red reflex (tomato catsup fundus) in the involved eye in contrast to the normal reflex in the opposite pupil [81].

On ophthalmoscopy a diffuse red-orange thickening of the posterior choroid is seen mainly in the macular area (Fig. 15.27). Cystoid degeneration in the overlying retina with retinal pigment epithelial disruption commonly occurs (Fig. 15.28). In comparison to circumscribed choroidal hemangioma, the diffuse choroidal hemangioma is frequently large and often extends anterior to the equator.

15.5.6 Diagnosis

Ultrasonography demonstrates a markedly thickened choroid with medium to high internal reflectivity with an overlying retinal detachment (Fig. 15.29). FFA reveals widespread early phase hyperfluorescence with diffuse leakage. On MRI, the tumor is relatively hyperintense in T1 weighted images and isointense to the vitreous in T2 weighted images. The tumor shows a marked enhancement with gadolinium (Fig. 15.30). Choroidal thickening corresponding to the lesion can be identified on OCT (Fig. 15.31). Subtle tumors can be identified and delineated on OCT (Fig. 15.32). Irregular vascular network distinct from the normal choroid can be appreciated on OCTA (Fig. 15.33).

MRI brain is recommended in patients between 3 and 6 months of age as it is difficult to detect them in first 3 months.

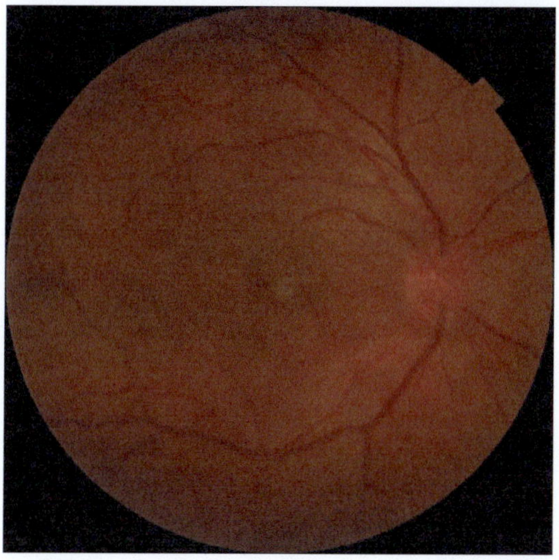

Fig. 15.27 Fundus photograph of an eye with diffuse choroidal hemangioma, showing orange red discoloration of the macula

15.5.7 Differential Diagnosis

Benign reactive lymphoid hyperplasia of choroid.

Leukemic choroidal infiltration.

Diffuse posterior scleritis.

Uveal effusion syndrome.

15.5.8 Histopathology

Diffuse choroidal hemangioma is characterized by an intermixed proliferation of small and large blood vessels and is usually classified as a mixed hemangioma. Fibrous transformation of the proliferated retinal pigment epithelium is observed in over 50% of diffuse choroidal hemangiomas in SWS.

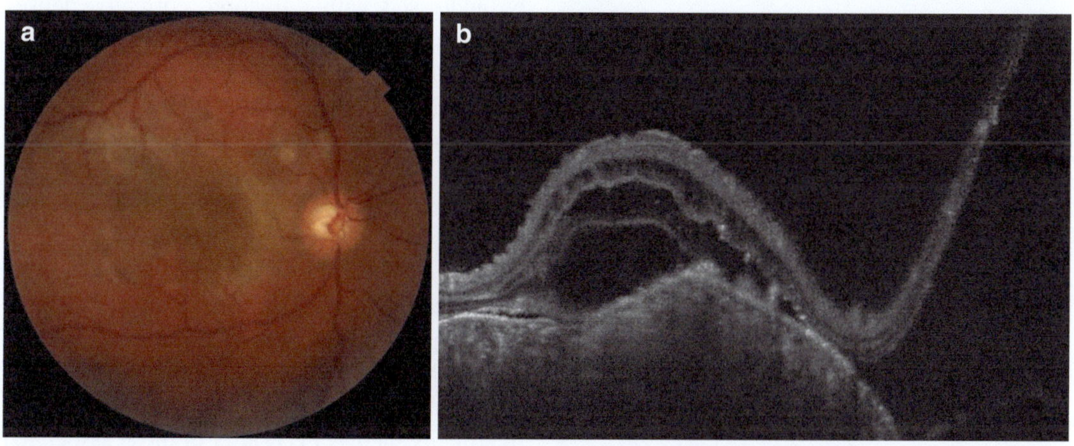

Fig. 15.28 Fundus photograph (**a**) and OCT (**b**) of an eye with diffuse choroidal hemangioma showing cystoid degeneration in the overlying retina with retinal pigment epithelial disruption and gliosis

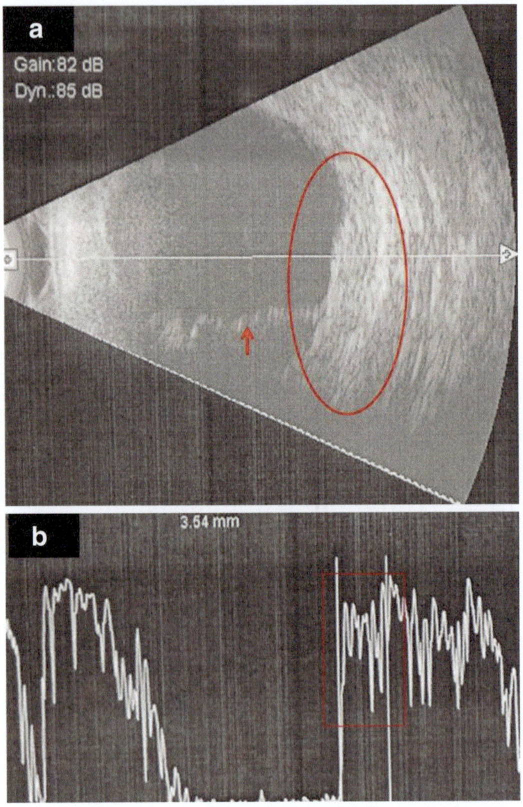

Fig. 15.29 B scan (**a**) and A scan (**b**) images of eye in Fig. 15.27 demonstrating a markedly thickened choroid (within circle) with medium to high internal reflectivity (within square) with an overlying retinal detachment (arrow)

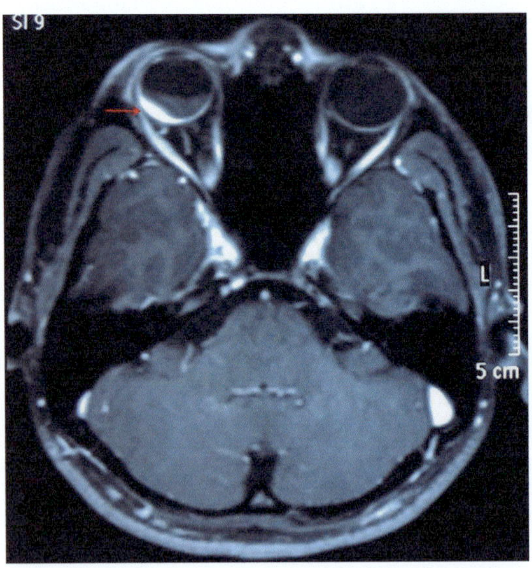

Fig. 15.30 Contrast enhanced MRI of diffuse choroidal detachment showing intense enhancement (arrow)

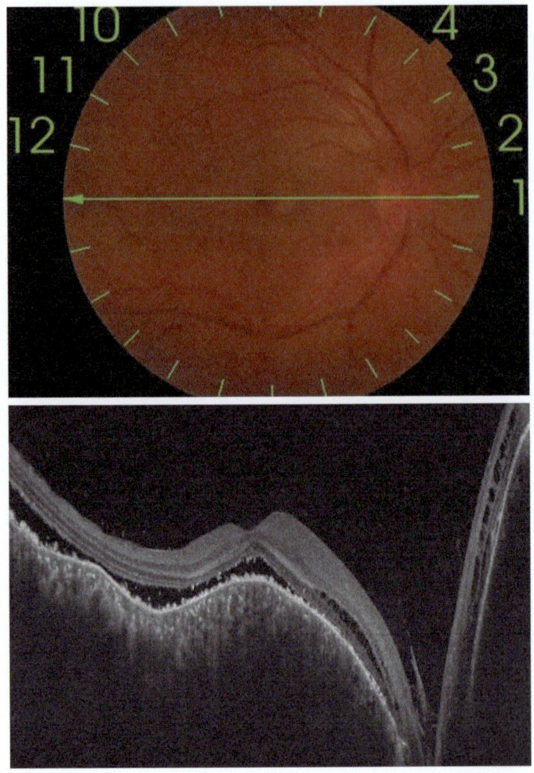

Fig. 15.31 OCT of eye in Fig. 15.27 showing choroidal thickening corresponding to the lesion. Subfoveal fluid is seen

15.5.9 Treatment

Diffuse choroidal hemangioma is a difficult condition to manage. Hyperopic refractive error can be addressed with refraction, corrective lenses and amblyopia therapy [82].

Photodynamic therapy is the preferred option to treat diffuse choroidal hemangioma with minimal subretinal fluid which would allow therapy. A single spot over the thickest part of the tumor or multiple non-overlapping spots of single or multiple sessions has resulted in resolution of exudative retinal detachment and regression of the tumor [83].

External beam radiation therapy in the dose of 1250–2000 cGy in divided fractions can be used to treat diffuse tumors that are too large for focal treatments such as PDT, laser or those associated with exudative retinal detachment that precludes visualization of the tumor [84]. Radiation leads

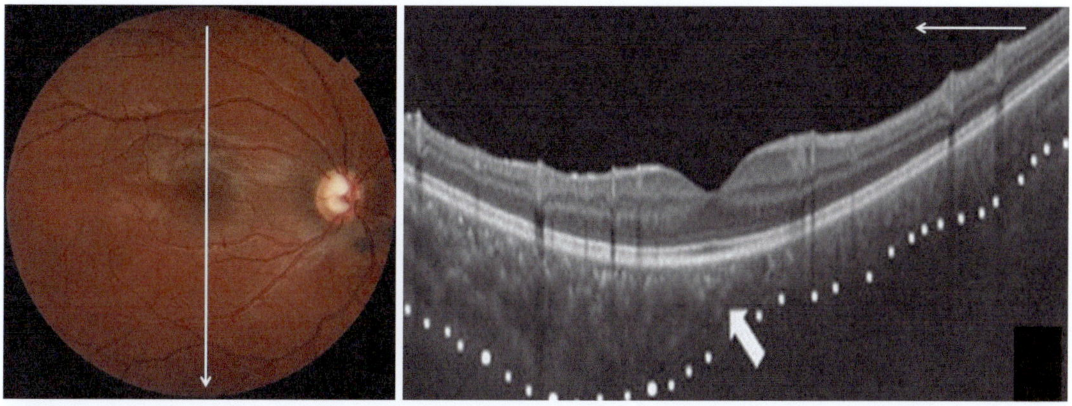

Fig. 15.32 Fundus photo and OCT of the eye in Fig. 15.25. Subtle orange hue is seen in inferior macula on color photo. But OCT shows choroidal thickening with a sharp delineation from normal choroid confirming the presence of diffuse choroidal hemangioma

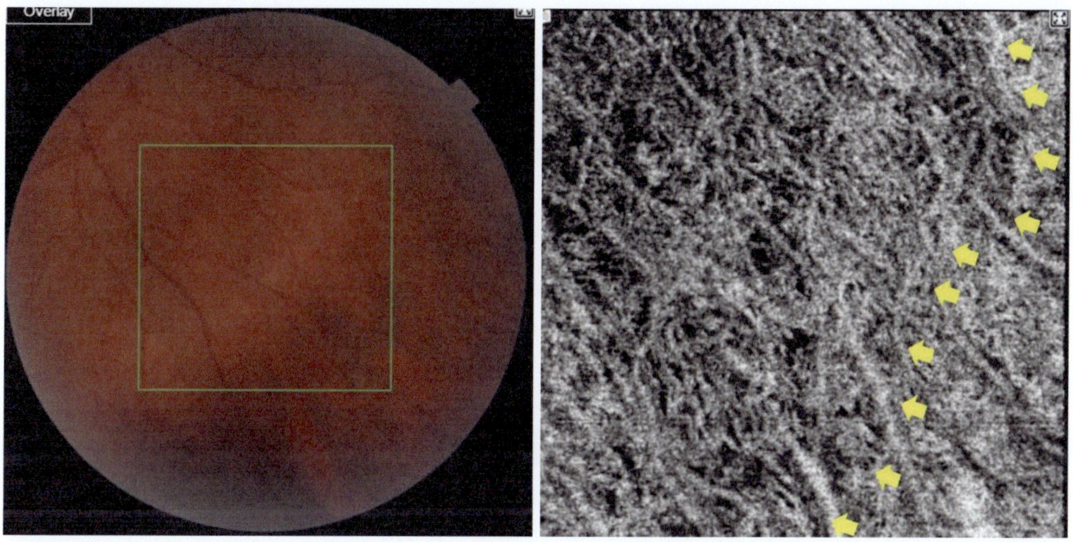

Fig. 15.33 OCTA of subtle diffuse choroidal hemangioma. Part of OCTA to the left of arrows shows irregular choroidal vascular pattern distinct from normal choroid. Normal choroid is seen on the right side

to resolution of the retinal detachment in most cases and control of glaucoma in some cases (Figs. 15.34 and 15.35).

Plaque brachytherapy can also be employed to treat eyes with the plaque being centered on the thickest part of the tumor [85]. (Fig. 15.36).

Propranolol, a nonselective β blocker in the dosage of 2 mg/kg/day has been noted to cause accelerated absorption of the exudative retinal detachment in some cases. The mechanism of action is unclear. Propranolol interferes with endothelial cells, vascular tone, angiogenesis, apoptosis and may lead to the resolution of the retinal detachment [86].

A single intravitreal bevacizumab injection resulted in sustained resolution of exudative retinal detachment in Sturge-Weber syndrome over 20 months in a single case [87].

We treated diffuse choroidal hemangioma with bullous retinal detachment resistant to systemic propranolol and brachytherapy, with drainage of subretinal fluid and intra-operative transpupillary thermotherapy (TTT), resulting in resolution of the retinal detachment, regression of the tumor

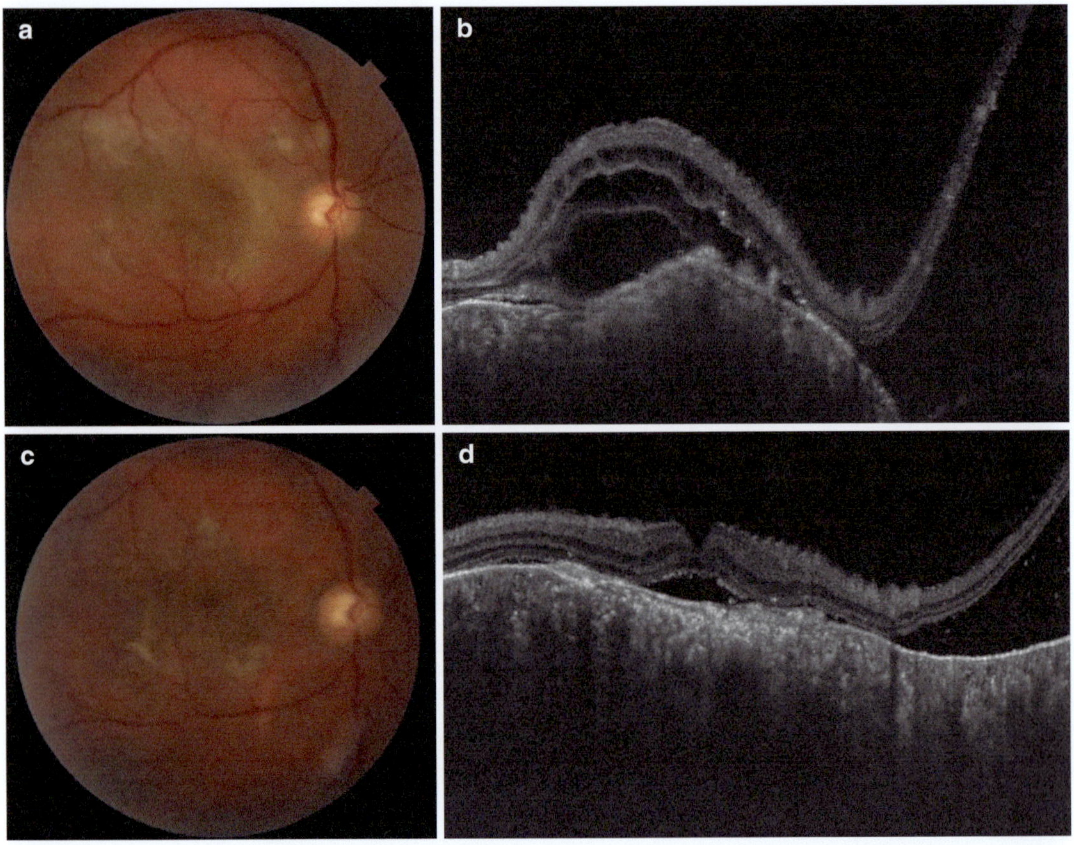

Fig. 15.34 Pre-treatment color photograph and OCT of diffuse choroidal hemangioma (**a**, **b**). Flattening of choroid, decrease in subretinal fluid and intra retinal fluid (**c**, **d**) is evident after external beam radiation (EBRT)

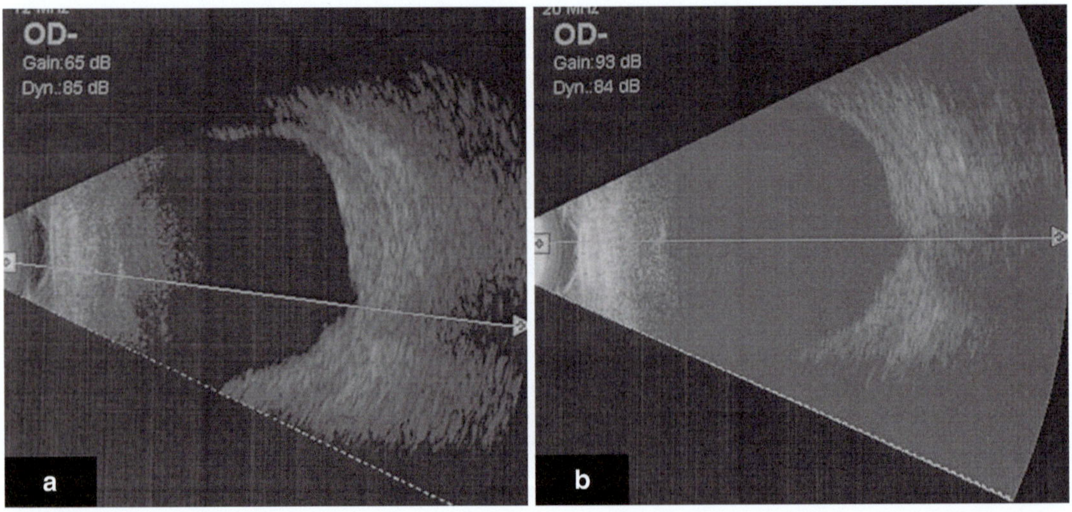

Fig. 15.35 Pre-treatment (**a**) and post treatment (EBRT) (**b**) ultrasound images of diffuse choroidal hemangioma. Decrease in choroidal thickness is evident

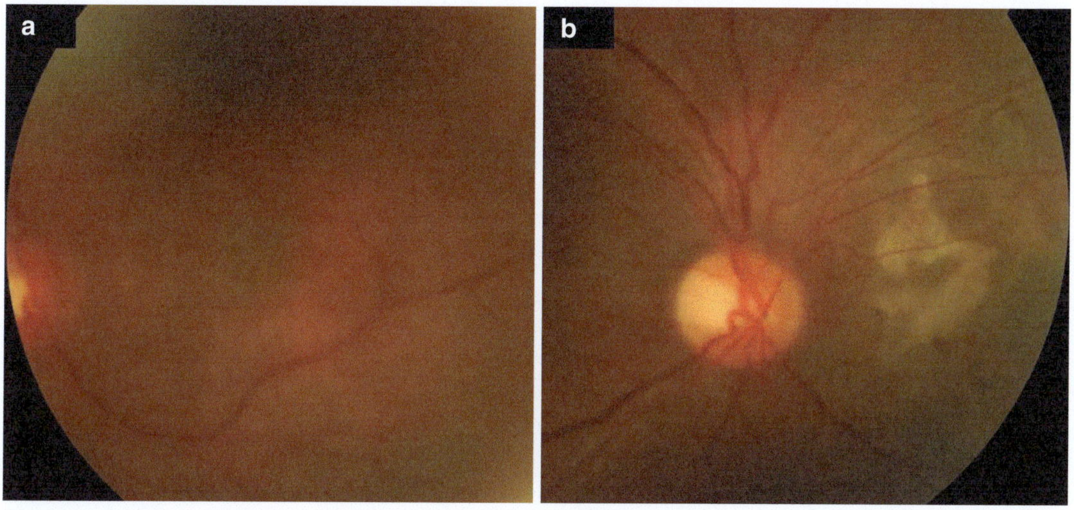

Fig. 15.36 Pre-treatment (**a**) and post treatment (plaque brachytherapy) (**b**) color photograph of choroidal hemangioma in a patient with SWS. Decrease in tumor height with gliosis is evident

and control of associated glaucoma. In TTT, infrared laser is employed to raise the internal tumor temperature above 45 °C but below 60 °C [88]. The chorioretinal scar observed after treatment is less pronounced in comparison to photocoagulation. Concomitant ICG can be used to augment the effect of TTT [89]. Transpupillary thermotherapy can result in complications such as cystoid macular edema, preretinal fibrosis, and retinal vascular occlusion making TTT unsuitable for subfoveal and peripapillary tumors [90].

Management of glaucoma is also complicated. Medical management is not sufficient in management of glaucoma associated with SWS. Risk of serous or hemorrhagic choroidal detachments is high with glaucoma filtering surgery in patients with diffuse choroidal hemangioma. Drainage devices may be necessary to control intraocular pressure. In resistant cases, cyclodestructive procedures such as cyclocryotherapy or cyclophotocoagulation may be necessary. Prostaglandin analogues in shown to be effective in decreasing the intraocular pressure in Sturge-Weber syndrome [91, 92] but should be used with caution as it increases the risk of uveal effusion [93, 94].

15.5.10 Prognosis

Visual prognosis depends on the location of the tumor (predominantly submacular tumor results in hyperopic amblyopia), age at onset of glaucoma (early age—poorer prognosis), presence of exudative retinal detachment, response to treatment (resolution of exudative retinal detachment and IOP control) and macular changes post treatment (pigmentary changes involving the macula or macular atrophy).

Poor systemic outcome is associated with early onset of seizures, extensive leptomeningeal angioma, development of hemiparesis and progressive cortical atrophy and deterioration of cognitive function.

15.6 Tuberous Sclerosis

Tuberous sclerosis complex (TSC) is a genetic disorder characterized by presence of multiple hamartomas involving the central nervous system, eye, skin, kidneys, heart, lung and liver.

15.6.1 Epidemiology

Incidence is 1 in 5000–6800. Prevalence is 1 in 10,000 (50–84% sporadic).

15.6.2 Genetics and Pathogenesis

Inheritance—Autosomal dominant.

TSC is caused by mutations in TSC1 or TSC2 genes located on 9q34 and 16p13 encoding hamartin and tuberin, respectively. TSC1 and TSC2 are tumor suppressor genes [95]. The hamartin–tuberin complex, is a critical negative regulator of mTORC1 (mammalian target of rapamycin complex 1). As mTORC1 activity controls anabolic processes to promote cell growth, loss of its inhibition promotes uncontrolled cell growth [96].

15.6.3 Systemic Features

Clinical features and management of systemic manifestations of TSC is summarized in Tables 15.6 and 15.7 [97–101].

15.6.3.1 Diagnostic Criteria

Tuberous Sclerosis Complex

Definite diagnosis: 2 major features or 1 major + 2 minor features.

Possible diagnosis: 1 major feature
or
1 major and 1 minor feature
or
≥2 minor features

Major Criteria

1. Hypomelanotic macules (≥3, at least 5 mm diameter)
2. Angiofibroma (≥3) or fibrous cephalic plaque (Fig. 15.37)
3. Shagreen patch
4. Ungual fibroma (≥2)
5. Multiple retinal hamartoma
6. Subependymal nodule (≥2) (Fig. 15.38)
7. Cortical dysplasia (≥3)
8. Subependymal giant cell astrocytomas
9. Cardiac rhabdomyoma
10. Lymphangioleiomyomatosis
11. Angiomyolipomas (≥2)

Minor criteria

1. Confetti skin lesions
2. Dental enamel pits (≥3)
3. Intraoral fibroms (≥2)
4. Retinal achromatic patch
5. Multiple renal cysts
6. Nonrenal hamartoma

Tuberous Sclerosis Complex (Genetic Diagnosis)

Identification of either a TSC1 or TSC2 pathogenic mutation in DNA from normal tissue is diagnostic.

15.6.4 Surveillance

Surveillance of individuals with TSC is essential in order to identify and monitor the visceral lesions. Recommendations of the 2012 International Tuberous Sclerosis Complex Consensus Conference is summarized in Tables 15.8 and 15.9 [101].

15.6.5 Ocular Features

Around 50% of patients with tuberous sclerosis have astrocytic hamartoma. It may be the first manifestation of the disease and is one of the major criteria for diagnosis of tuberous sclerosis [102, 103].

15.6.5.1 Symptoms

Patients are often asymptomatic with the lesion being detected on fundus examination.

15.6.5.2 Signs

Astrocytic hamartomas are glial tumors arising from the optic nerve head or the retina. Though these tumors have a predilection to the posterior pole they may occur anywhere on the retina. The tumor may manifest in two clinical forms: as a glistening, white-yellow calcified tumor with well-defined borders and multiple small excrescences (mulberry or fish egg lesions; "old tuberous bodies") (Fig. 15.39) or as a flat, grey-white tumor that is round or oval and has a smooth surface (young tuberous bodies) (Fig. 15.39). Perilesional circular reflex and the location near a vessel aid in identification of these "young tuberous bodies" that may be difficult to identify oth-

Table 15.6 Clinical features of systemic manifestations of TSC

	Cardiac rhabdomyoma	Pulmonary Lymphangioleiomyomatosis	Renal angiomyolipoma (AML)	Neurological	Cutaneous
Prevalence	61% in less than 5 years 36% in older children	Almost exclusively in women of child bearing age 1–3% of TSC 30% of middle aged women with TSC	80% of TSC	80% of TSC	Ash leaf macule: most common manifestation (92%)
Mean age at presentation	3 months in cases diagnosed in post-natal period	Variable, 30–40 years based on geographic area	11.3 years	1 year	Ash leaf macules: Birth Facial angioma: 2–5 years of age Shagreen patches: Increases with age Molluscum pendulum: First decade Forehead fibrous plaque: Birth to infancy Periungual fibroma: Puberty Confetti like lesions: Second decade
Location	Solid tumors in ventricular myocardium (94%), rarely in atrium and valves Multiple in few cases	Abnormal smooth muscle cells infiltrate airways and cause lung cysts and pneumothorax	Multiple and bilateral Cysts in 30% 3% mimic autosomal dominant polycystic kidney disease	Cortical tuber at junction of grey and white matter, often radiate to deep white matter and ventricles Subependymal gaint cell astrocytoma (SEGA) (10–15%) in the region of foromen of monro	Ash leaf macules: Trunk Facial angioma: centrofacial area sparing upper lip Shagreen patches: Dorsal body surface, especially lumbosacral area Molluscum pendulum: Neck, rarely axilla and groin Forehead fibrous plaque: Forehead or scalp Periungual fibroma: More commonly toes than in fingers Confetti like lesions: extremities

Table 15.7 Clinical feature, course and management of systemic manifestations of TSC

	Cardiac rhabdomyoma	Pulmonary Lymphangioleiomyomatosis	Renal angiomyolipoma (AML)	Neurological	Cutaneous
Clinical features	Usually found in routine antenatal ultrasound or during evaluation in patients of suspected tuberous sclerosis Rarely cause cardiac inflow and outflow obstruction and heart failure Arrhythmias	Insidious onset dyspnea, followed by fatigue, cough and chest pain 63% of patients can develop pneumothorax	Spontaneous hematuria, may be life threatening Flank pain Few patients develop end stage renal failure by replacement of renal parenchyma by AML Renal cell carcinoma	Infantile spasms (30%) TSC-associated neuropsychiatric disorders (TAND): Cognitive and behavioral impairment (25%)	Cosmetic blemish
Clinical course	Usually regress over time Only 10% undergo malignant transformation	Progressive, causes significant morbidity and mortality	Progressive, important cause of morbidity in these patients		
Treatment	Asymptomatic cases: Observation Symptomatic: Surgical resection mTOR inhibitors, sirolimus has been tried	Moderate to severe lung disease or rapid progression: mTOR inhibitors Advanced disease: Lung transplantation	Acute hemorrhage: Embolization followed by corticosteroids Growing angiomyolipoma measuring larger than 3 cm in diameter: mTOR inhibitor	Asymptomatic SEGA: Frequent MRI Acutely symptomatic SEGA: Surgical resection Growing but asymptomatic SEGA: Surgical resection or mTOR inhibitors TAND: Educational program Infantile spasm: Vigabatrin, ACTH, Epilepsy surgery for medically refractive seizures	Rapidly changing, disfiguring lesions: Surgical excision, laser, or possibly topical mTOR inhibitor

erwise. Intermediate lesions with both characteristics can also be seen [102].

Peripapillary and epipapillary lesions may range between ½ and 4 disc diameters in size. Rarely giant astrocytomas may occur in tuberous sclerosis (Fig. 15.40).

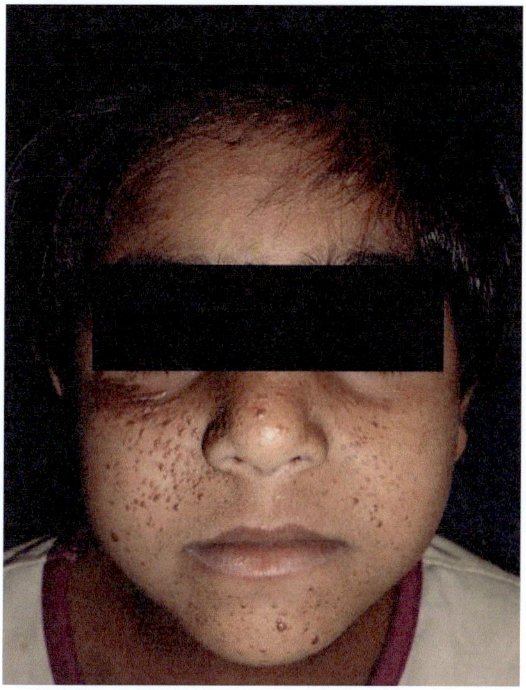

Fig. 15.37 Face photo of a patient with TSC showing multiple angiofibroma

Involvement of the macula or the optic disc by the astrocytic hamartoma or macular exudation may result in vision loss [104].

Progressive enlargement of the lesion can result in visual field loss and loss of vision. Rarely astrocytic hamartoma can lead to vitreous hemorrhage [105].

Retinal pigment epithelial abnormalities such as hyperpigmentation and "punched-out" hypopigmentation such as seen in combined hamartoma of the retina and retinal pigment epithelium may also be seen in patients with tuberous sclerosis. Palpebral angiofibromas, non-paralytic strabismus, refractive errors, iris depigmentation, cataract and choroidal colobomas are other associated findings [106].

Ash-leaf shaped iris atrophy, corneal leukoma, megalocornea, primary and secondary glaucoma, optic nerve atrophy, papilledema, and VI nerve palsy are other rarely reported findings in tuberous sclerosis [107].

Ultrasonography of calcified large astrocytic hamartoma show well demarcated, oval mass with a sharp anterior border, acoustic solidity and lack of choroidal excavation. There may be orbital shadowing.

The calcified astrocytic hamartoma may demonstrate autofluorescence in pre injection photographs of fluorescein angiography. There is diffuse hyperfluorescence in the late phases due to leakage from the tumor vessels.

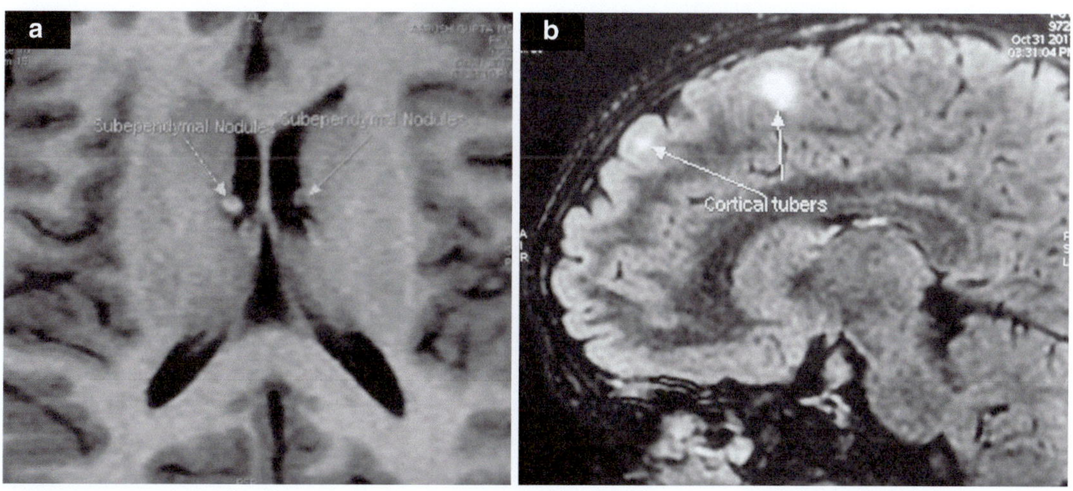

Fig. 15.38 MRI brain of a patient with TSC. Subependymal nodules (**a**) and cortical tubers (**b**). (Image courtesy: Dr. Vikas Khetan)

Table 15.8 Surveillance for newly diagnosed or suspected TSC

	Recommendation
Genetics	Three-generation family history Screening of family members Offer genetic testing • For counselling • In suspected cases
Brain	MRI brain Evaluate for TSC associated neuropsychiatric disorder educate parents to recognize infantile spasms Baseline electroencephalogram (EEG)
Kidney	MRI abdomen Blood pressure Renal function tests including glomerular filtration rate (GFR)
Lung	Baseline pulmonary function tests High resolution chest CT in females 18 years or older (even if asymptomatic) and in symptomatic males
Skin	Detailed dermatological exam
Teeth	Detailed dental exam
Heart	Echocardiogram, if younger than 3 years Electrocardiogram in all ages to assess conduction defects
Eye	Detailed examination including dilated fundus evaluation

Table 15.9 Surveillance for already diagnosed TSC

	Recommendation	Frequency
Genetics	Offer genetic testing in individuals of reproductive age or those considering children	
Brain	MRI brain in patients younger than 25 years	1–3 yearly
	Screening for TSC-associated neuropsychiatric disorders	Annually
	EEG in individuals with known or suspected seizure	Determined by clinical need
Kidney	MRI abdomen to assess progression of angiomyolipoma and renal cystic disease	1–3 yearly
	Renal function tests including glomerular filtration rate (GFR)	Yearly
Lung	Clinical screening for lymphangioleiomyomatosis (LAM) symptoms	Each visit
a. Individuals without lung cyst	HRCT	5–10 yearly
b. Individuals with lung cysts	Pulmonary function tests	Yearly
	HRCT	2–3 yearly
Skin	Detailed dermatological exam	Yearly
Teeth	Detailed dental exam	6 monthly
	Panoramic radiograph	7 years of age
Heart	Echocardiogram in asymptomatic kids	1–3 yearly until regression of cardiac rhabdomyoma
	ECG in asymptomatic patients of all ages	3–5 yearly
Eye	Detailed examination including dilated fundus evaluation	Yearly

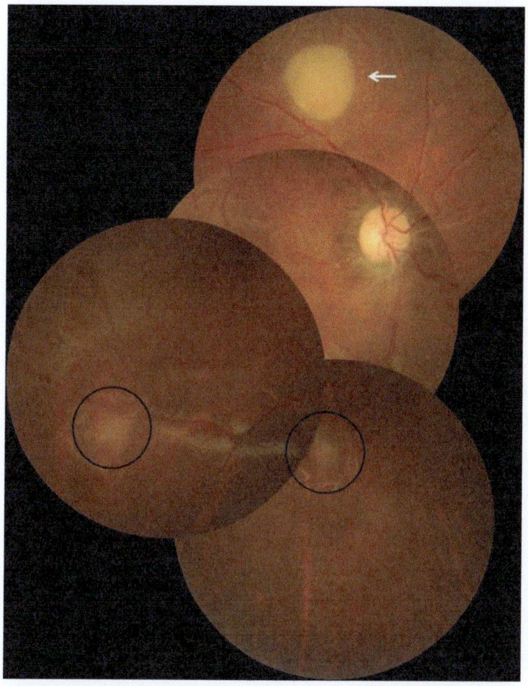

Fig. 15.39 Fundus photograph of a patient with TSC. Old tuberous body is seen as glistening, white-yellow calcified tumor with well-defined border (arrow). Young tuberous bodies are seen as a flat, grey-white tumor and have a smooth surface (within circles)

On OCT, astrocytomas are characterised by the presence of hypereflective and round, confluent, moth-eaten empty spaces with posterior shadowing on the surface of the tumor with disorganization of inner retinal layers (Fig. 15.41). Shallow elevation of the adjacent retina, macular edema and vitreoretinal traction over the tumor are other findings that can be found on OCT of astrocytomas [108]. Younger lesions may be localized to the nerve fiber layer with intact deeper retinal layers and RPE (Fig. 15.42) while older lesions show hyperreflectivity of the inner retinal layers with masking of the underlying retinal layers [109].

Lesions indistinct on fundus examination may be picked up on OCT. [110]

15.6.6 Histopathology

Retinal hamartomas are composed of fibrotic astrocytes with small oval nucleus and long cytoplasmic extensions.

15.6.7 Treatment

Ten percentage of flat lesions may progress and some may resolve spontaneously.

Astrocytic hamartoma are relatively stable and rarely affect visual acuity. Hence routine treatment is unnecessary. In cases with exudation with no spontaneous resolution direct laser photocoagulation or photodynamic therapy may aid in resorption of macular exudates [111–113].

In tumors associated with tumor neovascularization and macular edema, intravitreal bevacizumab can result in regression of the macular edema, tumor neovascularization and decrease in tumor size [114].

A rare subset of retinal astrocytoma associated with tuberous sclerosis may behave aggressively demonstrating progressive growth and complications such as exudative total retinal detachment, vitreous hemorrhage and neovascular glaucoma [115].

These patients may have multiple tumors, but the tumor near the optic disc shows growth. The aggressive retinal astrocytomas are composed of plump spindle cells and giant cells, giving them the name “Giant cell astrocytoma”. They demonstrate intense immunoreactivity for vimentin, GFAP and neuron-specific enolase [115].

Giant cell astrocytomas may need treatment. Laser photocoagulation is employed if associated with minimal subretinal fluid. Progressive growth, neovascularization and extensive subretinal fluid may need more aggressive treatment in the form of intravitreal anti-VEGF agents, PDT and subretinal fluid drainage [116].

Vitrectomy may be necessary for treating vitreous hemorrhage, epiretinal membrane and retinal detachment [117].

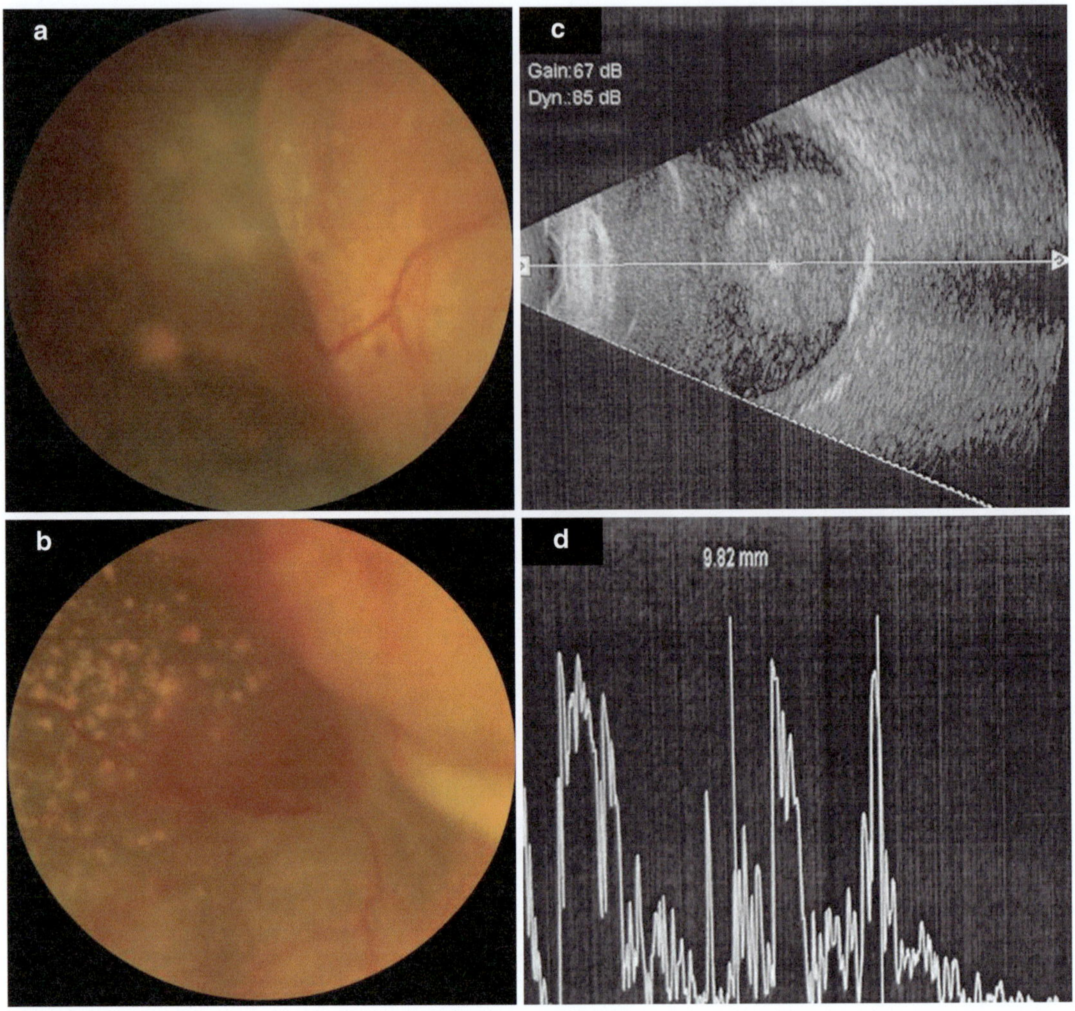

Fig. 15.40 Fundus photograph of a patient with TSC (**a**, **b**). Giant yellow white tumor with retinal detachment is seen. Ultrasound image (**c**, **d**) of the same tumor showing areas of calcification

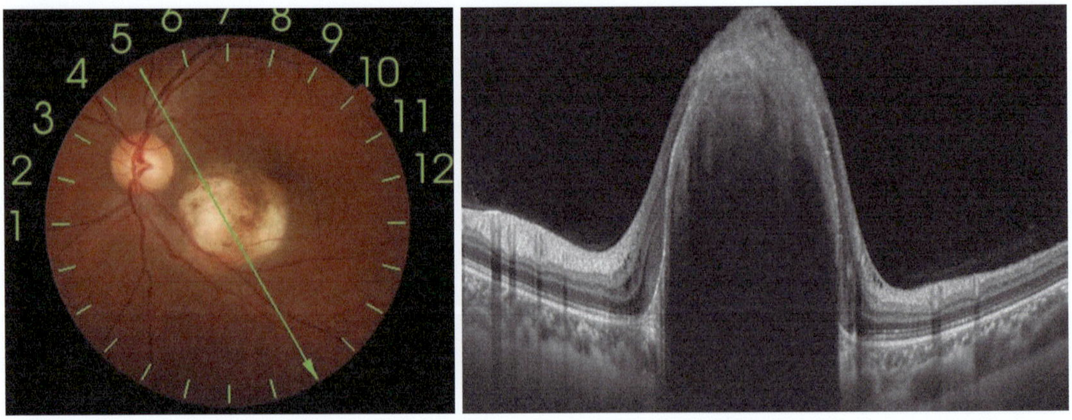

Fig. 15.41 OCT of older astrocytic hamartoma. Posterior shadowing with disorganization of inner retinal layers

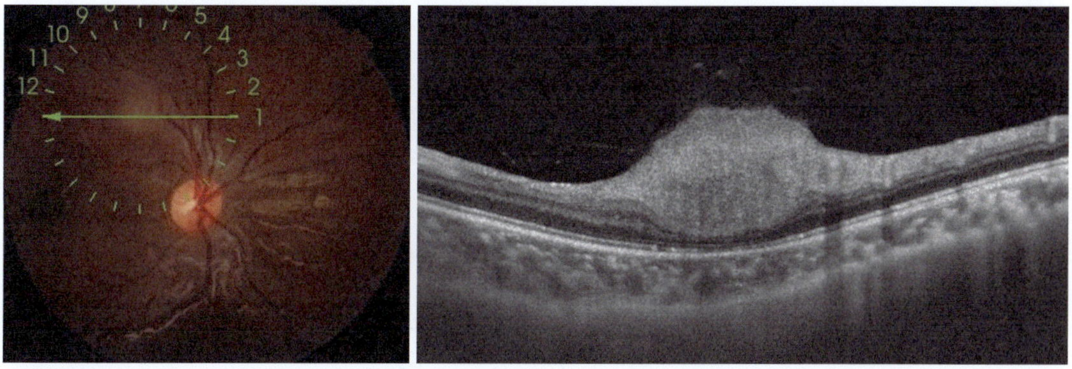

Fig. 15.42 OCT of younger astrocytic hamartoma. Tumor is localized to the nerve fiber layer with intact deeper retinal layers and RPE

Table 15.10 Systemic features of NF 1

Musculoskeletal	Cutaneous	CNS	Peripheral nervous system
Sphenoid bone dysplasia Congenital hydrocephalus Scoliosis Meningocele Dural ectasia Bowing of long bones Unilateral overgrowth of limbs	Cafe au lait spots Axillary and inguinal freckles Dermal neurofibroma	Epilepsy Cognitive and learning disability Attention deficit hyperactivity disorder	Neurofibroma Schwannoma

15.7 Neurofibromatosis 1

Neurofibromatosis type 1 (NF1) is a complex multi-system disorder with cutaneous, musculo-skeletal, neurological and ocular manifestations [118].

15.7.1 Epidemiology [119–122]

There is no gender, sex, race or geographical area predilection.

Prevalence—1:3000 people.

15.7.2 Genetics and Pathogenesis

Inheritence: Autosomal dominant with complete penetrance and variable expressivity.

NF 1 occurs due to the mutation in neurofibromin gene (NF1) located on chromosome 17p11.2. In 50% of individuals, the mutation occur de novo [122].

15.7.3 Systemic Features

Systemic features of NF1 are summarized in Table 15.10.

15.7.3.1 Diagnostic Criteria [123]

Two of these seven clinical features are required for diagnosis

1. Six or more café-au-lait spots over 5 mm in greatest diameter in pre-pubertal individuals and over 15 mm in greatest diameter in post-pubertal individuals. Note that multiple café-au-lait spots alone are not a definitive diagnosis of NF-1 as these spots can be caused by a number of other conditions.
2. Two or more neurofibromas of any type or 1 plexiform neurofibroma
3. Freckling in the axillary (Crowe sign) or inguinal regions
4. Optic glioma
5. Two or more Lisch nodules (pigmented iris hamartomas)

6. A distinctive osseous lesion such as sphenoid dysplasia, or thinning of the long bone cortex with or without pseudoarthrosis.
7. A first degree relative (parent, sibling, or off-spring) with NF-1 by the above criteria.

15.7.4 Ocular Features

Bilateral Lisch nodules of the iris are the classic manifestation of NF1. Lisch nodules appear by 2 years of age and 50% of children present with nodules. Lisch nodules are found in >90% of adults with NF1 [124–127].

Lisch nodules appear creamy white in dark irides and brown in light irides. They may appear as dome shaped nodules or as confluent masses with ragged borders, projecting from the iris surface (Fig. 15.43) [125].

Dome shaped elevated or flat placoid posterior pole choroidal nodules may be noted in NF1. These are seen well on OCT. They are composed of neuronal and melanocytic components. Overlying retinal vascular malformations may also occur. Rarely, multiple retinal capillary hemangiomas, astrocytic hamartomas and combined hamartoma of the retina and retinal pigment epithelium have been noted in NF1 [128–130].

Neurofibromatosis 1 patients are at an increased risk for developing uveal melanoma.

The number of Lisch nodules appears to correlate with that of the choroidal nodules.

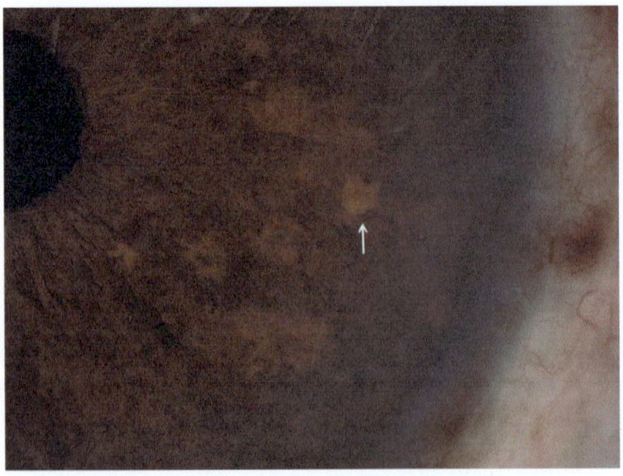

Fig. 15.43 Slit lamp photograph of iris showing Lisch nodules. (Image courtesy: Dr. Vinaya Kumar Konana)

Optic nerve glioma, plexiform neurofibromas of the orbit, microphthalmos, enophthalmos, conjunctival neurofibroma, hypertrophic corneal nerves, glaucoma are other associated ocular findings in NF1.

15.7.5 Histopathology

Lisch nodules are pigmented hamartomatous nodular aggregate of dendritic melanocytes.

15.7.6 Treatment

Lisch and choroidal nodules in NF1 do not need treatment and aid as a marker to the diagnosis of NF1.

15.8 Syndromes Associated with Combined Hamartoma of the Retina and Retinal Pigment Epithelium (CHRRPE)

Combined hamartoma of the retina and retinal pigment epithelium is a benign lesion commonly involving the juxtapapillary and macular region and less commonly the periphery.

15.8.1 Etiology

They are believed to be congenital lesions that are noticed in infants and young children. There is no sexual predilection. Caucasian race may be more affected.

15.8.2 Clinical Features

Combined hamartoma of the retina and retinal pigment epithelium appear as a slightly elevated black or charcoal gray mass involving the retinal pigment epithelium, retina and overlying vitreous [131].

It is usually unilateral and bilateral cases have been reported rarely.

CHRRPE causes vision loss due to macular distortion and epiretinal membrane (ERM). Patients may present with strabismus, floaters, leukocoria and ocular pain. Direct involvement of optic nerve and papillomacular bundle may reduce visual acuity.

Base of each lesion is composed of a relatively flat sheet of highly pigmented tissue and the outer more pigmented portion of tumor is covered centrally by gray-white retinal and preretinal tissue. Contraction of inner surface of the lesion is associated with distortion and displacement of adjacent retina and retinal blood vessels toward the center of the lesion. It blends imperceptibly with the surrounding RPE with absence of RPE or choroidal atrophy at the margin (Fig. 15.44).

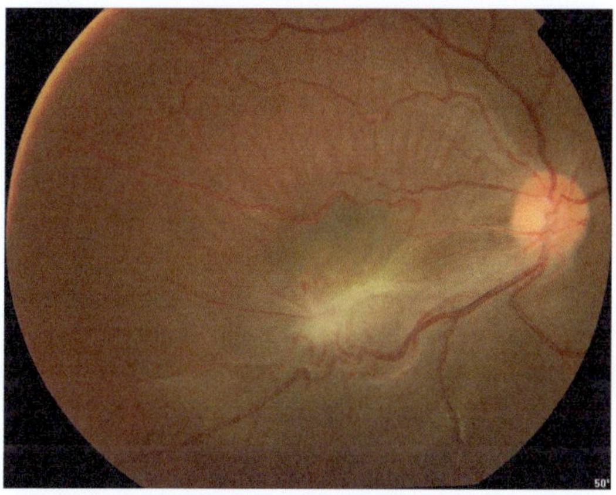

Fig. 15.44 Fundus photograph of CHRRPE

15.8.3 Diagnosis

In early-phase fluorescein angiography, hyperpigmentation of the tumor results in hypofluorescence. Tractional distortion of the retina leads to marked vascular tortuosity and telangiectasia. Vascular anomalies are more evident in the mid and the late phase and are hyperfluorescenct due to leakage from the tortuous vessels. ICG may show patchy hyperfluorescence corresponding to the location of the tumor in late phases.

OCT shows the distinct ERM with retinal striae and folds. Mini-peaks or saw tooth appearance of the inner retina, attenuation of outer retina with minimal attenuation or normal photoreceptor layer is typical of CHRRPE (Fig. 15.45).

15.8.4 Differential Diagnosis

Choroidal melanoma.
 Choroidal nevus.
 Adenoma or adenocarcinoma of RPE.
 Melanocytoma.
 Morning glory anomaly.

15.8.5 Complications

Combined hamartoma of the retina and retinal pigment epithelium may be associated with superficial hemorrhages, retinal capillary non-

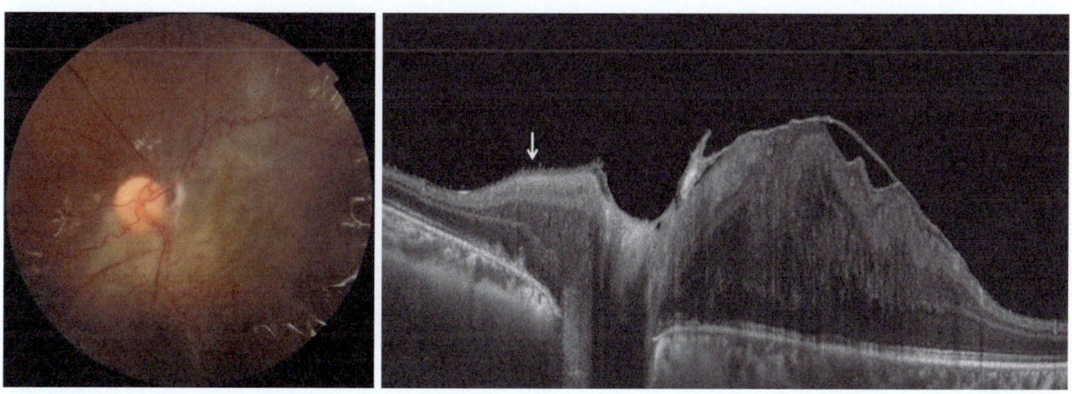

Fig. 15.45 OCT of CHRRPE showing mini-peaks or saw tooth appearance (arrow) of the inner retina, attenuation of outer retina with minimal attenuation or normal photoreceptor layer

perfusion with preretinal neovascularization resulting in vitreous hemorrhage [132–134].

Other complications such as choroidal neovascularization and macular hole may result in visual loss [135–137].

Less commonly retinal exudation, macular edema, retinoschisis may also occur in CHRRPE.

15.8.6 Histopathology

Combined hamartomas of the retina and retinal pigment epithelium characteristically contain pigment epithelium, vascular, and glial components [138].

15.8.7 Treatment

In those cases with visual loss due to traction involving the fovea, vitrectomy and membrane peeling can be attempted to improve visual acuity [139–141]. (Fig. 15.46).

A functional component of amblyopia may be superimposed on visual loss caused by structural abnormalities. In some cases this can be treated [142].

Subfoveal CNV associated with combined hamartoma of the retina and RPE has been surgically excised with good visual recovery in one patient [143].

CHRRPE can be seen in association with [144–149]

- Neurofibromatosis 1 and 2
- Incontinentia pigmentii
- Tuberous sclerosis
- Gorlin Goltz syndrome
- Poland anomaly
- Branchio-oculo-facial syndrome
- Branchio-oto-renal syndrome
- Juvenile nasopharyngeal angiofibroma.

15.8.8 Prognosis

Progressive vision loss may occur due to tumor growth or complications associated with the tumor.

15.9 Syndrome Associated with Congenital Hypertrophy of Retinal Pigment Epithelium (CHRPE): Gardner Syndrome

Gardner syndrome, is characterized by the presence of multiple polyps in the colon and extracolonic tumors including osteomas of the skull, thyroid cancer, epidermoid cysts, fibromas, desmoid tumors and CHRPE.

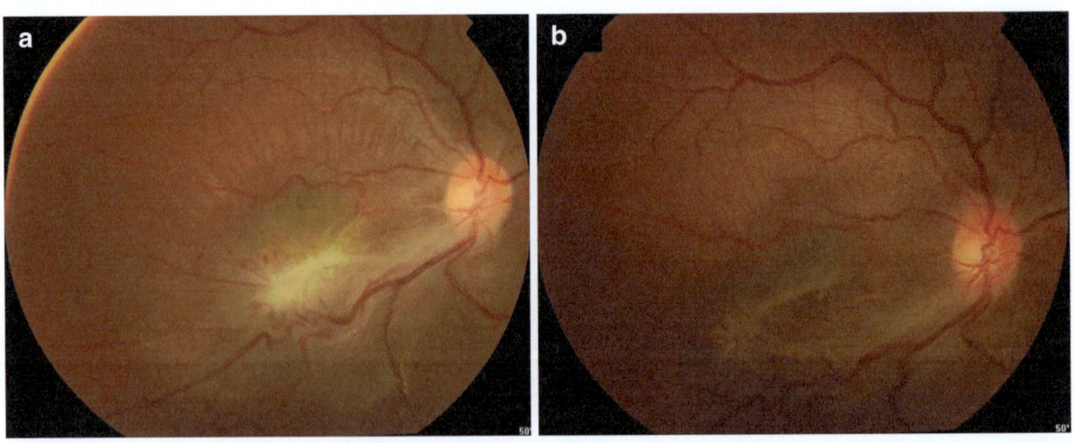

Fig. 15.46 Fundus photograph of CHRRPE with distortion of retina (**a**). Fundus photograph after epiretinal membrane peeling (**b**). But the patient developed re-proliferation of membrane with formation of macular hole

15.9.1 Epidemiology

Incidence: 1 in 7500 live births.

80% familial.

15.9.2 Genetics

Inheritance: autosomal dominant.

No sexual predilection.

Gardner syndrome is caused by mutation in the adenomatous polyposis coli (APC) gene, located in chromosome 5q21

15.9.3 Systemic Features [150]

Adenomatous polyps of the gastrointestinal tract.

Desmoid tumours.

Osteomas.

Epidermoid cysts.

Lipomas.

Dental abnormalities.

Periampullary carcinomas.

Gastric and duodenal polyps.

Thyroid carcinoma.

15.9.4 Ocular Features

Solitary, acquired CHRPE occurs late in life and is not associated with systemic disease. Multiple or grouped CHRPE may however be associated with systemic disease.

Multifocal haphazardly arranged small (4–5 mm), round or tear-drop shaped, flat, darkly pigmented RPE lesions with irregular borders, simulating bear-tracks are an indicator to Gardner's syndrome. They are situated in the mid periphery and are autofluorescent.

Four or more such pigmented fundus lesions in each eye is a reliable indication that the patient may eventually develop colorectal cancer. These lesions are hamartomas of RPE composed of tall, columnar densely pigmented RPE surrounded by halo of depigmented RPE cells. Malignant transformation to adenocarcinoma has rarely been reported [151].

15.10 Conclusions

Detection of tumors such as a retinal angioma, astrocytoma, atypical CHRPE or combined hamartoma of the retina and retinal pigment epithelium may be the first clue to an underlying multisystem disease. While the intraocular tumors associated with the syndromes discussed here are benign, the associated systemic disease as in von-Hippel Lindau disease, tuberous sclerosis and neurofibromatosis may be associated with life-threatening underlying conditions requiring screening and referral. The vascular lesions such as retinal and choroidal hemangiomas and some astrocytomas may need treatment to alleviate vision loss. Vitreoretinal surgical techniques may at times be needed to stabilize and improve vision.

References

1. Hardwig P, Robertson DM. Von Hippel-Lindau disease: a familial, often lethal, multi-system phakomatosis. Ophthalmology. 1984;91:263–70.
2. Maher ER, Iselius L, Yates JR, Littler M, Benjamin C, Harris R, Sampson J, et al. Von Hippel-Lindau disease: a genetic study. J Med Genet. 1991;28:443–7.
3. Lonser RR, Glenn GM, Walther M, Chew EY, Libutti SK, Linehan WM, et al. von Hippel-Lindau disease. Lancet. 2003;361(9374):2059–67.
4. Turturro F. Beyond the Knudson's hypothesis in von Hippel-Lindau (VHL) disease- proposing vitronectin as a "gene modifier". J Mol Med (Berl). 2009;87(6):591–3.
5. Nordstrom-O'Brien M, van der Luijt RB, van Rooijen E, van den Ouweland AM, Majoor-Krakauer DF, Lolkema MP, et al. Genetic analysis of von Hippel-Lindau disease. Hum Mutat. 2010;31(5):521–37.
6. Chan CC, Vortmeyer AO, Chew EY, Green WR, Matteson DM, Shen DF, et al. VHL gene deletion and enhanced VEGF gene expression detected in the stromal cells of retinal angioma. Arch Ophthalmol. 1999;117(5):625–30.
7. Kaelin WG Jr. The von Hippel-Lindau gene, kidney cancer, and oxygen sensing. J Am Soc Nephrol. 2003;14(11):2703–11.
8. Maher ER, Yates JR, Harries R, Benjamin C, Harris R, Moore AT, et al. Clinical features and natural history of von Hippel-Lindau disease. MAQ. J Med. 1990;77(283):1151–63.
9. Singh A, Shields J, Shields C. Solitary retinal capillary hemangioma: hereditary (von Hippel-Lindau

disease) or nonhereditary? Arch Ophthalmol. 2001;119(2):232–4.
10. Richard S, Chauveau D, Chrétien Y, Beigelman C, Denys A, Fendler JP, et al. Renal lesions and pheochromocytoma in von Hippel-Lindau disease. Adv Nephrol Necker Hosp. 1994;23:1–27.
11. Varshney N, Kebede AA, Owusu-Dapaah H, Lather J, Kaushik M, Bhullar JSJ, et al. A review of Von Hippel-Lindau syndrome. J Kidney Cancer VHL. 2017;4(3):20–9.
12. Kanno H, Kobayashi N, Nakanowatari S, et al. Pathological and clinical features and management of central nervous system hemangioblastomas in von Hippel-Lindau disease. J Kidney Cancer VHL. 2014;1(4):46–55.
13. Maher ER, Neumann HP, Richard S. Von Hippel-Lindau disease: a clinical and scientific review. Eur J Hum Genet. 2011;19(6):617–23.
14. Wing GL, Weiter JJ, von Kelly PJ. Hippel-Lindau disease. Angiomatosis of the retina and central nervous system. Ophthalmology. 1981;88:1311–4.
15. Singh AD, Nouri M, Shields CL, Shields JA, Smith AF. Retinal capillary hemangioma: a comparison of sporadic cases and cases associated with von Hippel-Lindau disease. Ophthalmology. 2001;108(10):1907–11.
16. Shields JA, Shields CL, Deglin E. Retinal capillary haemangioma in Marshall-Stickler syndrome. Am J Ophthalmol. 1997;124:120–2.
17. Shields JA, Shields CL. A textbook and atlas. Philadelphia: W. B. Saunders; 1992.
18. Saitta A, Nicolai M, Giovannini A, Mariotti C. Juxtapapillary retinal capillary hemangioma: new therapeutic strategies. Med Hypothesis Discov Innov Ophthalmol. 2014;3:71–5.
19. Gass JD, Braunstein R. Sessile and exophytic capillary angiomas of the juxtapapillary retina and optic nerve head. Arch Ophthalmol. 1980;98:1790–7.
20. Shields CL, Materin MA, Shields JA. Review of optical coherence tomography for intraocular tumors. Curr Opin Ophthalmol. 2005;16(3):141–54.
21. Chin EK, Trikha R, Morse LS, Zawadzki RJ, Werner JS, Park SS. Optical coherence tomography findings of exophytic retinal capillary hemangiomas of the posterior pole. Ophthalmic Surg Lasers Imaging. 2010;9:1–5.
22. Lang SJ, Cakir B, Evers C, Ludwig F, Lange CA, Agostini HT. Value of optical coherence tomography angiography imaging in diagnosis and treatment of hemangioblastomas in von Hippel-Lindau disease. Ophthalmic Surg Lasers Imaging Retina. 2016;47:935–46.
23. Champion KJ, Guinea M, Dammai V, Hsu T. Endothelial function of von Hippel-Lindau tumor suppressor gene: control of fibroblast growth factor receptor signaling. Cancer Res. 2008;68(12):4649–57.
24. Frantzen C, Klasson TD, Links TP, Giles RH, Adam MP, Ardinger HH, et al. Von Hippel-Lindau syndrome. Seattle: University of Washington; 2000. p. 1993–2017.
25. Maher ER. Von Hippel-Lindau disease. Curr Mol Med. 2004;4:833–42.
26. Schmidt D, Natt E, Neumann HP. Long-term results of laser treatment for retinal angiomatosis in von Hippel-Lindau disease. Eur J Med Res. 2000;28:47–58.
27. Singh AD, Nouri M, Shields CL, Shields JA, Perez N. Treatment of retinal capillary hemangioma. Ophthalmology. 2002;109:1799–806.
28. Parmar DN, Mireskandari K, McHugh D. Transpupillary thermotherapy for retinal capillary hemangioma in von Hippel-Lindau disease. Ophthalmic Surg Lasers. 2000;31:334–6.
29. Garcia-Arumi J, Sararols LH, Cavero L, Escalada F, Corcostegui BF. Therapeutic options for capillary papillary hemangiomas. Ophthalmology. 2000;107:48–54.
30. Kreusel KM, Bornfeld N, Lommatzsch A, Wessing A, Foerster MH. Ruthenium-106 brachytherapy for peripheral retinal capillary hemangioma. Ophthalmology. 1998;105:1386–92.
31. Russo V, Stella A, Barone A, Scott IU, Noci ND. Ruthenium-106 brachytherapy and intravitreal bevacizumab for retinal capillary hemangioma. Int Ophthalmol. 2012;32:71–5.
32. Raja D, Benz MS, Murray TG. Salvage external beam radiotherapy of retinal capillary hemangiomas secondary to von Hippel-Lindau disease: visual and anatomical outcomes. Ophthalmology. 2004;111:150–3.
33. Schmidt-Erfurth UM, Kusserow C, Barbazetto IA, Laqua H. Benefits and complications of photodynamic therapy of papillary capillary hemangiomas. Ophthalmology. 2002;109(7):1256–66.
34. Farah ME, Uno F, Höfling-Lima AL, Morales PH, Costa RA, Cardillo JA. Transretinal feeder vessel ligature in von Hippel-Lindau disease. Eur J Ophthalmol. 2001;11(4):386–8.
35. McDonald HR, Schatz H, Johnson RN. Vitrectomy in eyes with peripheral retinal angioma associated with traction macular detachment. Ophthalmology. 1996;103:329–35.
36. Ziemssen F, Voelker M, Inhoffen W, Bartz-Schmidt KU, Gelisken F. Combined treatment of a juxtapapillary retinal capillary haemangioma with intravitreal bevacizumab and photodynamic therapy. Eye (Lond). 2007;21(8):1125–6.
37. Wong WT, Liang KJ, Hammel K, Coleman HR, Chew EY. Intravitreal ranibizumab therapy for retinal capillary hemangioblastoma related to von Hippel-Lindau disease. Ophthalmology. 2008;115(11):1957–64.
38. Muthukumar N, Sundaralingam MP. Retinocephalic vascular malformation: case report. Br J Neurosurg. 1998;12(5):458–60.
39. Wyburn-Mason R. Arteriovenous aneurysm of midbrain and retina, facial nevi and mental changes. Brain Dev. 1943;66:163–203.
40. Ponce FA, Han PP, Spetzler RF, Canady A, Feiz-Erfan I. Associated arteriovenous malformation of

the orbit and brain: a case of Wyburn-Mason syndrome without retinal involvement. Case report. J Neurosurg. 2001;95(2):346–9.
41. Albert DM, Jakobiec FA, editors. Phakomatoses. In: Principles and practice of ophthalmology, 2nd ed. Philadelphia: W. B. Saunders; 2000. p. 3779.
42. Goh D, Malik NN, Gilvarry A. Retinal racemose haemangioma directly communicating with a intramuscular facial cavernous haemangioma. Br J Ophthalmol. 2004;88(6):840–2.
43. Luo CB, Lasjaunias P, Bhattacharya J. Craniofacial vascular malformations in Wyburn-Mason syndrome. J Chin Med Assoc. 2006;69(12):575–80.
44. Wyburn-Mason R. Arteriovenous aneurysm of midbrain and retina, facial naevi and mental changes. Brain. 1943;66:163–203.
45. Theron J, Newton TH, Hoyt WF. Unilateral retinocephalic vascular malformations. Neuroradiology. 1974;7:186–96.
46. Archer DB, Deutman A, Ernest JT, et al. Arteriovenous communications of the retina. Am J Ophthalmol. 1973;75:224–41.
47. Bernth-Petersen P. Racemose haemangioma of the retina. Report of three cases with long term follow-up. Acta Ophthalmol. 1979;57(4):669–78.
48. Mansour AM, Wells AM, Jampol LM, et al. Ocular complications of arteriovenous communications of the retina. Arch Ophthalmol. 1989;107:232–6.
49. Schatz H, Chang LF, Ober RR, et al. Central retinal vein occlusion associated with retinal arteriovenous malformation. Ophthalmology. 1993;100:24–30.
50. Papageorgiou KI, Ghazi-Nouri SM, Andreou PS. Vitreous and subretinal haemorrhage; an unusual complication of retinal racemose haemangioma. Clin Exp Ophthalmol. 2006;34:176–7.
51. Barreira AK Jr, Nakashima AF, Takahashi VK, Marques GA, Minelli T, Santo AM. Retinal racemose hemangioma with focal macular involvement. Retin Cases Brief Rep. 2016;10:52–4.
52. Gass JDM. Cavernous hemangioma of the retina. A neuro-oculocutaneous syndrome. Am J Ophthalmol. 1971;71:799–814.
53. Dubovsky J, Zabramski JM, Kurth J, et al. A gene responsible for cavernous malformations of the brain maps to chromosome 7q. Hum Mol Genet. 1995;4:453–8.
54. Gunel M, Awad IA, Finberg K, et al. A founder mutation as a cause of cerebral cavernous malformation in Hispanic Americans. N Engl J Med. 1996;334:946–51.
55. Gunel M, Awad IA, Finberg K, et al. Genetic heterogeneity of inherited cerebral cavernous malformation. Neurosurgery. 1996;38:1265–71.
56. Wallner EF, Moorman LT. Hemangioma of the optic disc. Arch Ophthalmol. 1955;53:115–7.
57. Sarraf D, Payne AM, Kitchen ND, Sehmi KS, Downes SM, Bird AC. Familial cavernous hemangioma: an expanding ocular spectrum. Arch Ophthalmol. 2000;118(7):969–73.
58. Lewis RA, Cohen MH, Wise GN. Cavernous haemangioma of the retina and optic disc. A report of three cases and a review of the literature. Br J Ophthalmol. 1975;59(8):422–34.
59. Drigo P, Mammi I, Battistella PA, et al. Familial cerebral, hepatic, and retinal cavernous angiomas: a new syndrome. Childs Nerv Syst. 1994;10:205–9.
60. Weskamp C, Cotlier I. Angioma del cerebro y de la retina con malformaciones capilares de la piel. Arch Oftalmol B Aires. 1940;15:1–10.
61. Zografos L, Gonvers M. Ocular melanocytosis and cavernous haemangioma of the optic disc. Br J Ophthalmol. 1994;78:73–4.
62. Gunduz K, Ozbayrak N, Okka M, et al. Cavernous hemangioma with cone dysfunction. Ophthalmologica. 1996;210:367–71.
63. Naftchi S, la Cour M. A case of central visual loss in a child due to macular cavernous haemangioma of the retina. Acta Ophthalmol Scand. 2002;80(5):550–2.
64. Yamaguchi K, Tamai M. Cavernous hemangioma of the retina in a pediatric patient. Ophthalmologica. 1988;197(3):127–9.
65. Bottoni F, Canevini MP, Canger R, Orzalesi N. Twin vessels in familial retinal cavernous hemangioma. Am J Ophthalmol. 1990;15:285–9.
66. Haller JA, Knox DL. Vitrectomy for persistent vitreous hemorrhage from a cavernous hemangioma of the optic disk. Am J Ophthalmol. 1993;116(1):106–7.
67. Shanmugam MP, Ramanjulu R, Dwivedi S, Barigali A, Havanje A. Therapeutic surprise! Photodynamic therapy for cavernous hemangioma of the disc. Indian J Ophthalmol. 2017;65:754–7.
68. Thomas-Sohl KA, Vaslow DF, Maria BL. Sturge-Weber syndrome: a review. Pediatr Neurol. 2004;30(5):303–10.
69. Shirley MD, Tang H, Gallione CJ, Baugher JD, Frelin LP, Cohen B, et al. Sturge-Weber syndrome and port-wine stains caused by somatic mutation in GNAQ. N Engl J Med. 2013;368(21):1971–9.
70. Rochkind S, Hoffman HJ, Hendrick EB. Sturge-Weber syndrome: natural history and prognosis. J Epilepsy. 1990;3:293–304.
71. Zanzmera P, Patel T, Shah V. Diagnostic dilemma: Sturge-Weber syndrome, without facial nevus. J Neurosci Rural Pract. 2015;6(1):105–7.
72. Piram M, Lorette G, Sirinelli D, Herbreteau D, Giraudeau B, Maruani A. Sturge-Weber syndrome in patients with facial port-wine stain. Pediatr Dermatol. 2012;29:32–7.
73. Ch'ng S, Tan ST. Facial port-wine stains - clinical stratification and risks of neuro-ocular involvement. J Plast Reconstr Aesthet Surg. 2008;61:889–93.
74. Higueros E, Roe E, Granell E, Baselga E. Sturge-Weber syndrome: a review. Actas Dermosifiliogr. 2017;108(5):407–17.
75. Zhao Y, Tu P, Zhou G, Zhou Z, Lin X, Yang H, et al. Hemoporfin photodynamic therapy for port-wine stain: a randomized controlled trial. PLoS One. 2016;11:e0156219.

76. Enjolras O, Riche MC, Merland JJ. Facial port-wine stains and Sturge-Weber syndrome. Pediatrics. 1985;76(1):48–51.
77. Mantelli F, Bruscolini A, La Cava M, Abdolrahimzadeh S, Lambiase A. Ocular manifestations of Sturge-Weber syndrome: pathogenesis, diagnosis, and management. Clin Ophthalmol. 2016;10:871–8.
78. Weiss JS, Richt R. Glaucoma in phakomatoses. The glaucomas. St. Louis: C. V. Mosby; 1996. p. 899–924.
79. Stevenson RF, Morin JD. Ocular findings in nevus flammeus. Can J Ophthalmol. 1975;10:136–9.
80. Sullivan TJ, Clarke MP, Morin JD. The ocular manifestations of the Sturge-Weber syndrome. J Pediatr Ophthalmol Strabismus. 1992;29(6):349–56.
81. Susac JO, Smith JL, Scufo RJ. The "tomato catsup fundus" in the Sturge Weber syndrome. Arch Ophthalmol. 1974;92:69–70.
82. Addison PK, Papadopoulos M, Nischal KK, Hykin PG. Serous retinal detachment induced by topical bimatoprost in a patient with Sturge Weber syndrome. Eye (Lond). 2011;25:124–5.
83. Tsipursky MS, Golchet PR, Jampol LM. Photodynamic therapy of choroidal hemangioma in Sturge-Weber syndrome, with a review of treatments for diffuse and circumscribed choroidal hemangioma. Surv Ophthalmol. 2011;56:68–85.
84. Alberti W. Radiotherapy of choroidal haemangioma. Int J Radiat Oncol Biol Phys. 1986;12:122–3.
85. Arepalli S, Shields CL, Kaliki S, Emrich J, Komamicky L, Shields JA. Diffuse choroidal hemangioma management with plaque radiotherapy in 5 cases. Ophthalmology. 2013;120:2358–9.
86. Arevalo JF, Arias JD, Serrano MA. Oral propranolol for exudative retinal detachment in diffuse choroidal hemangioma. Arch Ophthalmol. 2011;129:1373–5.
87. Shoeibi N, Ahmadieh H, Abrishami M, Poorzand H. Rapid and sustained resolution of serous retinal detachment in Sturge-Weber syndrome after single injection of intravitreal bevacizumab. Ocul Immunol Inflamm. 2011;19:358–60.
88. Garcia-Arumi J, Ramsay LS, Guraya BC. Trans pupillary thermotherapy for circumscribed choroidal hemangiomas. Ophthalmology. 2000;107:351–7.
89. Kamal A, Watts AR, Rennie IG. Indocyanine green enhanced transpupillary thermotherapy of circumscribed choroidal haemangioma. Eye (Lond). 2000;5:701–5.
90. Gunduz K. Transpupillary thermotherapy in the management of circumscribed choroidal hemangioma. Surv Ophthalmol. 2004;49(3):316–27.
91. Ong T, Chia A, Nischal KK. Latanoprost in port wine stain related paediatric glaucoma. Br J Ophthalmol. 2003;87:1091–3.
92. Yang CB, Freedman SF, Myers JS, et al. Use of latanoprost in the treatment of glaucoma associated with Sturge-Weber syndrome. Am J Ophthalmol. 1998;126:600–2.
93. Sakai H, Sakima N, Nakamura Y, Nakamura Y, Hayakawa K, Sawaguchi S. Ciliochoroidal effusion induced by topical latanoprost in a patient with Sturge-Weber syndrome. Jpn J Ophthalmol. 2002;46(5):553–5.
94. Gambrelle J, Denis P, Kocaba V, Grange JD. Uveal effusion induced by topical travoprost in a patient with Sturge-Weber-Krabbe syndrome. J Fr Ophtalmol. 2008;31(9):e19.
95. Wiederholt WC, Gomez MR, Kurland LT. Incidence and prevalence of tuberous sclerosis in Rochester, Minnesota, 1950 through 1982. Neurology. 1985;35(4):600–3.
96. Huang J, Manning BD. The TSC1-TSC2 complex: a molecular switchboard controlling cell growth. Biochem J. 2008;412(2):179–90.
97. Cohen MM, Pollock-BarZiv S, Johnson SR. Emerging clinical picture of lymphangioleiomyomatosis. Thorax. 2005;60(10):875–9.
98. Cohen MM, Pollock-BarZiv S, Johnson SR. Tuberous sclerosis complex-associated kidney angiomyolipoma: from contemplation to action. Nephrol Dial Transplant. 2013;28(7):1680–5.
99. Pirson Y. Cutaneous manifestations of tuberous sclerosis. Ochsner J. 2010;10:200–4.
100. Franz DN, Bissler JJ, McCormack FX. Tuberous sclerosis complex: neurological, renal and pulmonary manifestations. Neuropediatrics. 2010;41(5):199–208.
101. Krueger DA, Northrup H, International Tuberous Sclerosis Complex Consensus Group. Tuberous sclerosis complex surveillance and management: recommendations of the 2012 International Tuberous Sclerosis Complex Consensus Conference. Pediatr Neurol. 2013;49(4):255–65.
102. Rowley SA, O'Callaghan FJ, Osborne JP. Ophthalmic manifestations of tuberous sclerosis: a population based study. Br J Ophthalmol. 2001;85(4):420–3.
103. Nyboer JH, Robertson DM, Gomez MR. Retinal lesions in tuberous sclerosis. Arch Ophthalmol. 1976;94(8):1277–80.
104. Brown CG, Shields JA. Tumors of the optic nerve head. Surv Ophthalmol. 1985;29:239–64.
105. Atkinson A, Sanders MD, Wong V. Vitreous haemorrhage in tuberous sclerosis. Br J Ophthalmol. 1973;57:773–9.
106. Lopez JP, Ossandón D, Miller P, Sánchez L, Winter A. Unilateral eyelid angiofibroma with complete blepharoptosis as the presenting sign of tuberous sclerosis. J AAPOS. 2009;13(4):413–4.
107. Robertson DM. Ophthalmic manifestations of tuberous sclerosis. Ann N Y Acad Sci. 1991;615:17–25.
108. Shields CL, Benevides R, Materin MA, Shields JA. Optical coherence tomography of retinal astrocytic hamartoma in 15 cases. Ophthalmology. 2006;113(9):1553–7.
109. Soliman W, Larsen M, Sander B, Wegener M, Milea D. Optical coherence tomography of astrocytic hamartomas in tuberous sclerosis. Acta Ophthalmol Scand. 2007;85(4):454–5.

110. Xu L, Burke TR, Greenberg JP, Mahajan VB, Tsang SH. Infrared imaging and optical coherence tomography reveal early-stage astrocytic hamartomas not detectable by fundoscopy. Am J Ophthalmol. 2012;153(5):883–9.
111. Vrabec TR, Augsburger JJ. Exudative retinal detachment due to small noncalcified retinal astrocytic hamartoma. Am J Ophthalmol. 2003;136(5):952–4.
112. Bloom SM, Mahl CF. Photocoagulation for serous detachment of the macula secondary to retinal astrocytoma. Retina. 1991;11:416–22.
113. Mennel S, Hausmann N, Meyer CH, Peter S. Photodynamic therapy for exudative hamartoma in tuberous sclerosis. Arch Ophthalmol. 2006;124(4):597–9.
114. Saito W, Kase S, Ohgami K, Mori S, Ohno S. Intravitreal anti-vascular endothelial growth factor therapy with bevacizumab for tuberous sclerosis with macular oedema. Acta Ophthalmol. 2010;88(3):377–80.
115. Shields JA, Eagle RC Jr, Shields CL, Marr BP. Aggressive retinal astrocytomas in 4 patients with tuberous sclerosis complex. Arch Ophthalmol. 2005;123(6):856–63.
116. Eskelin S, Tommila P, Palosaari T, Kivelä T. Photodynamic therapy with verteporfin to induce regression of aggressive retinal astrocytomas. Acta Ophthalmol. 2008;86(7):794–9.
117. Tomida M, Mitamura Y, Katome T, Eguchi H, Naito T, Harada T. Aggressive retinal astrocytoma associated with tuberous sclerosis. Clin Ophthalmol. 2012;6:715–20.
118. Jett K, Friedman JM. Clinical and genetic aspects of neurofibromatosis 1. Genet Med. 2010;12(1):1–11.
119. Riccardi VM. Neurofibromatosis: past, present, and future. N Engl J Med. 1991;324(18):1283–5.
120. Hirbe AC, Gutmann DH. Neurofibromatosis type 1: a multidisciplinary approach to care. Lancet Neurol. 2014;13(8):834–43.
121. Neurofibromatosis. Conference statement. National Institutes of Health Consensus Development Conference. Arch Neurol. 1988;45(5):575–8.
122. Carey JC. Neurofibromatosis-Noonan syndrome. Am J Med Genet. 1998;75(3):263–4.
123. Huson MS, Hughes CRA. The neurofibromatoses: a pathogenetic and clinical overview. London: Chapman & Hall; 1994.
124. Abdolrahimzadeh S, Felli L, Plateroti R, Plateroti AM, Giustini S, Calvieri S, et al. Morphologic and vasculature features of the choroid and associated choroid-retinal thickness alterations in neurofibromatosis type 1. Br J Ophthalmol. 2015;99(6):789–93.
125. Recupero SM, Plateroti R, Abdolrahimzadeh S, et al. Lisch nodules in neurfibromatosis type 1: relationship to age and cutaneous neurfibromas. Ann Ophthalmol Glaucoma. 1996;28(3):178–83.
126. Ragge NK, Falk RE, Cohen WE, Murphree AL. Images of Lisch nodules across the spectrum. Eye (Lond). 1993;7:95–101.
127. Cassiman C, Legius E, Spileers W, Casteels I. Ophthalmological assessment of children with neurofibromatosis type 1. Eur J Pediatr. 2013;172(10):1327–33.
128. Destro M, D'Amico DJ, Gragoudas ES, Brockhurst RJ, Pinnolis MK, Albert DM, et al. Retinal manifestations of neurofibromatosis. Diagnosis and management. Arch Ophthalmol. 1991;109(5):662–6.
129. Ruggieri M, Pavone P, Polizzi A, Di Pietro M, Scuderi A, Gabriele A, et al. Ophthalmological manifestations in segmental neurofibromatosis type 1. Br J Ophthalmol. 2004;88(11):1429–33.
130. Abdolrahimzadeh S, Piraino DC, Plateroti R, Scuderi G, Recupero SM. Ocular alterations in a rare case of segmental neurofibromatosis type 1 with a non-classified mutational variant of the NF-1 gene. Ophthalmic Genet. 2016;37(2):214–6.
131. Font RL, Moura RA, Shetlar DJ, Martinez JA, McPherson AR. Combined hamartoma of sensory retina and retinal pigment epithelium. Retina. 1989;9(4):302–11.
132. Helbig H, Niederberger H. Presumed combined hamartoma of the retina and retinal pigment epithelium with preretinal neovascularization. Am J Ophthalmol. 2003;136(6):1157–9.
133. Moschos M, Ladas ID, Zafirakis PK, Kokolakis SN, Theodossiadis GP. Recurrent vitreous hemorrhages due to combined pigment epithelial and retinal hamartoma: natural course and indocyanine green angiographic findings. Ophthalmologica. 2001;215(1):66–9.
134. Kahn D, Goldberg MF, Jednock N. Combined retinal-retina pigment epithelial hamartoma presenting as a vitreous hemorrhage. Retina. 1984;4:40–3.
135. Schachat AP, Shields JA, Fine SL, et al. Combined hamartomas of the retina and retinal pigment epithelium. Ophthalmology. 1984;91:1609–15.
136. Mason JO, Kleiner R. Combined hamartoma of the retina and retinal pigment epithelium associated with epiretinal membrane and macular hole. Retina. 1997;17:160–2.
137. Verma L, Venkatesh P, Lakshmaiah CN, Tewari HK. Combined hamartoma of the retina and retinal pigment epithelium with full thickness retinal hole and without retinoschisis. Ophthalmic Surg Lasers. 2000;31(5):423–6.
138. Ryan SJ. Combined hamartoma of the retina and retinal pigment epithelium. In: Retina. St. Louis: Mosby; 2001. p. 640–6.
139. McDonald HR, Abrams GW, Burke JM, Neuwirth J. Clinicopathologic results of vitreous surgery for epiretinal membranes in patients with combined retinal and retinal pigment epithelial hamartomas. Am J Ophthalmol. 1985;100:806–13.
140. Sappenfield DL, Gitter KA. Surgical intervention for combined retinal-retinal pigment epithelial hamartoma. Retina. 1990;10(2):119–24.
141. Stallman JB. Visual improvement after pars plana vitrectomy and membrane peeling for vitreoretinal traction associated with combined hamartoma of

the retina and retinal pigment epithelium. Retina. 2002;22(1):101–4.
142. Kushner BJ. Functional amblyopia associated with organic ocular disease. Am J Ophthalmol. 1981;91:39–45.
143. Inoue M, Noda K, Ishida S, Yamaguchi T, Nagai N, Shinoda K, et al. Successful treatment of subfoveal choroidal neovascularization associated with combined hamartoma of the retina and retinal pigment epithelium. Am J Ophthalmol. 2004;138(1):155–6.
144. Vianna RN, Pacheco DF, Vasconcelos MM, de Laey JJ. Combined hamartoma of the retina and retinal pigment epithelium associated with neurofibromatosis type-1. Int Ophthalmol. 2001;24(2):63–6.
145. De Potter P, Stanescu D, Caspers-Velu L, Hofmans A. Photo essay: combined hamartoma of the retina and retinal pigment epithelium in Gorlin syndrome. Arch Ophthalmol. 2000;118(7):1004–5.
146. Stupp T, Pavlidis M, Bochner T, Thanos S. Poland anomaly associated with ipsilateral combined hamartoma of retina and retinal pigment epithelium. Eye (Lond). 2004;18(5):550–2.
147. Demirci H, Shields CL, Shields JA. New ophthalmic manifestations of branchio-oculo-facial syndrome. Am J Ophthalmol. 2005;139(2):362–4.
148. Arepalli S, Pellegrini M, Ferenczy SR, Shields CL. Combined hamartoma of the retina and retinal pigment epithelium: findings on enhanced depth imaging optical coherence tomography in eight eyes. Retina. 2014;34(11):2202–7.
149. Fonseca RA, Dantas MA, Kaga T, Spaide RF. Combined hamartoma of the retina and retinal pigment epithelium associated with juvenile nasopharyngeal angiofibroma. Am J Ophthalmol. 2001;132(1):131–2.
150. Tulchinsky H, Keidar A, Strul H, et al. Extracolonic manifestations of familial adenomatous polyposis after proctocolectomy. Arch Surg. 2005;140(2):159–63.
151. Amin AR, Jakobiec FA, Dreyer EB. Ocular syndromes associated with systemic malignancy. Int Ophthalmol Clin. 1997;37:281–302.

16 Post Enucleation Orbital Implants

C. Umadevi and Bipasha Mukherjee

16.1 Introduction

Enucleation may be a life-saving procedure in patients with unsalvageable retinoblastoma, but it is also a life-changing experience for a child and the parents. The soft tissue component of the orbit is a crucial determinant of orbital bony growth hence, adequate volume replacement following enucleation is a major factor contributing to orbital development in children [1]. The ocular prosthesis is also considered to be an important factor in minimizing orbital growth retardation and thus preventing further facial asymmetry. A natural appearing prosthesis is essential to improve the self-esteem and prevent psychological trauma. In the recent past numerous technical developments and refinements have taken place in the field of anophthalmic socket surgery with regard to implant material and design.

16.2 Historical Perspective

Egyptians and Romans used ocular prostheses as early as 500 B.C.. Different materials like ivory, cork, cartilage, fat, bone, platinum, aluminum, silver, and gold have been used to make orbital implants. The first spherical implant made of glass, into an eviscerated globe, was done by Mules in 1885 [2].

16.3 Characteristics of an Ideal Implant [3] (According to Baino et al.)

1. Non-degradable (the orbital implant is regarded as being permanent).
2. Biocompatible (i.e. non-toxic, non-allergenic and non-carcinogenic).
3. Does not produce foreign-body reaction (inflammation or encapsulation).
4. Can be sterilized easily without degradation of material.
5. Exhibit adequate mechanical resistance to allow safe manipulation during surgery.
6. Capable of bonding with (or being colonized by) soft vascularized tissue.
7. Inexpensive.
8. Easily shaped into the desired form.
9. Offers excellent motility to be transferred to the ocular prosthesis.

16.4 Considerations in Orbital Implant Selection

It is mandatory to replace the globe with an orbital implant after enucleation, as absence of an implant will lead to a contracted socket and facial asymmetry, due to lack of stimulus for orbital

C. Umadevi · B. Mukherjee (✉)
Orbit, Oculoplasty, Reconstructive and Aesthetic Services, Medical Research Foundation, Sankara Nethralaya, Chennai, India
e-mail: drbpm@snmail.org; drbpm@gmail.org

V. Khetan (ed.), *Intraocular Tumors*, https://doi.org/10.1007/978-981-15-0395-5_16

growth. In case an implant cannot be placed during primary surgery a secondary ball implantation should be scheduled as soon as possible.

Approximately 70–80% of the volume of a normal globe should be replaced by the implant to avoid post-enucleation socket syndrome (PESS) [2]. A globe with an axial length of 24 mm has a volume of approximately 7 mL. An 18 mm sphere has a volume of 3.1 mL; a 20 mm sphere has a volume of 4.2 mL [4]. The remaining volume is replaced by the prosthesis (2–2.5 mL). The axial length of the contra lateral eye (or age matched controls in a bilateral affliction) minus 2 mm (Or—3 if the implant is wrapped with sclera) estimates the ideal implant diameter for optimal volume replacement [5].

16.5 Selection of Orbital Implant in Children

The selection of orbital implants is influenced by the surgeon's own preference, personal experience and training, design and the cost.

The fastest growth rate of the eye and orbit is seen during the first year of life. By 4 years of age the volume of the globe reaches 70% and 90% by age seven. It has been seen that facial development is affected by the volume of the orbits. Studies have indicated that facial asymmetries are due to enucleation at an early age rather than orbital irradiation [6].

We advocate the use of a non-porous silicone/PMMA implant in the paediatric population due to the economic price, low rate of complications, and ease of removal for subsequent implant exchange, if required. Mourits et al. concluded that outcomes are better with acrylic implants compared to the Hydroxyapatite implants [7]. On imaging, hydroxyapatite implants are radio-opaque; this might interfere with identification of calcification associated with recurrent retinoblastoma. On imaging, an ideal implant should have a well-circumscribed appearance and intermediate signal intensity, not to interfere with the diagnosis of tumour recurrence [8–10].

16.6 Classification of Orbital Implants [2]

Orbital implants can be classified according to the material as porous or nonporous:

1. Porous implant: An implant with numerous interconnected pores or channels throughout its structure that permit fibrovascular ingrowth. E.g. hydroxyapatite (HA), aluminum oxide, porous polyethylene (PE).
2. Nonporous implant: An implant that is solid and does not allow fibrovascular ingrowth. E.g. polymethylmethacrylate (PMMA), silicone (Fig. 16.1).

Implants can also be classified according to the design or connection of the implant to the overlying prosthesis.

1. Buried implant: An implant that has been placed within the anophthalmic socket with an overlying closed, smooth, uninterrupted conjunctival surface completely covering the implant.
2. Exposed implant: An implant that does not have an overlying closed, smooth, uninterrupted surface covering it.
3. Non-integrated implant: An implant that has been placed within the anophthalmic socket that has no connection with the overlying prosthetic eye.
4. Integrated implant: An implant that is directly coupled to the overlying prosthetic eye.
5. Semi-integrated implant: A buried implant with an irregular anterior surface, allowing indirect coupling ("quasi-integration") to the posterior surface of an overlying, modified prosthesis (e.g., Allen, Iowa, Universal, MEDPOR© Quad implants).

16.7 Biomaterials for Orbital Implants

1. *Autologous or biogenic implant*: Dermis fat graft (DFG) - is recommended for its growth potential [11].

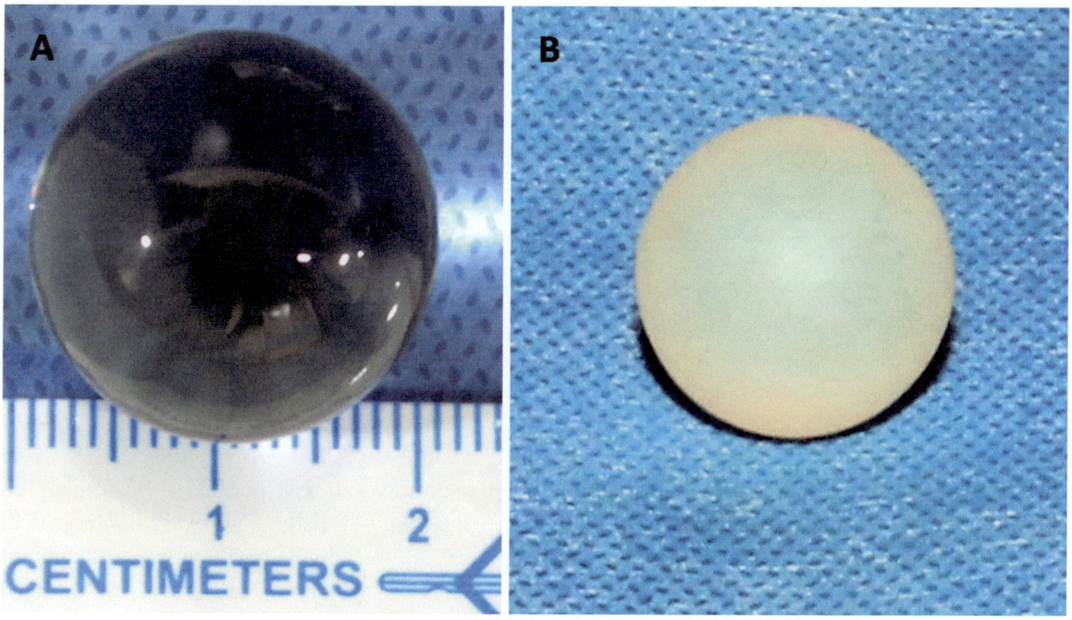

Fig. 16.1 Spherical non porous PMMA and silicone implants

The upside is that implant extrusion is a virtual impossibility in autografts.

DFG is preferred in the following scenarios:

- As a secondary procedure after extrusion or exposure of ball implant
- Deficient surface lining along with volume deficit in contracted socket
- As a primary procedure in children, since it has been reported to expand with the growth of the child [12].

Bosniak et al. reported very good socket movements and deeper fornices with primary autogenous dermis-fat orbital implants than synthetic ball implants [13]. Disadvantages of dermis-fat grafts include unpredictable rate of absorption especially in an irradiated socket resulting in orbital volume deficiency and donor site morbidity.

2. *Synthetic*:
   (a) Polymeric orbital implants: Silicone, polymethylmethacrylate (PMMA), polyethelene (PE), polytetrafluroethelene (PTFE), copolymer of methyl methacrylate.
   (b) Expandable implants—these implants expand in situ and thus are specifically useful in cases of children where a stimulus for orbital growth is required.
   - Silicon balloon expanders
   - Hydrogel expanders (N-vinyl pyrrolidine, polyacrylamide gel)

   (c) Ceramic implants
   (d) Composite implants
   (e) Magnetic implants

(a) *Polymeric implants* are widely used especially in the Asia-Pacific region.
Silicone is a commonly used spherical nonporous orbital implant. It is Inert, relatively pliable with well-established biocompatibility. Direct suture placement through the implant without wrapping is possible due to the soft and pliable nature of the material. However, foreign body reaction causing a dense, fibrous capsule surrounding the implant has been noted.

PMMA is another widely-used polymer due to its excellent biocompatibility. They owe their popularity to the low cost, availability, ease of handling and by and large good clinical outcomes.

Limitations: Fibro vascular in-growth is not possible hence exposure of implant is less amenable to conservative treatment and almost always results in extrusion of the implant.

PMMA implants

Allen type family PMMA implants underwent significant redesigning to reduce complications. Advantages -"lock-and-key" coupling system -supports the ocular prosthesis, thereby enhancing its motility.

Drawbacks—complex surgical procedure, exposure of the implant entails mandatory removal of the implant.

Iowa implant manufactured by injection-moulding a methyl methacrylate resin had four peripheral mounds located on its anterior surface designed to match four corresponding depressions on the posterior surface of the custom made prosthesis. The mounds create two channels so that the horizontal and vertical muscle stumps can be easily sutured together. Retrospective studies have shown low exposure and extrusion rates.

The drawback is possible necrosis of tissues covering the mounds of the implant.

Universal Implant has the advantage of Iowa's motility, but with smaller and rounded mounds, potentially decreasing the rate of complications [14].

Castroviejo implant—a variation of the Allen-type device, which offers motility to the ocular prosthesis. Anteriorly, it has a central depression surrounded by four bridges; the four recti muscles are accommodated in the tunnels situated directly beneath the bridge, and the ends of the opposed muscles are sewn so as to overlap each other. The implant is completely buried under the conjunctiva.

Synthetic porous polyethylene (PE) implants have been extensively accepted as an alternative to hydroxyapatite (HA) [8, 15]. Porous polyethylene implants, (MEDPOR®), although less biocompatible than HA, are usually well tolerated by orbital soft tissue. The smoother surface allows easier implantation and potentially less irritation of the overlying conjunctiva. These implants have a high tensile strength, but are malleable enough to allow for sculpting of the anterior surface of the implant. They may be used with or without a wrapping material.

Porous polyethylene implants are available in spherical, egg, conical, and mound shapes (MEDPOR Quad implant®). The anterior surface can also be manufactured with a smooth, nonporous surface to prevent abrasion of the overlying tissue (*MEDPOR smooth surface tunnel implant—SST®*) while retaining a larger pore size posteriorly to potentially facilitate fibrovascular ingrowth and suture tunnels to allow easy attachment of recti muscles [16]. Woog et al. used Medpor SST implants after enuleation with good motility with good cosmesis without complications [17]. Mahoney et al. reported that the exposure rate of MEDPOR SST® was significantly lower (3.3%) than other porous implants (7.1% over a 2-year follow-up) in 150 enucleated patients [18] (Fig. 16.2).

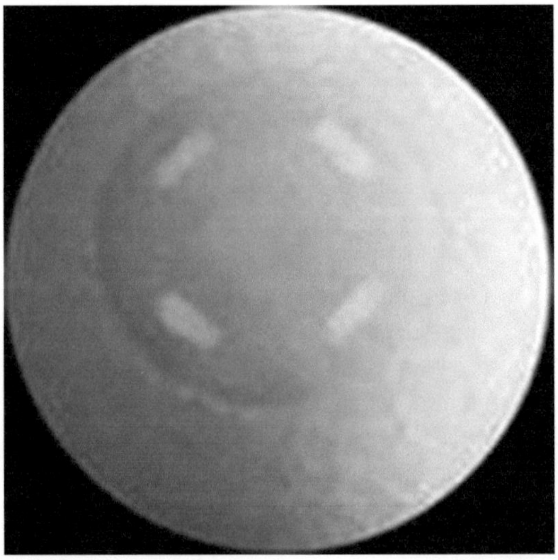

Fig. 16.2 MEDPOR SST implant (http://www.stryker.com/latm/products/Craniomaxillofacial/MEDPOR/MEDPOROculoplasticImplants)

The new version of PE porous devices is *MEDPOR Quad*™® implant, which is made of porous PE instead of PMMA.

Alpha Sphere—Poly (2-hydroxyethyl methacrylate) spherical implants have been introduced for the management of primary enucleation [19].

Advantages—Extraocular muscles can be directly sutured to the implant as is malleable and relatively soft; the smooth surface prevents conjunctival breakdown; and it undergoes anterior orbital fibrovascular in-growth (as the anterior hemisphere is porous).

The possible side effects are implant disintegration, fragmentation and partial extrusion.

(b) *Hydrogel* formulation is obtained by the copolymerization of methyl methacrylate and N-vinyl pyrrolidone. Hydrogel has been used in the form of both spherical orbital implants and small injectable pellets which can expand in situ for orbital volume augmentation [20] (Fig. 16.3).

(c) *Ceramic implants*

Porous ceramic implants have gained increasing popularity since their highly interconnected pore network allows fibrovascular ingrowth with low complication rates, while enhancing motility of the prosthesis, when pegging is done [8].

Bio-ceramic implant (Alumina®) made of Aluminum oxide is an alternative porous orbital implant available for use (FDA approved in April 2000) [21]. It is lightweight, reduces pressure over the upper lid, structurally strong, and has uniform evenly distributed pores and excellent pore interconnectivity enhancing host fibrovascular ingrowth, and much less expensive than HAp or PE implants.

Limitations-discharge, exposure, socket discomfort, and conjunctival thinning.

Jordan et al. reported the incidence of exposure associated with the Bioceramic implant (2.0%) is lower than that reported for HA implants [1].

Bio-active glass (bio-silicate, Na, Ca)-used to fabricate as well as salvage procedures to fill the peg tracts and re pegging with less inflammation.

(d) *Composite implants*

The anterior portion of the implant is made of synthetic porous HA to allow tissue integration which is connected to a posterior silicone hemisphere/cone. The muscles are sutured cross-wise in front of the implant to ensure better stability and motility (Guthoff implant®).

(e) *Magnetic implants*

Implant movement is transferred to the prosthesis by a couple of magnets with opposite poles incorporated on the posterior surface of the prosthesis and the anterior surface of the implant, the conjunctiva being sandwiched between the two elements [22].

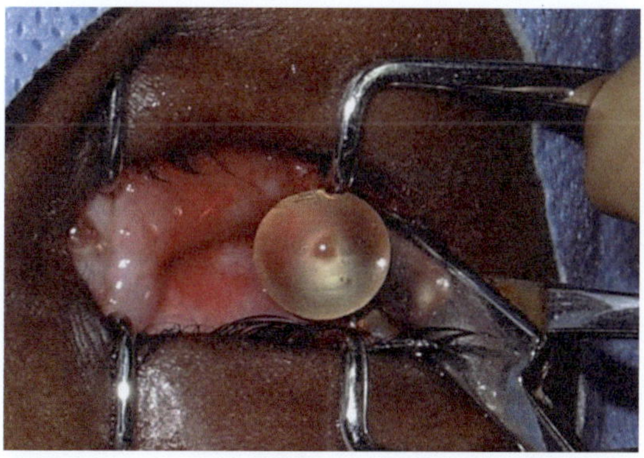

Fig. 16.3 Hydrogel implant being inserted through lateral conjunctival fornix in to the intraconal retrobulbar space

16.8 Common Complications Seen After Placement of Orbital Implants [3]

1. Conjunctival thinning
2. Ectropion/Entropion
3. Encapsulation
4. Enophthalmos
5. Exposure (Fig. 16.4)
6. Extrusion
7. Inflammation/infection
8. (Pseudo)Ptosis
9. Pyogenic granuloma
10. Superior sulcus deformity (Fig. 16.5)

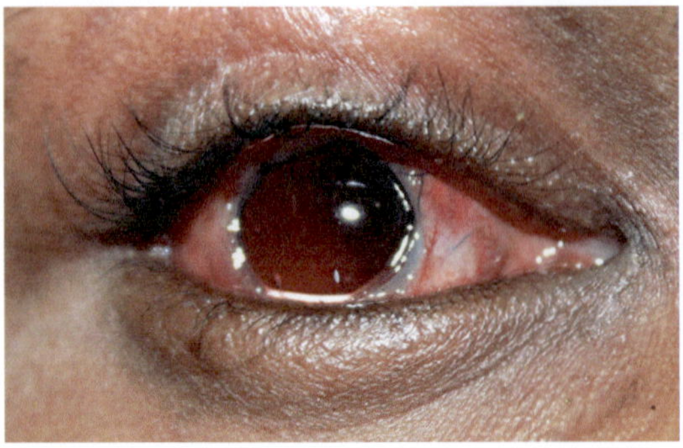

Fig. 16.4 Exposure of PMMA implant

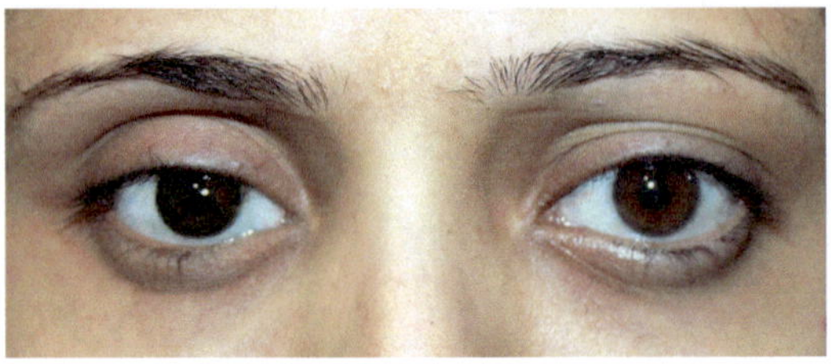

Fig. 16.5 Superior sulcus deformity due to inadequate volume replacement after enucleation

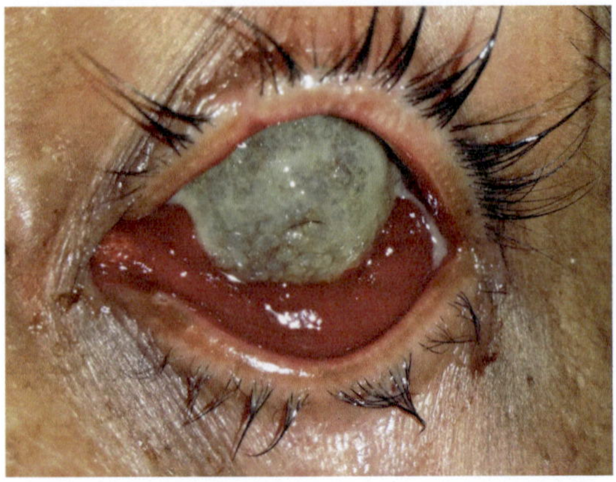

Fig. 16.6 Exposure of indigenous porous implant

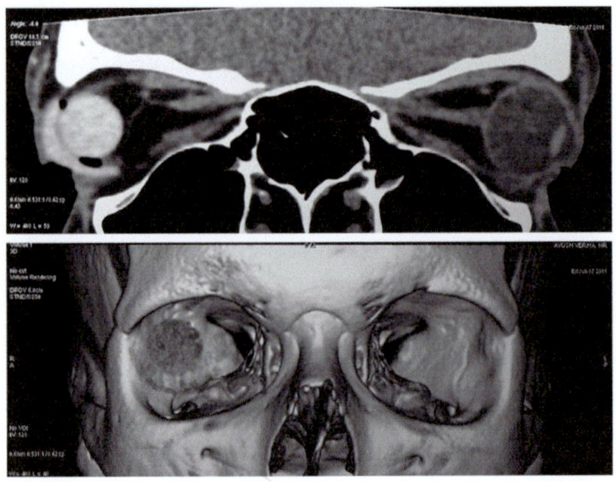

Fig. 16.7 Implant migration

Implant exposure rates after primary enucleation range from 0 to 21.6% [2, 23]. Significantly higher rates of implant exposure with porous implants have been reported, which may lessen after wrapping the implants [24] (Fig. 16.6).

Implant migration ranges from 0% to 61% (Fig. 16.7). Nikolaos et al. reported a significantly greater proportion of orbital implant migration in patients with a nonporous spherical implant than a porous implant [25]. Per operative orbital irradiation did not seem to increase implant migration and exposure. However, implant exposure was noted in a substantially greater proportion of patients who received perioperative systemic chemotherapy. According to Nikolaos et al., the effects of systemic chemotherapy on the conjunctiva and subconjunctival connective tissue over the implant predispose to exposure [25].

Kassaee et al. states that both sclera and Mersilene mesh are safe for wrapping HA orbital implant. Mersilene mesh may be the preferred choice as there is no possibility of disease transmission, easily available, economical, shorter surgery time with insignificant soft tissue complications [26]. However, the long-term efficacy and safety of Mersilene mesh needs to be assessed in a larger series of patients with longer follow-up.

16.9 Experimental Strategies and Future Research on Orbital Implants

The experimental strategies are that of surface modifications for implants and prostheses with coatings with Cu^{2+}, Ag^{+} ions in order to promote fibrovascularization as well as to provide an antibacterial effect. The nature of the material used as orbital implant has to be considered cautiously as they have to act as long-lasting devices for the patient's lifetime. Bioactive glass implants seem to be promising as they have reasonable bonding with the orbital soft tissues and are economical compared to other bioceramics such as HA and alumina [3].

16.10 Conclusion

Anophthalmic surgery is no longer merely restricted to treating the diseased eye and restoring the cosmesis. The research goals in this field, especially in case of children, are to minimize the likely complications, improve cosmesis, and provide maximal prosthetic motility after the enucleation. Meticulous surgery, proper implant selection with volume replacement, custom made prostheses, and regular follow up are needed to achieve an excellent cosmetic appearance in a growing child.

References

1. Jordan DR, Klappler SR. Chap. 18: Orbital implants. In: Clinical ophthalmic oncology, Orbital tumours. 2nd ed. Philadelphia: Lippincott Williams & Wilkins; 2014. p. 209–16.
2. Jordan DR, Stephen R, et al. Smith and Nesi's ophthalmic plastic and reconstructive surgery, vol. 68. 3rd ed. New York: Springer; 2012. p. 1105–28.
3. Francesco B, Isabel P. Orbital implants: state-of-the-art review with emphasis on biomaterials and recent advances. J Mater Sci Eng. 2016;69:1410–28.
4. Custer PL, Trinkaus KM. Volumetric determination of enucleation implant size. Am J Ophthalmol. 1999;128:489–94.
5. Kaltreider SA, Lucarelli MJ. A simple algorithm for selection of implant size for enucleation and evisceration. Ophthal Plast Reconstr Surg. 2002;18:336–41.
6. Bentley RP, Sgouros S, Natarajan K, et al. Normal changes in orbital volume during childhood. J Neurosurg. 2002;96:742–6.
7. Mourits DL, Moll AC, Bosscha MI, et al. Orbital implants in retinoblastoma patients: 23 years of experience and a review of the literature. Acta Ophthalmol. 2016;94:165–74.
8. Shields CL, Shields JA, De Potter P. Hydroxyapatite orbital implant after enucleation: experience with initial 100 consecutive cases. Arch Ophthalmol. 1992;110:333–8.
9. De Potter P, Shields CL, Shields JA, et al. Role of magnetic resonance imaging in the evaluation of the hydroxyapatite orbital implant. Ophthalmology. 1992;99:824–30.
10. David S, Steven Y, Robert P. Perspective on orbital enucleation implants. Surv Ophthalmol. 2007;52:245–65.
11. Nentwich M, Schebitz K, et al. Dermis fat grafts as primary and secondary orbital implants. Orbit. 2014;33:33–8.
12. Francesco Q, Sabrina S, Pietro R, et al. Dermis-fat graft in children as primary and secondary orbital implant. Ophthal Plast Reconstr Surg. 2016;32:214–9.
13. Bosniak SL, Nesi F, Smith BC, et al. A comparison of motility: autogenous dermis-fat vs synthetic spherical implants. Ophthalmic Surg. 1989;20:889–91.
14. Jordan DR, Anderson RL, Nerad JA. A preliminary report on the Universal Implant. Arch Ophthalmol. 1987;105:1726–31.
15. Huang D, Xu B, Yang Z. Fibrovascular ingrowth into porous polyethylene orbital implants (Medpor) after modified evisceration. Ophthal Plast Reconstr Surg. 2015;31:138–42.
16. Naik MN, Murthy RK, Honavar SG, et al. Comparison of vascularization of Medpor and Medpor-plus orbital implants: a prospective, randomized study. Ophthal Plast Reconstr Surg. 2007;23:463–7.
17. Woog JJ, Dresner SC, Lee TS, et al. The smooth surface tunnel porous polyethylene enucleation implant. Ophthalmic Surg Lasers Imaging. 2004;35:358–62.
18. Mahoney NR, Grant MP, Iliff NT, et al. Exposure rate of smooth surface tunnel porous polyethylene implants after enucleation. Ophthal Plast Reconstr Surg. 2014;30:492–8.
19. Shevchenko L, Boss J, Shah CT. Alpha sphere as a successful ocular implant in primary enucleation and secondary orbital implant exchange. Orbit. 2013;32:161–5.
20. Vagefi MR, McMullan TF, Burroughs JR, et al. Orbital augmentation with injectable calcium hydroxyapatite for correction of post enucleation/evisceration socket syndrome. Ophthal Plast Reconstr Surg. 2011;27:90–4.
21. David R, Steven G, Louise A. The bioceramic orbital implant: experience with 107 implants. Ophthalmic Plast Reconstr Surg. 2003;19:128–35.
22. Tomb EH, Gearhart DF, et al. A new magnetic implant. Arch Ophthalmol. 1954;52:763–8.
23. Suter AJ, Molteno ACB, Bevin T, et al. Long term follow up of bone derived hydroxyapatite orbital implants. Br J Ophthalmol. 2002;86:1287–92.
24. Custer PL, Kennedy RH, Woog JJ, et al. Orbital implants in enucleation surgery: a report by the American Academy of Ophthalmology. Ophthalmology. 2003;110:2054–61.
25. Nikolaos T, Augsburger JJ. Enucleation with unwrapped porous and nonporous orbital implants: a 15-year experience. Ophthal Plast Reconstr Surg. 2005;21:331–6.
26. Kassaee A, Mohsen B, Mohammadreza P. Mersilene mesh versus sclera in wrapping hydroxyapatite orbital implants. Ophthal Plast Reconstr Surg. 2006;22:41–4.

Post Enucleation Socket Management

17

Mangesh Dhobekar and Bipasha Mukherjee

17.1 Introduction

The management of the post enucleation anophthalmic socket remains a challenging one for the ophthalmic plastic surgeon and the ocularist. The best functional and cosmetic result depends upon the surgical techniques at the time of primary enucleation surgery and it should be performed very meticulously to avoid the postoperative socket deformities.

A functionally and cosmetically acceptable anophthalmic socket should have all of the following components [1]:

- A central, well-covered and biocompatible implant of adequate volume
- A socket lined with healthy conjunctiva or mucous membrane with deep fornices
- Eyelids with normal position, adequate tone and appearance
- A supra tarsal eyelid fold that is symmetric with that of the contra lateral eyelid
- Good transmission of motility from the implant to the overlying prosthesis
- A comfortable ocular prosthesis that looks similar to the sighted, contra lateral globe
- Any change in one of these components may lead to suboptimal cosmesis and function. It is emphasized to have the good coordination between the ophthalmic plastic surgeon and the ocularist in order to examine the anophthalmic socket preoperatively, to plan the surgical and conservative procedures and for the follow up examinations postoperatively at regular intervals.

17.2 Enucleation and Orbital Growth

The size and shape of the orbit is the result of the balance between variety of genetic and environmental factors that may function on a systemic, regional or local basis. Kaiser stated that the eye increases in volume after birth only threefold and that approximately 70% of its volume is reached by the age of 4 years [2]. The effect of enucleation on orbital growth and development with and without implant has been of great deal of concern over the years (Fig. 17.1a, b). Taylor reported the effect of enucleation in childhood on facial development and observed that enucleation performed before the age of 5 years led to a retardation of the bony growth of the orbit up to as much as 15% less than the normal unaffected side. The wearing of prosthesis had no influence on the development of the bony orbit but it probably

M. Dhobekar
Orbit, Oculoplasty and Ocular Prosthetic Services, Shri Ganapati Netralaya, Jalna, Maharashtra, India

B. Mukherjee (✉)
Orbit, Oculoplasty, Reconstructive and Aesthetic Services, Medical Research Foundation, Chennai, India
e-mail: drbpm@snmail.org

V. Khetan (ed.), *Intraocular Tumors*, https://doi.org/10.1007/978-981-15-0395-5_17

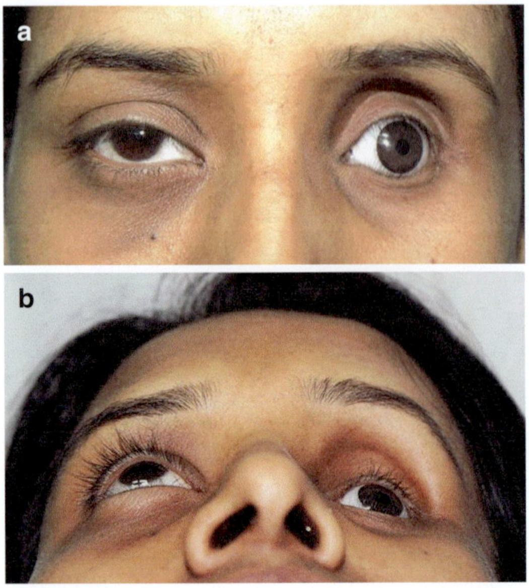

Fig. 17.1 (**a**) A 23 years old female patient following an enucleation and irradiation to the socket at the age of 2 years. No orbital implant was placed in leading to retarded growth of left orbit (**b**) Severe volume deficiency and superior sulcus deformity

exerted an influence on the development of orbital soft tissues [3]. A committee of the Ophthalmological Society of the United Kingdom reported in 1898 that the disadvantage of a simple enucleation performed early in life was the retardation of the orbital and facial growth on the involved side [4].

17.3 Post Enucleation Socket Syndrome (PESS)

The anophthalmic socket is different, both anatomically and physiologically, from an orbit containing an eye. Postoperative changes affect not only the cosmetic appearance but also the function of the socket. Post enucleation socket syndrome is the result of orbital volume deficiency and soft tissue changes post initial surgery (Fig. 17.2a–d) [5]. The term was introduced by Tyers and Collin with the following clinical features:

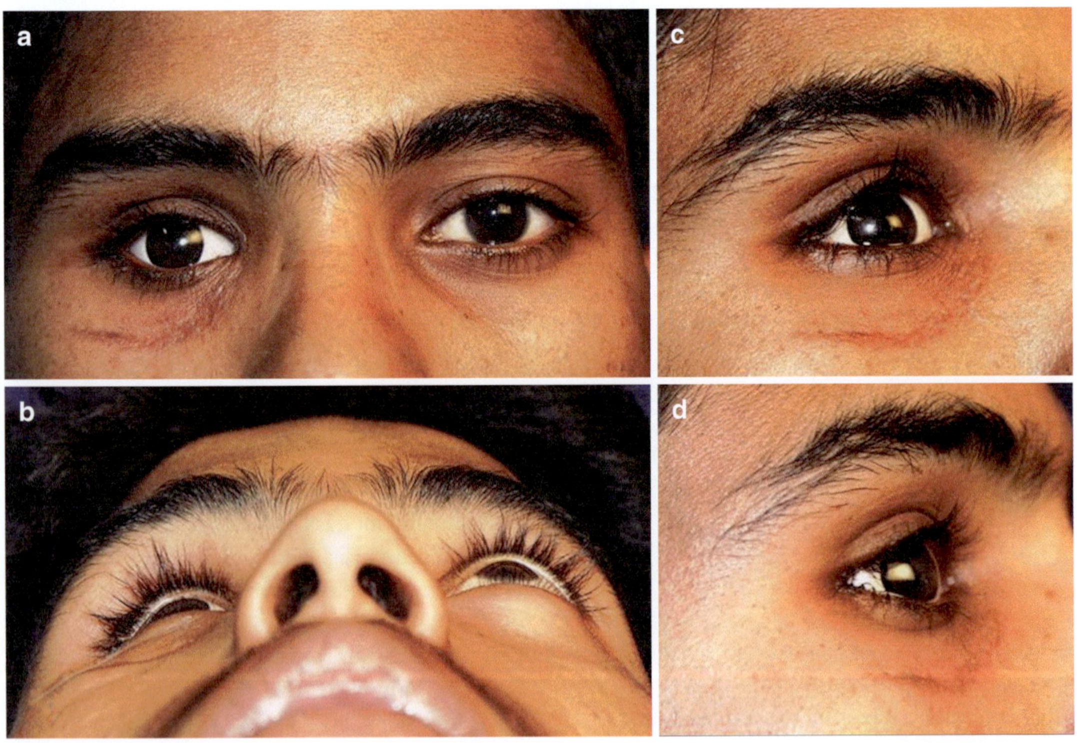

Fig. 17.2 (**a**, **b**) showing a young male patient who has the typical features of a right post-enucleation socket syndrome (PESS). No orbital implant was placed in this patient following an enucleation. (**c**, **d**) Showing a view of the patient demonstrating a typical backward tilt to the prosthesis

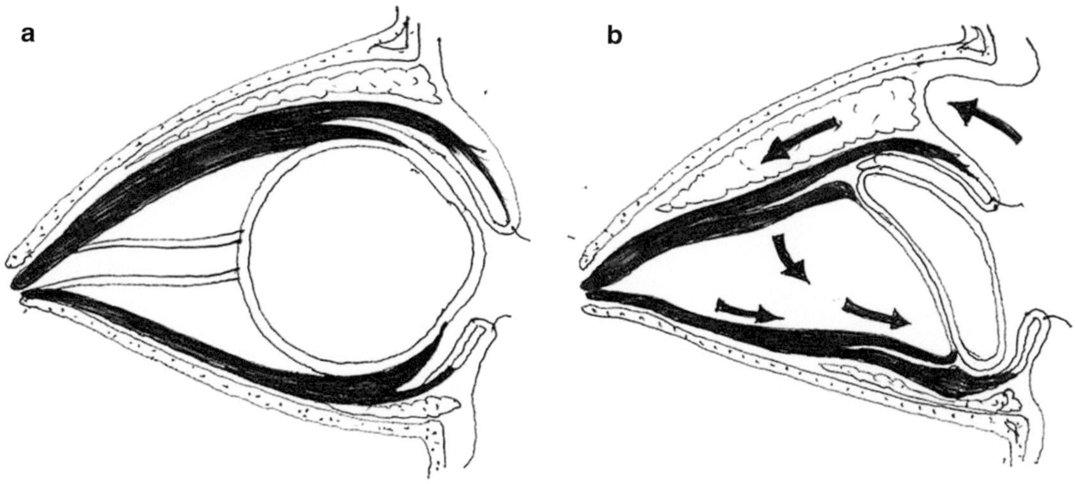

Fig. 17.3 (**a**, **b**) Anophthalmic socket soft tissue changes leading to post enucleation socket syndrome

- Enophthalmos
- Deep superior eyelid sulcus
- Ptosis or lid retraction
- Lower lid laxity
- Shallow inferior fornix

Post enucleation changes in orbital soft tissue like superior-to-posterior and posterior-to-inferior rotation leading to backward tilting of the ocular prosthesis were observed by the Smit and added later to the PESS (Fig. 17.3a, b) [6]. It was also observed that these orbital soft tissues changes associated with volume deficiency and not only orbital fat atrophy are responsible for the development of a PESS [7].

17.4 Pathophysiology

An enucleation surgery without the orbital implant leads to subsequent volume deficit and causes enophthalmos and a deep superior eyelid sulcus. The eye is no longer there to support superior rectus and levator muscle complex which drops to a variable degree giving rise to ptosis, or rarely, lid retraction. Lid retraction probably occurs due to the disinserted superior rectus muscle contracting and pulling on the levator complex via the common sheath. The inferior rectus muscle is no longer pushed down by the presence of the eye and it tends to rise in the socket. The inferior fornix becomes shallow due to associated elevation of lower lid retractors and their connections. The fat within the orbit tends to collect inferiorly with the gravity. There is posterior and anticlockwise rotation of the orbital content. If a small artificial eye is inserted into an enucleated socket with none or an inadequately sized implant, the upper part of the eyelid tends to tilt backwards leading to enophthalmic appearance, deep upper eyelid sulcus with obvious ptosis. If the artificial eye is increased in size, it initially improves these features but then the lower lid sags under the weight seeming lower than the other side or 'dropped socket appearance'. The artificial eye becomes unstable due to lax lower lid and shallow lower fornix (Fig. 17.4a–d) [5].

17.4.1 Basic Principles to Avoid PESS

The features of the PESS can be primarily avoided if suitable sized orbital implant is inserted at the time of the enucleation (Fig. 17.5a–d). A preoperative assessment of the axial lengths of the eye to be removed and the contralateral eye is a useful tool to determine the proper implant volume at the time of enucleation. But it has been observed that there is a considerable variation in axial length and globe volume with globe volumes varying between 6.9 and 9.0 mL [8]. For

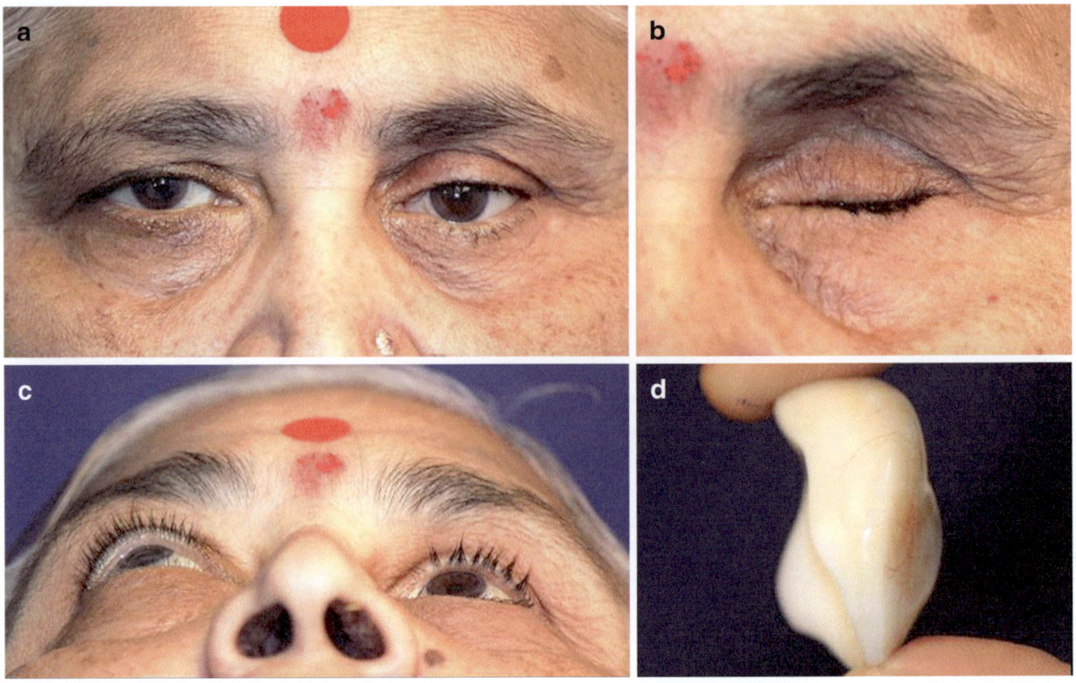

Fig. 17.4 (**a**, **b**) showing a female patient who has the typical features of a right post-enucleation socket syndrome (PESS). (**c**) Patient has severe enophthalmos as no orbital implant was placed in following an enucleation. (**d**) To restore a volume to the socket, a thick and heavy ocular prosthesis was fitted in but it will lead to decreased ocular movements and lower lid sagging

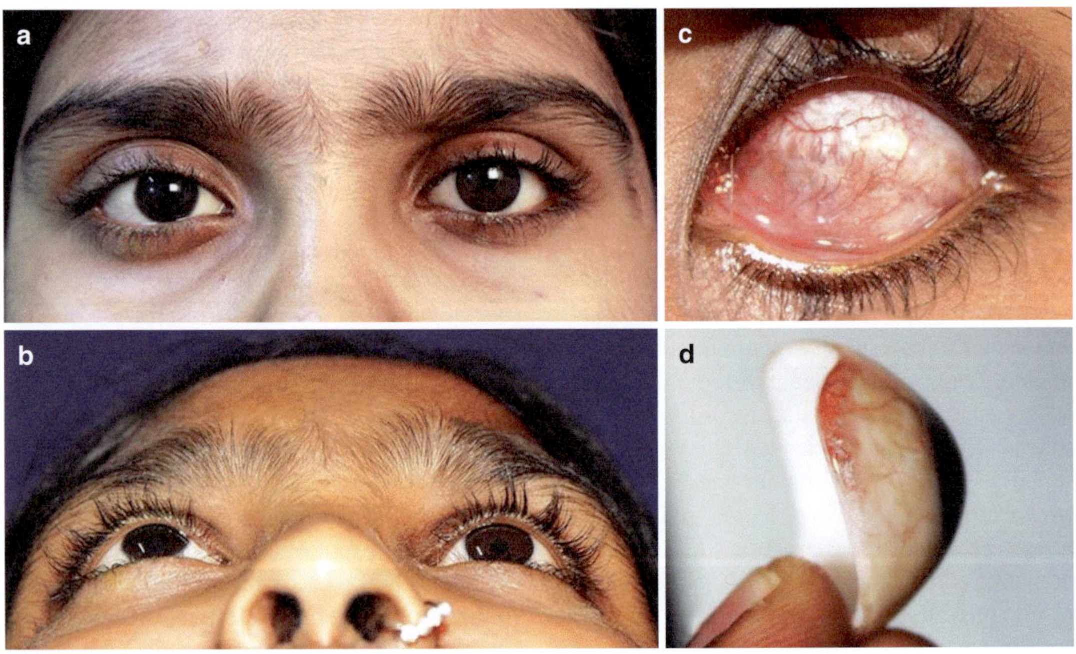

Fig. 17.5 (**a**) A 15 year old female patient following an enucleation and adequate sized orbital ball implant with good symmetry. (**b**) Both eyes are at same plane with no enophthalmos (**c**) a healthy socket with good volume restoration (**d**) A thin and light weight ocular prosthesis will impart good ocular movements

orbital volume restoration at the time of enucleation, we use the formula: Axial length of the eye—2 mm = Implant diameter [9]. An appropriate sized implant can also be determined by the volume of fluid displaced by an enucleated eye when placed in a graduated cylinder [10].

An orbital implant should replace approximately 70–80% of the volume of the enucleated eye and ocular prosthesis should restore the residual volume. An ideal prosthetic volume for the good excursion and movement is 2.0–2.5 mL [11]. Prosthetic volumes larger than 4.0 mL, often leads progressive lower lid laxity and malposition and limited excursion [9]. An ideal implant size can also be determined by the formula: volume of the enucleated eye in mL minus 2.0–2.5 mL [10]. Approximately an18-mm sphere equals 3.1 mL in volume, a 20-mm sphere 4.2 mL, and a 22-mm sphere 5.6 mL. An orbital implant larger than 22 mm may lead to exposure and difficulty in fitting an ocular prosthesis [8, 9]. Generally we use 18–20 mm orbital implants in paediatric patients and 20–22 mm spherical implants in adults.

17.5 Post Enucleation Complications

17.5.1 Orbital Implant Exposure and Extrusion

The porous as well as nonporous orbital implants may lead to an early or late implant exposure and subsequent implant extrusion. It was observed that nonporous orbital implants carry lower risk of implant exposure than porous orbital implants in spite of fibrovascular ingrowth associated with these types of implants. The porous orbital implants with exposure rates varying from 0 to 50%, can lead thinning of the overlying conjunctiva, persistent discharge, granulomatous reaction, infection and persistent pain [12].

A variety of factors may predispose to implant exposure and subsequent extrusion and include conjunctival wound closure under tension, implant larger than 22 mm, use of non-absorbable sutures, delayed wound healing, surface infection, irritation from the irregular surface of the porous implant, delayed fibrovascular ingrowth, ill-fitting prosthesis and improper care of prosthesis (Fig. 17.6a–d) [13].

Early implant exposure in porous as well as nonporous implants can be managed with re-approximating the wound if not under tension as early as possible. If wound is under tension, a scleral patch graft can be used. For late porous implant exposures less than 3 mm, modification of prosthesis with vaulting of the posterior surface in area of exposure to promote the conjunctival re-epithelization can be done. If no improvement within 8 weeks and for late exposures more than 3 mm, surgical intervention in the form of various flaps or patch grafts should be considered [14]. For late non-porous implant exposures, implant exchange and secondary orbital implant surgery remains a choice. In case of spontaneous implant exposure, if socket is allowed to heal without any intervention soft tissue contracture occurs and subsequent socket reconstruction may pose a difficulty resulting in suboptimal cosmesis [15].

17.5.2 Migration of the Orbital Implant

Post enucleation disturbances in orbital soft tissue and subsequent fibrosis may lead to orbital implant migration. Implant migration occurs more commonly in nonporous implants owing to poor surgical techniques and non-attachment of the extraocular muscles compared to porous implants due to extraocular muscle attachment and fibrovascular ingrowth [16]. An implant wrapping with attachment of the extraocular muscles in nonporous implant may help prevent implant migration. Implant migration in nonporous implants is seen in the area of least resistance, particularly in inferotemporal direction (Fig. 17.7a, b). A shallow inferior fornix due to anterior and inferotemporal implant migration hinders the proper positioning of the customised ocular prosthesis leading to poor motility and suboptimal cosmesis. Allen described refitting the new prosthesis with "modified impression technique" to impart additional motility and to improve the comfort [17].

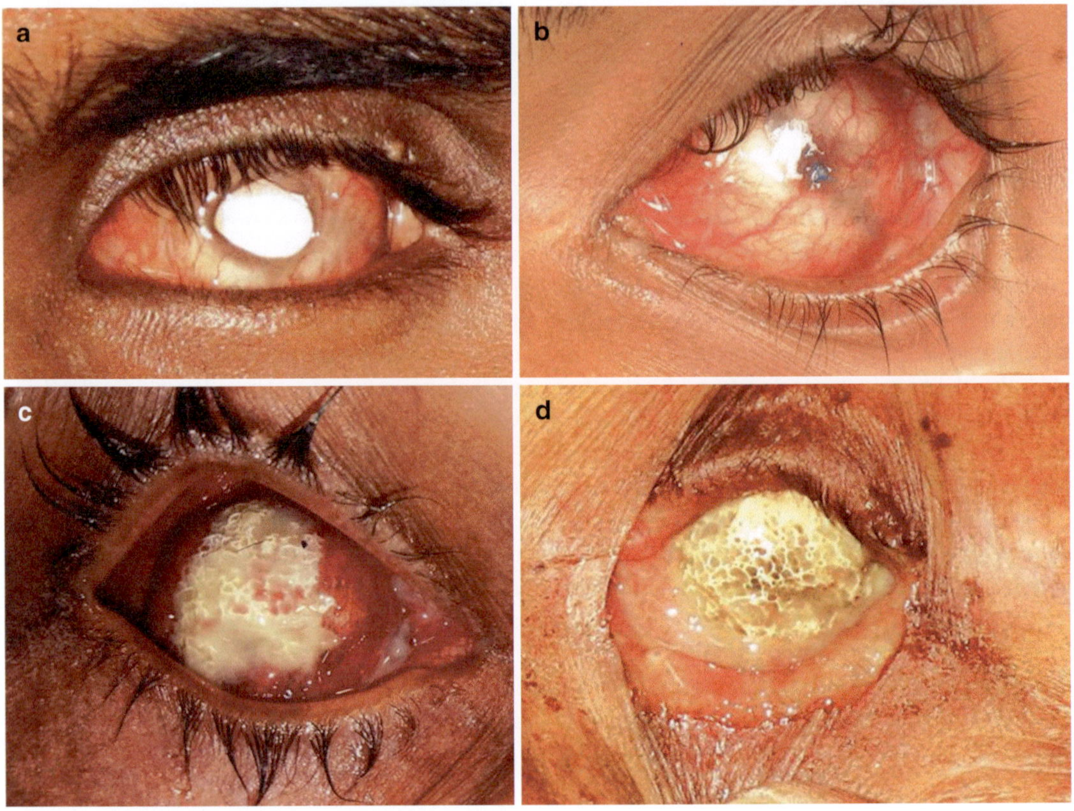

Fig. 17.6 (**a**) Exposed polymethylmethacrylate implant (**b**) Use of non-absorbable sutures leads to progressive conjunctival thinning and late implant exposure (**c**) Exposed porous polyethylene implant (**d**) Exposed and infected porous implant

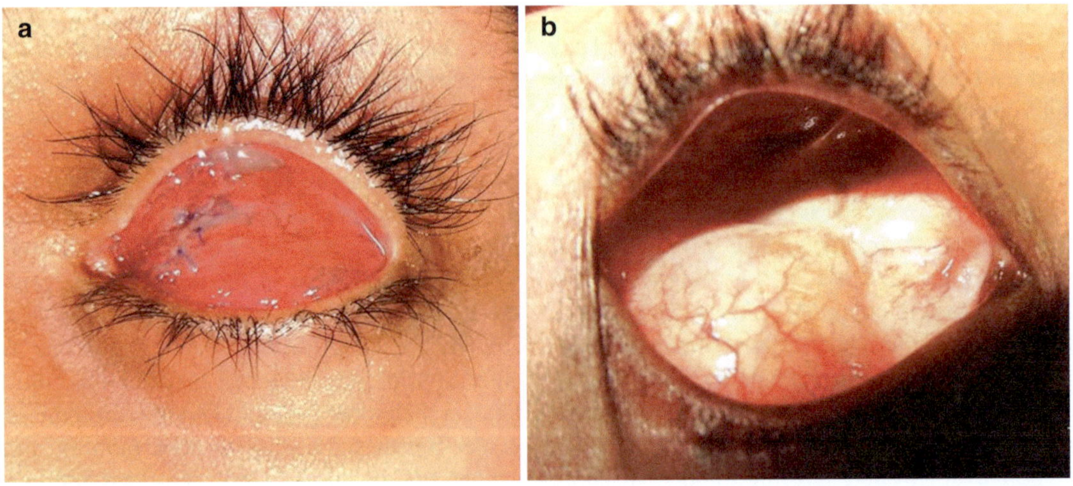

Fig. 17.7 (**a**) An inferior migration of an orbital implant with shallow inferior fornix in early postoperative period following enucleation (**b**) An inferior migration of orbital ball implant in late postoperative period

The management of the migrated implants includes implant removal and replacement of new implant with proper positioning and reattachment of the extraocular muscles to improve the movement and fitting of the customised ocular prosthesis. An implant removal and socket reconstruction with dermis fat graft can also be done in recurrent implant migration.

17.5.3 Volume Deficit and Superior Sulcus Deformity

Post enucleation volume deficit and superior sulcus deformity occurs as a result of inadequate volume restoration, no use of orbital implant or very small orbital implant, redistribution of the orbital soft tissues and progressive orbital fat atrophy (Fig. 17.1a, b) [16]. Volume deficit/enophthalmos and superior sulcus deformity can be corrected surgically in a staged approach. Placement of an adequate sized spherical orbital implant at the time of enucleation should be emphasized. An orbital floor subperiosteal implant placement and superior sulcus fat grafting can be performed to achieve the additional volume restoration and sulcus augmentation (Fig. 17.8a–d). A Superior sulcus deformity can be, alternatively corrected with hyaluronic acid gel with promising results [18].

17.5.4 Eyelid Malposition

An intraoperative injury or progressive dehiscence of levator aponeurosis and migration of the orbital implant may lead to upper eyelid ptosis.

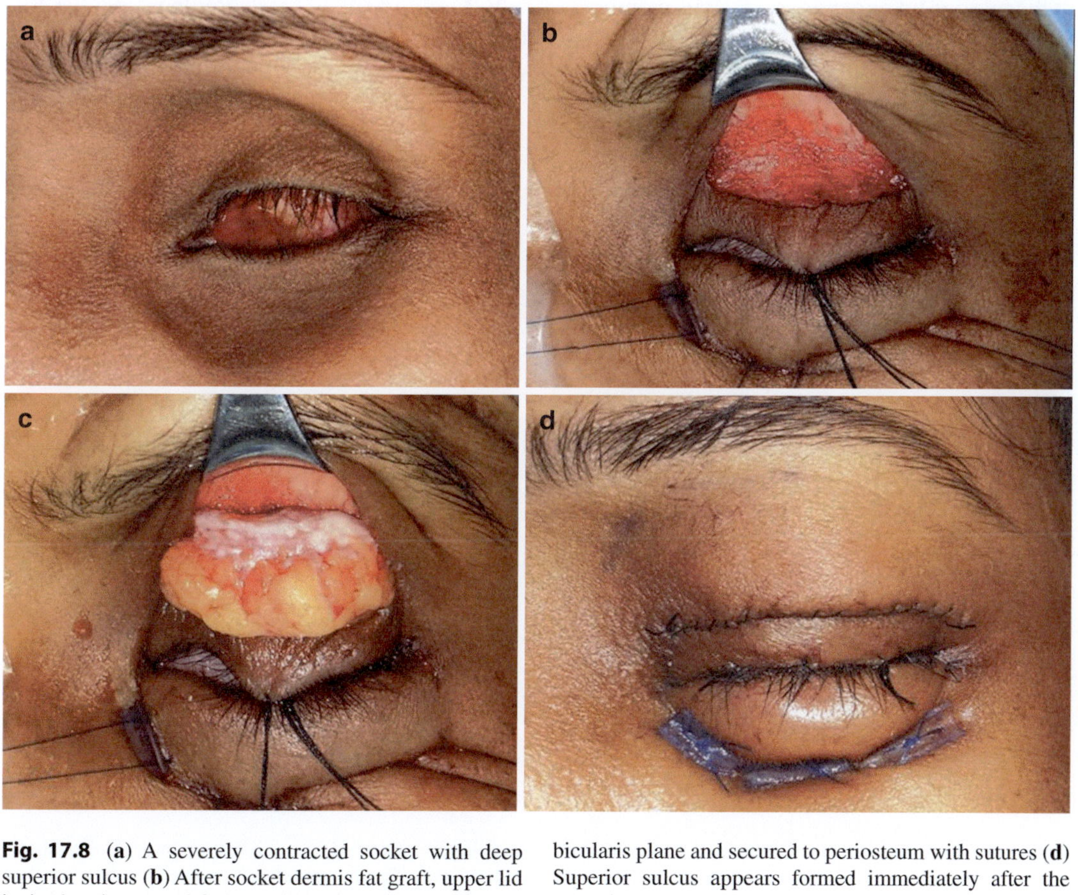

Fig. 17.8 (**a**) A severely contracted socket with deep superior sulcus (**b**) After socket dermis fat graft, upper lid incised and prepared for superior sulcus dermis fat graft (**c**) The dermis fat graft was placed in a preseptal suborbicularis plane and secured to periosteum with sutures (**d**) Superior sulcus appears formed immediately after the procedure

Upper lid ptosis can be improved conservatively with modification of the ocular prosthesis. A ptosis 'shelf' in the prosthesis may decrease the ptosis and improve the appearance. Surgical repair of the levator should be the next consideration if conservative method fails. In all such cases, the levator is usually of normal strength and overcorrection of ptosis may occur if levator strength is underestimated.

Post enucleation lower lid laxity, shortening of the posterior lamella, shallow inferior fornix, dehiscence of the inferior lid retractors and weight of the prosthesis can lead to ectropion or entropion of the lower eyelid (Fig. 17.9a–d). To correct the lower lid position conservatively, a part of volume can be removed from the area immediately below the lower limbus, creating a reverse prosthetic curvature inferiorly. If this does not correct the ectropion, horizontal tightening procedures, lateral tarsal strip, advancement of the inferior lid retractors or mucous membrane graft with deepening of inferior fornix are usually successful.

17.5.5 Painful Socket and Persistent Discharge

Ill-fitting ocular prosthesis and improper prosthesis care are the common factors responsible for the socket tenderness and persistent discharge from the socket. Prosthesis should be evaluated to rule out the improper fitting, sharp edges and irregular surfaces, presence of stock shell with pooling of mucoid secretions behind the prosthesis. The socket should be examined for the signs of ocular surface inflammation, giant papillary conjunctivitis, presence of granulomas, eyelid malpositions and shallow fornices and anterior conjunctival cysts (Fig. 17.10a, b). An orbital implant should be examined for the signs of implant exposure and implant migration. An orbital imaging should be ordered in case of intractable pain to rule out any recurrent orbital mass lesion, sinoorbital and intracranial pathology. To minimize all these problems, regular follow up examinations with ophthalmic plastic surgeon and ocularist are recommended.

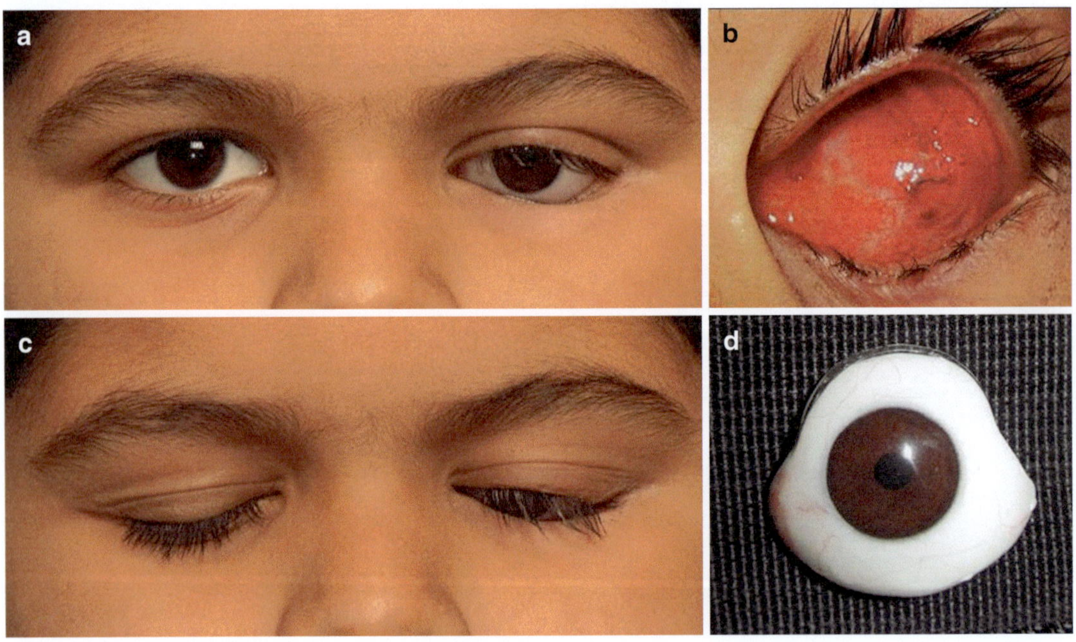

Fig. 17.9 (**a**) A young male patient with left anophthalmic socket has lower lid entropion and (**b**) Lagophthalmos (**c**) A socket shows shallow superior and inferior fornices with inflammation (**d**) A modification in ocular prosthesis did not show improvement and he needs further surgical intervention

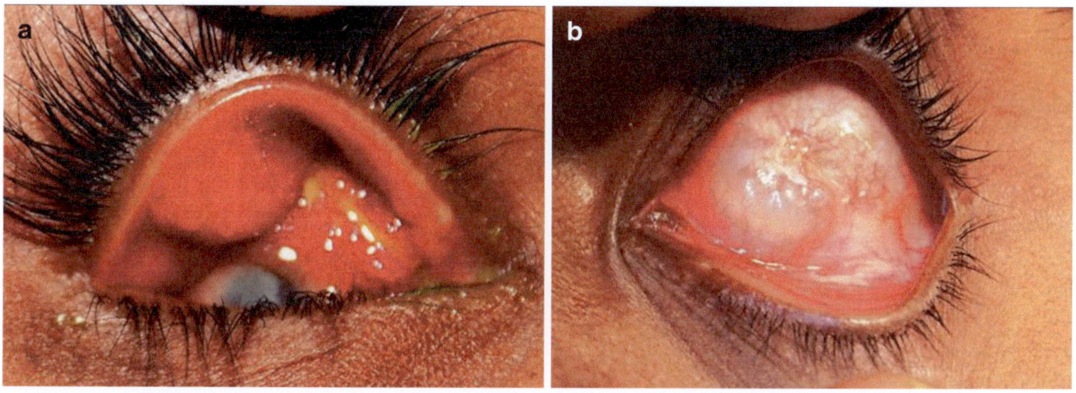

Fig. 17.10 (**a**) An inflammed socket with giant papillary conjunctivitis (**b**) A socket showing anterior conjunctival cysts

17.5.6 Contracted Socket

Contracted socket is one of the important aspects of the post-enucleation socket management. It is characterised by contracture of orbital soft tissues and bony parts associated with shallowing of the fornices, surface and volume deficit leading to an inability to retain prosthesis [19]. Poor initial surgical techniques, non-preservation of the conjunctiva, excessive use of the cautery, orbital radiation and compromised vascular supply, implant exposure and extrusion, no or very small orbital implant, no use of conformer or prosthesis, ill-fitting prosthesis and recurrent socket inflammation are the common factors responsible for the development of contracted socket.

Gopal Krishna has classified the contracted socket [20]:

Grade 1:	A shallow or shelved inferior fornix
Grade 2:	Shallow superior and inferior fornices
Grade 3:	Shallow superior, inferior, medial and lateral fornices
Grade 4:	All fornices shallow associated with decreased palpebral aperture in horizontal and vertical dimensions
Grade 5:	Recurrence of socket contracture even after multiple surgeries

Alternatively contracted socket can be classified as:

Mild:	Shallowing of only one fornix and posterior lamellar shortening of the lids
Moderate:	Shallow superior and inferior fornices
Severe:	Shallowing of all the fornices associated with palpebral aperture phimosis
Malignant contracted socket:	A severely contracted socket as result of extensive trauma or multiple surgeries [21]

17.5.7 Evaluation of the Contracted Socket

Preoperative clinical evaluation of the contracted socket should be performed with emphasis on the following:

Cosmesis with prosthesis with respect to fellow eye—good/fair/poor

- Colour match—good/fair/poor
- Movements—good/fair/poor
- Lagophthalmos—absent/present (in mm)
- Pseudoptosis—absent/present
- Enophthalmos—absent/present
- Discolouration—absent/present
- Deposits—absent/present
- Edges—sharp/blunt
- Surface—smooth /rough/scratches

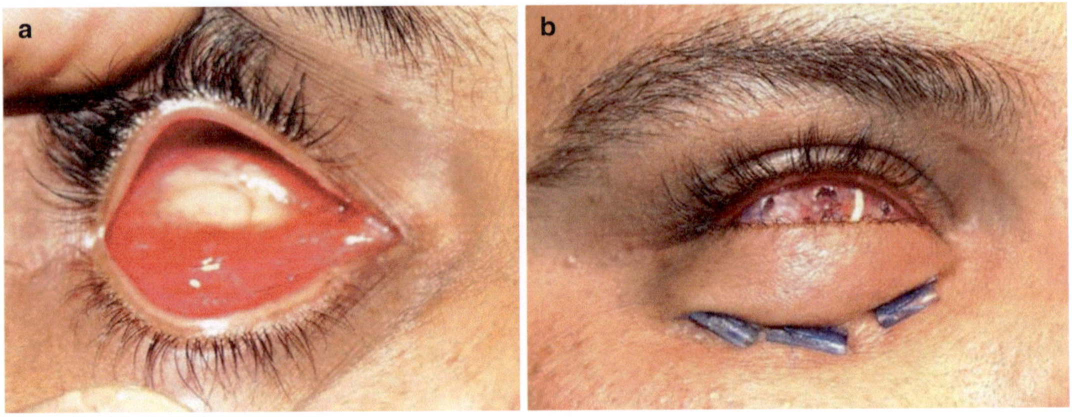

Fig. 17.11 (a) A contracted socket with a shallow inferior fornix (b) Inferior fornix forming sutures with bolsters

Socket: healthy/congested/papillae/granuloma/cicatricial bands/dry/wet

- Volume—adequate/deficit
- Implant—present/absent
- Implant position—central/migrated
- Implant exposure—present/absent
- Superior fornix—well-formed/shallow/absent
- Inferior fornix—well-formed/shallow/absent
- Medial fornix—well-formed/shallow/absent
- Lateral fornix—well-formed/shallow/absent
- Bony contracture—present/absent

17.5.8 Management of Contracted Socket

The aim of the management of contracted socket is to identify and correct underlying cause and to achieve the best possible cosmesis, prosthesis movement and comfort of the patient. A proper coordination between the ophthalmic plastic surgeon and ocularist is essential in the management of such challenging cases. The treatment options, prognosis of the surgery, staged approach for the socket reconstruction and realistic outcomes of achievable cosmesis should be well discussed with the patient beforehand.

17.5.9 Mild Socket Contracture

It involves shallowing of only one fornix and posterior lamellar shortening of the lids. A Shallow inferior fornix can be addressed by deepening the fornix with the help of fornix forming sutures in a closed or open method.

In a closed method, three horizontal mattress sutures, 4-0 non-absorbable, initially passed deep into the inferior fornix, advanced through the orbital rim periosteum and then exteriorized from the lower lid skin. A conformer is placed into the socket and sutures are secured and tied over the silicon bolsters. These sutures are removed after 4 weeks and fitting of the ocular prosthesis is then attempted (Fig. 17.11a, b).

In an open method, instead of closed method, a horizontal inferior forniceal trans-conjunctival incision is placed at least 10 mm inferior to the lower eyelid margin and deeper dissection is continued up to the lower orbital rim periosteum. Three horizontal mattress sutures are placed through the edge of posterior conjunctiva, through the orbital periosteum and then back through the anterior conjunctival edge [22].

Associated posterior lamellar shortening can be corrected with the help of the scleral or cartilage spacer graft. A lateral tarsal strip procedure may be required in case of significant lower lid laxity or lower lid entropion.

17.5.10 Moderate Socket Contracture

Moderate socket contracture is characterised by the shallow superior and inferior fornices associated with moderate surface and volume deficiency. Initially inferior fornix is affected followed by the contracture changes in the superior fornix limiting the movement of the lid and prosthesis. A variety of surgical techniques for the surface and volume augmentation in contracted socket have been described.

17.6 Mucous Membrane Graft (MMG)

A mucous membrane graft is the most commonly used tissue in the management of moderate to severe contracted socket with significant surface deficit [23]. Mucous membrane grafts are harvested from the lower lip or buccal mucosa. The mouth washes with betadine should be started 2 weeks prior to surgery in all cases. A size of the mucous membrane graft should be approximately 40–50% larger than the defect area to allow for subsequent tissue contracture. An appropriate marking taking into account the host defect should be done before the infiltration of mucosal area with 2% xylocaine with epinephrine 1:100,000. An incision over the marked area is placed with a no. 15 Bard Parker blade and the full thickness mucosal graft is then harvested using the scissors. A layer of fat and submucosal tissue should be trimmed off from the mucosal graft. The donor area on the lower lip is allowed to granulate while defect on the buccal mucosa should be closed with 4-0 absorbable sutures.

A Mucous membrane graft can be placed either in the fornices to increase the surface area and deepen the fornices along with the fornix forming sutures or it can be used alternatively in the center of the contracted socket to restore the surface (Fig. 17.12a–d). Quilting sutures to the mucosal

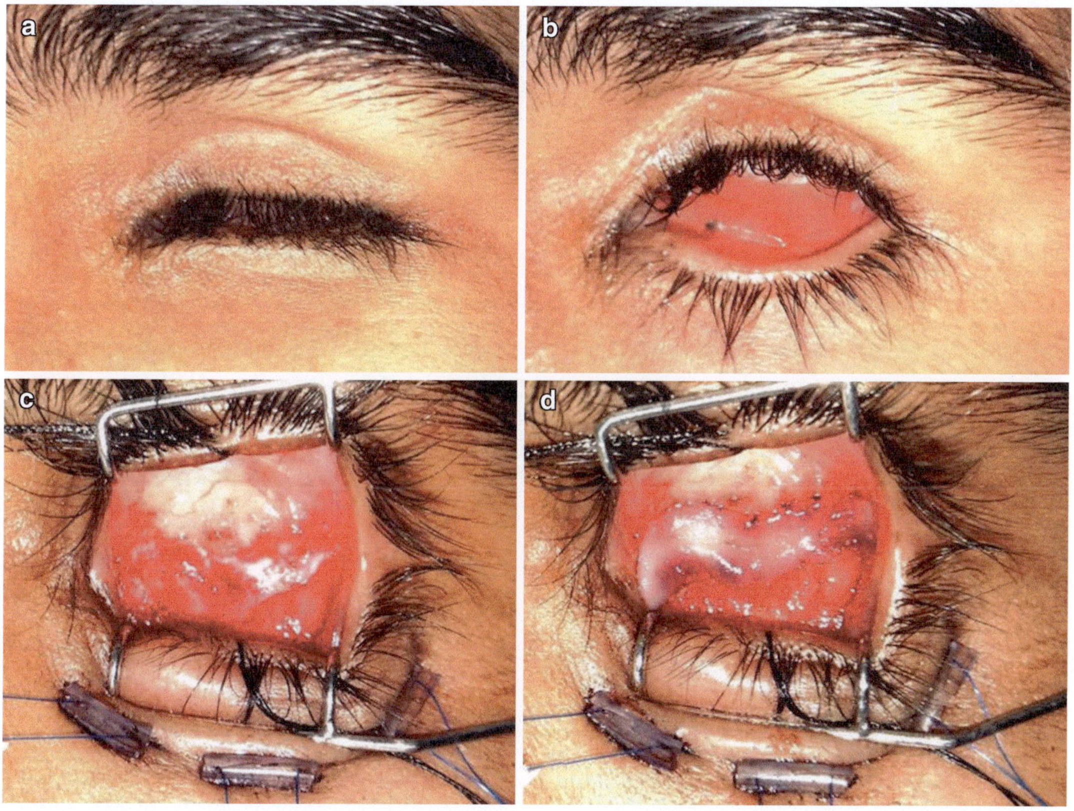

Fig. 17.12 (**a**) A 17 years old female patient with left side contracted anophthalmic socket (**b**) A socket with shallow inferior fornix and surface deficit. (**c**) A horizontal incision is given over the conjunctiva and inferior fornix forming sutures are placed (**d**) A mucous membrane graft is placed over the recipient bed with a central defect

graft are useful to ensure better opposition of the graft to the host bed [24]. A Mucous membrane graft, a "substitute graft" is preferred to the amniotic membrane, a "substrate graft" in the management of the contracted socket with surface deficit [25].

17.7 Secondary Orbital Implantation

Socket reconstruction with secondary orbital implantation is mainly indicated in moderately contracted socket with volume deficit but with an adequate surface area. It helps achieve volume restoration, correct superior sulcus deformity and improve the motility of the ocular prosthesis. Secondary orbital implantation can also be performed as a part of the implant exchange procedure indicated for implant migration, exposure and extrusion of the implant and small implant with difficulty in fitting of the ocular prosthesis. Secondary orbital implantation is more difficult than primary surgery owing to disturbances and subsequent fibrosis of the orbital soft tissues. Identification of the recti muscles and placement of the implant into the intraconal region help to improve motility and decrease the chances of implant migration.

In a secondary orbital implant surgery, a conjunctiva is incised in a horizontal direction and the previous implant is removed. Nonporous implants can be removed without any difficulty but porous implants are not straightforward to remove. After removal of the implant, a pseudocapsule is then gently dissected and removed (Fig. 17.13a–d). The central Tenon's layer is dissected further with blunt instruments to expose

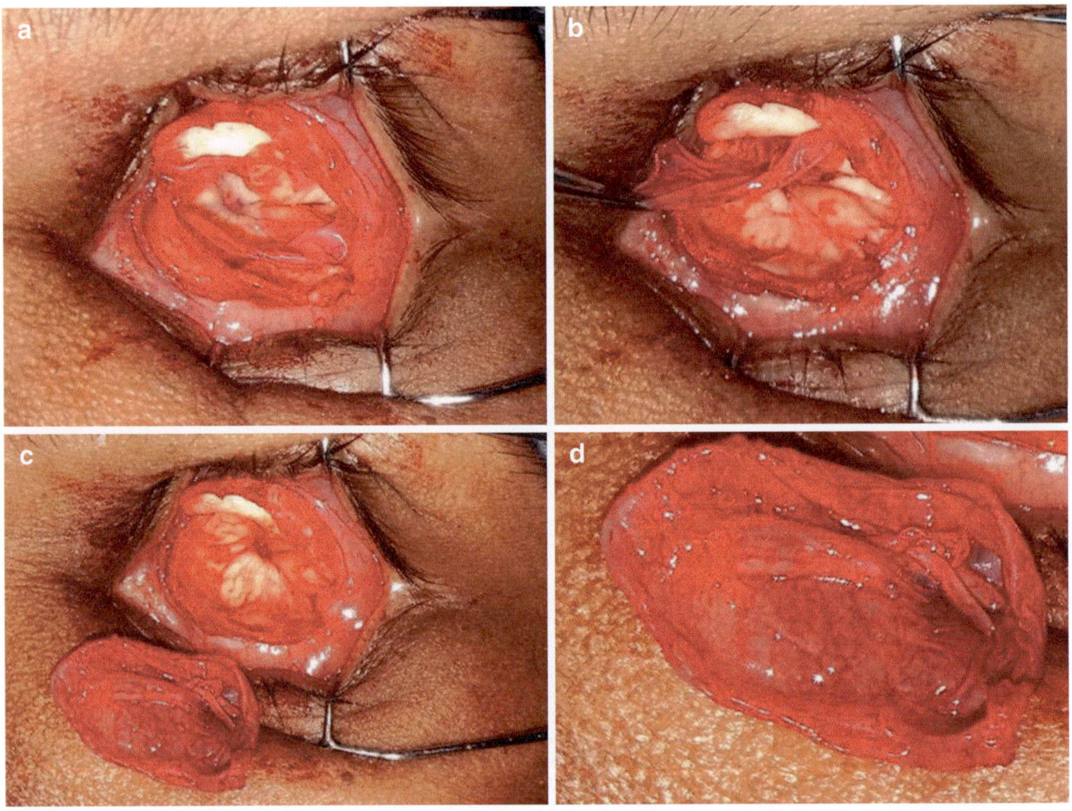

Fig. 17.13 (**a**) An intraoperative photograph of a patient with post-evisceration anophthalmic socket with spontaneously extruded nonporous ball implant showing residual scleral cavity and implant pseudocapsule. (**b**) An implant pseudocapsule is removed gently. (**c**) A pseudocapsule removed completely before further deeper dissection (**d**) Closure view of a glistening, pinkish and fibrous pseudocapsule

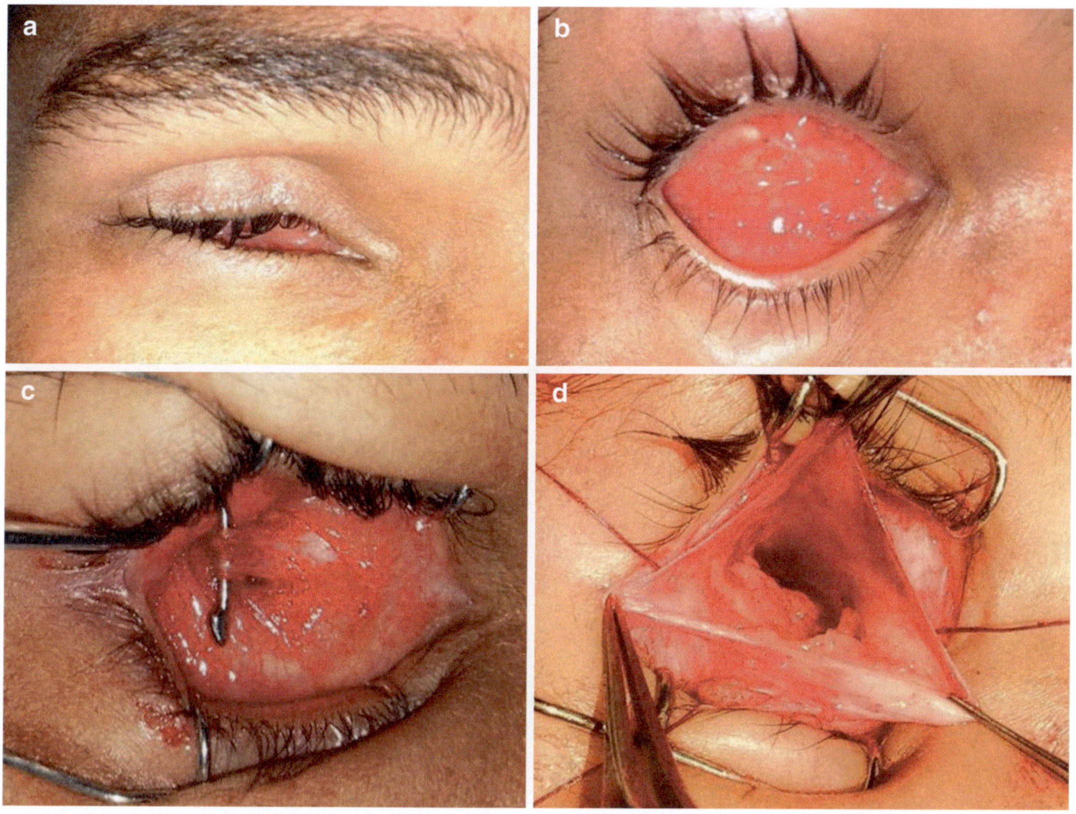

Fig. 17.14 (**a**) A patient without an orbital implant who has a typical post enucleation socket syndrome referred for secondary orbital ball implantation. (**b**) An appearance of his contracted anophthalmic socket with minimal inflammation and shallow inferior fornix. (**c**) A conjunctiva-Tenon's layer incised and position of extra-ocular muscles is assessed. (**d**) Further blunt dissection done to expose the intraconal space

the intraconal fat. A finger is inserted into the socket to ascertain whether any intraorbital adhesions are present. Further blunt dissection through the orbital tissues is carried out to identify connective tissue channels and thereby to localize the recti muscles and intraconal space for the secondary implantation. (Fig. 17.14a–d) [15]. A closure of conjunctiva and Tenon's layer is done with absorbable sutures. Additionally, inferior fornix forming sutures and mucous membrane graft can be placed along with secondary orbital implant if mild to moderate surface deficit and shallow fornices are present (Fig. 17.15a–d).

17.7.1 Dermis Fat Graft

Socket reconstruction with dermis fat graft is indicated in a moderate to severely contracted socket to correct volume and surface deficiency [26]. A de-epithelialized dermis with an underlying subcutaneous fat tissue constitutes the dermis fat graft, an autologous transplant. It is harvested from relatively non-hair bearing area of upper and outer part of gluteal region. It is relatively not a weight bearing part. Initially, a circle with about 25 mm diameter is marked on the donor site and then skin over the donor site is infiltrated with 2% xylocaine with epinephrine 1:100,000. A superficial incision with no. 15 Bard Parker blade is placed over the marked area and epidermis is excised from the underlying dermis. A stab incision is then made with no. 11 blade through the underlying dermis and subcutaneous fat and dermis fat graft is harvested from the donor site. A closure of subcutaneous tissue is done with interrupted 4-0 absorbable sutures placed through fat and subcutaneous tissue and skin closure is

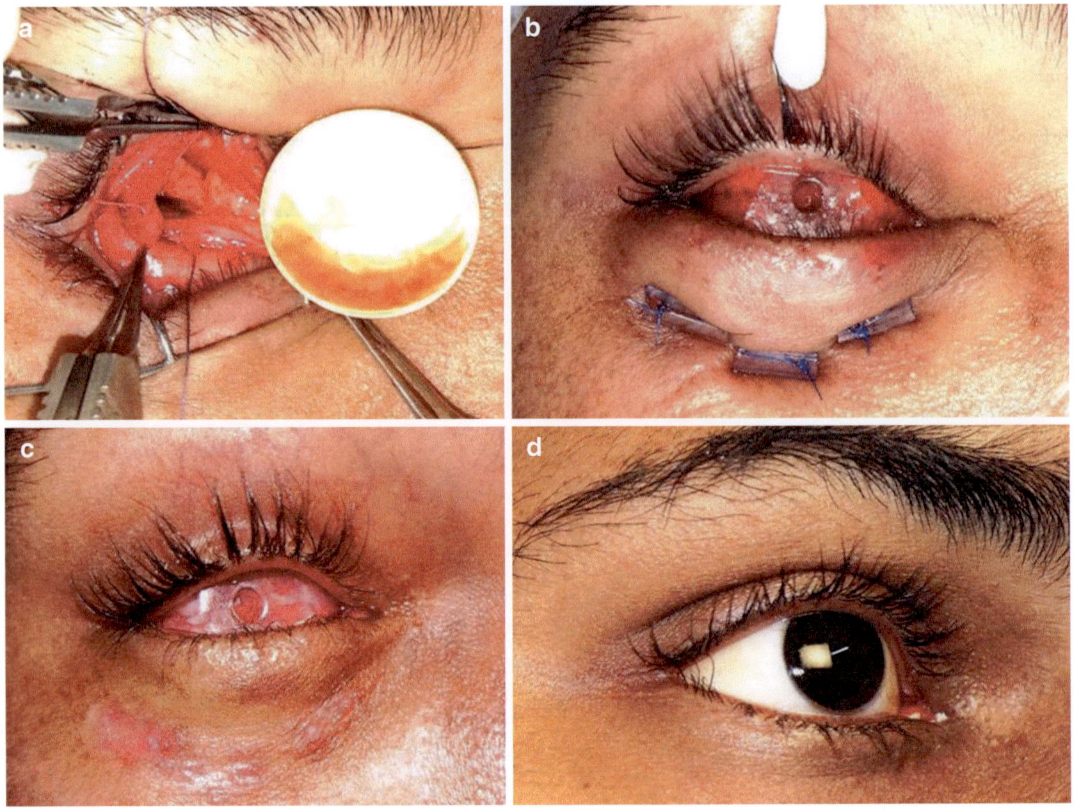

Fig. 17.15 (**a**) An appropriate sized ball implant placed in intraconal space and layered closure done. (**b**) Inferior fornix deepening sutures were placed to address the shallow inferior fornix and conformer was placed inside. (**c**) An Appearance of socket after removal of fornix deepening suture after 4 weeks. (**d**) A customised ocular prosthesis was fitted in after 8 weeks with satisfactory output

done with 4-0 non-absorbable mattress sutures (Fig. 17.16a–d).

A horizontal conjunctival incision from medial to the lateral canthus is placed to prepare the host bed. Further dissection in subconjunctival and deeper plane is performed with blunt scissors to create a space for the graft to accommodate. A dermis fat graft harvested from the donor site is then implanted into the host area without any undue pressure over the graft. A graft is approximated to the edges of the conjunctiva with interrupted 6-0 absorbable sutures. A conformer is placed inside and temporary suture tarsorrhaphy is done. Dressing is left undisturbed for next 2–3 days (Fig. 17.17a–d).

Dermis-fat graft is a promising option in the management of contracted socket with minimal soft tissue fibrosis and good vascular supply of the orbit. Complications associated with dermis fat graft donor site include delayed wound healing, unhealthy scar, wound infection and hematoma formation. Post dermis fat graft socket complications include wound dehiscence, graft ulceration and central necrosis, surface keratinization, granulomas, retention and growth of the cilia, graft atrophy and subsequent volume loss, excessive dermis-fat growth and graft failure (Fig. 17.18a–c) [27].

17.7.2 Severe Socket Contracture

In the severely contracted socket, all the fornices are extremely shallow or obliterated along with narrow palpabral aperture and may not retain even a small prosthesis. All such patients often experience discharge from the socket, irritation

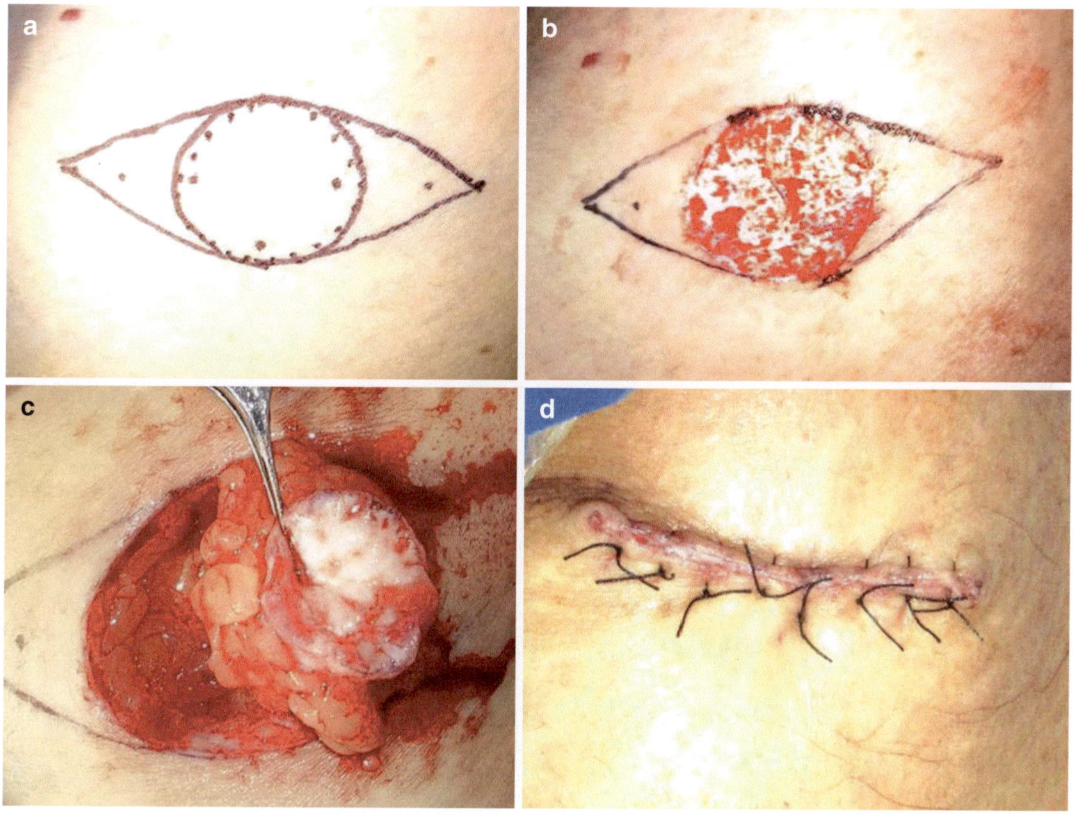

Fig. 17.16 (**a**) An outline of a dermis fat graft to be harvested. (**b**) The appearance of the dermis following removal of epidermis. (**c**) The dermis fat graft is being harvested (**d**) A donor area is closed in layers

and discomfort. Management of the severely contracted socket remains a challenging one and patient should be well counselled beforehand about the prognosis of the surgery, multiple staged approach for the reconstruction and realistic outcomes of achievable suboptimal cosmesis.

In severely contracted socket with good vascular supply, Putterman has described a surgical technique for the reconstruction using the mucous membrane graft, custom conformer and custom prosthesis with good outcomes [28].

Severely contracted socket with poor vascular supply often presents even more difficulty to achieve an acceptable cosmesis. In such sockets, a variety of surgical techniques including temporalis muscle or fascial flaps, radial forearm free flaps, a short pedicle thoracodorsal artery trilobed adiposal flap have been reported with variable success rates [29–32]. Lopez-Arcas recently described a retroauricular island flap technique for the socket reconstruction in children with promising results [33].

17.7.3 Management of Malignant Contracted Socket

In all such sockets additional surgical interventions may not benefit the patient to achieve an acceptable cosmesis. Dortzbach and Callahan have advised exenteration of the residual socket and then fitting of the orbital prosthesis with a reasonable appearance [34].

17.7.4 Care of the Custom Ocular Prosthesis

An ocularist fabricates the custom ocular prosthesis as per the socket dimensions. All the

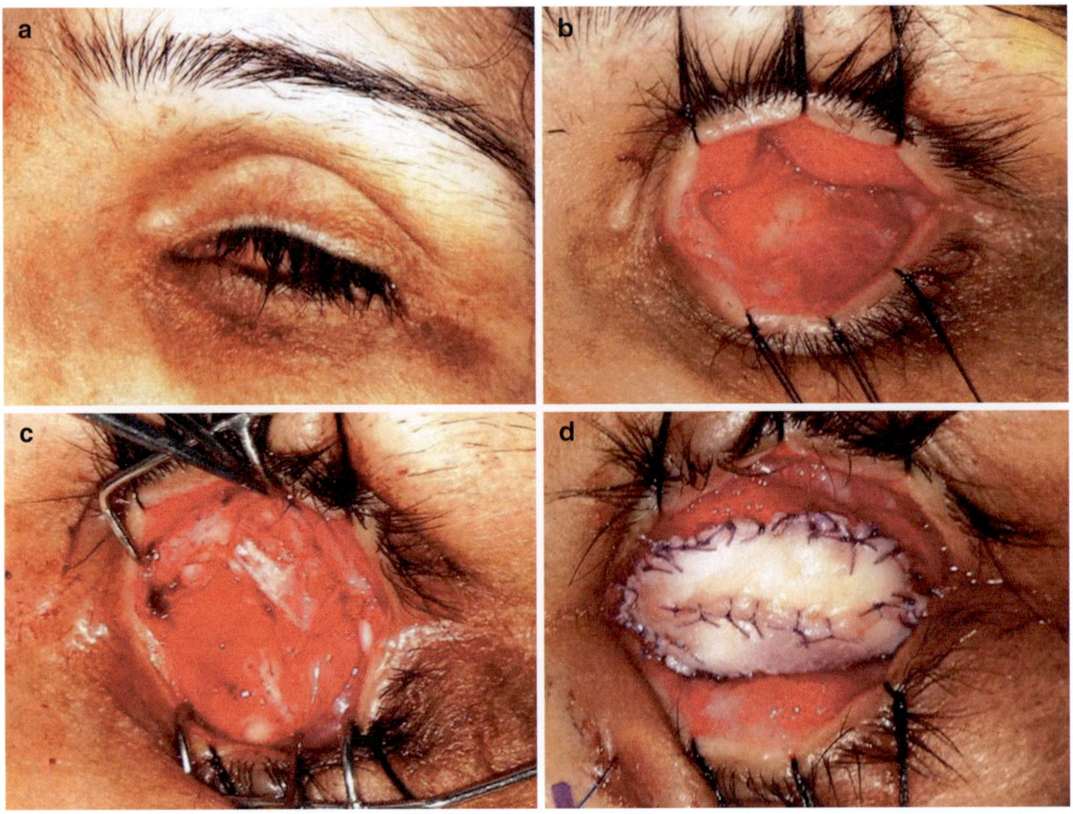

Fig. 17.17 (**a**) A patient with moderate to severe contracted anophthalmic socket. (**b**) A contracted socket with shallow inferior and superior fornices with volume and surface deficit. (**c**) A horizontal incision is placed over the conjunctiva and deeper dissection done to expose the intraconal fat. (**d**) The dermis fat graft sutured to conjunctiva and Tenon's layer with vicryl sutures

patients are advised about the care and maintenance of the ocular prosthesis in a systematic way. Patients are encouraged to learn insertion and removal of the prosthesis correctly. They are advised to use the prosthesis all the time including night while sleeping. Patients are asked to continue with their daily activities including facial and periocular hygiene. Frequent handling and removal of the prosthesis is discouraged to avoid injury to the surface of the prosthesis. Patient should use the prescribed topical lubricant medications to improve the socket comfort. Prosthesis can be cleaned with mild soap and water and then gently dried with a soft cloth. Cleaning with alcohol should be discouraged as it damages the polished surface of prosthesis. If not to be used, prosthesis should be stored in soft contact lens solution.

The patient should follow up every 6 months with ocularist for the prosthesis polishing and minor modification if any to improve the fitting and appearance. A regular polishing of the prosthesis provides a smoother surface and allows for smoother movement reducing irritation and discharge from the socket. All the prostheses have limited movement in extreme gazes. The ocularist should help patient use turning head and shoulders, not eyes, in the direction of gaze in order to maintain the primary gaze and minimize the ocular asymmetry. All the prosthetic wearing patients must be encouraged to use the full frame polycarbonate glasses for the protection of the remaining functional eye. Lightly tinted glasses can be used to reduce the minor ocular asymmetries. Magnifying or minifying lenses, cylindrical

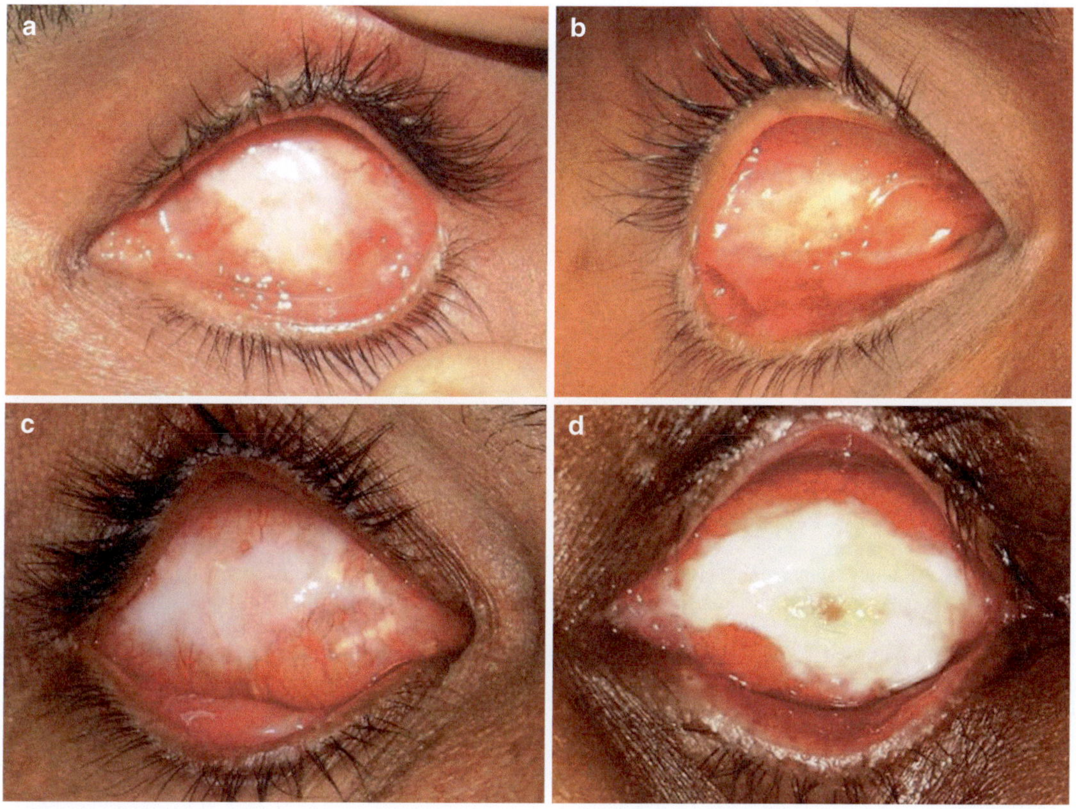

Fig. 17.18 (**a**) Well healed dermis fat graft (**b**) Fat graft atrophy (**c**) Excessive dermis fat growth (**d**) Fat necrosis leading to graft failure

lenses and prisms may be used in the spectacles to improve the position, size and appearance of the prosthesis.

The management of the post enucleation socket remains challenging and includes variety of surgical techniques. A fine coordination between the ophthalmic plastic surgeon and expert ocularist is essential to achieve an optimal cosmesis with near normal appearance, socket comfort and to rebuild the patient's lost confidence.

References

1. Gougelmann HP. The evolution of the ocular motility implant. Int Ophthalmol Clin. 1976;10:689–711.
2. Kaiser JH. Size and growth of cornea in children. Arch Ophthalmol. 1925;116:288.
3. Taylor WOG. The effect of enucleation of one eye in childhood upon the subsequent development of the face. Trans Ophthalmol Soc. 1939;59:361.
4. Byers WGM. Report of the committee of the Ophthalmological Society on Excision. Trans Ophthalmol Soc. 1898;18:256.
5. Tyers AG, Collin JRO. Orbital implants and post enucleation socket syndrome. Trans Ophthal Soc. 1982;102:90–2.
6. Smit AJGM. Computed tomography in the assessment of the post enucleation socket syndrome. Ophthalmology. 1990;97:1347–51.
7. Hintschich C, Zonneveld F, Koornneef L. Normal orbital volumes and its pathology in orbital socket surgery. Oper Tech Oculoplast Orbital Reconstr Surg. 2001;4:3–14.
8. Thaller VT. Enucleation volume measurement. Ophthal Plast Reconstr Surg. 1997;13:18–20.
9. Kaltreider SA, Lucarelli MJ. A simple algorithm for selection of implant size for enucleation and evisceration. Ophthal Plast Reconstr Surg. 2002;18:336–41.
10. Custer PL, Trinkaus KM. Volumetric determination of enucleation implants size. Am J Ophthalmol. 1999;128:489–94.
11. Kaltreider SA. The ideal ocular prosthesis: analysis of prosthetic volume. Ophthal Plast Reconstr Surg. 2000;16:388–92.
12. Custer PL, Trinkaus KM. Porous implant exposure: incidence, management, morbidity. Ophthal Plast Reconstr Surg. 2007;23:1–7.

13. Jordan DR, Klapper SR. Anophthalmic orbital implants: current concepts and controversies. Compr Ophthalmol Update. 2005;6(6):287–96.
14. Soporkar CNS, Patrinely JR. Tarsal patch flap for orbital implant exposure. Ophthal Plast Reconstr Surg. 1998;6:391–7.
15. Jordan DR. Localization of extraocular muscles during secondary orbital implantation surgery. The tunnel technique: experience with 100 patients. Ophthalmology. 2004;111:1048–54.
16. Smit TJ, et al. Primary and secondary implants in the anophthalmic orbit: preoperative and postoperative computed tomographic appearance. Ophthalmology. 1991;98(1):106–10.
17. Allen L. Modified impression fitting. Int Ophthalmol Clin. 1970;10:747–62.
18. Morley AMS, Taban M, Malhotra R, Goldberg R. Use of hyaluronic acid gel for upper eyelid filling and contouring. Ophthal Plast Reconstr Surg. 2009;25:440–4.
19. Nesi FA, Lisman RD, Levine MR. Evaluation and current concepts in the management of anophthalmic socket. In: Smith's ophthalmic plastic and reconstructive surgery. 2nd ed. St. Louis: Mosby; 1998. p. 1079–124.
20. Krishna G. Contracted sockets - I (Aetiology and types). Indian J Ophthalmol. 1980;28:117–20.
21. Vistnes L. The eye socket. In: Repair and reconstruction in the orbital region, vol. 335. 3rd ed. Edinburgh: Churchill Livingstone; 1991.
22. Ma'luf RN. Correction of the inadequate lower fornix in the anophthalmic socket. Br J Ophthalmol. 1999;83:881–2.
23. Molgat YM, Hurwitz JJ, Webb MC. Buccal mucous membrane graft in the management of the contracted socket. Ophthal Plast Reconstr Surg. 1993;9:267–72.
24. Naugle TC, Lee WW, Couvillion S. Use of quilting sutures in ophthalmic plastic surgery. Ophthal Plast Reconstr Surg. 2004;20:237–9.
25. Bajaj MS, Pushker N, Kumar KS, Chandra M, Ghose S. Evaluation of amniotic membrane grafting in the reconstruction of contracted socket. Ophthal Plast Reconstr Surg. 2006;22(2):116–20.
26. Aryasit O, Preechawai P. Indications and results in anophthalmic socket reconstruction using dermis-fat graft. Clin Ophthalmol. 2015;9:795–9.
27. Shore JW, McCord CD Jr, Bergin DJ, Dittmar SJ, Maiorca JP, Burks WR. Management of complications following dermis-fat grafting for anophthalmic socket reconstruction. Ophthalmology. 1985;92(10):1342–50.
28. Putterman AM, Karesh JW. A surgical technique for the successful and stable reconstruction of the totally contracted ocular socket. Ophthalmic Surg. 1988;19(3):193–201.
29. Mu X, Dong J, Chang T, et al. Correction of the contracted eye socket and orbitozygomatic hypoplasia using post-auricular skin flap and temporalis fascial flap. J Craniofac Surg. 1999;10(1):11–7.
30. Tessier P, Krastinova D. Transplantation of the temporalis muscle into an anophthalmic orbit. Ann Chir Plast. 1982;27:211–20.
31. Aihara M, Sakai S, Matsuzaki K, Ishida H. Eye socket reconstruction with free flaps in patients who have had postoperative radiotherapy. J Craniomaxillofac Surg. 1998;26:301–5.
32. Koshima I, Narushima M, Mihara M, et al. Short pedicle thoracodorsal artery perforator (TAP) adiposal flap for three dimensional reconstruction of contracted orbital cavity. J Plast Reconstr Aesthet Surg. 2008;61:e13–7.
33. Lopez-Arcas JM, Martin M, Gomez E, et al. The Guyuron retroauricular island flap for eyelid and eye socket reconstruction in children. Int J Oral Maxillofac Surg. 2009;38:744–50.
34. Dortzbach RK, Callahan A. Advances in socket reconstruction. Am J Ophthalmol. 1970;70:800–13.

Intraocular Tumors: Imaging

18

Veena Noronha

Abbreviations

FRFSE	Fast relaxing fast spin echo
FSE	Fast spin echo
FSPGR	Fast spoiled gradient-echo
FLAIR	Fluid attenuated inversion recovery
Gd-DTPA	Gadolinium—diethylinetriamine penta-acetic acid
ONH	Optic nerve head

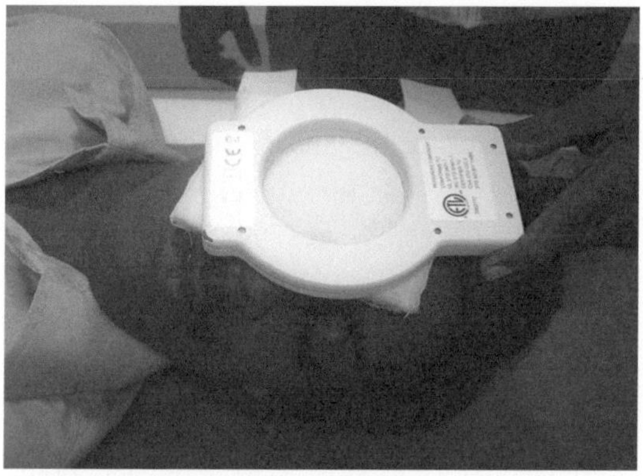

Fig. 18.1 Surface coil technique

18.1 Introduction

The advent of high field strength MRI and surface coils has greatly revolutionised ocular imaging. The refinement in technology and high resolution coils has greatly enhanced the accuracy of the diagnosis. Ultrasound and MRI complement each other and help the radiologist in making a reliable diagnosis and thereby better patient management.

18.2 Technique and Protocols

1.5 T or 3 T MRI with surface coil is recommended for ocular imaging. Patient cooperation, use of proper imaging technique and protocol is most important to get good quality images. The patient's head is immobilised using straps and pads. The 3 in. coil is placed on the eye to be examined with cotton spacer between the coil and the eye to avoid direct contact of the coil with the patient body (Fig. 18.1).

Recommended protocol: Surface coil study

- Axial T1 FSFGR with fat saturation and T2 FRSE—1–1.5 mm slice thickness from the orbital floor to the roof parallel to the optic nerve.
- Coronal T1 FSE and T2 FRFSE—1–1.5 mm slice thickness perpendicular to the optic nerves
- Oblique sagittal T2 FRFSE

Brain screening: Axial FLAIR and Diffusion weighted imaging.

Post contrast—Axial, Coronal and Sagittal T1 3D FSPGR with fat suppression.

V. Noronha (✉)
VRR Scan Chennai and Sankara Nethralaya, Chennai, India

V. Khetan (ed.), *Intraocular Tumors*, https://doi.org/10.1007/978-981-15-0395-5_18

18.3 Intraocular Tumors: Adults

18.3.1 Melanoma

It is the most common intraocular malignancy encountered in clinical practice. Common sites are choroid, ciliary body and iris. The posterior uveal melanoma is usually well- defined dome shaped lesion and can occur anywhere from the ciliary body to the posterior pole. Factors that predict an unfavorable prognosis are tumor size, extraocular extension, extension to the ciliary body and intense pigmentation. The choroidal melanoma is dome or mushroom shaped. Liver is the most common site for metastases, hence tumor work up should include liver imaging.

18.3.2 Imaging Features

18.3.2.1 Computed Tomography

- Melanoma is usually a well defined dome shaped hyperdense lesion and homogeneously enhance with contrast.
- It is difficult to characterize the lesion as other intraocular lesions such as choroidal hemangioma and metastases have similar CT features.

18.3.2.2 Magnetic Resonance Imaging

- Uveal melanoma has characteristic MRI appearance. It is typically dome or mushroom shaped and have characteristic T1 hyperintense andT2 hypointense signal with respect to vitreous (Fig. 18.2). The T1 hyperintense signal is attributed to the T1 shortening property of melanin [1].
- This property helps in differentiating it from other intraocular tumors as they usually display intermediate signal in T1 WI and isointense signal in T2 weighted images with respect to the vitroeus.
- Amelanotic melanoma usually pose a diagnostic challenge as it lacks the characteristic T1 hyperintense signal.
- Contrast enhanced MRI is done to look at the enhancement pattern, identify extraocular extension (Fig. 18.3) and intracranial lesions.

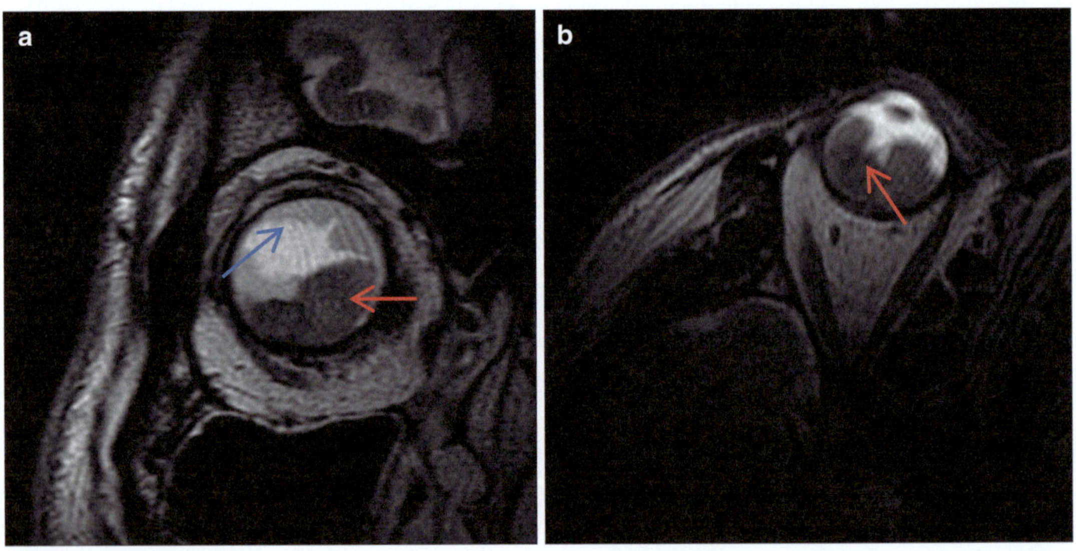

Fig. 18.2 Surface coil images of the eye (**a**) Coronal T2 FRFSE, (**b**) axial T2 FRFSE, (**c**) coronal T1 non contrast, (**d**) post contrast coronal T1 FSPGR showing a large lobulated T1 hyperintense and T2 hypointense intraocular lesion (red arrow) with associated retinal detachment (blue arrow)

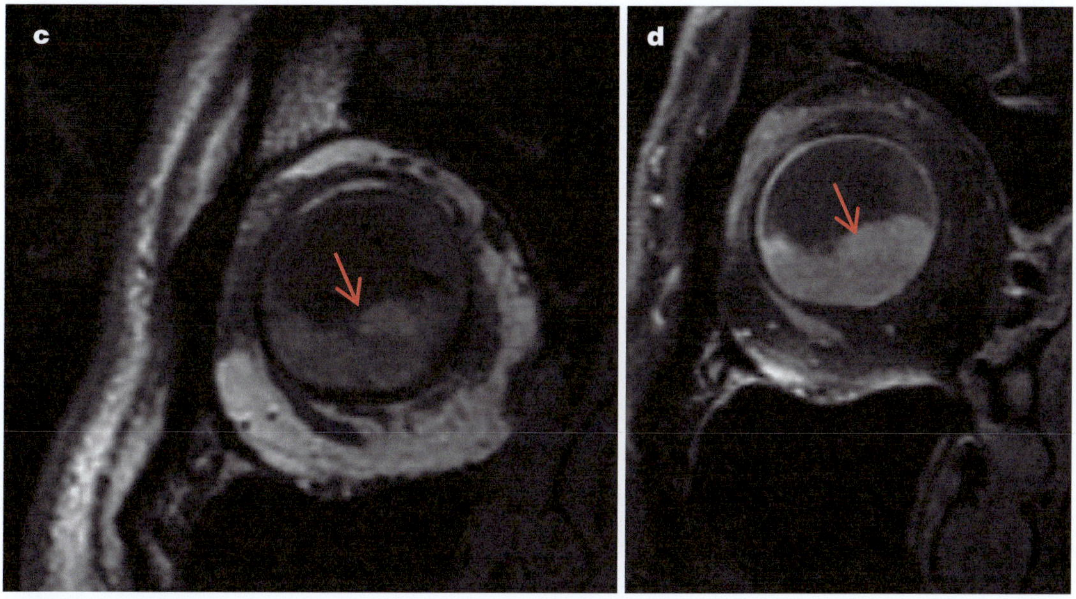

Fig. 18.2 (continued)

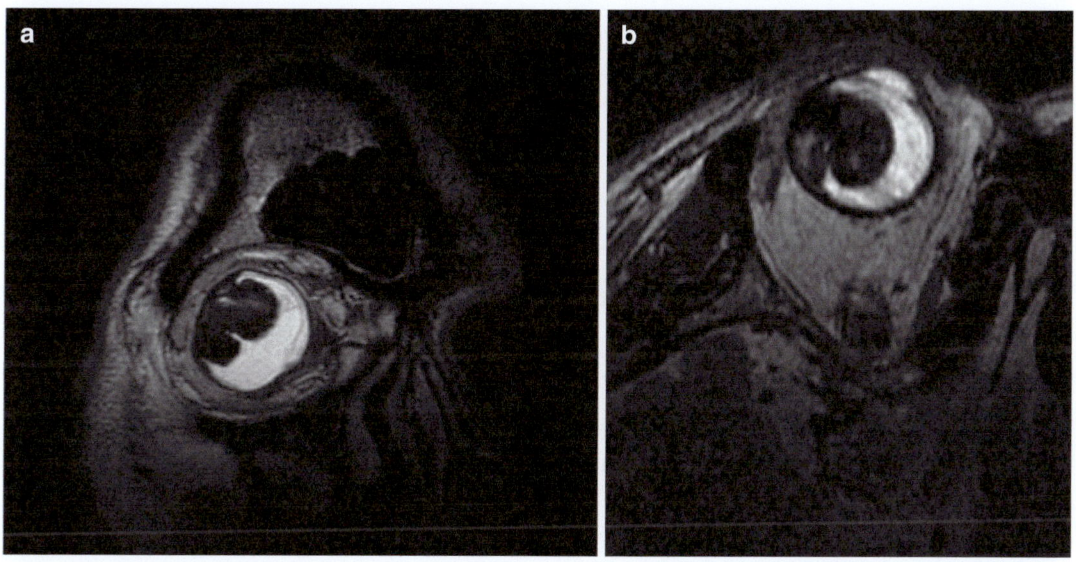

Fig. 18.3 (**a**) Coronal T2 FRFSE, (**b**) axial T2 FRFSE, (**c**) axial T1 SE, (**d**) coronal T1 SE Surface coil images of the right eye showing a large mushroom shaped choroidal lesion in the temporal quadrant of the right eye. There is scleral thinning and extrascleral extension of the lesion (arrow). The lesion is hyperintense in T1 weighted image and hypointense in T2 weighted image consistent with melanoma

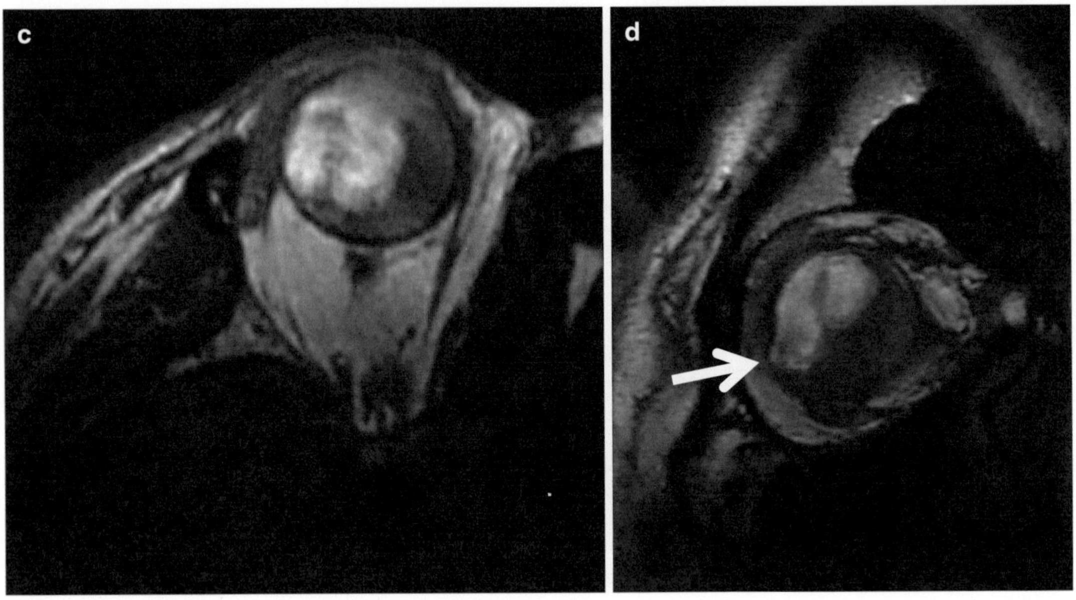

Fig. 18.3 (continued)

- Studies have been done to look at the enhancement pattern and identify the malignant lesions based on the intensity of enhancement. It also helps to see the response to treatment [2].
- Post brachytherapy they found reduction in the contrast enhancement.
- Doppler study can also be done to look for tumor vascularity. The non-malignant lesions usually demonstrate poor flow.

18.3.2.3 Differential Diagnosis

- Subretinal haemorrhage—subacute haemorrhage will have the same signal as a uveal melanoma. Clinical findings, contrast and follow up study will help in differentiating subretinal hemorrhage from uveal melanoma
- Metastases—metastases from mucin producing tumors may have similar signal as an uveal melanoma.

18.4 Choroidal Hemangioma

Choroidal hemagiomas are congenital vascular hamartomas seen in middle age to elderly patients. They are two types

1. Solitary well circumscribed dome shaped lesion seen posterior to the equator and confined to the choroid
2. The diffuse type seen in Sturge Weber syndrome are seen circumferentially in the choroid and may also involve ciliary body, iris, and also the episclera, conjunctiva, and limbus.

18.4.1 Imaging Features

- On Computed Tomography they are isodense in the non-contrast study and show intense contrast enhancement especially in high dose contrast.

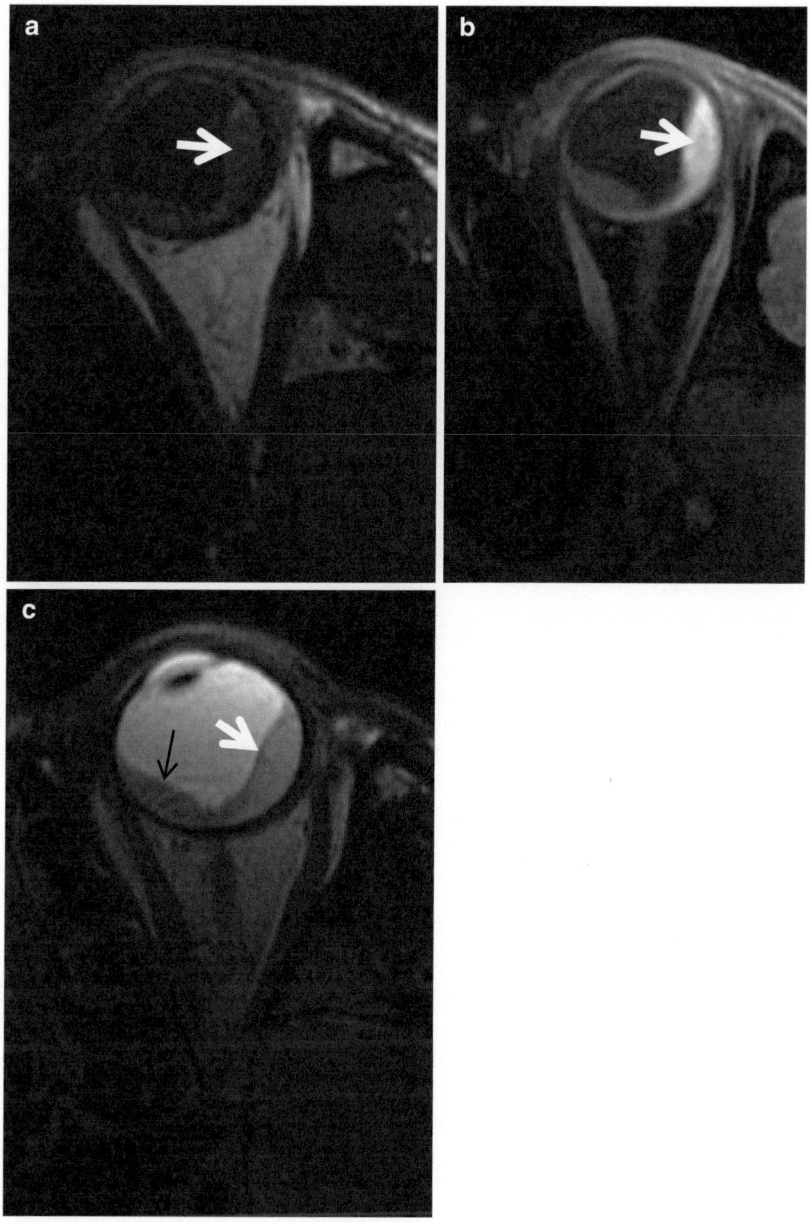

Fig. 18.4 (**a**) Axial T1 pre contrast, (**b**) axial T1 post contrast and (**c**) axial T2 surface coil images of the left eye showing a well circumscribed dome shaped choroidal lesion in the temporal quadrant, intermediate signal in T1 and T2 WI w.r.t vitreous and brilliant homogenous enhancement in the post contrast study (arrow). Note the associated retinal detachment (black arrow)—Choroidal hemangioma

- MRI they are typically isointense to hyperintense to the vitreous in T1 and isointense in T2 WI and therefore may not be well delineated. Contrast enhanced MRI is mandatory to identify these lesions (Fig. 18.4). They show brilliant contrast enhancement [3].

18.4.2 Metastases

Uveal metastases result from hematogenous dissemination and reach the globe via the posterior ciliary artery and commonly involve the posterior half of the globe. The primary lesions that most com-

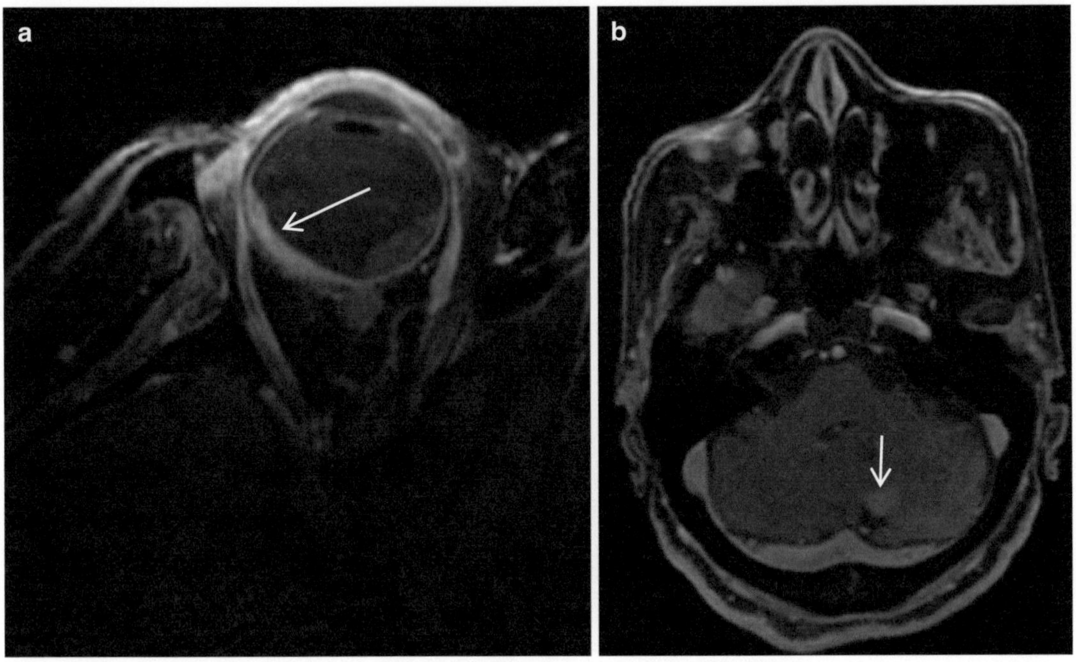

Fig. 18.5 (**a**) Axial post contrast T1 WI surface coil image of the right eye showing a elevated, enhancing and bumpy choroidal lesion in the temporal quadrant with associated retinal detachment. (**b**) Axial post contrast image of the brain showing an enhancing lesion in the cerebellum (arrow) suggestive of metastases

monly metastasize are breast (47%), lung (21%), and the gastrointestinal tract (4%). Both eyes are affected in about one-third of cases. These are usually dome shaped with a bumpy surface. Metastases, especially those from breast and lung carcinomas, also may involve extraocular muscles [4–6].

18.4.3 CT

- CT lacks sensitivity due to its poor soft tissue resolution
- They may be seen as small elevated slightly hyperdense lesions that enhance with contrast.
- Post contrast imaging of the brain should be performed to look for intracranial metastases

18.4.4 MRI

- Gadolinium enhanced MRI is the investigation of choice
- They are usually small elevated lesions with bumpy surface. They display iso to hyperintense signal in T1 WI with respect to the vitreous (Figs. 18.5 and 18.6).
- The T2 signal is usually hypointense with respect to the vitreous.
- Mucinous adenocarcinoma may mimic melanoma as they demonstrate T1 hyperintense signal due to mucin
- Metastases from renal cell carcinoma may mimic haemorrhage
- Post gadolinium they demonstrate enhancement which may be similar to the primary tumor.

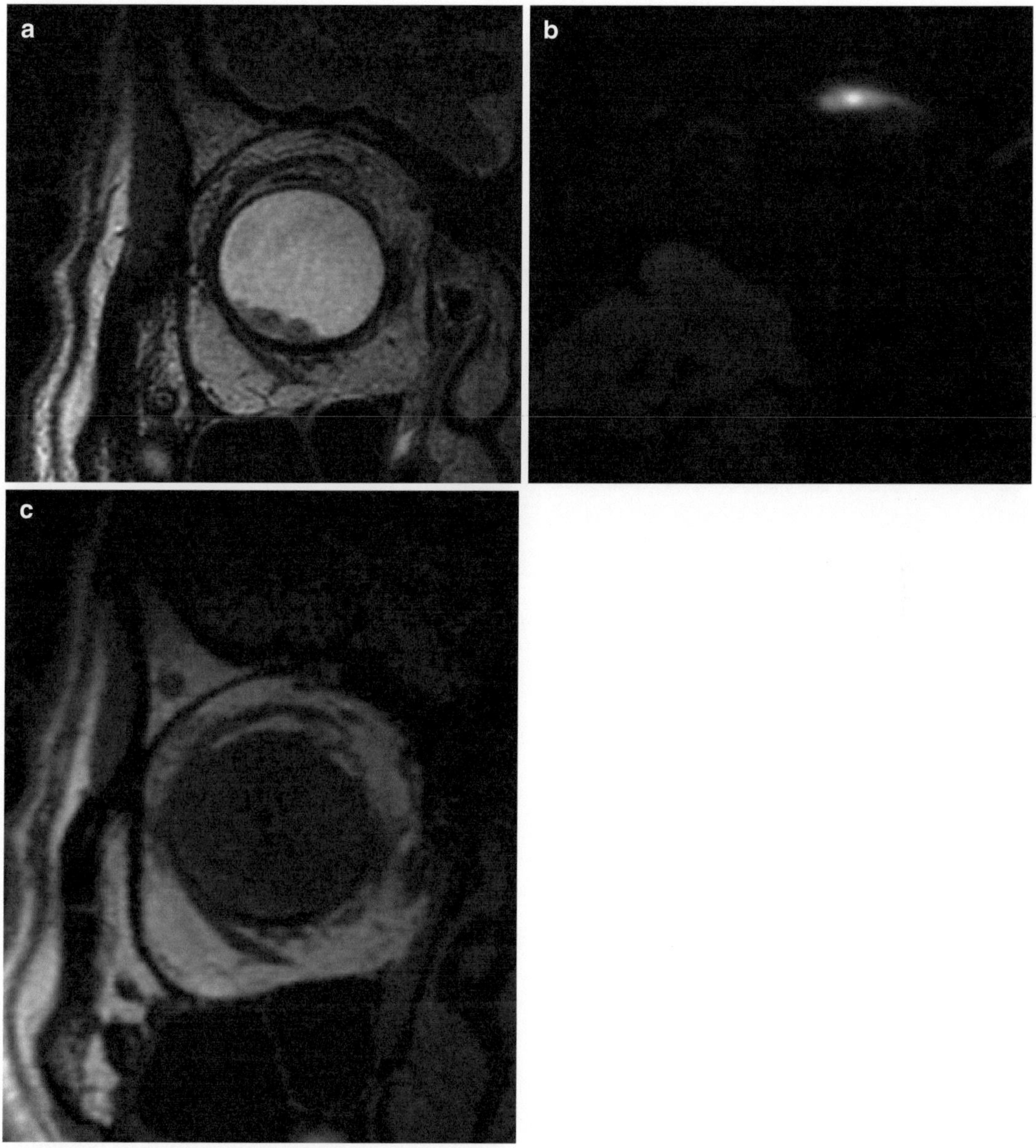

Fig. 18.6 (**a**) Coronal T2 FRFSE surface coil image of the right eye. (**b**) Axial diffusion weighted image. (**c**) Coronal T1 WI. There is a bumpy choroidal lesion in the inferior quadrant of the right eye. It displays hypointense signal in T2 WI and intermediate signal in T1 WI w.r.t vitreous and restricted diffusion

18.5 Melanocytoma

Melanocytoma, also known as hyperpigmented magnocellular nevus. It is a variant of melanocytic nevus that has typical clinical and histopathologic features. Melanocytoma of the ONH is a hamartoma which consists of large round or oval heavily pigmented melanocytes packed closely and located among axons in the optic disc, anterior optic nerve and in the peripapillary retina. Melanocytoma is commonly seen at the optic disc or optic nerve head. It can also be found in the uveal tract, including the iris, ciliary body, and choroid. Approximately 50% of melanocytomas occur in black race, whereas the inci-

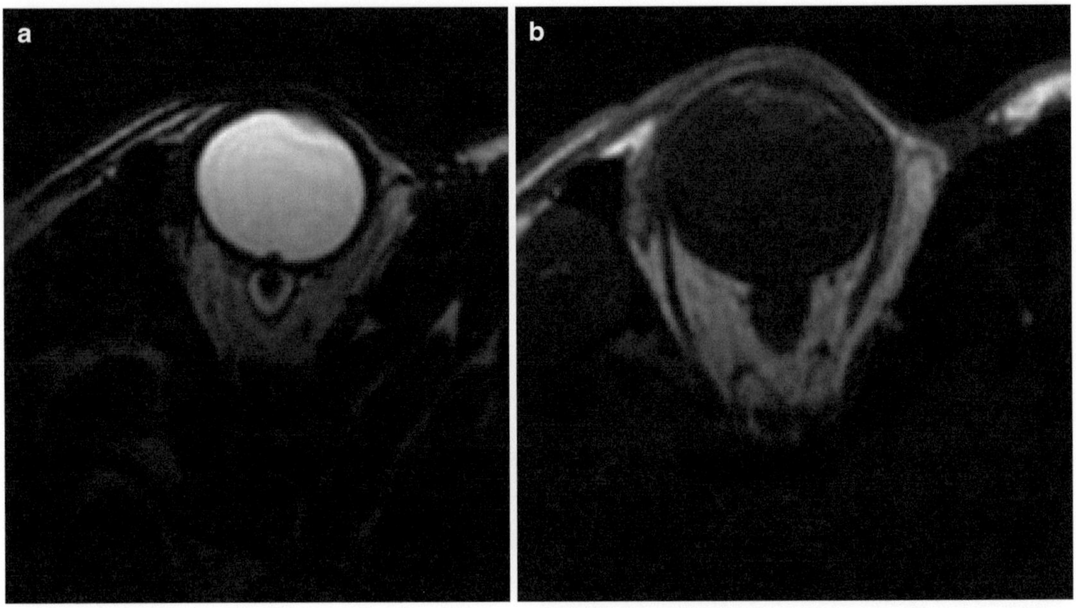

Fig. 18.7 Surface coil MRI images of the right eye showing a small nodular lesion at the right optic disc. It is not appreciable in the T1 WI (**b**) and is hypointense in T2 WI (**a**)—Melanocytoma

dence of uveal malignant melanoma is less than 1% in black race [7, 8].

18.5.1 MR Imaging

- MRI may not be helpful in differentiating choroidal melanoma from melanocytoma.
- There is most commonly located at the optic disc and small. The melanin content of melanocytoma is seen as a hyperintense signal on TIW images and hypointense signal on T2W images with respect to vitreous (Fig. 18.7)
- There is minimal enhancement seen after Gd—DTPA administration.

18.6 Primary Intraocular Lymphoma

Primary intraocular lymphoma (PIOL) is an ocular malignancy that is a subset of primary central system lymphoma (PCNSL). Approximately one-third of PIOL patients will have concurrent PCNSL at presentation, and 42–92% will develop PCNSL within a mean of 8–29 months. The majority of PIOL is diffuse large B-cell lymphoma. Vitreoretinal lymphoma is the most common type of ocular lymphoma related to PCNSL. Uveal tract lymphoma are low grade tumors and therefore have better prognosis [9].

These tumors have a tendency to mimic choroiditis and vasculitis and hence the diagnosis can be delayed.

18.6.1 Imaging

The vitreo-retinal lesions are small and quite often not appreciated even in the high resolution surface coil study. They are usually small elevated lesions and display iso to intermediate signal in T1 weighted images and hypointense in T2 weighted images (Fig. 18.9). Post contrast they homogeneously enhance.

As they are associated with concurrent PCNSL, it is mandatory to have the brain imaging with contrast. The spectrum of CNS findings are varied ranging from periventricular enhancing lesion, dural based enhancing lesions, leptomeningeal thickening to diffuse parenchymal infiltration (Fig. 18.8) that does not show significant contrast enhancement.

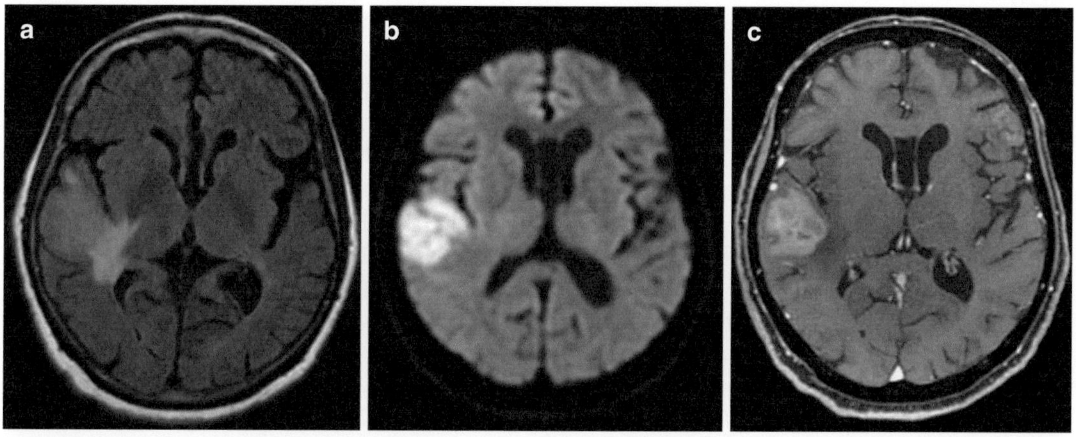

Fig. 18.8 (**a**) Axial FLAIR, (**b**) axial DWI and (**c**) axial post contrast images of the brain showing an ill-defined lesion in the right temporal lobe displaying hyperintense signal in FLAIR and restricted diffusion in DWI and heterogeneous contrast enhancement in a known case of intraocular lymphoma

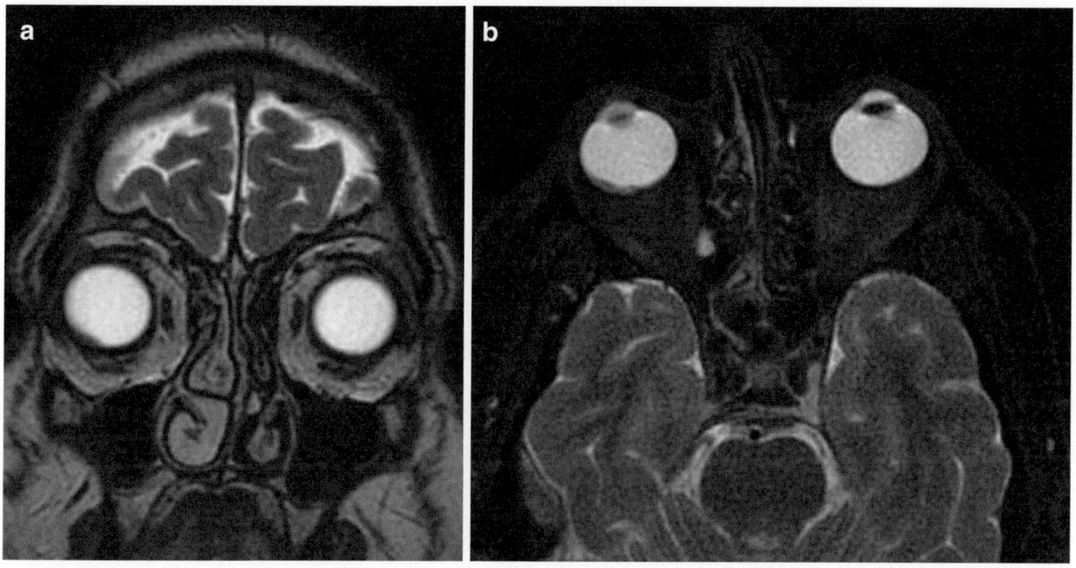

Fig. 18.9 (**a**) Coronal T2 FRFSE and (**b**) axial T2 FRSE images of the orbit showing a small elevated lesion in the infero-temporal quadrant of the right eye. The brain imaging was normal

The atypical CNS lesions should have a biopsy for definitive diagnosis if CSF is negative.

18.7 Leiomyoma

Uveal leiomyoma is a rare benign tumor of the smooth muscle origin which can arise in the iris, ciliary body, or choroid.

18.7.1 Clinical Features

- They it tends to occur in younger patients with female predilection.
- On ophthalmoscopy it appears as yellowish elevated highly vascularized elevated mass.
- The tumor may simulate amelanotic choroidal melanoma on the basis of clinical appearance [10].

18.7.2 MR Features

- Leiomyoma appears as a hyperintense mass with respect to the vitreous on the non-enhanced T1W images & hypointense on T2W images (isointense to brain parenchyma in T1 and T2 weighted images). The tumor is not as hyperintense as a melanoma on T1 weighted images (Fig. 18.10).
- On Gd-DTPA enhanced T1W images the tumor showed marked enhancement [11].

18.8 Retinal Astrocytoma

Retinal astrocytic hamartoma is a yellow-white rare benign retinal tumor that is frequently associated with tuberous sclerosis complex (TSC) or Bourneville's disease, neurofibromatosis or in isolation. Early retinal astrocytoma looks exactly like an early retinoblastoma and may present before any neurologic or dermatologic manifestations of tuberous sclerosis appear [12–14].

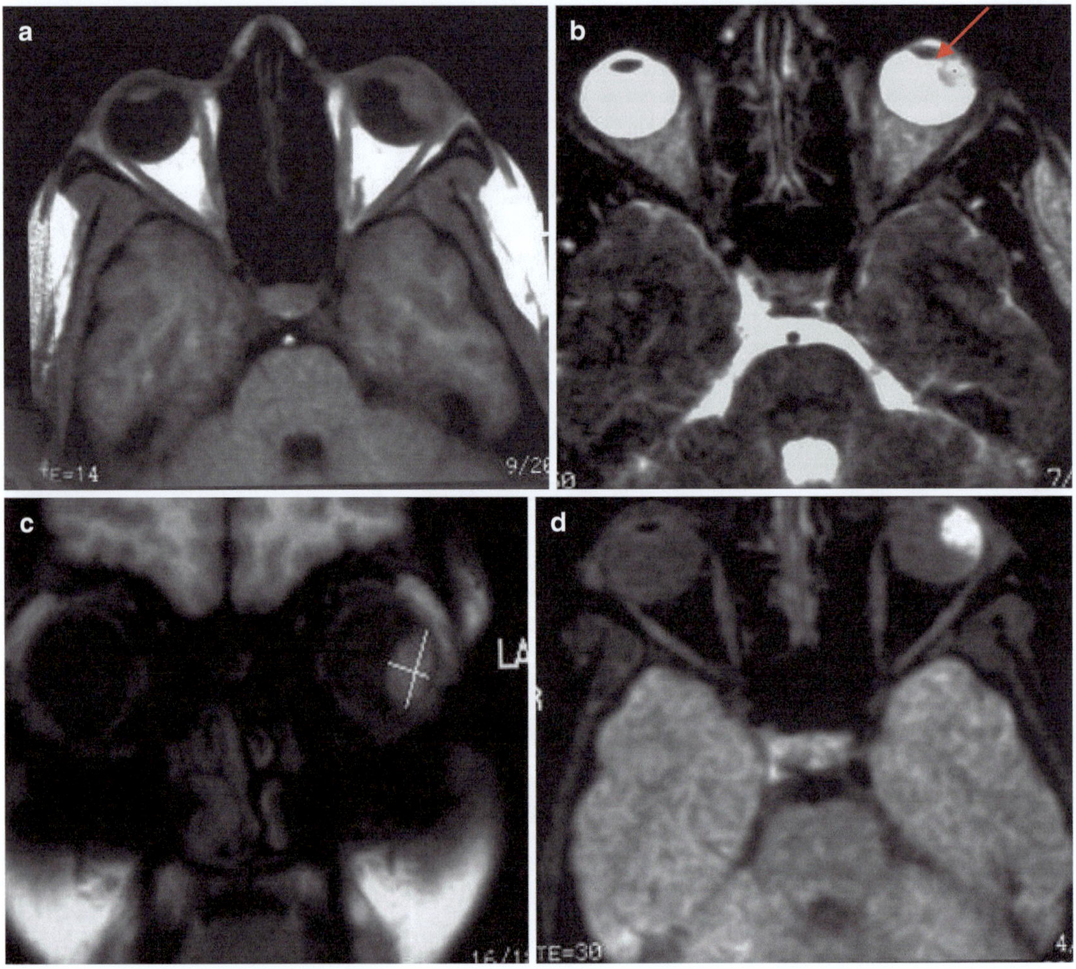

Fig. 18.10 A 19 years old female presented with ciliary body lesion. (**a**) Axial T1 weighted image showing a well circumscribed minimally hyperintense mass arising from the ciliary body and extending posteriorly up to the equator. (**b**) Axial T2 weighted imaging showing the lesion as predominantly hyperintense. (**c**) Post contrast coronal T1 weighted image showing moderate contrast enhancement. (**d**) axial STIR image showing the hyperintense lesion more clearly against the hypointense vitreous

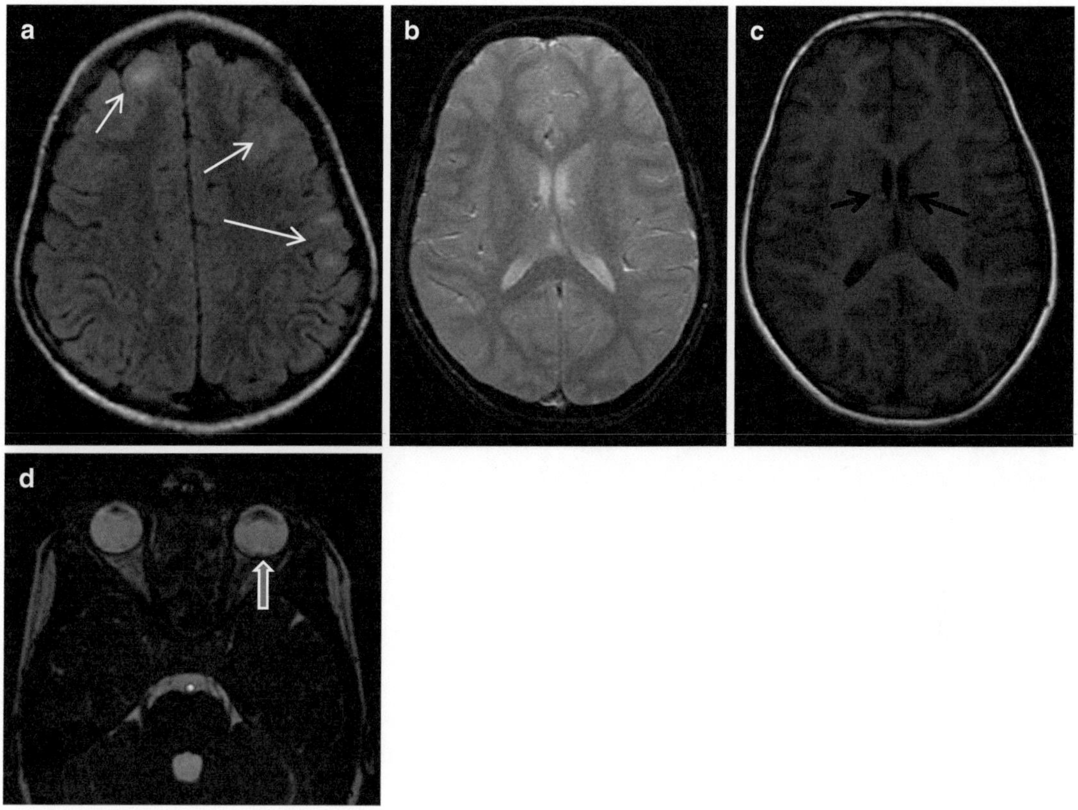

Fig. 18.11 (**a**) Axial FLAIR, (**b**) axial gradient, (**c**) axial T1 WI images of the brain showing cortical T2 hyperintense lesions in the bifrontal region in axial FLAIR (white arrow). Subependymal nodules seen along the lateral ventricles (black arrow). (**d**) Axial FIESTA image of the orbit showing a small elevated lesion temporal to the left optic disc (block arrow) – retinal astrocytoma with cortical tubers and subependymal nodules

- These tumors may appear in the retina or in the optic nerve.
- They appear as single or multiple nodules elevated 1 or 2 mm above the surface of the retina (Fig. 18.11).
- MRI will help in identifying the cortical tubers (Fig. 18.11)

Clinical findings and their imaging help in confirming the diagnosis.

18.8.1 Imaging

- These are seen as well defined elevated dome shaped lesions at the posterior pole.
- CT may be useful in these patients to identify the calcification in the astrocytoma and calcified sub ependymal nodules.
- If the typical features of tuberous sclerosis are absent then differentiating from other ocular lesions such as retinoblastoma may be difficult on imaging.

18.9 Pediatric Intraocular Tumors

Imaging in pediatric patients is a challenge due to long scanning times and noise of the MR equipment, quite often requiring sedation. Magnetic Resonance imaging has almost completely replaced computed tomography for imaging intraocular tumors due to the radiation risk especially in retinoblastoma children and sensitivity of MRI is identifying non—calcified retinoblastoma, optic nerve invasion, intracranial disease and lesions simulating retinoblastoma.

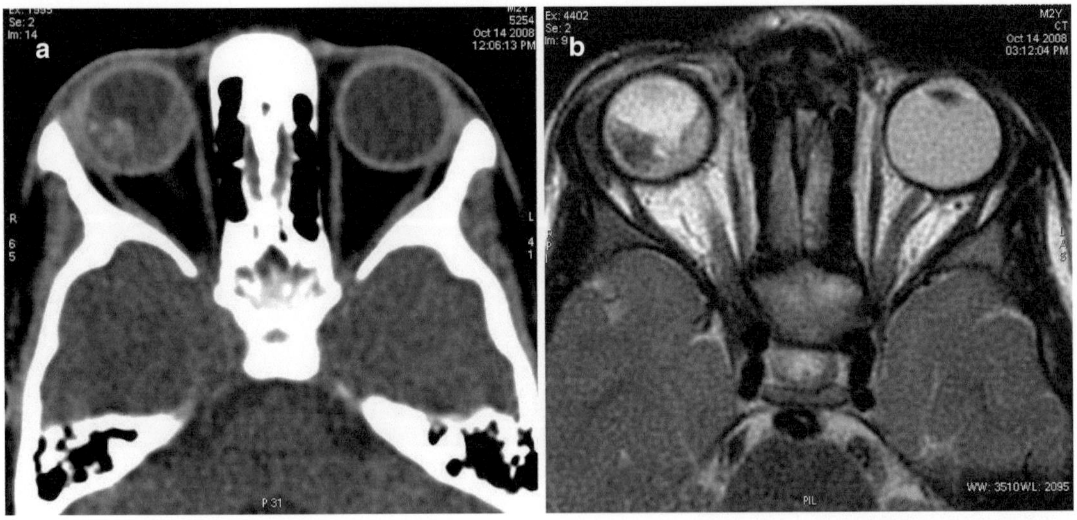

Fig. 18.12 (**a**) Axial CT scan of the orbit showing a hyperdense mass in the temporal quadrant of the right eye. Multiple specks of calcification are seen within and associated retinal detachment. (**b**) Axial T2 weighted image showing T2 hypointense mass lesion corresponding to the CT image and calcifications are seen as low signal intensity specks. Note the associated retinal detachement is hyperintense w.r. t the mass lesion

MRI should include dedicated orbit imaging with or without surface coil and entire brain imaging. Surface coil study gives high resolution images of the eye, however is usually not necessary in children especially in retinoblastoma as the depth of the coil is limited or unless the lesion is very small.

18.10 Retinoblastoma

It is the most common orbital tumor in childhood. The incidence of retinoblastoma is 1 in 15,000–20,000 live births. Retinoblastoma usually occur in children under the age of 5 years; the median age of diagnosis is 2 years of age for unilateral retinoblastoma and 9–12 months for bilateral retinoblastoma. The disease is unilateral in 60% of cases and bilateral in 40%. All bilateral and 15% of unilateral retinoblastomas are hereditary.

The most common clinical presentation is Leukocoria. They may also present with strabismus, amblyopia, cellulitis and proptosis.

18.10.1 Imaging

Diagnosis of retinoblastoma is clinical. MRI has largely replaced CT as the diagnostic modality, mainly due to its lack of radiation and superior soft tissue resolution that enables us to visualise the intraocular tumor, extraocular extension, optic nerve invasion and trilateral tumors and intracranial metastases (Fig. 18.12). Imaging should include the orbit and brain both pre and post contrast.

18.10.2 Computed Tomography

- CT scan was widely used to image patients suspected to have retinoblastoma, because of its sensitivity to detect calcium.
- The mass is hyperdense w.r.t vitreous and the calcifications can be single or multifocal; clump like or speckled (Fig. 18.13)

18.10.3 MRI Findings

- The imaging features depend on the three patterns of tumor growth—endophytic, exophytic and diffuse infiltrating types.
- They typically display hypointense signal in T2 that is similar to the gray matter.
- Calcification is usually seen as low intensity areas within the tumor (Fig. 18.12)
- Due to their cellular content the active tumor displays restricted diffusion.

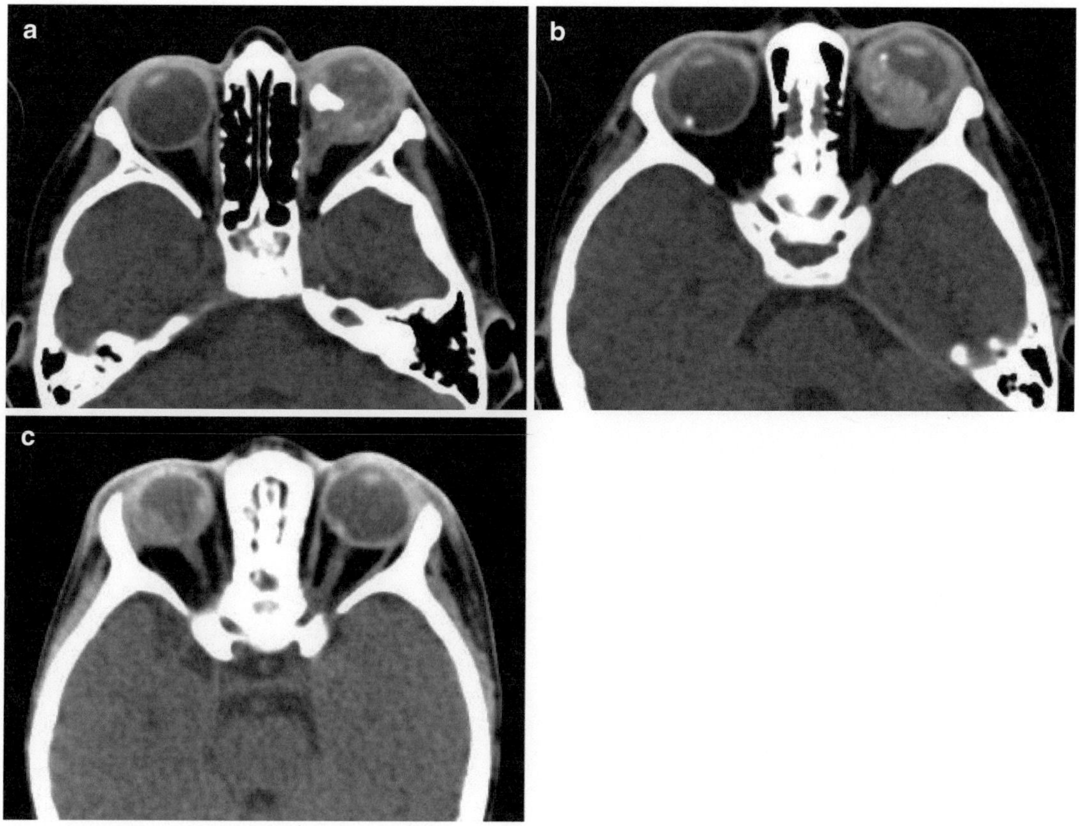

Fig. 18.13 Axial CT scans of the orbit of different patients showing the types of calcification seen in retinoblastoma. (**a**) Clump like. (**b**) Multifocal speckled. (**c**) Single dense

- Diffusion weighted imaging can be useful to differentiate the active and necrotic tumor and response to therapy [15].
- Retinal detachment is usually an associated finding. The subretinal fluid is usually exudative hence will have hyperintense signal in T1 weighted images and variable signal in T2 weighted images.
- Optic nerve invasion may vary from subtle T2 hyperintense signal to gross thickening of the nerve and enhancement (Fig. 18.14).
- Contrast enhanced MRI will help to identify the non-necrotic component and intracranial metastases.
- Leptomeningeal deposits in the brain and spine are best appreciated in the contrast enhanced MRI (Fig. 18.15).
- Trilateral retinoblastoma is an intracranial midline mass in the presence of unilateral or bilateral retinoblastoma. It occurs in 1.5–5% of the retinoblastoma patients. The most common is pineal tumor [16, 17]. They are usually cystic. Enlarged pineal gland with cyst and irregular wall or solid component should be considered suspicious and closely followed up—every 3 months (Fig. 18.16).
- Quadrilateral retinoblastoma is presence of suprasella or parasellar mass.
- MRI helps to differentiate retinoblastoma and other simulating lesions

18.10.4 Lesions Simulating Retinoblastoma

- Coats' disease
- Persistent hyperplastic primary vitreous
- Toxocara

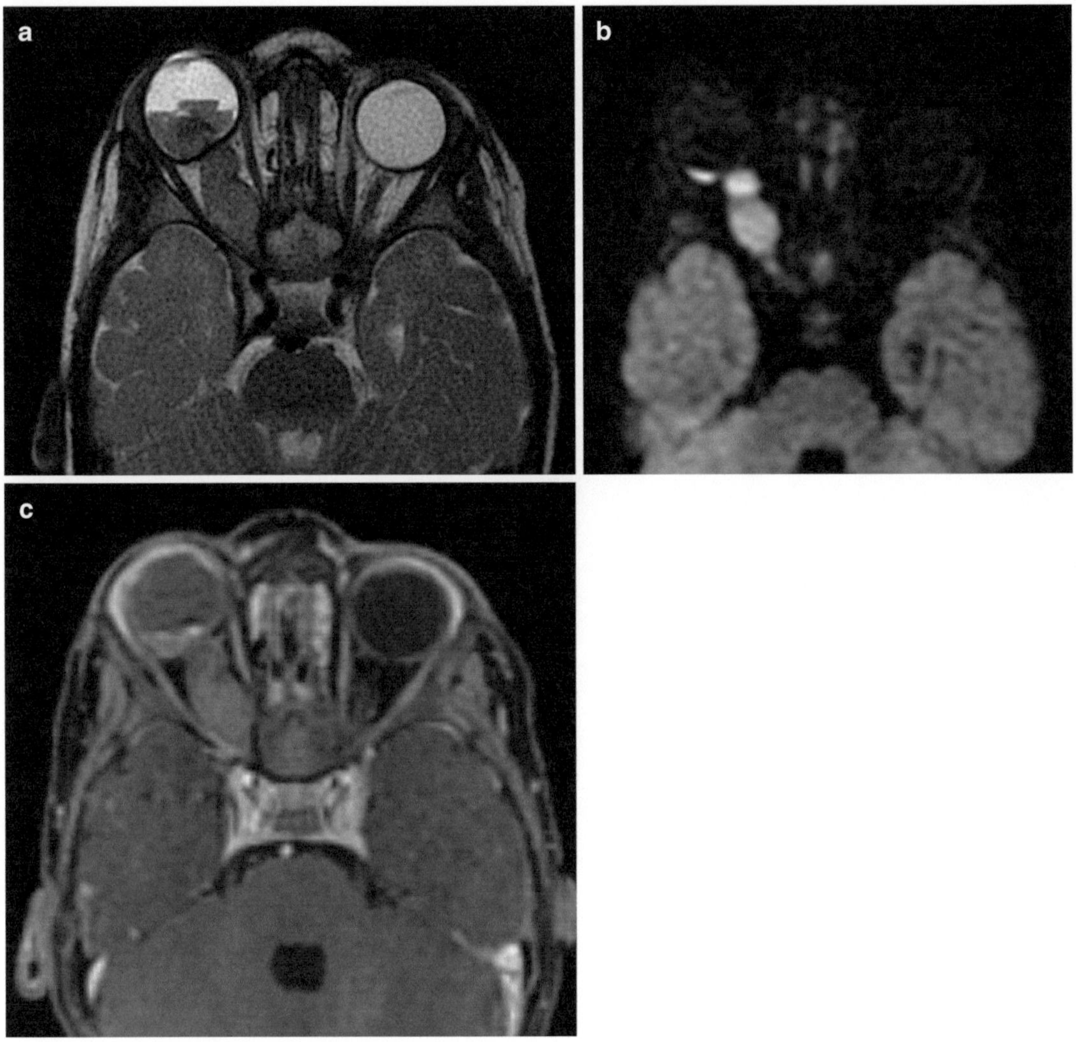

Fig. 18.14 Retinoblastoma with optic nerve invasion. (**a**) Axial T2 weighted image showing enlarged right globe, an irregular T2 hypointense intraocular mass lesion and gross invasion of the optic nerve. (**b**) Axial diffusion weighted image showing restricted diffusion in the active and cellular part of the intraocular lesion and optic nerve. (**c**) Contrast enhanced fat suppressed T1 weighted image showing enhancement in the active part of the tumor and optic nerve

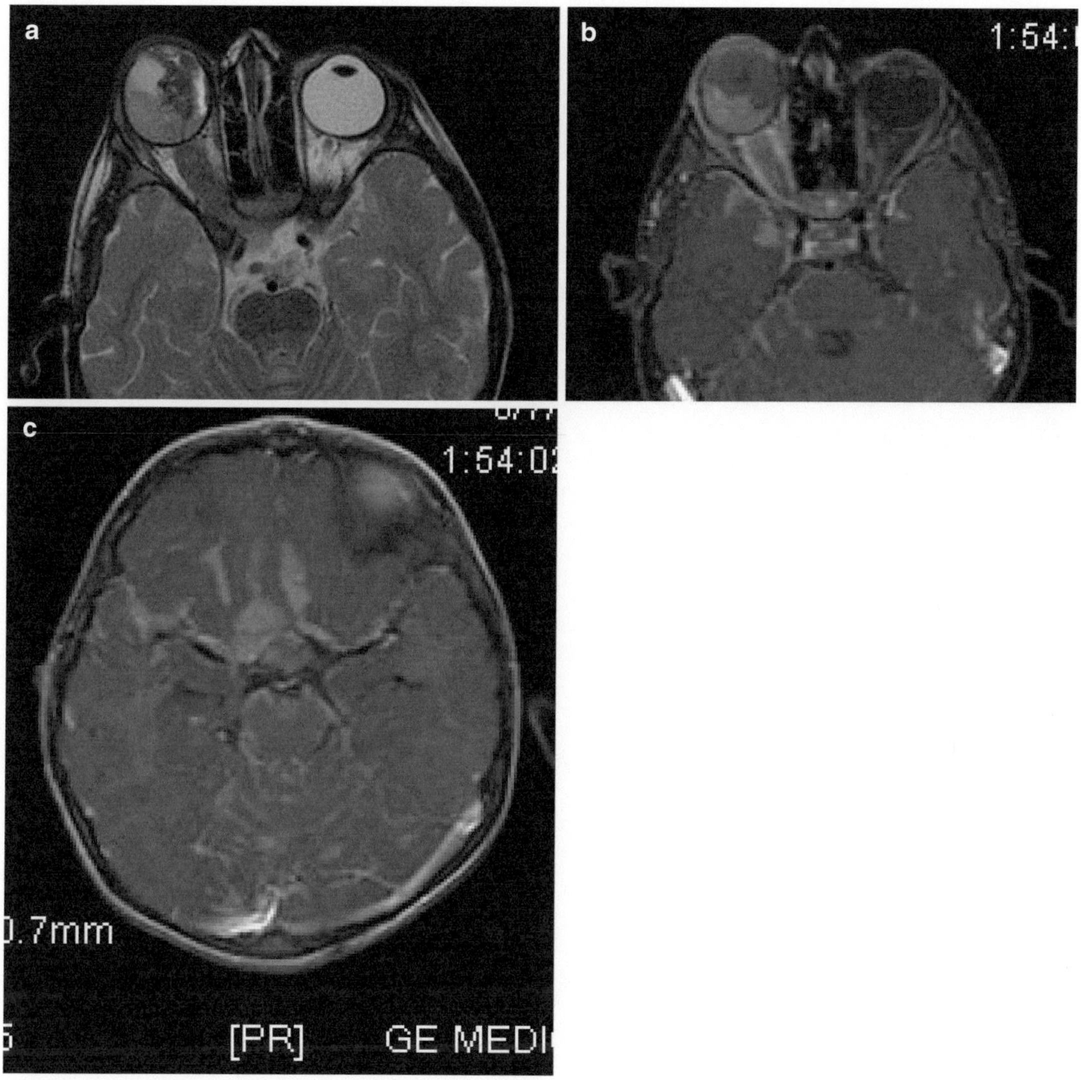

Fig. 18.15 Retinoblastoma with optic nerve invasion and subarachnoid metastases. (**a**) Axial T2 weighted image showing enlarged right globe, an irregular T2 hypointense intraocular mass lesion, retinal detachment and gross invasion of the optic nerve. (**b**) Axial post contrast T1 fat suppressed image showing enhancement in the active and cellular part of the intraocular lesion and perioptic and cerebral subarachnoid space. (**c**) Contrast enhanced fat suppressed T1 weighted image of the brain showing leptomeningeal enhancement

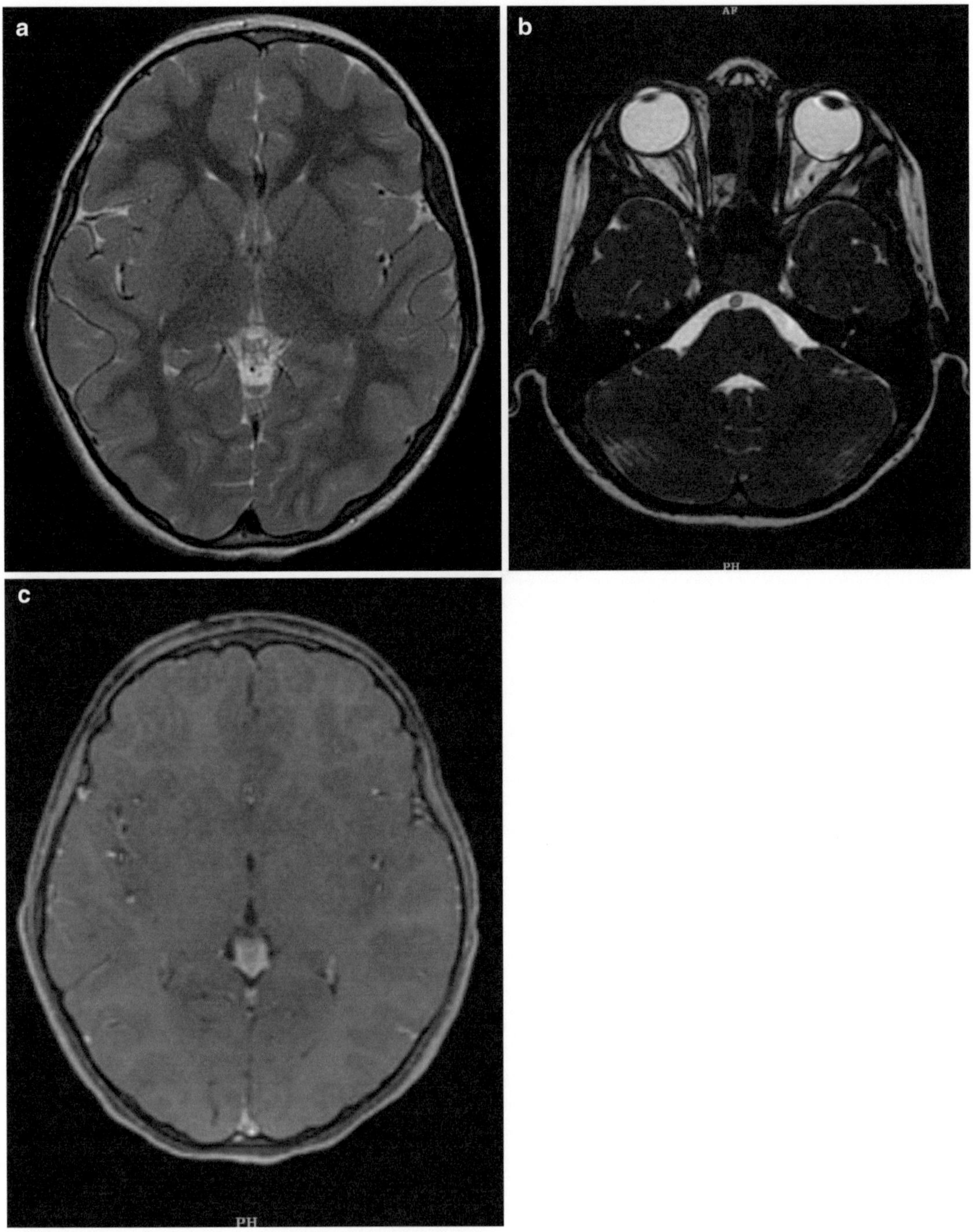

Fig. 18.16 A case of left eye retinoblastoma with pineal mass. (**a**) Axial T2 weighted image showing mild enlargement of the pineal gland and heterogenous signal. (**b**) Post contrast axial T1 weighted image showing heterogenous enhancement in the pineal gland. (**c**) Axial FIESTA image showing a small intraocular lesion in the left eye

- Cellulitis
- Retinopathy of prematurity
- Astrocytic hamartoma

18.11 Medulloepithelioma (Diktyoma)

Medulloepithelioma, usually occur in the first decade of life. It is a non-pigmented, vascular mass and usually arises from the ciliary body. Very rarely it can arise in the retina or optic nerve. The morphology of the tumor is characteristic solid and cystic [18].

18.11.1 Imaging

- MRI using surface coil technique is usually preferred due to its high signal to noise ratio as this is an anteriorly located tumor.
- It is mixed solid and cystic and therefore are usually isointense to the vitreous in T1 WI and mixed signal in T2 WI (Figs. 18.17 and 18.18).
- The cystic component is usually isointense to the vitreous.
- Marked enhancement of the solid component is seen following administration of gadolinium.

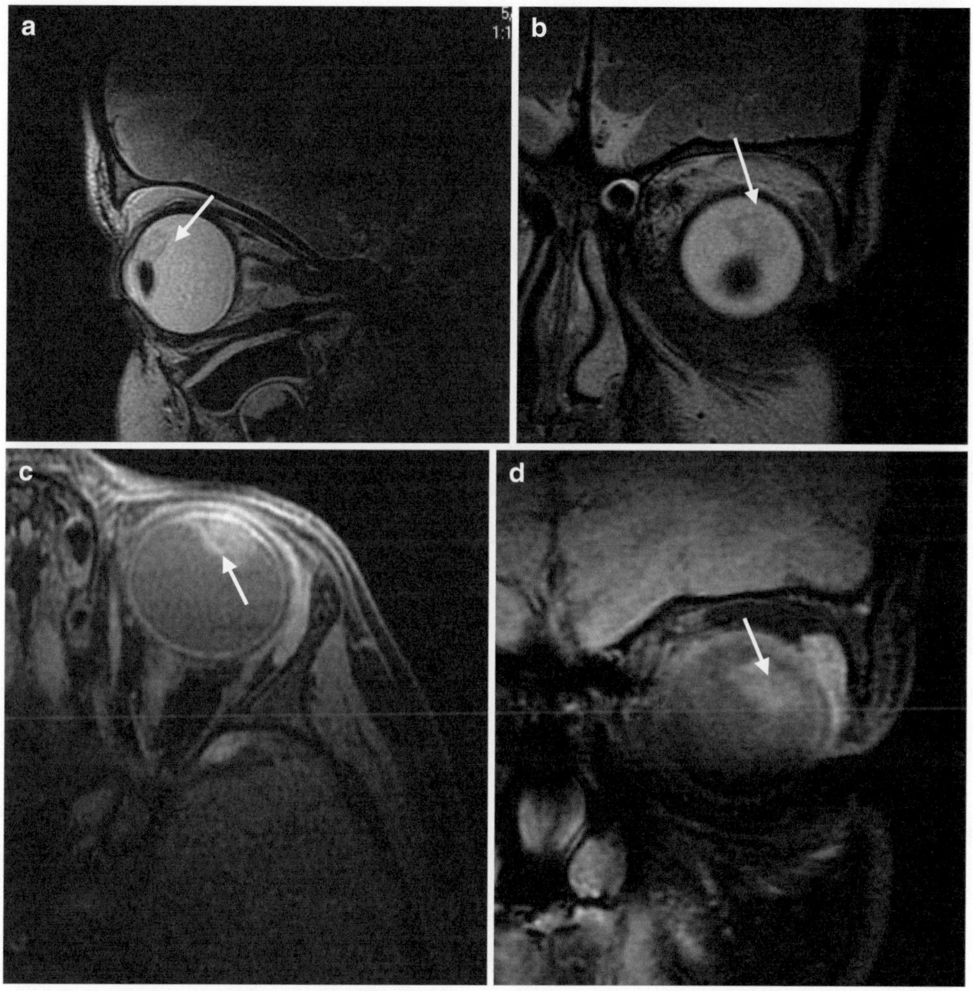

Fig. 18.17 (**a**, **b**) 3 years old child presented with redness, watering and white lesion in the eye-Sagittal and coronal T2 weighted surface coil image respectively showing ill-defined lesion mixed hypo and hyperintense ciliary body lesion superior to the lens s/o mixed solid and cystic nature of the lesion. (**c**, **d**) Non contrast axial and coronal T1 FSPGR fat sat images show the lesion to be hyperintense with respect to vitreous (white arrow)

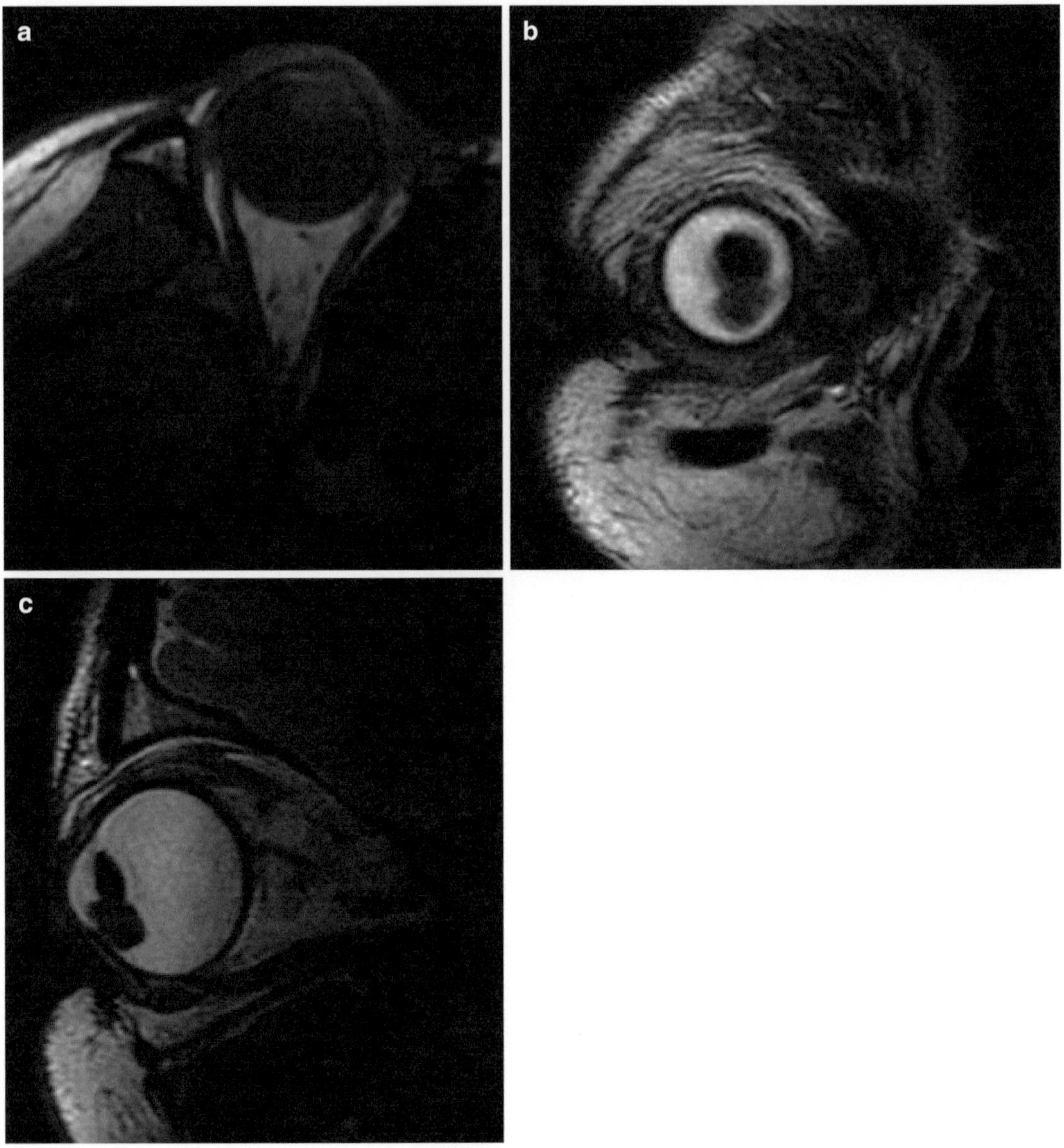

Fig. 18.18 Medulloepithelioma. (**a**) Axial T1 weighted surface coil study of the right eye showing an intermediate signal intensity ciliary body lesion. (**b**) Coronal T2 weighted image showing a hypointense lesion inferior to the lens. (**c**) Sagittal T2 weighted image clearly defining the tumor location and morphology

References

1. Mihara F, Gupta KL, Murayama S, Lee N, Bond JB, Haik BG. MR imaging of malignant uveal melanoma: role of pulse sequence and contrast agent. AJNR Am J Neuroradiol. 1991;12(5):991–6.
2. Wei W, Jia G, von Tengg-Kobligk H, Heverhagen JT, Abdel-Rahman M, Wei L, Christoforidis JB, Davidorf F, Knopp MV. Dynamic contrast-enhanced magnetic resonance imaging of ocular melanoma as a tool to predict metastatic potential. J Comput Assist Tomogr. 2017;41(5):823–7.
3. Smoker WR, Gentry LR, Yee NK, Reede DL, Nerad JA. Vascular lesions of the orbit: more than meets the eye. Radiographics. 2008;28(1):185.
4. Shields CL, Shields JA, Gross NE, Schwartz GP, Lally SE. Survey of 520 eyes with uveal metastases. Ophthalmology. 1997;104(8):1265–76.
5. Cohen VML. Ocular metastses. Eye (Lond). 2013;27(2):137–41.

6. Lemke AJ, Hosten N, Wiegel T, Prinz RD, Richter M, Bechrakis NE, Foerster PI, Felix R. Intraocular metastases: differential diagnosis from uveal melanomas with high-resolution MRI using a surface coil. Eur Radiol. 2001;11(12):2593–601.
7. LoRusso FJ, Boniuk M, Font RL. Melanocytoma (magnocellular nevus) of the ciliary body: report of 10 cases and review of the literature. Ophthalmology. 2000;107(4):795–800.
8. Reidy JJ, Apple DJ, Steinmetz RL, Craythorn JM, Loftfield K, Gieser SC, Brady SE. Melanocytoma: nomenclature, pathogenesis, natural history and treatment. Surv Ophthalmol. 1985;29(5):319–27.
9. Sagoo MS, Mehta H, Swampillai AJ, Cohen VML, Amin SZ, Plowman N, Lightman S. Primary intraocular lymphoma. Surv Ophthalmol. 2014;59:503.
10. Jellie HG, Gonder JR, Willis NR, Green L, Tokarewicz AC. Leiomyoma of the iris. Can J Ophthalmol. 1989;24(4):169–71.
11. Oh KJ, Kwon BJ, Han MH, Hwang PG, Kim CJ, Na DG, Chang KH. MR imaging findings of uveal leiomyoma: three cases. AJNR Am J Neuroradiol. 2005;26:100–3.
12. Sharma A, Ram J, Gupta A. Solitary retinal astrocytoma. Acta Ophthalmol (Copenh). 1991;69(1):113–6.
13. Bhende P, Babu K, Kumari P, Krishnakamar S, Biswas J. Solitary retinal astrocytoma in an infant. J Pediatr Ophthalmol Strabismus. 2004;41(5):305–7.
14. Margo CE, Barletta JP, Staman JA. Giant cell astrocytoma of the retina in tuberous sclerosis. Retina. 1993;13(2):155–9.
15. de Graaf P, Pouwels PJW, Rodjan F, Moll AC, Imhof SM, Knol DL, Sanchez E, van der Valk P, Castelijns JA. Single-shot turbo spin-echo diffusion-weighted imaging for retinoblastoma: initial experience. Am J Neuroradiol. 2012;33(1):110–8.
16. James SH, Halliday WC, Branson HM. Trilateral retinoblastoma. Radiographics. 2010;30(3):833.
17. Rodjan F, de Graaf P, Brisse HJ, Göricke S, Maeder P, Galluzzi P, Aerts I, Alapetite C, Desjardins L, Wieland R, Popovic MB, Diezi M, Munier FL, Hadjistilianou T, Knol DL, Moll AC, Castelijns JA. Trilateral retinoblastoma: neuroimaging characteristics and value of routine brain screening on admission. J Neuro-Oncol. 2012;109(3):535–44.
18. Brennan RC, Wilson MW, Kaste S, Helton KJ, McCarville MB. Ultrasound and MRI of pediatric ocular masses with histopathologic correlation. Pediatr Radiol. 2012;42(6):738–49.

19 Retinoblastoma: A Journey of 60 Years

Claire Hartnett and M. Ashwin Reddy

Retinoblastoma is a malignant tumour of the retina that is diagnosed in approximately 8000 children worldwide each year and although it is the most common primary eye cancer to affect children, it is considered rare in high resource countries with low birth rates [1–3].

19.1 Reducing Paediatric Mortality

In the 1950s retinoblastoma was associated with high mortality throughout the world. It is a paediatric cancer and so has a higher incidence in countries with high birth rates. As high resource countries have less children, the burden of retinoblastoma now falls upon low and middle resource countries e.g. in Nigeria it is the most common paediatric cancer in under 5 s [4]. Whilst there have been many medical advances in high resource countries noted over the last 6 decades, the high survival rate of greater than 95% stems from increased awareness of signs by the parents and guardians and the development of specialized centres for the treatment of the condition. It is no surprise that in countries without universal screening strategies, mortality rates have been documented of up to 60% [5, 6].

19.1.1 Lag Time

Delay in diagnosis is a pejorative term to describe the time interval between the onset of symptoms/signs and presentation to a service that can diagnose and treat the condition in a timely manner [7]. It has been demonstrated that increased lag time is associated with increased mortality for retinoblastoma [8]. This is the case in low/medium resource countries. However, in the UK it has been shown that increased lag time is no longer associated with a poorer outcomes [9] compared to three decades beforehand [10]. This is a similar finding to the US [11]. It is becoming more apparent that individual tumour biology is relevant in countries where the median lag time is around 1 month [9] and mortality is rare [11].

There have been concerted efforts to universally screen for retinoblastoma often at the same time as congenital cataracts. This is effective in

C. Hartnett
The Judith Kingston Retinoblastoma Service, Royal London Hospital, Barts Health NHS Trust, London, UK

Department of Ophthalmology, University Hospital Limerick, Limerick, Ireland

M. A. Reddy (✉)
The Judith Kingston Retinoblastoma Service, Royal London Hospital, Barts Health NHS Trust, London, UK

National Institute for Health Research Biomedical Research Centre at Moorfields Eye Hospital NHS Foundation Trust and UCL Institute of Ophthalmology, London, UK
e-mail: ashwin.reddy1@nhs.net; Ashwin.reddy@bartshealth.nhs.uk

V. Khetan (ed.), *Intraocular Tumors*, https://doi.org/10.1007/978-981-15-0395-5_19

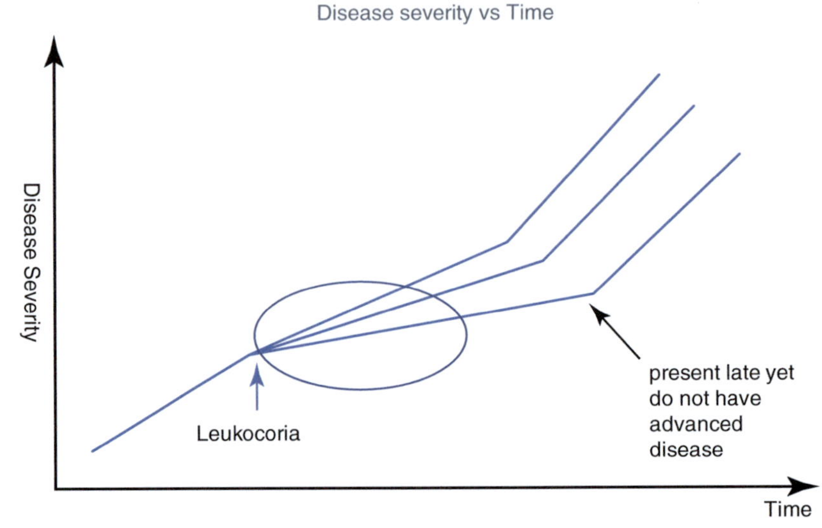

Fig. 19.1 This hypothetical chart shows that disease severity is independent of lag time in countries where the lag time is short (circled)

reducing mortality but not avoiding enucleation as early RB (Groups A, B and C) can only be detected by ophthalmologists with children under anaesthesia and this is not cost effective for the general population [12]. Kaliki et al. [13] found that only 21% of Indian patients with high-risk Rb (adverse histopathology) presented after 6 months of signs being noted which is surprising, as one would expect the vast majority to be presenting at such a late time. This suggests other factors are at play for the majority who are presenting relatively early to the service. For countries with established primary care systems, a linear relationship does not exist between lag time and retinoblastoma and individual tumour biology has become more relevant to invasiveness (Fig. 19.1).

19.1.2 Communication

In addition to presenting in a timely manner, the parents and guardians need to accept the advice given for treatment. As enucleation remains the mainstay of treatment in groups C, D and E in low/middle resource countries, refusal for enucleation is a cause of increased mortality. However, in specialised centres there is an opportunity for the families to speak to non-health care professional patient support groups (e.g.: The Childhood Eye Cancer Trust in the UK). These support workers often have relatives affected with retinoblastoma and can be instrumental in persuading families that enucleation can save a child's life with good cosmesis.

Conversely, poor communication between health care professionals will increase the risk of poor outcomes. In avoiding enucleation or systemic chemotherapy, units may use innovative treatments and this may increase the risk of metastases and therefore mortality [14]. Such decisions need to be discussed within a multidisciplinary environment including an open discussion with the families.

19.1.3 Orbital Disease

Until recently, orbital retinoblastoma was considered fatal with very little that could be done to prolong the child's life. However, a concerted multidisciplinary approach involving systemic chemotherapy, external beam radiation and enucleation can improve survival to 90% (18 of 20 cases) [15]. These are cases without intracranial involvement on MRI scanning nor metastases at presentation, but can still provide hope to clinicians and patients in countries that often see patients presenting in this manner.

19.1.4 Pinealoblastoma

In high resource countries death from retinoblastoma is rare, but mortality may be seen with children who have pinealoblastoma in addition to retinoblastoma. The survival for children who develop pinealoblastoma due to being *RB1* carriers is poor compared to those with sporadic pinealoblastoma [16].

19.2 Shift from Radiation

The first attempt to treat retinoblastoma with X-ray occurred in 1903 and was carried out by H.l. Hilgartner in Austin, Texas [17]. In 1919, Schoenberg described the use of radiation therapy in a 2-year-old girl with bilateral retinoblastoma. The eye with the larger tumour was enucleated and the less involved eye was treated by radium therapy. The tumour in the latter eye regressed and 3 years after first commencing treatment, the child was healthy with good vision [18]. Enucleation of the worse eye and radiation of the least affected eye represented standard treatment of retinoblastoma for the next 70 years. If diagnosed early enough, both eyes could be cured by X-ray irradiation [18]. Foster Moore in 1929 in London and Martin & Reese in 1936 [17] in New York confirmed that ionizing radiation could treat this type of tumour and also identified patterns of regression. Although success with externally applied radiation became apparent, ophthalmic complications were frequent. They began working with radiologists to progressively reduce the dose from 20,000 rads (cGy) to present day 3500–4500 cGy levels in order to attempt to preserve useful vision [19].

Kupfer in 1953 was the first ophthalmologist to combine chemotherapy, using a nitrogen mustard agent intravenously, with radiation therapy [20]. He believed that this would result in a reduction in the overall dose of radiation required to treat intraocular retinoblastoma. This technique was later abandoned due to the recorded immediate side effects of this chemotherapeutic agent; in some cases children died.

Forrest first wrote about the observations of second cancers in patients previously treated with irradiation for retinoblastoma in 1961 [21]. More evidence emerged confirming these finding in the years and decades that followed. Abramson wrote of similar findings in 1976 [22] and later wrote of the incidences of sarcomas and other cancers in these patients in 1997 [23].

19.2.1 Recognition of Oncology Risks to Adult Survivors

Much attention for retinoblastoma care was dedicated to saving the lives of children. However, there is increasing awareness of the risk to survivors of retinoblastoma.

It became widely recognized that patients with constitutional mutation of the *RB1* gene are at increased life-long risk of developing other specific second cancers. This risk is increased with exposure to radiation (a 50% risk of developing cancer by the age of 50 years of age if they received EBRT compared to 27% risk if they did not). These include osteosarcoma, leiomyosarcoma, malignant melanoma, lung cancer and bladder cancer [24]. Lifestyle counselling can educate survivors on ways to reduce their risk of developing a second cancer by avoiding unnecessary radiation (such as UV light) and carcinogens (such as smoking and alcohol) and obesity. They should also promptly report any suspicious unexplained lesions [25] and there have been awareness campaigns to make doctors aware of the risk to retinoblastoma survivors (Case Study).

Case Study

Caroline Aherne was a famous comedian in the UK. She had familial retinoblastoma and after treatment for retinoblastoma including External Beam Radiotherapy at St Bartholomew's Hospital in London, she was left partially sighted in one eye. Unfortunately, she suffered from bladder cancer as an adult, and later in 2014 she embarked on a programme of treatment for lung cancer. She died aged 52.

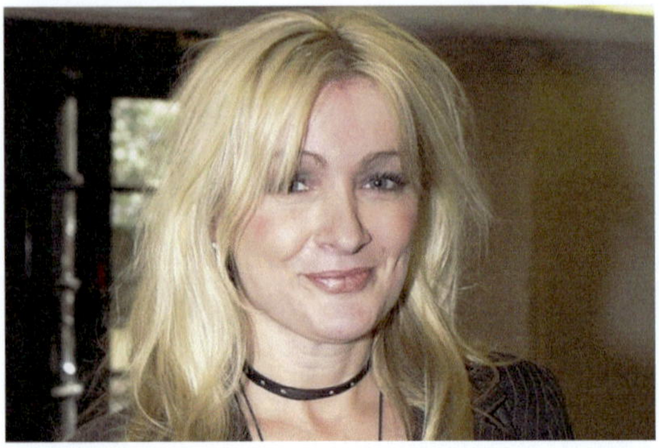

The risk of second primary cancers within the radiation field in children with germline *RB1* mutation is significant when the infant is irradiated under the age of 1 year [26]. Therefore, radiation is no longer a primary therapy for retinoblastoma.

19.3 A More Relevant Classification System

In the late 1950s Ellsworth and Reese developed a classification system for retinoblastoma. This was devised to predict prognosis and outcomes when intraocular retinoblastoma was treated with external beam radiotherapy (EBRT). It did allow international investigators and clinicians to compare results to treatment of tumour based on size for the first time.

With the advent of new therapies and the shift from radiotherapy to intravenous chemotherapy as a primary treatment for retinoblastoma, several classification systems [27, 28] developed to reflect prognosis with chemotherapy [29]. Unfortunately, they use the same nomenclature (Groups A–E) with variations of diagnostic features and therefore make comparison of publications and consensus regarding treatment difficult [30].

The TNM cancer classification system is another system used for retinoblastoma staging and was published in 2010 [31]. A revised system was published in 2016 and incorporates heritability into the classification [32]. According to this classification Group D retinoblastoma is cT2a (>5 mm subretinal fluid from the base of the tumour) and cT2b (tumours with any vitreous or subretinal seeding). It remains to be seen if this system will be used consistently by units in the future.

19.4 Increased Understanding of Genetics

The empiric risk for relatives of retinoblastoma was all that was known in the 1970s and 1980s. Offspring of patients with a family history of retinoblastoma or bilateral tumours have a 50% risk of inheriting the mutant allele and a 45% risk of developing retinoblastoma, due to incomplete penetrance. It was first reported by Knudson and later shown conclusively that 15% of patients with unilateral retinoblastoma have a germline mutation [33].

However the most accurate way to predict who will develop retinoblastoma in a family is to test them for the precise *RB1* mutant allele found in the proband. In many countries genetic testing began on retinoblastoma patients in the mid-1990s. This was gradually expanded and genetic testing offered to retinoblastoma patients in high-income and middle-income countries from the late 1990s and the turn of the century. This has been a huge advancement for patients and families.

Genetic testing of infants born at risk of retinoblastoma can be performed on DNA from amniotic fluid or from cord blood samples taken at birth. These at risk infants are examined regularly to detect early tumours. Examination without anaesthesia may be performed initially (as tumours often are within the posterior pole and mid-equatorial region) but after 2–3 months of age anesthesia is required to detect small tumours with visualization of the ora serrata essential. All children at risk should undergo multiple examinations under anaesthesia in the first 3 years life in accordance with agreed protocols. Each unit should stratify risks according to the sensitivity of screening for the *RB1* gene and previous audits of tumour detection [34]. Tables 19.1 and 19.2 demonstrate the screening strategy for offspring

Table 19.1 Screening protocol for at risk children with affected parents

	Low risk screening (risk < 1%)	High risk screening (risk 1–100%)
Starting age	Within 4 weeks	Within 2 weeks
Screening frequency		
Up to 6 months	EUA at 3 and 6 months Awake at 4.5 months	4 weekly
6–12 months	EUA at 9 and 12 months	4–6 weekly
1–2 years	At 16 and 22 months	2 monthly until 18 months 3 monthly until 2 years
2–3 years	6 monthly	4 monthly
Stop screening age	3 years	3 years at retinoblastoma unit 3–5 years: screening to be performed every 6 months by local ophthalmologist Children who have a mutation should be seen annually at a retinoblastoma unit until 16 years of age

Table 19.2 Screening protocol for children with affected sibling

	Low risk screening (risk < 1%)	High risk screening (risk 1–100%)
Starting age	Within 4 weeks	Within 2 weeks
Screening frequency		
Up to 6 months	At 3 and 6 months	4 weekly
6 months to 1 year	4 monthly	4–6 weekly
1–2 years	6 monthly	2 monthly until 18 months 3 monthly until 2 years
2–3 years	6 monthly	4 monthly
Stop screening age	3 years	3 years at retinoblastoma unit 3–5 years: Screening to be performed every 6 months by local ophthalmologist Children who have a mutation should be seen annually at a retinoblastoma unit until 16 years of age

and siblings in the UK. Recently, it has been shown that survivors of retinoblastoma (particularly women) have fewer children if the risk is unknown or they do not understand the implications of the genetic testing. This emphasizes the importance of providing information to families in a manner that they can understand [35].

19.5 The Role of Enucleation

All eyes with features suggestive of imminent extraocular extension (IIRC Group E) still require immediate enucleation. The reason for this is that there is an increased chance of high-risk retinoblastoma on histopathology with secondary glaucoma and iris neovascularization, which are deemed Group E retinoblastoma in all classification systems [13]. Kaliki et al. compared 145 cases with high risk features and compared with 258 cases without high risk features. As expected secondary glaucoma increased the risk, but only 63% developed high risk features so that 37% did not have high risk features and therefore had no increase in the risk of metastases. Similarly only 53% with iris neovascularization had concomitant high-risk features on histopathology so almost half did not. As retinoblastoma surgeons are unsure as to which eyes harbor the adverse histopathology at present, it is safer to enucleate these eyes.

Historically, many children were not fitted with an orbital implant following enucleation, as it was felt that it would interfere with the detection of tumour recurrence by not allowing for palpation of the orbit [36]. However the emergence of MRI allowed for the imaging of the orbit despite the presence of an implant. In addition, a good cosmetic outcome is achieved by replacement of the volume of the eye with an implant deep in the orbit and has also been proven to be beneficial for orbital growth [37].

Changes in the techniques of enucleation and the types of implants used have changed over the last few decades. Expensive porous implants that become vascularized with the muscles sutured to the implant had been used extensively in the past. However, they were noted to be susceptible to infection and extrusion over the years. Equal artificial eye motility has been shown with the use of the cheaper polymethyl methacrylate (PMMA) implants and muscles sutured to the conjunctival fornices (myoconjunctival technique) rather than on front of the implant [38, 39]. The role of the prosthetist is very important in achieving the motility in the studies and it has been difficult to achieve the results in children of other ethnicities who do not have the well-formed posterior tenon's that Indian children possess. Additionally, the use of a prosthetic eye conformer at the time of the enucleation results in a positive psychological benefit to the parents and child and these conformers have been adopted internationally more recently. This is particularly relevant in countries with high mortality such that compliance with this treatment becomes acceptable.

As discussed below, some units may enucleate more children for valid reasons taking into account risk factors for metastasis. The role of child play specialists cannot be understated for these children and, if possible, it is important that long term follow-up is provided so that psychosocial concerns are addressed in a timely manner. An excellent way of providing this includes children teaching younger children about prosthesis management (http://www.bbc.co.uk/programmes/p05d4m8d).

19.6 Systemic Chemotherapy

The use of the nitrogen mustard group of chemotherapeutic agents, particularly triethylenemelamine was largely abandoned in the late 1960s [19]. However, systemic chemotherapy became important again for primary treatment of intraocular disease in the 1970s when drugs that had been shown to be effective in metastatic disease (cyclophosphamide, vincristine and doxorubicin) were also noted to have a dramatic effect on reducing the size of the intraocular lesions. It was noted though that the lesions regrew after stopping the chemotherapy treatment. However, alternatives to external beam irradiation were sought in the 1990s [40].

From 1996 [41], the first-line treatment to control Murphree IIRC Groups B, C and D retinoblastoma has been intravenous chemotherapy with different combinations, doses, schedules and durations of carboplatin, etoposide and vincristine (CEV) followed by focal therapy with cryotherapy or laser, applied to consolidate chemotherapy responses [42] and to destroy any recurrent tumour [41, 43]. CEV is generally given every 3 weeks through a central venous line. Intravenous chemotherapy alone eradicates the retinoblastoma completely and regular, frequent examinations under anaesthesia are necessary to observe for relapses or recurrences following completion of chemotherapy treatment [44, 45].

19.7 Focal Therapy

Focal therapy is the local application of treatment to the eye under direct visualization i.e.: laser, cryotherapy or plaque. It has become the primary treatment for IIRC Group A eyes and is also used to consolidate responses of IIRC Group B, C and D eyes following intravenous or intra-ophthalmic arterial chemotherapy.

19.7.1 Laser

In Germany in the 1950s, Gerd Meyer-Schwickerath developed photocoagulation using a xenon arc beam [17]. It was noted that this could be used for small retinoblastoma tumours (1–4 mm in diameter) and it was called light coagulation. It was also used to treat recurrences following plaque or EBRT during this time [17].

Its use continued through the following decades and currently still plays an important role in treatment of IIRC Group A and B eyes and to those tumours that have been initially shrunk by chemotherapy. As with many treatments for retinoblastoma, the evidence for laser in patients having chemotherapy is not robust [42] yet it is standard treatment for many centres. Transpupillary thermotherapy involves directing 810 nm diode laser through the dilated pupil to heat the tumour for 3–5 min per spot. Photocoagulation therapies with 532 nm, 810 nm or continuous-wave 1064 nm laser beams are directly applied by multiple short burns. The power is gradually increased until the tumour is coagulated and grey to white.

19.7.2 Cryotherapy

Cryotherapy was introduced by Harvey Lincoff et al. in the 1960s [18] and became an important adjunct in the treatment of peripheral or anteriorly-located small retinoblastomas [17]. It can be used for more posterior tumours where central visual damage will not result. Cryotherapy involves freezing the tumour through the sclera with a nitrous oxide probe. The tumour cells die during the thawing stage and therefore a full 1 min interval between each freeze cycle is important. A triple-freeze thaw technique is used.

In general, focal therapies are repeated 2–3 weekly until the tumour is completely atrophic.

Whilst a flat scar can be easily achieved using cryotherapy, repetitive laser sessions are necessary to create a scar after chemotherapy and laser (dependent on the size of the original tumour). As a result it has been advocated that certain phenotypes that do not flatten with post chemotherapy laser (e.g. cavitary retinoblastoma) do not require repetitive laser after chemotherapy [46].

19.7.3 Radioactive Plaque Therapy

Stallards' collaboration with Innes in 1964 led to the development of Cobalt-60 applications of varying size which could deliver a dose of 4000 rads to the apex of the tumour in 7 days at St Bartholomew's Hospital, London [19]. This was the beginning of modern-day brachytherapy and plaque therapy later began in the United States in 1969.

Episcleral radioactive plaques such as the iodine or the ruthenium plaque have become another form of focal therapy option. Plaque focal radiation is effective at treating single recurrences after chemotherapy or EBRT had failed. In some instances, where a single tumour of less than 13 mm in diameter exists, not adjacent to the optic disk or macula, it may be treated with a plaque as a primary treatment. Its use has recently declined as it is recognized that it may result in haemorrhages and retinal detachment if used prior to intra-ophthalmic arterial chemotherapy [47].

19.8 Intra-Ophthalmic Artery Catheterization (IAC)

Intra-arterial catheterization has been used for eye salvage therapy in Japan since the 1990s using a balloon to block the carotid artery and direct chemotherapy flow to the ophthalmic artery. In 2006, Abramson and colleagues modified this technique to achieve a more selective delivery to the eye via catheterization of the ophthalmic artery (intra-ophthalmic artery chemotherapy). Reported results were encouraging with high eye salvage rates [48–50]. Indications for IAC use soon expanded to include primary treatment. One study demonstrated overall globe salvage was 74% when IAC was used as first-line treatment and 67% when used as second-line treatment [50]. Additional chemotherapeutic agents were added later including topotecan and carboplatin.

The early adopters of this treatment may have given this treatment to group E eyes with a 50% risk of high risk features and as a result children may have died. Therefore, it is not universally adopted [51]. Another concern is vision (see below) when used for non-macula tumours.

19.9 Widespread Use of Intravitreal Chemotherapy

Historically, one of the most difficult features to control in the treatment of retinoblastoma was that of vitreous seeding, and it was one of the main causes of failure of primary treatment [52]. Again intravitreal chemotherapy was performed for decades in Japan before a safety enhanced method was introduced by Munier et al. in 2012 [53]. Following the use of this methodology, it has been acceptable to virtual all units.

Encouraging results have been emerging over the last 3 years [53, 54]. Vitreous seed median time regression has been reported at 0.6, 1.7 and 7.7 months for dust, spheres and cloud seeds respectively. The median number of injections required to reach regression was 3, 5 and 8 injections for the respective seed groups [55, 56]. Metastatic spread has been shown in a systematic review to be a rare occurrence [57]. Topotecan is another agent recently being used for recurrent seeds [58].

19.10 The Battle for Group D Eyes

Virtually all units will salvage Groups A, B and C eyes and enucleate Group E eyes with certain phenotypic characteristics. Controversies arise for Group D eyes with some advocating enucleation in all unilateral cases and some advising salvage at all times. Unfortunately, there is no consensus on the definition of a Group D eye (as discussed above) and this makes comparison between different centres difficult.

19.10.1 Discussion with Parents

The discussion with parents is essential. Generally, parents would like to save the eye if it is safe to do so. Uncommonly parents may be keen for enucleation, e.g. a recent relative has died from chemotherapy for a non-retinoblastoma cancer and they would like to minimize the use of chemotherapy. Parents need to be aware of the risk of enucleation after the attempt to salvage, visual potential and the treatment burden in terms of number of examinations under anaesthesia.

In London, the success rate for salvage for Group D eyes is 63% with 55 months median follow-up and no children receiving first line IAC nor suffering metastases [59]. Children who undergo enucleation have three times fewer EUAs compared to those who have salvage treatment [60]. This is important information as parents are concerned about the risk of multiple anaesthetics on their children particularly neurodevelopment [61]. Unfortunately, even if enucleation was to take place and adverse histopathology identified with appropriate adjuvant chemotherapy, there is still a risk of metastases of up to 4% [13, 62].

19.10.2 Type of Treatment: Systemic vs Intra-Ophthalmic Arterial Chemotherapy

13% of Group D eyes [27] are associated with high risk features [63]. Interestingly vitreous seeding appears to be a good sign for the avoidance of high risk features in the 10 of 62 eyes exhibiting this feature. All patients were treated with systemic chemotherapy and none developed metastases. IAC may also be used to treat Group D eyes but metastases have been noted in 3% (3/103) [64]. None of the children who had metastases died.

Our approach is to advocate first line IAC for children with group D eyes and vitreous seeding and to use systemic chemotherapy for Group D eyes without vitreous seeding.

19.11 The Role of Vision

With more eyes being saved, the retinoblastoma specialist must now also consider long-term visual acuity when choosing therapies and counselling families. It has been shown that up to 58% of eyes maintain vision of better than 6/12 (20/40)

[65, 66] when they are old enough to perform Snellen visual acuities. However, the reports relate to eyes independently and it is important to be aware that early support for visually impaired infants from any cause will provide life-long benefits [67]. As a result a delay in assessing vision in infants and sending to the appropriate visual rehabilitative service can have far reaching effects. Therefore, it is essential that vision is assessed in pre-verbal children using appropriate paediatric ophthalmological tests.

Visual potential is an important consideration in the discussion with the family regarding enucleation of an eye or attempts at salvage. With particular relevance for Group D eyes, half had better vision than 6/60 (20/200) and 7 of 32 (22%) had better than 6/12 (20/40) vision [68].

It is also relevant for new treatments. Rather than wait until young children being treated are old enough to perform tests suited for adults, it is important to identify complications early and address the causes. This means the assessment of pre-verbal children by appropriate tests and the use of visual evoked potentials. Retinoblastoma units were initially tentative in their use of IAC due to complications including choroidal ischaemia and visual loss [47]. Vision in previously seeing eyes was initially lost in 42% of patients [69] which was thought to be due to the learning curve for interventional neuro-radiologists. However, Reddy et al. [70] showed that patients with similar catheterization complications yet a reduced dose of melphalan did not lose vision.

19.11.1 Patient Centred Approach

The vast majority of patients are under 5 years of age and therefore a patient centred approach needs to consider that these are children not adults. Until recently there was little consideration of the non-medical concerns of children with retinoblastoma. However, there is now a desire to address psychological issues, particularly regarding the parents [71] and make the multiple EUAs that they have to endure as painless as possible. Families benefit from the presence of a patient support group representative (e.g. The Childhood Eye Cancer Trust in the UK) at diagnosis and subsequent visits to address non-medical concerns but also to raise questions that they feel they cannot ask the health care professionals. As a result, it is important for the psychologist and patient support group representative to be part of the multi-disciplinary meeting so that psychosocial concerns can be addressed. This integrated team approach can optimize patient care.

19.12 Conclusion

Over the last 60 years, the management of retinoblastoma has been revolutionized with the advent of novel therapeutic modalities, diagnostic imaging, improved chemotherapeutic agents and approach to children. The gradual shift from EBRT to systemic chemotherapy has improved survival and also helped with greater rates of eye salvage. The survival rate of retinoblastoma in high resource countries was 90% in 1997 and that rate is now over 95% in 2017. The adaptation of intra-ophthalmic artery chemotherapy and intravitreal chemotherapy has also improved eye salvage rates and the retention of vision.

Significant challenges remain however. Retinoblastoma in low-income countries is associated with low patient survival of approximately 30–40%. This is a statistic that needs to be improved. The creation of toolkits (Fig. 19.2) and international collaborations can and will improve survival.

Retinoblastoma Management: Resource Manual: Sept 2017

A RESOURCE MANUAL

FOR THE

MANAGEMENT

OF

RETINOBLASTOMA

IN

LOW & MIDDLE
RESOURCE SETTINGS

UPDATED SEPTEMBER 2017

RETINOBLASTOMA NETWORK, ICEH

This Resource manual is a product of the work of the Retinoblastoma Network, part of the Commonwealth Eye Health Consortium at the International Centre for Eye Health, LSHTM, London.

The Retinoblastoma Network currently consists of a partnership of many individuals and institutions from a number of African, Asian and European countries involved in improving the management of Retinoblastoma with an emphasis on low and middle income countries.

Fig. 19.2 The development of a toolkit to assist in the development of a Retinoblastoma Service

References

1. Seregard S, Lundell G, Svedberg H, Kivela T. Incidence of retinoblastoma from 1958 to 1998 in northern Europe: advantages of birth cohort analysis. Ophthalmology. 2004;11:1228–32.
2. Kivela T. The epidemiological challenge of the most frequent eye cancer: retinoblastoma, an issue of birth and death. Br J Ophthalmol. 2009;93:1129–31.
3. Broaddus E, Topham A, Singh AD. Incidence of retinoblastoma in the USA: 1975-2004. Br J Ophthalmol. 2009;93:21–3.
4. Ochicha O, et al. Pediatric malignancies in Kano, Northern Nigeria. World J Pediatr. 2012;8(3):215–9.
5. Waddell KM, et al. Improving survival of retinoblastoma in Uganada. Br J Ophthalmol. 2015;99:937–42.
6. Owoeye JF, et al. Retinoblastoma—a clinic-pathological study in Ilorin, Nigeria. Afr J Health Sci. 2006;13(1–2):117–23.
7. Barr RD. "Delays" in diagnosis: a misleading concept, yet providing opportunities for advancing clinical care. J Pediatr Hematol Oncol. 2014;36(3):169–72.
8. Ribeiro KC, Antoneli CB. Trends in eye cancer mortality among children in Brazil, 1980-2002. Pediatr Blood Cancer. 2007;48:296–305.
9. Posner, et al. Lag time for retinoblastoma in the UK revisited: a retrospective analysis. BMJ Open. 2017;7:e015625. https://doi.org/10.1136/bmjopen-2016-015625.
10. Goddard AG, Kingston JE, Hungerford JL. Delay in diagnosis of retinoblastoma: risk factors and treatment outcome. Br J Ophthalmol. 1999;83:1320–3.
11. Butros LJ, et al. Delayed diagnosis of retinoblastoma: analysis of degree, cause and potential consequences. Pediatrics. 2002;109:E45.
12. Khan AO, Al-Mesfer S. Lack of efficacy of dilated screening for retinoblastoma. J Pediatr Ophthalmol Strabismus. 2005;42:205–10.
13. Kaliki S, Srinivasan V, Gupta A, et al. Clinical feature predictive of high-risk retinoblastoma in 403 Asian Indian patients: a case-control study. Ophthalmology. 2015;122:1165–72.
14. Abramson DH, et al. Intra-arterial chemotherapy (ophthalmic artery chemosurgery) for Group D retinoblastoma. PLoS One. 2016;11(1):e0146582.
15. Honavar SG, Singh AD. Management of advanced retinoblastoma. Ophthalmol Clin N Am. 2005;18:65–73.
16. Plowman PN, Pizer B, Kingston JE. Pineal parenchymal tumours: II. On the aggressive behavior of pinealoblastoma in patients with an inherited mutation of the RB1 gene. Clin Oncol (R Coll Radiol). 2004;16(4):244–7.

17. Bedford MA, Bedotto C, MacFaul PA. Retinoblastoma. A study of 139 cases. Br J Ophthalmol. 1971;55:19–27.
18. Albert DM. Historic review of retinoblastoma. Ophthalmology. 1987;94:654–62.
19. Abramson DH. Retinoblastoma in the 20th century: past success and future challenges. Invest Ophthalmol Vis Sci. 2005;46:2684–91.
20. Kupfer C. Retinoblastoma treated with intravenous nitrogen mustard. Am J Ophthalmol. 1953;36:1721–3.
21. Forrest AW. Tumours following radiation about the eye. Trans Am Acad Ophthalmol Otolaryngol. 1961;65:694–717.
22. Abramson DH, Ellsworth RM, Zimmerman LE. Non-ocular cancer in retinoblastoma survivors. Trans Am Acad Ophthalmol Otolaryngol. 1976;81:454–7.
23. Wong FL, Boice JD, Abramson DH, et al. Cancer incidence after retinoblastoma radiation dose and sarcoma risk. JAMA. 1997;278:1262–7.
24. MacCarthy A, et al. Second and subsequent tumours among 1927 retinoblastoma patients diagnosed in Britain 1951-2004. Br J Cancer. 2013;108:2455–63.
25. Fletcher O, et al. Lifetime risks of common cancers among retinoblastoma survivors. J Natl Cancer Inst. 2004;96:357–63.
26. Abramson DH, Frank CM. Second non-ocular tumors in survivors of bilateral retinoblastoma: a possible age effect on radiation-related risk. Ophthalmology. 1998;105:573–9.
27. Murphree AL. Intraocular retinoblastoma: the case for a new group classification. Ophthalmol Clin N Am. 2005;18:41–53.
28. Shields CL, et al. The international classification of retinoblastoma predicts chemoreduction success. Ophthalmology. 2006;113:2276–80.
29. Just diagnosed: staging. Children's Oncology Group Website. 2011. https://www.childrensoncologygroup.org/index.php/newlydiagnosedwithretinoblastoma.
30. Scelfo C, et al. An international survey of classification and treatment choices for Group D retinoblastoma. Int J Ophthalmol. 2017;10(6):961–7.
31. Finger PT, et al. AJCC cancer staging manual. New York: Springer; 2010. p. 561–8.
32. Mallipatna AC, Gallie BL, Che'vez-Barrios P, et al. Retinoblastoma. In: Amin MB, Edge SB, Greene F, et al., editors. AJCC cancer staging manual. 8th ed. New York: Springer; 2017. p. 819–31.
33. Knudson AG. Mutation and cancer: statistical study of retinoblastoma. Proc Natl Acad Sci. 1971;68:820–3.
34. Price EA, Price K, Kolkiewicz K, et al. Spectrum of RB1 mutations identified in 403 retinoblastoma petients. J Med Genet. 2014;51:208–14.
35. Munier FL, Balmer A, Van Melle G, Gailloud C. Radial asymmetry in the topography of retinoblastoma. Clues to the cell of origin. Ophthalmic Genet. 1994;15:101–6.
36. De Potter P, Shields CL, Shields JA, et al. Use of the hydroxyapatite ocular implant in the pediatric population. Arch Ophthalmol. 1994;112:208–12.
37. Kaste SC, Chang G, Fontanesi J, et al. Orbital development in the long-term survivors of retinoblastoma. J Clin Oncol. 1997;15:1183–9.
38. Yadava U, Sachdeva P, Arora V. Myoconjunctival enucleation for enhanced implant motility. Result of a randomized prospective study. Indian J Ophthalmol. 2004;52:221–6.
39. Shome D, Honavar SG, Raizada K, Raizada D. Implant and prosthesis movement after enucleation: a randomized controlled trial. Ophthalmology. 2010;117:1638–44.
40. Ferris FL 3rd, Chew EY. A new era for the treatment of retinoblastoma. Arch Ophthalmol. 1996;114:1412.
41. Kingston JE, Hungerford JL, Madreperla JA, Plowman PN. Results of combined chemotherapy and radiotherapy for advanced intraocular retinoblastoma. Arch Ophthalmol. 1996;114(11):1339–43.
42. Fabian ID, et al. Focal laser treatment in addition to chemotherapy for retinoblastoma. Cochrane Database of Syst Rev. 2017;6:CD012366.
43. Gallie BL, et al. Chemotherapy with focal therapy can cure intraocular retinoblastoma without radiotherapy. Arch Ophthalmol. 1996;114:1321–8.
44. Gombos DS, Kelly A, Coen PG, Kingston JE, Hungerford JL. Retinoblastoma treated with primary chemotherapy alone: the significance of tumour size, location and age. Br J Ophthalmol. 2002;86:80–3.
45. Lee V, et al. Globe conserving treatment of the only eye in bilateral retinoblastoma. Br J Ophthalmol. 2003;87:1374–80.
46. Chaudhry S, Onadin Z, Sagoo MS, Reddy MA. The recognition of cavitary retinoblastoma tumours: Implications for management and genetic analysis. Retina. 2018;38:782–7. https://doi.org/10.1097/IAE.0000000000001597.
47. Muen WJ, et al. Efficacy and complications of super-selective intra-ophthalmic artery melphalan for the treatment of refractory retinoblastoma. Ophthalmology. 2012;119(3):611–6.
48. Berry JL, et al. Long-term outcomes of Group D eyes in bilateral retinoblastoma patients treated with chemoreduction and low-dose IMRT salvage. Pediatr Blood Cancer. 2013;60:688–93.
49. Gobin YP, Dunkel IJ, Marr BP, Brodie SE, Abramson DH. Intra-arterial chemotherapy for the management of retinoblastoma: four-year experience. Arch Ophthalmol. 2011;129:732–7.
50. Susuki S, Yamane T, Mohri M, Kaneko A. Selective ophthalmic arterial injection therapy for intraocular retinoblastoma: the long-term prognosis. Ophthalmology. 2011;118:2081–7.
51. Yousef YA, Soliman SE, Astudillo PP, et al. Intra-arterial chemotherapy for retinoblastoma: a systemic review. JAMA Ophthalmol. 2016;134:584–91. https://doi.org/10.1001/jamaophthalmol.2016.0244.

52. Manjandavida FP, Honavar SG, Reddy VA, Khanna R. Management and outcome of retinoblastoma with vitreous seeds. Ophthalmology. 2014;121:517–24.
53. Munier FL, et al. Intravitreal chemotherapy for vitreous disease in retinoblastoma revisited: from prohibition to conditional indications. Br J Ophthalmol. 2012;96:1078–83.
54. Shields CL, et al. Intravitreal melphalan for persistent or recurrent retinoblastoma vitreous seeds: preliminary results. JAMA Ophthalmol. 2014;132: 319–25.
55. Francis JH, et al. The classification of vitreous seeds in retinoblastoma and response to intravitreal melphalan. Ophthalmology. 2015;122:1173–9.
56. Munier FL. Classification and management of seeds in retinoblastoma. Ellsworth Lecture Ghent August 24th 2013. Ophthalmic Genet. 2014;35:193–207.
57. Smith SJ, Smith BD. Evaluating the risk of extraocular tumour spread following intravitreal injection therapy for retinoblastoma: a systematic review. Br J Ophthalmol. 2013;97(10):1231–6.
58. Rao R, Honavar SG, Sharma V, Reddy VA. Intravitreal toptecan in the management of refractory and recurrent vitreous seeds in retinoblastoma. Br J Ophthalmol. 2017;102:490–5. https://doi.org/10.1136/bjophthalmol-2017-310641.
59. Fabian ID, et al. Primary intravenous chemotherapy for Group D retinoblastoma: a 13 year retrospective analysis. Br J Ophthalmol. 2017;101:82–8.
60. Fabian ID, et al. Primary Enucleation for Group D retinoblastoma in the era of systemic and targeted chemotherapy: the price of retaining and eye. Br J Ophthalmol. 2017;0:1–5. https://doi.org/10.1136/bjophthalmol-2017-310624.
61. Loepke AW, Soriano SG. An assessment of the effects of general anesthetics on developing brain structure and neurocognitive function. Anesth Analg. 2008;106:1681–707.
62. Honavar SG, Singh AD, Shields CL, et al. Postenucleation adjuvant therapy in high-risk retinoblastoma. Arch Ophthalmol. 2002;120(7):923–31.
63. Fabian ID, et al. High-risk histopathology features in primary and secondary enucleated international intraocular retinoblastoma classification Group D eyes. Ophthalmology. 2017;124:851–8.
64. Abramson DH, Daniels AB, Marr BP, Francis JH, Brodie SE, Dunkel IJ, et al. Intra-arterial chemotherapy (ophthalmic artery chemosurgery) for Group D retinoblastoma. PLoS One. 2016;11(1):e0146582.
65. Narang, et al. Predictors of long-term visual outcome after chemoreduction for management of intraocular retinoblastoma. Clin Exp Ophthalmol. 2012;40(7):736–42.
66. Hall LS, Ceisler E, Abramson DH. Visual outcomes in children with bilateral retinoblastoma. J AAPOS. 1999;3(3):138–42.
67. Dale N, et al. Developmental outcome, including setback, in young children with severe visual impairment. Dev Med Child Neurol. 2002;44(9):613–22.
68. Fabian ID, et al. Long-term visual acuity, strabismus and nystagmus outcomes following multimodality treatment in Group D retinoblastoma eyes. Am J Ophthalmol. 2017;179:137–44.
69. Tsimpida M, et al. Visual outcomes following intra-ophthalmic artery melphalan for patients with refractory retinoblastoma and age appropriate vision. Br J Ophthalmol. 2013;97:1464–70.
70. Reddy MA, et al. Reduction of severe visual loss and complications following intra-arterial chemotherapy (IAC) for refractory retinoblastoma. BJO. 2017;101(12):1704–8. https://doi.org/10.1136/bjophthalmol-2017-310294.
71. Hamama-Raz Y, Rot I, Buchbinder E. The coping experience of parents of a child with retinoblastoma- malignant eye cancer. J Psychosoc Oncol. 2012;30(1):21–40.

20 Counselling Parents of Retinoblastoma Patients

Sonal S. Chaugule

Retinoblastoma is the most common primary intraocular malignancy encountered in paediatric age group, affecting 1 in 15,000–18,000 live births [1–4]. It is a heritable life as well as vision threatening disease. However, it is also believed to be perhaps the 'most curable paediatric cancer' [5]. Worldwide, survival parallels economic development as retinoblastoma survival is approximately 30% in Africa, 60% in Asia, 80% in Latin American, and 95–97% in Europe and North America [6]. The goals of management of retinoblastoma include: life salvage, globe and vision salvage as primary, secondary and tertiary preference respectively. The management modalities for retinoblastoma have evolved from enucleation and external beam radiation to more conservative systemic, focal and local methods aiming to achieve higher rates of globe as well as functional vision salvage over the last couple of decades.

Being a predominantly paediatric cancer, the subject of patient counselling are usually the parents of the affected child, except for the rare adult onset disease. The elements of informed consent include: clinical diagnosis, grouping and staging, treatment modalities, prognostication, cost factor, surveillance and need for long term follow up, treatment of metastatic disease, genetic counselling and screening of present as well as future children.

20.1 Diagnosis of Retinoblastoma

Retinoblastoma is one of the few malignancies which are diagnosed mainly on clinical evaluation as opposed to standard histopathological evidence, which is needed for most other malignancies. In fact, an interventional diagnostic procedure such as pars plana vitrectomy or fine needle aspiration biopsy are contraindicated in a child with suspected retinoblastoma. The clinical diagnosis is made after a detailed anterior segment and fundus examination under anaesthesia, ultrasound B scan, ultrasound biomicroscopy and neuroimaging (computed tomography [CT] and/or magnetic resonance imaging [MRI]) as and when needed. In case of dilemmas or uncertainty regarding diagnosis; it is highly recommended to seek a second expert opinion on the case before proceeding with intraocular biopsy.

20.2 Grouping and Staging

The grouping system is for tumor that is limited to the eye where globe salvage is the end point, whereas staging system predicts overall survival in a patient. The international classifi-

S. S. Chaugule (✉)
Ophthalmic Plastic Surgery, Orbit and Ocular Oncology, PBMA's H V Desai Eye Hospital, Pune, Maharashtra, India
e-mail: schaugule@eyecancercure.com

V. Khetan (ed.), *Intraocular Tumors*, https://doi.org/10.1007/978-981-15-0395-5_20

cation of intraocular retinoblastoma gave a logical flow of tumor grading that correlates with the outcome of newer treatment modalities [7] (Table 20.1). The recent American Joint Committee on Cancer (AJCC eighth Ed) TNMH (tumor, node, metastasis and hereditary trait) staging is comprehensive and includes clinical, histopathological as well as hereditary aspect of the tumor. It is also the first evidence-based-system for predicting overall prognosis of both eye(s) and patients [8] (Table 20.2).

Table 20.1 International Classification of Retinoblastoma (ICRB) [7]

Groups	Description
Group A Small tumors	Retinoblastoma<3 mm in size in basal dimensions or thickness
Group B Larger tumors	• Retinoblastoma >3 mm in basal dimensions or thickness • Macular location (<3 mm to foveola) • Juxtrapapillary location (<1.5 mm to disc) • Clear subretinal fluid <3 mm from margin
Group C Focal seeds	• C1 subretinal seeds <3 mm from retinoblastoma • C2 vitreous seeds <3 mm from retinoblastoma • C3 both subretinal and vitreous seeds <3 mm from retinoblastoma
Group D Diffuse seeds	• D1 subretinal seeds >3 mm from retinoblastoma • D2 vitreous seeds >3 mm from retinoblastoma • D3 both subretinal and vitreous seeds >3 mm from retinoblastoma
Group E Extensive retinoblastoma	• Occupying >50% globe or • Neovascular glaucoma • Opaque media from hemorrhage in anterior chamber, vitreous, or subretinal space • Invasion of post laminar optic nerve, choroid (>2 mm), sclera, orbit, anterior chamber

Table 20.2 TNMH Staging as per AJCC 8th Edition [8]

Stage	Description
cTX	Unknown evidence of intraocular tumor
cT0	No evidence of intraocular tumor
cT1 cT1a cT1b	Intraretinal tumor(s) with subretinal fluid <5 mm from the tumor base. No vitreous or subretinal seeding Tumors ≤3 mm in size and >1.5 mm away from the optic disc and fovea Tumors >3 mm in size and <1.5 mm away from the optic disc and fovea
cT2 cT2a cT2b	Tumors with retinal detachment/subretinal seeding/vitreous seeding Subretinal fluid >5 mm from the tumor base Tumors with vitreous seeding and/or subretinal seeding
cT3 cT3a cT3b cT3c cT3d cT3e	Advanced intraocular tumor(s) Phthisis or prephthisis bulbi Tumor invasion of choroid, pars plana, ciliary body, lens, zonules, iris, or anterior chamber Raised intraocular pressure with neovascularization and/or buphthalmos Hyphema and/or massive vitreous haemorrhage Aseptic orbital cellulitis
cT4	Extraocular tumor(s) involving orbit, including optic nerve
HX H0 H0* H1	Unknown or insufficient evidence of *RB1* constitutional mutation Normal *RB1* alleles in blood Normal *RB1* in blood with <1% residual risk mosaicism Bilateral retinoblastoma, trilateral retinoblastoma, family history of retinoblastoma, or molecular definition of constitutional *RB1* gene mutation
pTX	Unknown evidence of intraocular tumor
pT0	No evidence of intraocular tumor

Table 20.2 (continued)

Stage	Description
pT1	Intraocular tumor(s) without any local invasion, focal choroidal invasion, or pre- or intralaminar involvement of the optic nerve head
pT2 pT2a pT2b	Intraocular tumor(s) with local invasion Concomitant focal choroidal invasion and pre- or intralaminar involvement of the optic nerve head Tumor invasion of stroma of iris and/or trabecular meshwork and/or Schlemm canal
pT3 pT3a pT3b pT3c pT3d	Intraocular tumor(s) with significant local invasion Massive choroidal invasion (>3 mm in largest diameter, or multiple foci of focal choroidal involvement totaling >3 mm, or any full-thickness choroidal involvement) Retrolaminar invasion of the optic nerve head, not involving the transected end of the optic nerve Any partial-thickness involvement of the sclera within the inner two thirds Full-thickness invasion into the outer third of the sclera and/or invasion into or around emissary channels
pT4	Evidence of extraocular tumor: tumor at the transected end of the optic nerve, tumor in the meningeal spaces around the optic nerve, full-thickness invasion of the sclera with invasion of the episclera, adjacent adipose tissue, extraocular muscle, bone, conjunctiva, or eyelids

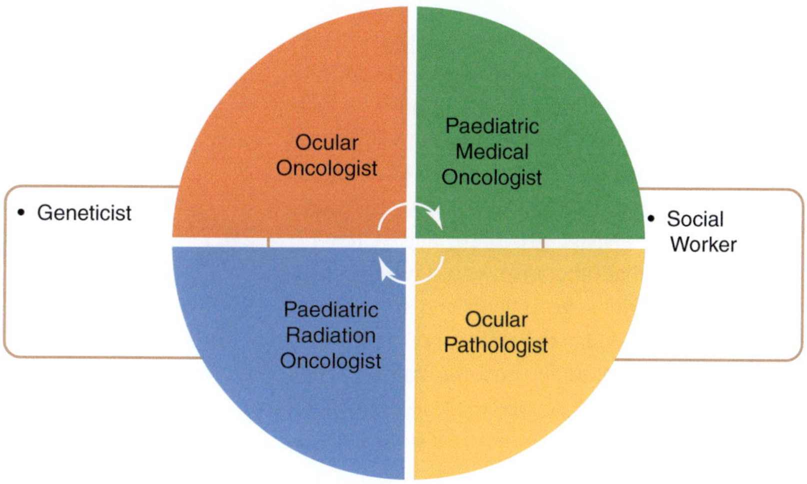

Fig. 20.1 Multi-disciplinary team efforts in management of retinoblastoma

20.3 Explaining the Diagnosis to the Parents

After reaching to the clinical diagnosis, grouping and staging of retinoblastoma the parents of the child need to be explained about the same. In my experience, a sit-down with the parents with results of imaging modalities e.g. RetCam and ultrasound images helps in their understanding of the pathology. They are explained about the normal anatomy of the eyeball (sclera, choroid, retina, lens, fovea and optic nerve) and its relation to the tumors location, size, number and their relation to those structures. In addition, the presence of retinal detachment, extra-ocular extension, optic nerve and frank orbital involvement, intracranial extension or presence of trilateral disease are discussed. The need for initial staging and systemic metastatic survey is also explained.

20.4 Choice of Treatment

As mentioned at the start of this chapter, the primary goal of retinoblastoma management is to save child's life followed by salvage of the eye and optimization of visual function. There are multiple treatment options available and the appropriate line of management depend upon the laterality, extent and systemic status of the child in question. This requires a multidisciplinary team approach which includes ocular oncologist, paediatric medical oncologist, radiation oncologist, geneticist and social worker to facilitate the optimized care (Fig. 20.1). It needs to be emphasized on the parents that mortality related to retinoblastoma occurs when the disease escapes the confines of the eyeball; the delayed diagnosis and treatment and excessive focus on saving a blind eye harbouring advanced form of the disease may put the child at risk for extraocular extension, metastasis and death [9].

The modalities available are: (a) Focal—cryotherapy, laser photocoagulation, transpupillary thermotherapy, transscleral thermotherapy, intravitreal chemotherapy and plaque brachytherapy; (b) Local—external beam radiotherapy and enucleation and (c) Systemic—intravenous and intra-arterial chemotherapy.

20.5 Primary Enucleation

Primary enucleation is considered definitive treatment for advanced unilateral retinoblastoma (TNMH cT3 [8] and ICRB group E [7]). It enables histopathological analysis and allows the child to return to normal life [10]. Enucleation is recommended for when the optic nerve is not visible and in presence of total retinal detachment (TNMH [8] cT2a, and ICRB [7] Group D eyes) or extensive vitreous seeds (TNMH [8] cT2b, and ICRB [7] Group D eyes) that otherwise would require invasive treatments over several years and are costly to the family to save the eye with poor vision [9]. Enucleation is strongly recommended when orbital or optic nerve involvement is suspected, when there is anterior segment invasion, neovascular glaucoma, intraocular haemorrhage, orbital cellulitis and no potential for useful vision [9].

20.6 Chemotherapy with Adjuvant Focal Treatment

Efforts to save the eye require a consideration of staging, visual potential and considerable discussion with the child's family. Small tumors (TNMH cT1a [8] and ICRB [7] Group A) can be managed with focal modalities (thermotherapy and/or cryotherapy) alone. Larger tumors or small ones those near to optic nerve and/or fovea (TNMH cT1b, cT2 [8] and ICRB [7] Group B, C, D) need consolidating chemotherapy along with adjuvant focal modalities. Chemotherapy can be systemic or intra-arterial.

Systemic chemotherapy (most commonly intravenous carboplatin, etoposide, and vincristine) is given over 6 cycles, every 3–4 weeks depending on the extent of disease. Chemotherapy reduces tumor size, and focal therapy on repeated follow-up EUAs destroys remnants of tumor [9].

Intra-arterial chemotherapy (IAC) with topotecan, melphalan and carboplatin has emerged as an important option for unilateral cT1b and cT2 (ICRB Gr C/D) eyes. Intra-arterial chemotherapy has become the standard of care in developed nations for these eyes. In developing countries like India, IAC is utilised to improve eye salvage for refractory and selected cases. Although it reportedly has high rates of globe salvage (66% of all eyes and 57% with advanced disease), the data for long term outcomes as visual acuity, extraocular disease, delayed metastasis and death is still limited. The literature is limited by different staging schemes, absence of defined long-term protocols and lack of follow up data [11].

20.7 Management of Vitreous Seeds

Vitreous seeds are generally resistant to systemic and intra-arterial chemotherapy mainly due to the avascular nature of the vitreous. Intravitreal chemotherapy (melphalan and/or topotecan) is used to control vitreous seeds.

20.8 Orbital Retinoblastoma

Orbital retinoblastoma poses a challenging situation. The protocol for management of orbital retinoblastoma includes: high dose neoadjuvant chemotherapy, surgery (enucleation or exenteration), external beam radiotherapy and adjuvant high dose chemotherapy. Orbital retinoblastoma has conventionally shown poor prognosis with mortality rates ranging from 25 to 100% [12].

20.9 Management of Metastatic Disease

The possibility of metastatic disease increases when the disease is in advanced stage at the time of presentation e.g. orbital retinoblastoma, advanced intraocular retinoblastoma with clinical high-risk factors. Initial metastatic survey with bone marrow and cerebrospinal fluid examination with/out positron emission tomography [PET/CT] rules out metastasis at presentation in above cases. Regular timely metastatic survey on treatment completion helps in early diagnosis of systemic metastasis. The prognosis for cases detected with systemic metastasis remains poor. The recommended management includes multidisciplinary team efforts to provide high dose chemotherapy, intrathecal chemotherapy and radiotherapy.

20.10 Genetic Testing and Counselling

Genetic testing and counselling are essential in management of retinoblastoma. This involves a laboratory with high sensitivity to detect *RB1* mutations [13]. *RB1* genetic testing of the proband may identify heritability, and at-risk family members may then undergo testing for the specific mutation. Children of a proband with bilateral retinoblastoma have a 50% risk of carrying the *RB1* mutation, whereas children of an untested unilateral proband have a 7.5% risk (50% × 15%), which can be accurately updated to either 100% or 0% by genetic testing of the proband and then the fetus if the proband is found to carry an *RB1* mutation [14]. The frequency of follow-up for children at risk of retinoblastoma is informed by the results of genetic testing and counselling [9].

20.11 Prenatal Screening

Children with a family history of retinoblastoma who carry *RB1* mutation are at risk of tumors at birth. Chorionic villus sampling (between 11–14 weeks' gestation) or amniocentesis (after 16 weeks' gestation) may be considered so parents have choices of how to manage the pregnancy if the fetus has the *RB1* mutation. Amniocentesis can also be offered at 33 weeks' gestation when the risks of miscarriage are lower and manageable [9, 15]. Examination for tumors as soon as possible after birth, followed by repeated EUA for the first few years of life, facilitates early detection of tumors that can be managed with less invasive interventions [16]. Infants who had prenatal *RB1* mutation detection followed by early full-term delivery (36–38 weeks' gestation) and coordinated retinal examination had smaller tumors at birth and improved visual outcomes [9].

Financial Disclosure None.

Conflict of Interest None.

References

1. Moll AC, Kuik DJ, Bouter LM, et al. Incidence and survival of retinoblastoma in The Netherlands: a register based study 1862-1995. Br J Ophthalmol. 1997;81:559–62.
2. Broaddus E, Topham A, Singh AD. Incidence of retinoblastoma in the USA: 1975-2004. Br J Ophthalmol. 2009;93:21–3.
3. Seregard S, Lundell G, Svedberg H, et al. Incidence of retinoblastoma from 1958 to 1998 in Northern Europe: advantages of birth cohort analysis. Ophthalmology. 2004;111:1228–32.
4. Krishna SM, Yu GP, Finger PT. The effect of race on the incidence of retinoblastoma. J Pediatr Ophthalmol Strabismus. 2009;46:288–93.
5. Abramson DH, Shields CL, Munier FL, Chantada GL. Treatment of retinoblastoma in 2015: agreement and disagreement. JAMA Ophthalmol. 2015;133(11):1341–7.
6. Kivela T. The epidemiological challenge of the most frequent eye cancer: retinoblastoma, an issue of birth and death. Br J Ophthalmol. 2009;93:1129–31.
7. Shields CL, Shields JA. Basic understanding of current classification and management of retinoblastoma. Curr Opin Ophthalmol. 2006;17:228–34.
8. Mallipatna A, Gallie BL, Chévez-Barrios P, et al. Retinoblastoma. In: Amin MB, Edge SB, Greene FL, editors. AJCC cancer staging manual. 8th ed. New York: Springer; 2017. p. 819–31.
9. AlAli A, Kletke S, Gallie B, Lam WC. Retinoblastoma for pediatric ophthalmologists. Asia Pac J Ophthalmol. 2018;7(3):160–8. https://doi.org/10.22608/APO.201870.
10. Mallipatna AC, Sutherland JE, Gallie BL, et al. Management and outcome of unilateral retinoblastoma. J AAPOS. 2009;13:546–50.
11. Yousef YA, Soliman SE, Astudillo PP, et al. Intra-arterial chemotherapy for retinoblastoma: a systematic review. JAMA Ophthalmol. 2016;134:584–91.
12. Honavar SG, Manjandavida FP, Reddy VA. Orbital retinoblastoma: an update. Indian J Ophthalmol. 2017;65(6):435–42.

13. Skalet AH, Gombos DS, Gallie BL, et al. Screening children at risk for retinoblastoma. Ophthalmology. 2018;125(3):453–8.
14. Roelofs K, Shaikh F, Astle W, et al. Incidental neuroblastoma with bilateral retinoblastoma: what are the chances? Ophthalmic Genet. 2018;39:410–3.
15. Soliman SE, Racher H, Zhang C, et al. Genetics and molecular diagnostics in retinoblastoma--an update. Asia Pac J Ophthalmol. 2017;6:197–207.
16. Soliman SE, Dimaras H, Khetan V, et al. Prenatal versus postnatal screening for familial retinoblastoma. Ophthalmology. 2016;123:2610–7.

Counseling for Patients with Choroidal Melanoma

21

Sonal S. Chaugule and Paul T. Finger

Choroidal melanoma is the most common primary intraocular malignancy in adults. The goals of primary treatment are: destruction or removal of the primary tumour to prevent metastatic spread, preservation of vision and retention of the affected eye. These goals should be tempered by the eye cancer specialist's experiential knowledge of what will be required to meet them. For example, the amount of patient discomfort involved and the side-effects of treatment as well as the long-term prognosis for vision and eye retention needs to be considered.

The main elements of informed consent involve: presenting the clinical and/or pathology elements that led to the diagnosis. Information concerning ocular, vision and prognosis for life. The need for subsequent systemic surveillance, the patient's relative risk and currently available treatments for metastatic disease. That said, this initial consultation should be comprehensive. It is the doctor's duty to inform the patient of the known risks and benefits of treatment, only limited by the patient ability to understand and doctor's knowledge. Together, the patient and the doctor should come to an understanding that will have a durable impact on the patient's quality of life.

21.1 Diagnosis of Choroidal Melanoma

With the advent of multimodal imaging techniques, the clinical diagnosis of choroidal melanoma has reached a high degree of accuracy [1]. Apart from clinical examination, office-based techniques that are useful are fundus photography, fluorescein angiography (FFA), autofluorescent imaging, optical coreference tomography (OCT), transillumination and ultrasound imaging. Orbital radiographic imaging (magnetic resonance imaging [MRI], computed tomography [CT] or positron emission tomography [PET/CT]) is needed in selected cases [1]. Intraocular tumor biopsy is indicated for atypical tumors, metastatic tumors, when the patient requires a pathology diagnosis, and for genetic/molecular analysis [2].

21.2 Explaining the Diagnosis to the Patient and Family

Patients are referred to the ocular oncologist by primary care providers, retina specialist general ophthalmologist or optometrists. They may be

S. S. Chaugule (✉)
Department of Ophthalmic Plastic Surgery, Orbit and Ocular Oncology, PMBA's H V Desai Eye Hospital, Pune, Maharashtra, India
e-mail: schaugule@eyecancercure.com

P. T. Finger
The Eye Cancer Foundation, Inc., The New York Eye Cancer Center, New York University School of Medicine, New York, NY, USA
e-mail: pfinger@eyecancer.com; http://eyecancer.com

V. Khetan (ed.), *Intraocular Tumors*, https://doi.org/10.1007/978-981-15-0395-5_21

given a diagnosis of choroidal melanoma, suspicious nevus or non-specific intraocular tumor. The relevant medical, surgical and family history are required before proceeding with clinical examination. It has been our experience that more than 99% of tumors can be clinically diagnosed using the aforementioned in-office tools. It is a routine practice at The New York Eye Cancer Center to have the patient and their accompanying relatives review their results of imaging (with the eye cancer specialist) on large (55–85″) high-definition (4K) screens. The intent of this display is to help the patient understand the diagnostic characteristics of their tumour, its relationship to critical ocular structures. They are educated about basic eye anatomy (sclera, choroid, retina, lens, fovea and optic nerve) and its relation to the tumors location, size, its proximity to those structures. In addition, the presence of retinal detachment, subretinal fluid, intra-tumoral haemorrhage and possibility of extraocular extension are discussed. Therapeutic challenges to local control and long-term vision retention are made clear prior to treatment. Each tumor is staged using the American Joint Commission on Cancer (eighth Edition, AJCC), TNM (tumor, node, metastasis) system. The indications and need for initial staging and follow up systemic surveys are discussed [3].

21.3 Choice of Treatment

Modalities of treatment for choroidal melanoma are varied and dependent on tumour specific factors, specialist preference and local availability of therapeutic choices. These include: observation, plaque brachytherapy (iodine-125 [^{125}I], palladium-103 [^{103}Pd] strontium-90 [90Sr] and ruthenium-106 [^{106}Ru]), proton beam radiotherapy, stereotactic photon beam irradiation, local tumor resection, phototherapy (transpupillary thermotherapy, photodynamic therapy), enucleation and exenteration [4]. Of these, the eye cancer specialist should present the most reasonable and available choices, while comparing and contrasting their likely side-effects. At The New York Eye Cancer Center, all patients are educated about the risks and benefits of observation, radiation (plaque and proton beam), laser photocoagulation, chemotherapy, resection and/or enucleation. They are informed of the Collaborative Ocular Melanoma Study's (COMS) medium-sized tumor trial, which found no difference in survival between those patients treated with iodine-125 plaque or primary enucleation [5].

Radiation therapy is the most widely used eye and vision-sparing alternative to enucleation. The eye cancer specialist's choice of treatment also depends upon the size, location and extent of the tumour as well as patient's need, preference and circumstances (e.g. travel restrictions, financial constraints and availability of health care facilities etc.).

21.3.1 Small T1 Choroidal Melanoma

Unlike cutaneous melanoma, eye cancer specialists are more likely to use observation for change or growth prior to treatment of select, small choroidal melanomas. This is because many small melanomas are in close proximity to the macula, fovea and optic nerve where irradiation is likely to cause loss of vision. In these cases, rapid change, growth or advancing exudative retinal detachment indicates that the tumor itself will cause loss of vision, thus tipping the scales and balancing the known radiation-related risks. The documented tumor growth helps establish that the tumor is malignant and reassures the patient that the sight-threatening treatment is indicated.

Observation as initial treatment is particularly helpful for patients with small choroidal melanomas close to fovea, one-eyed patients and systemically ill patients who cannot tolerate treatment. Serial observation with comparative photography, OCT and angiography at the time of each visit can be used to detect subtle changes in tumor features essential in such cases. Clearly, documented growth of suspicious nevi may offer clinical evidence that it is indeed a small melanoma; while observation may allow additional months or years of useful functional vision. However, several large evidence-based studies that have found statistically significant evidence that largest tumor diameter is associated with increased risk of metastatic death [5–7]. This proves that observation of small malignant melanoma growth increases the patient's potential risk of metastatic disease.

In addition, all patients [even with small choroidal melanoma] with small choroidal melanoma should be made aware that there exist effective eye and vision sparing treatments and that anti-VEGF medications play a vital role in supressing radiation retinopathy and optic neuropathy [8]. For example, in 2013 Semenova and Finger analysed 72 small melanomas treated with palladium-103 plaque brachytherapy with a mean follow up duration of 54 months. They reported almost half of the eyes developed radiation retinopathy while almost 20% had radiation optic neuropathy. But, with the advent of intravitreal anti-VEGF therapy, only 19% (4 of 21) affected patients lost >2 lines of visual acuity chart. Therefore, patients presenting with small melanoma should be made aware of the risks and potential benefits of observation and risks of conservative treatment prior to making a clinical decision. Specifically, if patient chooses to observe their small melanoma, he or she should be made aware of the potential risk of metastasis.

21.3.2 Medium/T2 Sized Melanoma

21.3.2.1 Plaque Radiotherapy

Socioeconomics largely drive the availability and selection of radionuclides used in treatment of intraocular tumours. For example, higher-cost, custom-assembled iodine-125 [^{125}I] or palladium-103 [^{103}Pd] episcleral plaques are widely used in the United States; while lower cost, factory-made ruthenium-106 [^{106}Ru] plaques are typically used in Europe and India. Low energy seeded, medical physicist-dependent plaque construction and dosimetry depends upon tumor data i.e. size, location and distances from the optic disc as well as fovea [9]. Ruthenium-106 plaque energy is typically based on a factory look-up table, where only plaque size and duration of treatment can be modulated. These sources also differ in intraocular and extraocular dose-distribution and their different rates of side effects. Seeded plaques can be constructed to treat almost any size (height or width) melanoma, whereas ^{106}Ru beta-irradiation is tumor-height limited in that it can only reach 5–6 mm into the eye.

Both types of plaque are surgically sutured onto the sclera overlying the tumor, left in place for 5–7 days and then surgically removed. Due to a high-energy component, patients with ^{106}Ru plaques must stay in the hospital. In contrast, at The New York Eye Cancer Center, low-energy ^{125}I or ^{103}Pd plaque patients can go home with instructions for having family members at least 3 feet away during this interval (according to their specific national radiation safety guidelines). Informed consent for plaque insertion surgery should include a detailed discussion: of the relative rates of local tumor control, secondary enucleation, ophthalmic complications and metastatic disease. (Table 21.1) This should include but not be limited to radiation retinopathy, optic neuropathy, cataract and glaucoma; including the possibility and relative efficacy of future laser photocoagulation and/or intravitreal anti-VEGF injections [8].

21.3.2.2 Proton Beam

Proton beam therapy is available at select institutions around the world but is unavailable in wide-parts of India. It has been shown to be effective for local tumor control, globe and functional vision preservation [18]. However, the beam typically deposits a large anterior entrance dose resulting in eye lash loss, dry eye, neovascular glaucoma, and cataract (not as commonly seen with plaques).

Further, unlike plaques which are sewn to, and thus move along with, the eye for the duration of treatment; protons are like a tube of radiation that is beamed into the eye. As the eye moves, the dose to the tumor and normal ocular structures suffer more unintended radiation [19].

21.3.3 Choroidal Melanomas that Touch or Surround the Optic Disc

Failure of choroidal melanoma local control has been associated with a 6.3 increased hazard of dying from metastatic disease. In order to maxi-

Table 21.1 Radiotherapy for choroidal melanoma

Authors	Radiation	Study group size	Mean dose (Gy)	Mean follow-up (months)	Recurrence (%)	Secondary enucleation (%)	Neovascular glaucoma (%)	Metastasis (%)	Visual acuity
COMS [5, 10]	I-125	657	>85 Gy to 5 mm	60	10	13	N/A	10 (5 year) 18 (10 year)	57% >20/200 at 3 year
Packer et al. [11]	I-125	64	91	64	7.8	17.2	10.9	15.6	45% better or 20/100 at 5.3 year
Fontanesi et al. [12]	I-125	144	79	46	2.3	9.7	5.5	5.5	41% better or 20/200 at 3.9 year
Lommatzsch [13]	Ru-106	205	100	80	15	26	1.3	20	N/A
Char et al. [14]	Helium	218	70	110	5	22	35	18.6 (5 year) 23.6 (10 year)	33%better or 20/200 at 10 year
Brovkina and Zarubei [15]	Proton	63	100–125	34	19	25	N/A	6	N/A
Gragoudas et al. [16]	Proton	128	70	64	3	6	N/A	20.5	42% better than 20/200 at 5.3 year
Finger et al. [17]	Pd-103	400	73	51	3	3.5	2.5	7.3 (5 year) 13.4 (10 year)	79% better or 20/200 at 5 year 69% better or 20/200 at 10 year

This table is based on data published in article—Finger PT, Chin KJ, Duvall G, et al. Palladium-103 ophthalmic plaque radiation therapy for choroidal melanoma: 400 treated patients. Ophthalmology 2009;116:790–796, 796.e1 (Reprint permission) mize local, "normal plaque position" was defined as including the tumor and 2–3 mm of normal appearing tissue within the irradiated zone [4]. This is particularly difficult in treatment of choroidal melanomas that are near, touch or surround optic disc. This is because the retrobulbar optic nerve sheath is 5 mm wide and circumferentially 1.5 mm wider than the intraocular disc. In an effort to "normalize" ophthalmic plaque placement for these tumors, Finger developed slotted plaques with a 8-mm wide and variably deep slots designed to incorporate the 5–6 mm orbital optic nerve in and this overcame the obstruction [20]. In contrast, typical 4-mm wide notched plaques are not only incapable of overcoming the optic nerve sheath diameter, it offsets the plaque and thus worsen geographic miss (plaque misapplication). Other published options for treating peripapillary tumors include: stereotactic radiotherapy, proton beam irradiation or plaque brachytherapy with adjunctive transpupillary thermotherapy [14, 21–23].

21.3.4 Large T3 and T4 Choroidal Melanoma

Large tumor size is not a contraindication for use of eye-sparing radiation therapy (Box 21.1) [4]. According to the 2014 American Brachytherapy Society (ABS) Ophthalmic Oncology Task Force Guidelines, suggested relative contraindications Include: extraocular extension that would alter plaque position, basal diameters that extend the limits of brachytherapy, blind painful eyes or those with no perception of light for vision [4]. That said, enucleation is typically reserved for the melanomas >20 mm in diameter, >16 mm in thickness, suspected optic nerve invasion, significant extra scleral extension, multifocal recurrence and at the patient's request [4].

21.3.5 Extraocular Tumor Extension

If the patient is diagnosed with extra-scleral extension of tumor at presentation; it is then classified into [24],

(a) Minimal—microscopic or encapsulated
(b) Moderate—localised unencapsulated nodule, or
(c) Massive—filling most part of the orbit

The minimal extension may be included within the irradiation zone or beneath the plaque; moderate and massive extension can be removed by enucleation with local orbital resection followed by external beam (typically 50Gy) or implant high-dose-rate radiation therapy (35Gy). Irradiation is added typically to address presumed residual subclinical disease [24]. For unresectable massive extension, orbital exenteration with post-operative radiotherapy is advised.

Box 21.1 American Brachytherapy Society (ABS) Guidelines for Ophthalmic Plaque Brachytherapy: Indications for Eye and Vision Conserving Plaque Radiation Therapy [4]

- Clinical diagnosis of uveal melanoma is adequate for treatment
- Histopathological verification is not required
- Small melanomas can be treated at the eye cancer specialist's discretion. AJCC T1, T2, T3 and T4a-d uveal melanoma patients can be treated after counseling about likely vision, eye retention and local tumor outcomes
- Patients with peripapillary and sub-foveal and those with exudative retinal detachments typically have poorer resultant vision and local control outcomes. They should be accordingly counselled.
- Tumors with T4e extraocular extension,[a] basal diameter that exceeds the limits of brachytherapy, blind painful eyes, and those with no light perception vision are not suitable for plaque therapy

[a] ^{106}Ru and ^{90}Sr plaques are less accommodating for nodular extra-scleral extension

This table is based on—The American Brachytherapy Society - Ophthalmic Oncology Task Force. The American Brachytherapy Society consensus guidelines for plaque brachytherapy of uveal melanoma and retinoblastoma. *Brachytherapy*. 2014; 13: 1–14

21.4 Metastases

At diagnosis, the patient and family can be informed that metastatic disease is discovered in less than 1% of T1 and T2-sized tumors and up to 4% of patients with T3 or T4-sized melanomas [25]. A history of weight loss, subcutaneous nodularity and/or abdominal pain at presentation should arouse suspicion and should be investigated thoroughly. Signs or symptoms of radicular or focal pain suggest possible osseous disease [26]. Multiple large and statistically significant studies have found that largest tumor diameter together with thickness can be used as a non invasive method to predict risk of metastasis [5, 7, 27] (Fig. 21.1).

21.5 Systemic Surveys

There are no available international consensus guidelines for pre/post-treatment and surveillance techniques for early detection of metastatic uveal melanoma. However, the COMS found that periodic hematologic screening (e.g. LFT's), a chest x-ray and physical examination will only detect advanced disease [7]. Radiographic imaging will allow for earlier detection, enrolment in a clinical trial or life-extension through palliative therapies.

21.5.1 Systemic Staging Before Treatment

Liver imaging and chest radiography are widely recommended to exclude both hepatic metastasis and a non-ocular primary tumor metastatic to the uvea [25, 28]. Largely based on socio-economic and governmental restrictions, abdominal ultrasound imaging or radiographic imaging of the liver is used to evaluate for systemic metastasis. However, in consideration that there exist multiple known sites of metastatic disease (e.g. liver, bone, skin, etc.) which can affect patient decisions related to undergoing ocular surgery and life planning, at The New York Eye Cancer Center initial systemic staging is performed utilizing a physical examination, a haematological survey and total body PET/CT scan. We have been informed that total body PET/CT scanning that reveals no evidence of metastasis provides psychologic relief to melanoma affected patients [24, 25]. However, they are counselled that even PET/CT scanning cannot reveal micro metastasis.

21.5.2 After Treatment

As liver is the most common presenting site of metastasis, it is common to examine patients one or two times a year with abdominal imaging (e.g. ultrasound, MRI imaging, and CT) [29]. In consideration of both preference and efficacy, abdominal MRI and CT are preferred over ultrasound. Author (PF) recommends follow up abdominal imaging (MRI or CT) every 6 months for 5 years and then annually for at least 5 additional years. (Fig. 21.2).

21.5.3 Management of Metastatic Disease

When the metastasis is limited to liver, local control or palliation of liver metastasis can be achieved with a range of techniques (e.g. hepatic resection, intra-arterial chemotherapy or radia-

Fig. 21.1 Classification of ciliary body and choroid uveal melanoma based on thickness and diameter (AJCC eighth Edition) [3] (Reprint permission)

Thickness (mm)	≤ 3.0	3.1-6.0	6.1-9.0	9.1-12.0	12.1-15.0	15.1-18.0	>18.0
>15.0					4	4	4
12.1-15.0				3	3	4	4
9.1-12.0		3	3	3	3	3	4
6.1-9.0	2	2	2	2	3	3	4
3.1.6.0	1	1	1	2	2	3	4
≤ 3.0	1	1	1	1	2	2	4

Largest basel diameter (mm)

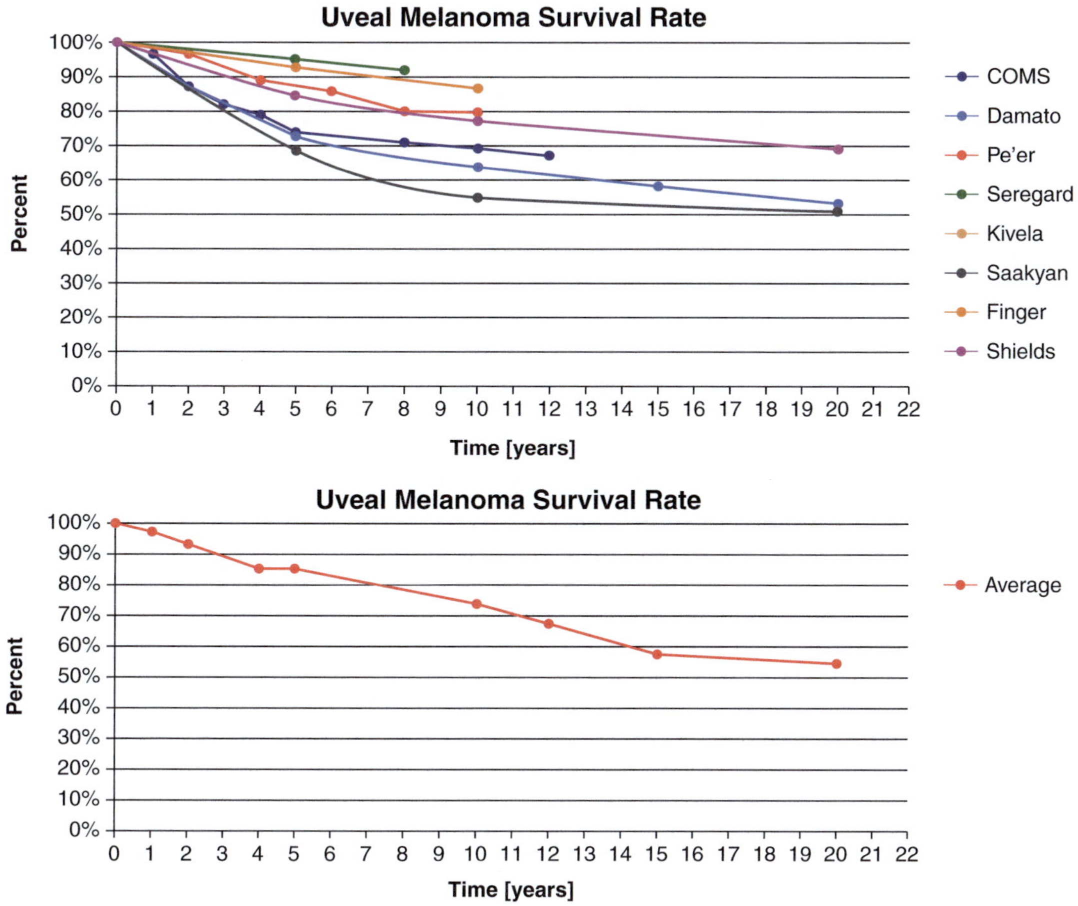

Fig. 21.2 Metastatic death from uveal melanoma. COMS, Diener-West et al. [7]; Damato et al. [30]; Kaiserman et al. [31], Bergman et al. [32]; Kujala et al. [33]; Saakyan et al. [34]; Finger, et al. [17]; Shields et al. [35]. Table curtesy of Ekatrina Semenova, MD. The data used to make the graph was culled from published literature) [25] (Reprint permission—Finger PT. Intraocular Melanoma, Cancer: Principles and Practice of Oncology, tenth edition, DeVita, Jr. VT, Lawrence TS, Rosenberg SA, (eds.) Wolters Kluwer, Lippincott, Williams and Wilkins, Philadelphia, 2014, 1770–1779)

tion embolization and/or radiofrequency ablation) [26]. Systemic immunotherapy has provided few durable responses [31]. Until there is an effective treatment, our primary recommendation is for patients with metastatic disease to enroll in a clinical trial.

21.6 Prognostic Factors

As available, the following prognostic factors can be used to explain metastatic, disease related and overall survival rates.

21.6.1 Clinical Prognostic Factors

- *Tumor size*—Largest tumor diameter has been the most reproducible biomarker for choroidal melanoma metastasis [3–5]. It is both practical, non-invasive and useful in that tumor measurements are typically available at the time of diagnosis [26]. Utilizing the COMS data, Diener-West et al. performed a meta-analysis of 5-year mortality among enucleated patients, providing weighted estimates of 5-year mortality after enucleation: 16% for small tumors, 32% for medium-sized tumors, and 53% for large tumors. This analysis also found older patient age was a significant risk factor for metastasis [7]. (Figure 21.1) The eighth edition American Joint Committee on Cancer (AJCC) and the Union International for Cancer Control (UICC) have recognized 2 registries collectively including over 10,000 patients which has shown tumor size can be used to stage risk for systemic metastasis [3].

- *Tumor location*—Ciliary body and ciliochoroidal melanomas carry a worse prognosis compared to melanomas confined only to choroid or iris [3]. Diffuse choroidal melanomas, low-lying tumors with indistinct margins are found difficult to treat (more likely to fail local control) and thus carry worse prognosis [26].
- *Extraocular extension*—The presence of extraocular extension is independently associated with higher metastatic risk [3].

21.6.2 Histopathologic, Genetic and Molecular Prognostic Factors

21.6.2.1 Intraocular Tumor Biopsy

The role of intraocular tumor biopsy still remains controversial in the management of choroidal melanoma. On one hand it provides cytopathological confirmation of diagnosis, cytogenetical analysis for prognostication and research opportunities; on the other hand, there are risks of intraocular hemorrhage, glaucoma, epiretinal membrane formation, retinal detachment and periorbital melanoma seeding in orbit. However, any increased chances of systemic metastasis secondary to tumor seeding are yet unquantified by long-term observation.

21.6.2.2 Methods of Tumor Biopsy

Fine needle aspiration biopsy (FNAB) is the most frequently used technique for biopsy of uveal melanoma. Excisional and incisional biopsy (in combination with vitrectomy) are also used in special circumstances at some centers [36]. The methods for performing intraocular tumor biopsy include: transcorneal (for anterior iris and iridociliary tumors), transscleral (for anterior as well as posterior tumors) and transvitreal (with or without vitrectomy) [37]. Out of these, transcorneal and transscleral are easier methods as compared to transvitreal where help from vitreoretinal surgeon may be sought. The technical limitations for FNAB include insufficient cellularity that compromises diagnostic yield, intratumoral heterogeneity and variability in the techniques which can affect the prognostication. In biopsy of small tumors.

Pre-treatment tumor biopsy typically yields melanoma-specific prognostic information. Although, the facilities for histopathology, genetic and molecular analysis are limited in developing countries, factors are described as per current knowledge for the benefit of readers.

21.7 Prognostic Information

- *Cell Type*— Spindle cell melanomas have been shown to predict the longest and epithelioid cell melanomas the shortest survival times [3].
- *Chromosomal analysis*—Monosomy 3, especially if combined with a frequently coexisting gain in chromosome 8q, is independently associated with metastatic risk [3, 38–43].
- *Gene Expression Profiling*—GEP class 2 (high grade) or equivalent is independently associated with higher metastatic risk [44, 45]. With respect to survival, class 1A predicts the longest survival, class 1B an intermediate survival, and class 2 the shortest survival time [3].
- *Mitotic count*—The mitotic count is independent predictor of metastatic risk. Higher counts are associated with shorter survival [3, 46].
- *Tumor Vascular Matrix Loops and Networks*—The presence of certain types of extravascular matrix patterns is independently associated with risk of metastasis [42]. Absence of both loops and networks is associated with the longest survival and presence of loops forming networks is associated with the shortest survival time [3].
- *Microvascular Density*—The number of immunopositive elements is labeled with a

marker for vascular endothelial cells (e.g., CD34 epitope, CD31 epitope, factor VIII–related antigen) and counted from areas of densest vascularization (typical field area, 0.31 mm^2). Higher counts are associated with shorter survival [3, 47].
- *Tumor-infiltrating Macrophages*—The higher number of tumor infiltrating macrophages are associated with shorter survival [3, 48, 49].

In sum, management of choroidal melanoma needs a multidisciplinary approach involving an ocular oncologist, medical oncologist and a radiation oncologist. There are a number of factors to be considered in deciding the appropriate treatment option for each case. Knowledge about evidence-based success, recurrence rates, associated metastasis risk and overall survival should be considered as well as the clinical factors and suitable treatment options. Informed consent and patient-centered decision making are essential to the management plan.

References

1. Accuracy of diagnosis of choroidal melanomas in the Collaborative Ocular Melanoma Study. COMS report no. 1. Arch Ophthalmol. 1990;108:1268–73.
2. Augsburger JJ, Shields JA. Fine needle aspiration biopsy of solid intraocular tumors: indications, instrumentation and techniques. Ophthalmic Surg. 1984;15:34–40.
3. Caines R, Eleuteri A, Kalirai H, et al. Cluster analysis of multiplex ligation-dependent probe amplification data in choroidal melanoma. Mol Vis. 2015;21:1–11.
4. Finger PT, Tena LB, Semenova E, et al. Extrascleral extension of choroidal melanoma: post-enucleation high-dose-rate interstitial brachytherapy of the orbit. Brachytherapy. 2014;13:275–80.
5. Collaborative Ocular Melanoma Study Group. The COMS randomized trial of iodine 125 brachytherapy for choroidal melanoma: V. Twelve-year mortality rates and prognostic factors: COMS report no. 28. Arch Ophthalmol. 2006;124:1684–93.
6. Kujala E, Damato B, Coupland SE, et al. Staging of ciliary body and choroidal melanomas based on anatomic extent. J Clin Oncol. 2013;31:2825–31.
7. Diener-West M, Reynolds SM, Agugliaro DJ, et al. Development of metastatic disease after enrollment in the COMS trials for treatment of choroidal melanoma: Collaborative Ocular Melanoma Study Group Report No. 26. Arch Ophthalmol. 2005;123:1639–43.
8. Semenova E, Finger PT. Palladium-103 radiation therapy for small choroidal melanoma. Ophthalmology. 2013;120(11):2353–7.
9. Wilson MW, Hungerford JL. Comparison of episcleral plaque and proton beam radiation therapy for the treatment of choroidal melanoma. Ophthalmology. 1999;106:1579–87.
10. Packer S, Stoller S, Lesser ML, et al. Long-term results of iodine 125 irradiation of uveal melanoma. Ophthalmology. 1992;99:767–73.
11. Fontanesi J, Meyer D, Xu S, Tai D. Treatment of choroidal melanoma with I-125 plaque. Int J Radiat Oncol Biol Phys. 1993;26:619–23.
12. Lommatzsch PK. Beta-irradiation of choroidal melanoma with 106Ru/106Rh applicators: 16 years' experience. Arch Ophthalmol. 1983;101:713–7.
13. Char DH, Kroll SM, Castro J. Ten-year follow-up of helium ion therapy for uveal melanoma. Am J Ophthalmol. 1998;125:81–9.
14. Brovkina AF, Zarubei GD. Ciliochoroidal melanomas treated with a narrow medical proton beam. Arch Ophthalmol. 1986;104:402–4.
15. Gragoudas ES, Seddon JM, Egan K, et al. Long-term results of proton beam irradiated uveal melanomas. Ophthalmology. 1987;94:349–53.
16. Fastenberg DM, Finger PT, Chess Q, Koizumi JH, Packer S. Vitrectomy retinotomy aspiration biopsy of choroidal tumors. Am J Ophthalmol. 1990;110:361–5.
17. Damato BE, Heimann H, Kalirai H, Coupland SE. Age, survival predictors, and metastatic death in patients with choroidal melanoma: tentative evidence of a therapeutic effect on survival. JAMA Ophthalmol. 2014;132(5):605–13.
18. Finger PT. Finger's "slotted" eye plaque for radiation therapy: treatment of juxtapapillary and circumpapillary intraocular tumors. Br J Ophthalmol. 2007;91:891–4.
19. Finn AP, Materin MA, Mruthyunjaya P. Choroidal tumor biopsy: A review of the current state and a glance into future techniques. Retina. 2017;38:S79–87.
20. Krema H, Somani S, Sahgal A, et al. Stereotactic radiotherapy in the treatment of juxtapapillary choroidal melanoma: 3-year follow-up. Br J Ophthalmol. 2009;93:1172–6.
21. Sagoo MS, Shields CL, Emrich J, et al. Plaque radiotherapy for juxtapapillary choroidal melanoma: tumor control in 650 consecutive cases. JAMA Ophthalmol. 2011;118:402–7.
22. Lane AM, Kin IK, Gragoudas ES. Proton irradiation for peripapillary and parapapillary melanomas. Arch Ophthalmol. 2011;129:1127–30.
23. The American Brachytherapy Society - Ophthalmic Oncology Task Force. The American Brachytherapy Society consensus guidelines for plaque brachytherapy of uveal melanoma and retinoblastoma. Brachytherapy. 2014;13:1–14.
24. Freton A, Chin KJ, Raut R, Tena LB, Kivelä T, Finger PT. Initial PET/CT staging for choroidal melanoma: AJCC correlation and second nonocu-

lar primaries in 333 patients. Eur J Ophthalmol. 2012;22(2):236–43.
25. Finger PT. Intraocular melanoma. In: DeVita Jr VT, Lawrence TS, Rosenberg SA, editors. Cancer: principles and practice of oncology. 10th ed. Philadelphia: Wolters Kluwer, Lippincott, Williams and Wilkins; 2014. p. 1770–9.
26. Eskelin S, Summanen P, Pyrhönen S, Tarkkanen A, Kivelä T. Screening for metastatic uveal melanoma revisited. Cancer. 1999;85:1151–9.
27. Kivelä T, Simpson ER, Grossniklaus HE, et al. Chapter 67: Uveal melanoma. In: Amin MB, Edge S, Greene F, editors. The AJCC cancer staging manual. 8th ed. New York: Springer; 2017. p. 805–17.
28. Gomez D, Wetherill C, Cheong J, et al. The Liverpool uveal melanoma liver metastases pathway: outcome following liver resection. J Surg Oncol. 2014;109(6):542–7.
29. Hawkins BS. Collaborative Ocular Melanoma Study Group. The Collaborative Ocular Melanoma Study (COMS) randomized trial of pre-enucleation radiation of large choroidal melanoma: IV. Ten-year mortality findings and prognostic factors. COMS report number 24. Am J Ophthalmol. 2004;138:936–51.
30. Bergman L, Seregard S, Nilsson B, Lundell G, Ringborg U, Ragnarsson-Olding B. Uveal melanoma survival in Sweden from 1960 to 1998. Invest Ophthalmol Vis Sci. 2003;44(8):3282–7.
31. Kaiserman I, Amer R, Pe'er J. Liver function tests in metastatic uveal melanoma. Am J Ophthalmol. 2004;137(2):236–43.
32. Shields CL, Kaliki S, Furuta M, et al. American Joint Committee on Cancer classification of posterior uveal melanoma (tumor size category) predicts prognosis in 7731 patients. Ophthalmology. 2013;120:2066–71.
33. Finger PT, Chin KJ, Duvall G, et al. Palladium-103 ophthalmic plaque radiation therapy for choroidal melanoma: 400 treated patients. Ophthalmology. 2009;116:790–796, 796.e1.
34. Saakyan SV, Panteleeva OG, Shirina TV. Metastatic disease characteristics and survival of patients with uveal melanoma depending on the method of treatment of the primary tumor. Russ Ophthalmol J. 2012;5(2):55–7.
35. Jampol LM, Moy CS, Murray TG, et al. The COMS randomized trial of iodine 125 brachytherapy for choroidal melanoma: IV. Local treatment failure and enucleation in the first 5 years after brachytherapy. COMS report no. 19. Ophthalmology. 2002;109:2197–206.
36. Singh AD, Medina CA, Singh N, et al. Fine-needle aspiration biopsy of uveal melanoma: outcomes and complications. Br J Ophthalmol. 2016;100:456–62.
37. Triozzi PL, Singh AD. Adjuvant therapy of uveal melanoma: current status. Ocul Oncol Pathol. 2015;1:54–62.
38. Cassoux N, Rodrigues MJ, Plancher C, et al. Genome-wide profiling is a clinically relevant and affordable prognostic test in uveal melanoma posterior uveal melanoma. Br J Ophthalmol. 2014;98(6):769–74.
39. Ewens KG, Kanetsky PA, Richards-Yutz J, et al. Chromosome 3 status combined with BAP1 and EIF1AX mutation profiles are associated with metastasis in uveal melanoma. Invest Ophthalmol Vis Sci. 2014;55(8):5160–7.
40. van Beek JG, Koopmans AE, Vaarwater J, et al. The prognostic value of extraocular extension in relation to monosomy 3 and gain of chromosome 8q in uveal melanoma. Invest Ophthalmol Vis Sci. 2014;55(3):1284–91.
41. Mäkitie T, Summanen P, Tarkkanen A, Kivelä T. Microvascular loops and networks as prognostic indicators in choroidal and ciliary body melanomas. J Natl Cancer Inst. 1999;91(4):359–67.
42. Shields CL, Ganguly A, Bianciotto CG, Turaka K, Tavallali A, Shields JA. Prognosis of uveal melanoma in 500 cases using genetic testing of fine-needle aspiration biopsy specimens. Ophthalmology. 2011;118(2):396–401.
43. Onken MD, Worley LA, Char DH, et al. Collaborative Ocular Oncology Group report number 1: prospective validation of a multi-gene prognostic assay in uveal melanoma. Ophthalmology. 2012;119(8):1596–603.
44. Onken MD, Worley LA, Ehlers JP, Harbour JW. Gene expression profiling in uveal melanoma reveals two molecular classes and predicts metastatic death. Cancer Res. 2004;64(20):7205–9.
45. Damato B, Dopierala JA, Coupland SE. Genotypic profiling of choroidal melanomas with multiplex ligation-dependent probe amplification. Clin Cancer Res. 2010;16(24):6083–92.
46. Chen X, Maniotis AJ, Majumdar D, Pe'er J, Folberg R. Uveal melanoma cell staining for CD34 and assessment of tumor vascularity. Invest Ophthalmol Vis Sci. 2002;43(8):2533–9.
47. Mäkitie T, Summanen P, Tarkkanen A, Kivelä T. Tumorinfiltrating macrophages (CD68(+) cells) and prognosis in malignant uveal melanoma. Invest Ophthalmol Vis Sci. 2001;42(7):1414–21.
48. Bronkhorst IH, Ly LV, Jordanova ES, et al. Detection of M2-macrophages in uveal melanoma and relation with survival. Invest Ophthalmol Vis Sci. 2011;52(2):643–50.
49. Finger PT. Radiation therapy for choroidal melanoma. Surv Ophthalmol. 1997;42:215–32.

Correction to: Various Syndromes with Benign Intraocular Tumors

Vikas Khetan

Correction to: M. S. Palanivelu, *Various Syndromes with Benign Intraocular Tumors*, https://doi.org/10.1007/978-981-15-0395-5

Chapter 15 was inadvertently published with some minor errors, and the following changes has been updated in this version.

- **Under Section 15.2.4.1 in the last paragraph of page number 193, the sentence-** 'Exophytic tumor appears as an orange-red lesion (Fig. 15.8). But the sessile and endophytic tumors…' **has been replaced with** 'Endophytic tumor appears as an orange-red lesion (Fig. 15.8). But the sessile and the exophytic tumors…'
- **In the figure legend 15.8, the sentence-** 'Fundus photograph of juxtapapillary RCHs. Endophytic form (a) and endophytic form (b)' **has been replaced with** 'Fundus photograph of juxtapapillary RCHs. Endophytic form (a) and exophytic form (b)'.

The updated online version of this chapter can be found at
https://doi.org/10.1007/978-981-15-0395-5_15

V. Khetan (ed.), *Intraocular Tumors*, https://doi.org/10.1007/978-981-15-0395-5_22

MIX
Papier aus verantwortungsvollen Quellen
Paper from responsible sources
FSC® C105338

If you have any concerns about our products,
you can contact us on
ProductSafety@springernature.com

In case Publisher is established outside the EU,
the EU authorized representative is:
Springer Nature Customer Service Center GmbH
Europaplatz 3, 69115 Heidelberg, Germany

Printed by Libri Plureos GmbH
in Hamburg, Germany